Drugs in Anaesthetic Practice

Sixth Edition

M. D. Vickers, MB BS (Lond.), DA, FFA RCS, FFA RACS (Hon.)
Professor of Anaesthetics, Welsh National School of Medicine

H. Schnieden, MB ChB, MD, MSc
Emeritus Professor of Pharmacology, Materia Medica and Therapeutics,
University of Manchester

F. G. Wood-Smith, MA, MB (Cantab.), FFA RCS
Formerly Senior Lecturer in Anaesthetics, Royal Postgraduate Medical School,
Consultant Anaesthetist, Hammersmith Hospital and the King's College Hospital Group, London

Butterworths
London Boston Durban Singapore Sydney Toronto Wellington

First published 1962
Second edition 1964
Third edition 1968
Reprinted 1970
Fourth edition 1973
Reprinted 1975
Fifth edition 1978
Reprinted 1979
Reprinted 1981
Sixth edition 1984
Reprinted 1985

British Library Cataloguing in Publication Data

Vickers, M. D.
Drugs in anaesthetic practice.—6th ed
1. Anesthesia adjuvants 2. Anesthetics
I. Title II. Schnieden, H.
III. Wood-Smith, F. G.
615'.1'024617 RD82

ISBN 0-407-15505-8

Library of Congress Cataloging in Publication Data

Vickers, M. D. (Michael Douglas), 1929-
Drugs in anaesthetic practice.

Rev. ed. of: Drugs in anaesthetic practice /
F. G. Wood-Smith. 5th ed. 1978
Bibliography: p.
Includes index.
1. Anesthetics. 2. Anesthesia adjuvants.
3. Preanesthetic medication. I. Schnieden, H.
II. Wood-Smith, F. G. (Francis Geoffrey)
III. Wood-Smith, F. G. (Francis Geoffrey).
Drugs in anaesthetic practice. IV. Title.
[DNLM: 1. Anesthetics. 2. Anesthesia adjuvants. QV 81 V637d]
RD82.V48 1983 615'.1'024617 83-7471

Photoset by Butterworths Litho Preparation Department
Printed by Anchor-Brendon Ltd., Tiptree, Essex

Additional contributions by

C. M. Conway, MBBS(Lond.), FFARCS
Professor of Anaesthetics, Westminster Hospital, London

Ronald F. Fletcher, PhD, MD, FRCP
Consultant Physician, Dudley Road Hospital, Birmingham
Senior Clinical Lecturer, University of Birmingham

P. J. Horsey, MBBS (Lond.), FFARCS
Consultant Anaesthetist, Southampton Hospital Group

J. D. Williams, MD(Liverp.), MRCPath
Professor of Medical Microbiology, The London Hospital Medical College

Preface to the first edition

The modern practice of anaesthesia necessitates a considerable knowledge of physiology and pharmacology. Not only should the anaesthetist know about the action and side-effects of those drugs that he uses himself, but also about those employed by his surgical and medical colleagues on the patients he is called upon to anaesthetize, as they may have a marked influence on the course of anaesthesia.

We have therefore included not only those drugs which produce anaesthesia and analgesia and those controlling their complications, but also others which may have some influence on their course. Some drugs have been included because of their historic interest or because they have become the yardstick by which other drugs are measured; even though they are not now used in clinical practice they may still be of experimental interest.

We hope that the book will be of assistance to students studying for higher examinations in anaesthesia and to practising anaesthetists who require a book of reference. We think surgical students will also find it useful as their ever increasing curriculum requires a knowledge of many of the drugs and problems discussed.

The classification of the drugs described has caused some difficulty. As far as possible they have been grouped according to their main actions and the purposes for which they are used. There have had to be some exceptions, as if a drug could be placed in one of several groups an arbitrary decision had to be made. Much of the information given is well known and references are not needed; where, however, recent research has brought new facts to light, or when well summarized accounts of certain problems have been quoted, appropriate references are included.

Each section is preceded by a general article on the drugs concerned, and this is followed by monographs on individual drugs. Other articles have been included to link up various sections, especially where the drugs concerned are described in other groups. It is suggested that whenever a monograph on an individual drug is consulted it should be read, if possible, in conjunction with the general article on the group. In the text, *BP, BPC*, or approved names of drugs are used throughout; chemical names, synonyms and trade names are given under the headings of individual drugs.

Although new drugs are continually being produced by pharmaceutical firms, few prove of sufficient value to pass the test of time. Older drugs, thought to be of therapeutic benefit on empirical grounds, may eventually prove to be ineffective, some even harmful. We have tried to keep up to date, and much of the script written earlier has been revised recently. We are, however, conscious of the fact that in the course of time reconsideration of the value of certain drugs, especially the newer ones, will be necessary.

We would like to extend our special thanks to Dr C. L. Cope for writing for us the section on Corticosteroids, and to Dr P. J. Horsey for that on Electrolytes and Infusion Fluids. Our thanks are also due to Dr J. B. E. Baker for his advice and assistance during the early stages of the book, and to Mr C. R. Day of May and Baker Ltd, whose help with the preparation of drafts, advice on pharmaceutical aspects of drugs and the production of facts and figures has been of great value.

It is with considerable pleasure that we also acknowledge the helpful criticism and advice of our many colleagues whom we have consulted, and the patience of Butterworths, our publishers, during the time that the book has been in preparation.

Finally, we want to thank Joan Wood-Smith for much secretarial help and for looking after us so patiently during our many meetings.

Geoffrey Wood-Smith
H. C. Stewart

Preface to the sixth edition

With this edition we welcome Professor Harold Schnieden as co-author and wish Professor Stewart a happy retirement. Professor Stewart has been associated with this book since its inception and a tower of strength in the preparation of earlier editions. We look forward to an equally fruitful association with Professor Schnieden. Harold Schnieden is an examiner in the Primary FFARCS and thus well acquainted with the needs of trainee anaesthetists. He has also undertaken much research in areas of pharmacological interest to anaesthetists.

We have been fortunate in being able to retain the help and advice of our existing collaborators, Professor C. M. Conway (chapter 4), Professor D. Williams (chapter 19), Dr R. Fletcher (chapter 18) and Dr P. Horsey (chapter 20), who have revised their respective contributions.

As usual, we have needed to introduce monographs or short notes on drugs introduced since the previous edition and have cut out a few which have now been removed from general circulation.

In this edition greater use has been made of illustrations, particularly in chapter 1 on General Pharmacology, and we are indebted to Dr Carpenter (University of Manchester) for drawing these. In an effort to prevent the book becoming unnecessarily large, we have introduced 'small print' sections, not as traditionally thought of for the arcane, exotic, or unimportant, but for drugs that closely resemble others on which full monographs are included, in an endeavour to pick up any minor differences. We have also reduced the number of references; enquiry reveals that our readers very rarely consult them. We hope, on balance, therefore, to provide better value for money with this edition.

With this edition we also bid farewell to Mr Day, who has undertaken the indexing, preparing the converters, and checking the pharmaceutical information since the inception of the book. We welcome Dr Rees, also of the University of Manchester, who has compiled the Appendix on drug name converters.

One particular problem that creates increasing difficulty in preparing new editions is the growing practice of pharmaceutical companies to promote (and journals to publish) studies on drugs ahead of general marketing. It is not uncommon for such studies to figure widely in the literature for several years before the drug is obtainable for routine use. Such drugs may be available in the UK long before being available in the USA or vice versa, due to differing attitudes of the relevant regulatory bodies. Examiners appear to expect candidates to be knowledgeable about these drugs, and there is often no hard information as to when the drug will be available and indeed no guarantee that it ever will be. Our approach has been to include a monograph when we are reasonably confident that the drug will be available during the life of the edition and to include a synopsis on what is currently known about such a drug at the time of preparation of the manuscript when the future is uncertain. It is an unfortunate fact of publishing life that the completion of the manuscript precedes publication by up to a year and we apologize in advance for any bad guesses in this respect.

Despite the numerous changes, the aims of the book remain unchanged, namely to provide a general textbook of pharmacology of special relevance to the practising anaesthetist, written particularly with the trainee in mind, and a reference source for the drugs that anaesthetists employ themselves or which are commonly given to their patients.

Professor Vickers gratefully acknowledges the assistance of Sara Marshall in undertaking numerous tasks associated with the preparation of the manuscript for the printers. Professor Schnieden is indebted to his secretary, Mrs V. Sillivan, for her word processing skills and her meticulous checking of the data presented to her.

M. D. Vickers
Geoffrey Wood-Smith

Contents

1

General pharmacology

The *Concise Oxford Dictionary* defines a drug as 'a medicinal substance'. Implicit in this definition is that a drug should be used for a therapeutic purpose. There are other definitions of a drug: for example, it has been defined as 'any chemical agent which affects living processes'. This is an all-embracing definition, for included in it would be environmental pollutants and food additives. To talk of 'the pharmacological action of a drug' is somewhat misleading as drugs do not really have actions: it is the tissues which have responses. Drugs commonly act by increasing or decreasing the normal physiological actions of a functioning tissue.

Mechanism of action of drugs

There are numerous ways in which drugs can produce their therapeutic effects. They can act on specific sites (receptors), initiating or impeding the normal response. They can raise or lower the concentration of a transmitter or modulator; for instance, a drug that inhibits the enzyme responsible for metabolizing a particular transmitter can effectively prolong its action. Some drugs by virtue of their physical properties act non-specifically. General anaesthetics are thought to act in this way.

Drugs usually have a single type of action on a tissue. In the intact organism, however, the direct response of a tissue to a drug may be modified by indirect actions due to drug effects on other tissues. Thus noradrenaline would increase cardiac rate by a direct action on the heart. However, if given intravenously to man heart rate falls due to a reflex bradycardia produced by the rise in mean arterial blood pressure – noradrenaline, by increasing peripheral resistance, causes the rise in blood pressure. Many drugs, especially those acting on the CNS, may have biphasic actions, initial stimulation being followed by depression.

Although many drugs are highly selective in their action, some are unfortunately not so selective, and their side effects may seriously upset the patient to the point of totally precluding their use. Toxic effects such as liver damage or agranulocytosis are even more serious, and patients taking drugs known to be likely to cause these complications must be carefully watched.

The response to a drug often varies in different individuals. The expected effect may not occur, there may be an abnormal response, or the drug may be without effect. These variations in effect may be due to the size of the dose, the route by which it is administered, the condition of the patient at the time, the presence of other drugs in the body, or sensitivity or resistance of the patient's tissues to the drug.

Although drugs with similar chemical structures often have similar actions, minor changes in structure may totally change the activity of a drug. Sometimes an antagonist of the original drug results, as when the methyl group of morphine is replaced by an allyl group to produce nalorphine. Optical isomers can vary considerably in their activity. Dexamphetamine, for example, is three to four times more active than its *laevo* isomer. Drugs with similar actions may have different chemical structures and antagonists may differ in gross chemical structure from their agonists, for example atropine and acetylcholine.

It is often forgotten that in addition to their pharmacological actions drugs can also exert an effect through psychological mechanisms. When drugs have weak or marginal actions these psychological effects can overshadow the true drug effects. In clinical trials it is common to use a control group of patients treated with an inert medicament or placebo to evaluate these psychological effects and estimate the number of 'placebo reactors'. Placebo reaction may be related to the personality of the patient, to the personality of the person prescribing or administering the drug, or to the extra attention a patient may receive during the trial of a new drug.

Drug allergy or individual hypersensitivity to certain drugs is becoming increasingly recognized as a problem in therapeutics. A drug that most patients can take with impunity may cause a violent reaction in a small number of patients, and the effects seen often bear no resemblance to the normal actions of that drug. Abnormal drug responses commonly resemble the allergic reaction of man to certain proteins to which hypersensitivity has been acquired, taking the form of skin rashes, swelling of mucous membranes, or fever. Experimental work has shown that during the initial exposure to a drug a drug–protein complex may be formed which can act as an antigen and promote antibody formation. Subsequent administration of the drug may cause severe antigen–antibody reactions. Benzylpenicillin can behave in this way. On first exposure the patient may experience no harmful effects. A subsequent exposure can induce a severe anaphylactic response. The patient may have severe bronchospasm and a pronounced fall in blood pressure due to the release of histamine and other substances, for example bradykinin, 5-hydroxytryptamine, and slow-reacting substance of anaphylaxis. This release is triggered by the antigen–antibody response.

A similar type of response called an anaphylactoid response can occur on *first* exposure to a drug; certain steroid anaesthetics, for example, can produce this effect. The mechanism for release is not due to the classic antigen–antibody reaction but involves the alternative complement pathway (Pearson, Freed and Taylor, 1981).

At a molecular level many drugs act specifically on an enzyme or group of enzymes. A drug that combines with the active centre of an enzyme may inhibit the specific activity of that enzyme. Enzyme activity may also be altered by modifying cofactors such as calcium or magnesium, coenzymes, or prosthetic groups.

Concept of a receptor

The drug receptor concept was introduced by Langley (1852–1925), a British physiologist, and by Ehrlich (1854–1915), a German chemist and physician who worked in the pharmaceutical industry. A receptor is a small region of a cell which combines with a drug. This drug–receptor complex initiates a biological response. Langley showed that nicotine stimulated muscles only when applied to certain small areas of the muscle surface, and he postulated that there was a receptive substance at these points. Ehrlich generalized the concept of drug receptors and extended this concept into the field of antigen–antibody reactions. The receptor theory explains why many drugs are effective in extremely low concentrations and why optical isomers may vary so greatly in their activity. A simple analogy is to regard the drug as a key and the receptor as a lock. Just as physically similar keys may open the same lock, so chemically similar drugs may combine with the same receptors. Receptors can become blocked just as a lock may be jammed.

Among the properties attributed to receptors are that they are selective, specific, and sensitive.

Selectivity

Selectivity exists if, for a given receptor type, responses can only be produced by a relatively small number of chemical substances that have similar physicochemical properties, for example members of a homologous series. Optical isomers may differ markedly in activity because there can be a marked difference in their 'goodness of fit' to the receptor site (*Figure 1.1*).

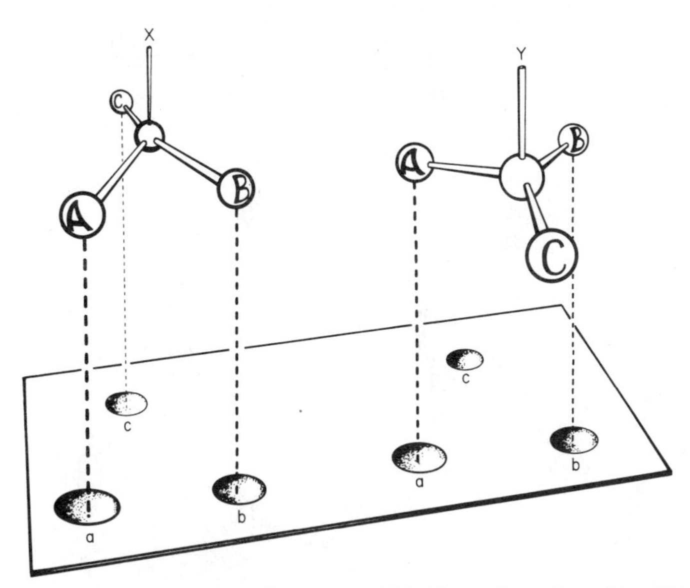

Figure 1.1 Diagrammatic representation of 'goodness of fit'. The conformation of drug X ideally fits that of its receptor, whereas Y, the optical isomer of X, is a poor fit

Specificity

If a drug initiates a response by interacting with a receptor, that response is always of the same type because it depends on the properties of the cell. For example, stimulation of β-adrenoceptors on cardiac muscle will cause contraction: it will never cause the release of antidiuretic hormone because that is not a property of cardiac cells.

Sensitivity

Many drugs can produce therapeutic responses in small doses. Isolated tissues can be shown to contract when the concentration of drug to which they are exposed is low, for example 10^{-8}M. The drug–receptor interaction must therefore act as a trigger. This could initiate the release of energy stored within the cell, for example ATP breakdown, or start a cascade process, the steps of which involve an amplification factor.

The nature of receptors

During the last decade our knowledge of receptors has dramatically increased. Using radioactive-labelled drugs it has been shown that drugs can bind with a high affinity to specific areas. For instance, using radioactive-labelled morphine it has been shown that selective binding occurs in the brain. This was a major stimulus in the search for a naturally occurring transmitter that would interact with opioid receptors. Cells that are targets for a specific drug contain specialized molecules (the receptors) that bind the drug and subsequently mediate its cellular response. The receptor has two roles: first, to distinguish a particular signal (a drug or natural transmitter) from the myriad of other signals impinging on the cell (for example hormones, other transmitters, and proteins) and, secondly, to transduce the signal so that the appropriate cellular response follows.

Several types of receptor have been recognized. Catecholamines, certain peptide hormones, and releasing factors act on receptors situated on the external surface of the cell. Steroid receptors initially are found in the soluble intracellular compartment of the cell. Following steroid binding, the modified hormone–receptor complex moves into the nucleus and attaches to the nuclear chromatin there. For thyroid hormones the nuclear chromatin appears to act as a receptor site (*Figure 1.2*). While steroids interact with intracellular receptors many drugs act as agonists for receptors on the cell surface.

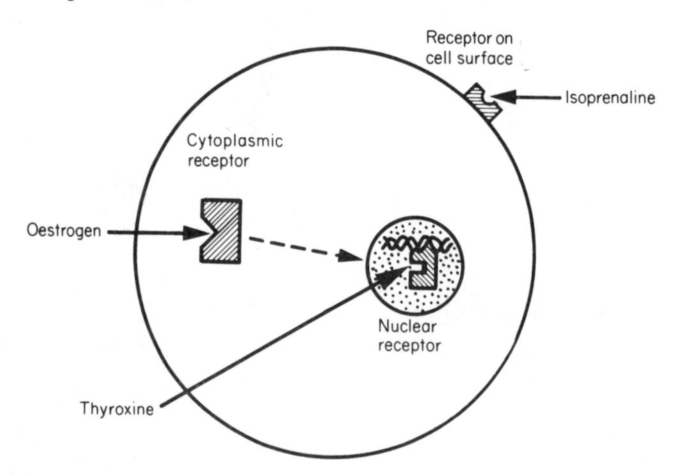

Figure 1.2 Receptors are found on the cell surface, in the cytoplasm, and in the nucleus

The mechanism(s) by which the signal is transmitted from the drug–receptor complex into the cell is still unclear. The following steps may occur. A conformational change occurs in the receptor protein structure. This leads to the opening of ion channels, for instance for sodium or calcium; calcium ions, probably acting through a protein called calmodulin, can modify adenyl cyclase activity. Alternatively the formation of the drug–receptor complex activates membrane adenyl cyclase by a different mechanism, a multistage process involving a

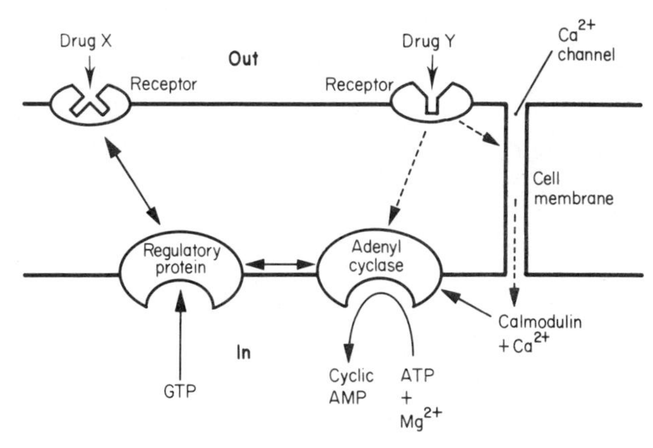

Figure 1.3 Two possible mechanisms by which adenyl cyclase can be activated: via regulatory protein (drug X) or via calmodulin (drug Y)

regulatory protein. Binding of drug to receptor allows guanosine triphosphate (GTP) to interact with a guanyl nucleotide regulatory protein. The complex formed then activates adenyl cyclase which converts ATP to cyclic AMP (*Figure 1.3*; Paton, 1970; Baxter and Funder, 1979).

Drug–receptor combination

For a drug to act at a receptor it must be bound there by physicochemical forces. 'The drug receptor is, in general, a pattern (R) of forces of diverse origin forming a part of some biological system and having roughly the same dimensions as a certain pattern (M) of forces presented by the drug molecule such that between patterns M and R a relationship of complementarity for interaction exists' (Schueler, 1960). If a drug is tightly bound (for instance, by covalent bonding) its effects are usually difficult to antagonize and its duration of action tends to be long (for example, days). If more loosely bound its duration of action is usually shorter and it is often easier to antagonize its action (*see Figure 1.4*). The following are the types of bonding that can exist between a drug molecule and a protein surface.

Covalent bonding

A covalent bond is formed by the sharing of a pair of electrons between atoms, and is the familiar strong bond of the organic chemist. It has a bond strength of 40–100 kcal/mol (167–418 kJ/mol), and because of its high stability plays little part in the reversible binding of drugs to receptors. Covalent bonding is involved in the inactivation of cholinesterase by organophosphate insecticides, and the prolonged α-adrenergic blockade produced by members of the β-haloalkylamine group, such as phenoxybenzamine. Covalent bonds are also involved in the sulphur binding of arsenical and mercurial compounds.

Ionic bonding

Ionic bonds arise from the electrostatic forces existing between groups of opposite charge, and have bond strengths of the order of 4–6 kcal/mol (16–25 kJ/mol). Acidic or basic drugs that are ionized at plasma pH may readily combine with the free charged groups of diamino or dicarboxylic amino acids contained in protein.

Hydrogen bonding

The hydrogen nucleus is strongly electropositive, and is able to accept an electron pair in part from each of two donor atoms, forming a bridge between them. Hydrogen bonds have a strength of 2–7 kcal/mol (8.4–29 kJ/mol). In drug–receptor interactions hydroxyl or amino groups can donate hydrogen to react with an electronegative carbonyl oxygen group.

Ion-dipole bonding

Areas of relative electropositivity and negativity can arise within a molecule due to an unequal distribution of electron density. Intermolecular bonding can then occur due to weak electrostatic forces between dipoles of opposite charge.

Van der Waals' forces

These are weak bonds occurring between any two atoms or groups of atoms of different molecules. The bond energy is only 0.5–2 kcal/mol (2–8.4 kJ/mol) and the attractive force is inversely proportional to the seventh power of the distance between the molecules. Although single bonds are weak, when the configuration between drug and receptor is so sterically close that a number of van der Waals' bonds can form, significant linkages with strengths of the order of 5 kcal/mol (21 kJ/mol) can be produced.

Kinetics of drug–receptor reaction

When a drug is administered a portion of the dose, by being bound to plasma protein, converted to an inactive form, or excreted, will be pharmacologically inert. A fraction of the drug, by processes of absorption, transport, diffusion, or conversion into a metabolically active form, may reach the biophase and there be in a position to react with receptors.

The combination of a drug with its receptor may be analysed in a similar fashion to that applied to the interactions of an enzyme and its substrate. A drug A can be considered to combine with a receptor R to form a drug–receptor complex AR, represented by the equation

$$A + R \underset{k_2}{\overset{k_1}{\rightleftharpoons}} AR$$

where k_1 and k_2 are the rate constants for each partial reaction. At equilibrium the forward and reverse reactions are equal. An affinity constant K_A (the reciprocal of the dissociation constant) can then be defined as

$$K_A = \frac{k_1}{k_2} = \frac{[AR]}{[A][R]}$$

Affinity can also be defined in terms of receptor occupancy (the proportion of receptors occupied) as

$$K_A = \frac{y}{A(1-y)}$$

where y is the fractional receptor occupancy. This equation can be rearranged to give

$$y = \frac{K_A A}{K_A A + 1}$$

This equation, the value of which approaches unity as A increases, bears considerable resemblance to the classic Michaelis–Menton equation of enzyme dynamics.

The equations above refer to the actions of an agonist. For an antagonist B

$$y = \frac{K_B B}{K_B B + 1}$$

For an agonist and competitive antagonist acting together, the fractional receptor occupancy is given by

$$y = \frac{K_A A x}{K_A A x + K_B B + 1} = \frac{K_A A}{K_A A + 1}$$

$$K_B = \frac{x - 1}{B}$$

where y is the proportion of receptors occupied by the agonist; A and B are concentrations respectively of agonist and antagonist in solution; K_A and K_B are respective affinity constants of agonist–receptor and antagonist–receptor complex; x is the dose ratio. Dose ratio is defined as the number by which the concentration of agonist must be multiplied to maintain a given response in the presence of an antagonist.

It was originally assumed that pharmacological response was directly proportional to the fraction of receptors occupied and that 100 per cent response meant 100 per cent receptor occupancy. This is no longer accepted. The limited proposition that equal pharmacological responses produced in the presence or absence of a competitive antagonist involve equal numbers of activated receptors is still accepted.

Dose–response relationship

For many drugs, if dose is plotted on an arithmetic scale against response, a sigmoid curve is obtained. At low doses no response is obtained. As dose increases a small effect is obtained. A further increase in dose results in a greater response. If dose is still increased, eventually a maximum response is obtained and further increases in dose do not produce an increase in response.

If, instead of using an arithmetic scale for the abscissa (x axis), a log scale is used so that log dose is compared with response, for responses between 16 and 84 per cent of maximum a straight-line relationship would exist between response and log dose. From either of these figures the ED_{50} (the dose of drug that will produce a half maximal response) can be calculated. Pharmacologists tend to plot log dose–response relationships for reasons that will become clearer later.

Although the dose–response relationships outlined above are very common, the reader should be aware that there are other possible relationships, for example a bell-shaped response and a biphasic response curve.

Drug antagonism

Drug antagonism can be of various kinds (*Table 1.1*).

Table 1.1 Characteristics of different types of drug antagonism

Type of antagonism	*Surmountable?*
Competitive	Yes
True non-competitive	No
Irreversible	No
Physiological	Yes
Chemical	Yes
Mixed	Yes (dependent on concentration)

Simple competitive antagonism

By inspection of *Figure 1.4* it can be seen that atropine causes a parallel rightward shift in the log dose–response curve for acetylcholine. A parallel shift is suggestive of competitive antagonism. If the log (dose ratio x−1) is plotted against −log molar concentration B, a regression line can be drawn (*Figure 1.5*). If drug B is a simple competitive antagonist of drug A then the line is linear with a slope of −1. Its intercept on the abscissa corresponds to log K_B.

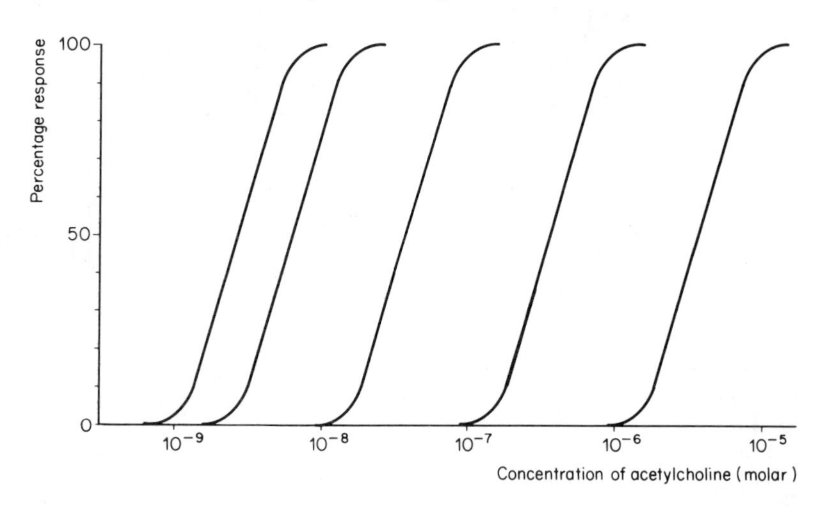

Figure 1.4 Parallel concentration–response curves for acetylcholine in the presence of increasing concentrations of atropine (on log scale). Tissue is guinea-pig ileum

Pharmacologists use the pA_2 to measure quantitatively the potency of an antagonist. The pA_2 of an antagonist is the negative logarithm of the molar concentration of antagonist which reduces the effect of a dose of agonist by 50 per cent. Where the antagonism is of the simple competitive type, $pA_2 = \log K_B$.

Two theories of drug action based upon the kinetics of drug–receptor combination have been advanced. The older theory, developed by Gaddum (1937), is known as the occupation theory, and holds that the response of a tissue to a drug depends on the proportion of receptors occupied.

A modification of the occupation theory involved the postulate that drugs have two properties. They have affinity and efficacy. Affinity is a measure of the ability of a drug to combine with its receptor. Efficacy is a measure of the ability of the drug–receptor complex to cause a pharmacological response. Mathematically, response R has been stated as

$$R = f(ey) = f\left(e \frac{K_A A}{K_A A + 1}\right)$$

where f is a function; e is efficacy; y is fraction of receptor occupied. Based on this theory, antagonists are drugs that have affinity but lack efficacy, and partial agonists are drugs that have less efficacy than full agonists.

Paton (1961) has suggested that the response depends on the rate of combination of drug with receptor – the rate theory.

Difficulty in accurately relating the measured effects of drugs to their

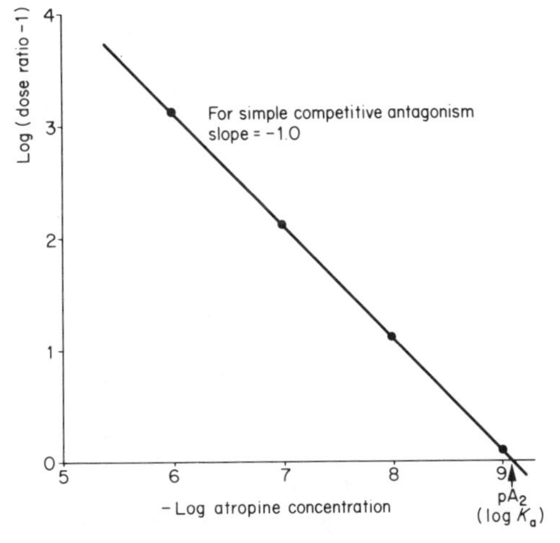

Figure 1.5 Derived from data from *Figure 1.4*. Dose ratio (often represented by x) = concentration of Ach in presence of atropine/concentration of Ach in absence of atropine for same response

concentrations introduces uncertainty in the use of experimental results to validate theoretical assumptions. The two theories are not necessarily mutually exclusive, and it has been suggested that both may be involved in drug actions, the response depending on receptor occupation with some drugs, but related to rate of occupation with others.

Competitive antagonism is one example of surmountable antagonism. Increasing the concentration of the antagonist at the receptor site will overcome (surmount) the presence of the agonist (*Figure 1.6*). Some agonists produce log dose–response curves that become increasingly flatter with increasing antagonist concentration. Eventually an antagonist concentration is produced where increasing the dose of agonist produces no effect. Gaddum used the term unsurmountable antagonism to describe this phenomenon (*Figure 1.7*).

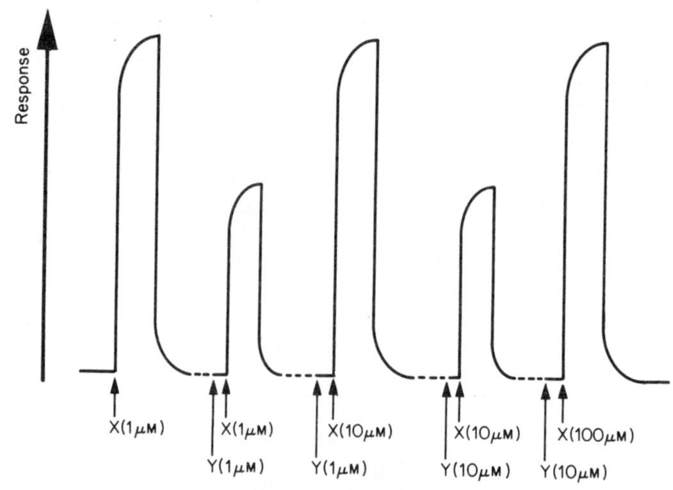

Figure 1.6 Drug X is an agonist which induces the responses shown in a particular tissue (for example, contractions of guinea-pig ileum). Y is a competitive antagonist of X. By increasing the concentration of X it is possible to overcome the effect of any particular concentration of Y

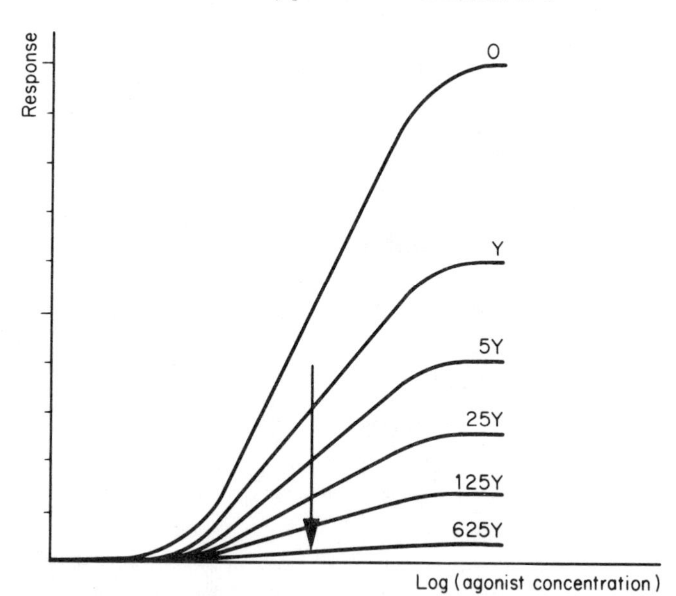

Figure 1.7 Log concentration–response curves for agonist in the presence of increasing concentrations (arrow) of 'unsurmountable' antagonist Y

True non-competitive antagonism

True non-competitive antagonists are a subgroup within the term unsurmountable antagonists. A true non-competitive antagonist acts reversibly at a different receptor site to that at which the agonist acts and blocks its effects. Some antagonists can form a strong bond with receptors, for example phenoxybenzamine. In such instances the rate of dissociation of the antagonist–receptor complex is very slow and can be regarded as zero. Such antagonism is not surmountable by increasing agonist concentrations. The antagonism for practical purposes is irreversible and such antagonism is called irreversible antagonism. It is sometimes loosely referred to as non-competitive antagonism.

Physiological antagonism
This is the term used to describe the antagonism that occurs when two drugs act on different receptors, each producing opposite responses to the other. For example, adrenaline relaxes bronchial muscle by acting on β_2-adrenoceptors present there, while histamine contracts bronchial muscle by acting on H_1 receptors which are also present. These two substances will antagonize one another.

Chemical antagonism
This is an unusual type of antagonism where the antagonist combines chemically with the agonist to form an inactive compound. A good example is the anticoagulant heparin, which is acidic and can be antagonized by the basic substance protamine sulphate.

Mixed antagonism
Some antagonist drugs exhibit mixed antagonism: at low concentrations they behave as competitive antagonists while at higher concentrations they may behave as non-competitive antagonists.

Before leaving the theory of drug–receptor interaction, reference should be made to multiple subunit models. In these the receptor is considered to be formed from a number of subunits, each of which may bind the drug. The important feature is not the multiple drug binding, but what effect this has on the subsequent interactions of the subunits. There are now believed to be pores in the cellular membrane which can allow the entry of ions. The passage of such ions is determined by the size of the pore. If the subunits in a membrane receptor surround a pore, binding of a drug could alter the shape of the molecule, increasing or decreasing its size, thus altering membrane permeability.

An example of a protein made up of subunits is haemoglobin. When this binds with oxygen its function and shape are altered. 2:2-Diphosphoglyceric acid binds at a different site to oxygen on the haemoglobin molecule, but by so altering the shape of the subunits it produces a decreased affinity of the subunits for oxygen. This is an example of allosteric inhibition. The acetylcholine receptor is probably a polymer made up of a number of subunits. There are a number of mathematical models showing how subunits can interact and how inhibitors may alter such actions. The interested reader is referred to Norman's review (1979). One model referred to is where the subunits can exist in one or two forms, the tense state (T) or relaxed state (R). A two-subunit model could therefore exist as TT or RR, but never as TR or RT. An important feature of such a model is that for a small change in agonist concentration a marked effect can be produced. It can explain a steeper dose–response curve than would be predicted by earlier classic theory.

Drug action not due to receptors

The effects of a number of drugs do not appear to involve attachment to specific receptors. The most important members of this class are the general anaesthetics, where there is no obvious relation between chemical structure and pharmacological activity. The theories advanced to explain the action of general anaesthetics are dealt with on page 122.

Drug interactions

Drug interactions are common. The anaesthetist should be aware of the mechanisms by which drug interactions can occur. Patients obtain drugs in three ways. They may be prescribed by a doctor; patients in hospital often receive 10–12 different drugs. They may indulge in self-medication, for example by purchasing vitamins, cold and cough mixtures, or antacids from their local pharmacist. Unbeknown to themselves they may be absorbing drugs from their environment, for instance penicillin which is present in the milk of cows treated with penicillin for bovine mastitis.

The theoretical size of the problem in hospital can be evaluated if a number of assumptions are made. Assuming that a doctor prescribes from a pool of 200 drugs and that the patient in hospital can receive six drugs from that pool, then football pool fanatics could easily calculate that the number of combinations of 6 from 200 is approximately 6×10^{13}. If the chance of a drug interaction is only 1 in 100 000 ($1:10^5$), the number of interactions possible is

$$\frac{6 \times 10^{13}}{10^5},$$

which equals 6×10^8 or six thousand million. Fortunately only a few of these interactions are therapeutically important, although it is likely that many more drug interactions will be described in the future as techniques for measuring drug plasma levels become more widely used.

When the effect of one drug is inhibited by another drug, antagonism has occurred. If the effect of one drug is enhanced by another and the effect is greater than the sum of their individual active effects, potentiation (or synergy) has resulted. Addition is the term used when the combined effect is equal to the sum of their individual effects. The reduced anaesthetic requirement for halothane when given together with nitrous oxide is an example of a therapeutically useful drug interaction, nitrous oxide usually having an additive effect with halothane to produce deeper anaesthesia.

Drug interactions can occur at different stages of drug action. In general, interactions may affect drugs by reactions before absorption occurs, by interfering with the binding, during biotransformation or excretion of a drug, or by an effect at receptors. An example of the first stage is the mixing of thiopentone and suxamethonium before administration. Likewise, antacids can bind tetracyclines and digoxin in the stomach and reduce the amount available for absorption.

Binding to plasma proteins occurs with most drugs. As only the unbound form is active, reduced binding will enhance drug action. The effects of coumarin anticoagulants, for example warfarin, are increased by salicylates, sulphonylureas, sulphonamides, phenylbutazone, and other acidic drugs that have a greater affinity for plasma proteins and increase the concentration of unbound coumarin. It should be noted that highly protein-bound drugs are in general more likely to produce hazardous drug interactions than those less bound (*Figure 1.8*).

Drug metabolism occurs mainly in the liver, the microsomal cytochrome P450 enzymes being responsible for the transformation of drugs to more polar substances. Many drugs are capable of stimulating the activity of these microsomal enzymes. There is no clear relationship between their ability to stimulate enzymes and their chemical structures or pharmacological effects. Among commonly used drugs, barbiturates, inhalational anaesthetics, analgesics, insecticides, and nicotine (from cigarette smoking) are well known to stimulate cytochrome P450 activity. The effects of coumarin anticoagulants can be greatly reduced by concomitant administration of phenobarbitone. Clinically important interactions can occur if phenobarbitone therapy is stopped or started in a patient stabilized on a coumarin anticoagulant. Women on oral contraceptives have been known to become pregnant when treated with rifampicin, an antituberculous drug which is a powerful enzyme inducer.

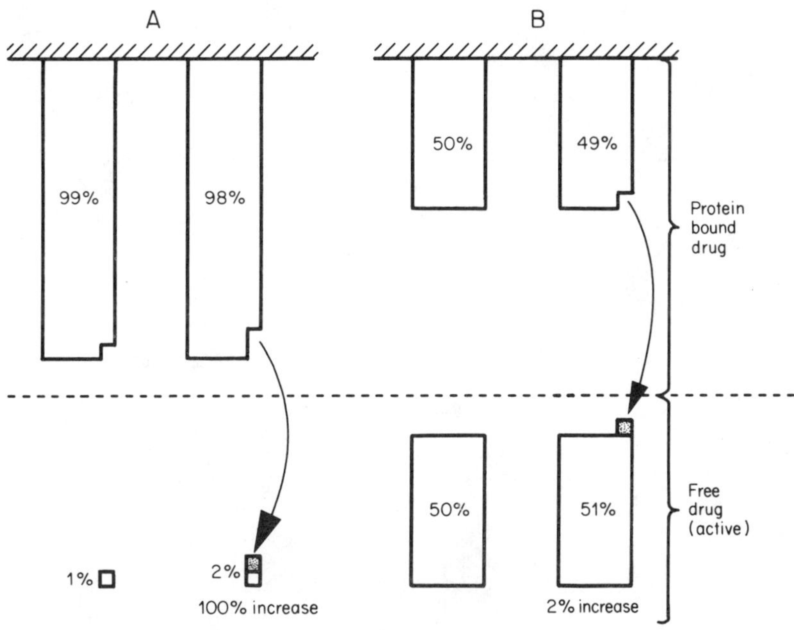

Figure 1.8 Diagrammatic representation of two drugs: drug A is 99 per cent bound to plasma protein, drug B is 50 per cent bound. A displacement of 1 per cent of drug bound will result for drug A in a 100 per cent increase in free (active) drug concentration but only a 2 per cent increase in free drug concentration for drug B

Repeated administration of a drug may cause induction of the enzymes responsible for its metabolism; this process is known as self-induction. Tolerance to barbiturates following chronic administration may be due to self-induction.

Enzyme inhibition can also occur, reducing the metabolism and therefore the excretion of drugs. Monoamine oxidase inhibitors (MAOIs) elevate levels of catecholamines and enhance the effects of indirectly acting sympathomimetic amines such as ephedrine and amphetamine. Foods such as cheese and meat extracts, which have a high tyramine content, can cause severe hypertension in patients on MAOI therapy. Many MAOIs also inhibit hepatic microsomes, which may explain the prolonged effects of pethidine and related narcotic analgesics in patients who are receiving MAOIs.

Enzyme inhibition has been utilized in therapeutics. About 95 per cent of an oral dose of levodopa (an antiparkinsonian agent) is metabolized to dopamine systemically by L-amino acid decarboxylase. This reduces the amount available for penetration of the brain as well as causing systemic side effects. Concurrent administration of carbidopa, an inhibitor of this enzyme in the periphery, reduces by 75 per cent the dose of levodopa necessary to produce the required central effect, as well as reducing the systemic effects.

Renal excretion is the most important method of drug elimination. Drug effects can be modified by alterations of active tubular secretion or of tubular reabsorption. Probenecid, by blocking tubular secretion, potentiates the actions of penicillin. Substances that affect urinary pH may profoundly affect reabsorption of drugs. This is made use of in the treatment of aspirin overdose by forced alkaline diuresis. In alkaline urine, aspirin is more ionized and less lipid soluble and thus its excretion is promoted.

Table 1.2 Drug interactions

Primary drug	*Secondary drug*	*Effect*
Tetracyclines	Methoxyflurane	Nephrotoxicity
	Antacids	Reduced antibiotic absorption
Aminoglycosides (gentamicin, streptomycin)	Competitive neuromuscular blocking agents	Enhanced neuromuscular block
	Cephalosporins	Nephrotoxicity
	Frusemide, ethacrynic acid	Ototoxicity
MAOIs	Indirectly acting sympathomimetic amines, food with high tyramine content	Excessive pressor response
	Oral hypoglycaemic agents	Prolonged hypoglycaemia
	Pethidine	Hypotension and coma
	Tricyclic antidepressants	Excitation
Suxamethonium	Propanidid, ecothiopate, cytotoxic drugs	Prolonged neuromuscular block
Benzodiazepines	Antithyroid drugs	Increased antithyroid activity
Coumarin anticoagulants	Oral antibiotics, salicylates	Enhanced anticoagulant effect
	Barbiturates, phenytoin, cigarette smoking, insecticides	Reduced anticoagulant effect
Tricyclic antidepressants	Adrenaline, ephedrine, amphetamine	Increased pressor effect

The actions of a drug at receptors may be altered in many ways. Competition for receptors is often used for therapeutic purposes, such as the antagonism of tubocurarine by anticholinesterases. Increased concentrations of acetylcholine at the motor end plate displace the muscle relaxant. Treatment of morphine overdose with naloxone is another example of competitive antagonism at a receptor level. Receptor responses can be modified, as when digitalis is given to a patient who is hypokalaemic following diuretic therapy. The concentration of a drug at receptors may be modified by other drugs. Tricyclic antidepressants may affect the actions of some antihypertensive drugs by blocking re-uptake of noradrenaline at nerve endings and preventing uptake of the antihypertensive agent into the nerve terminal.

The table of drug interactions (*Table 1.2*) is in no way comprehensive. Grogono (1974) has reviewed drug interactions that may be of importance in anaesthetic practice.

Tolerance

Tolerance to a drug can be said to occur when the dose administered has to be increased to produce the same pharmacological effect; for instance, if the dose of morphine given to a patient has to be increased from 10 mg to 30 mg to obtain the same degree of pain relief, tolerance to morphine has occurred.

Different mechanisms may produce tolerance. Tolerance can be produced if there is a change in the pharmacokinetics of the drug; for example, it may be metabolized faster. Tolerance to phenobarbitone can occur in this way. Receptor tolerance is another entity; changes in the number (and possibly response) of receptors may occur during chronic treatment. Morphine is believed to produce tolerance by this ill-understood mechanism. Physiological tolerance depends on the presence of physiological control loops; for instance, in the intact animal the failure of an α-adrenoceptor blocking agent to maintain its initial drop in blood pressure when given chronically is due to cardiovascular reflexes coming into play, resulting in an increase in cardiac output which counteracts the fall in blood pressure.

Cross-tolerance is said to occur when, tolerance having been established to one drug, it is found necessary to give higher doses than were previously necessary of pharmacologically related drugs.

Resistance

This is a term often used in relation to antimicrobial agents; for instance, strains of bacteria that were once sensitive to an antimicrobial agent become resistant to the drug. Bacteria can become resistant because of differential survival of sub-strains that produce enzymes that destroy the drug. Penicillinase production by staphylococci is a well-known example; or the strain may switch its metabolic pathway.

Transfer of drugs across membranes

In order to produce their pharmacological effects, drugs must attain an adequate concentration in the tissues upon which they act. Pharmacologists talk of biophase concentration, that is the concentration of a drug in the immediate vicinity of the receptor. In only a few cases are drugs applied directly; most drugs are administered at a point remote from their eventual sites of action and are transported to receptors at their site of action via the plasma and extracellular space. Drugs injected directly into the bloodstream reach tissues rapidly. When given by intramuscular or subcutaneous injection a drug is readily able to transverse the endothelium of capillaries or lymphatics to reach the plasma. Drugs given by other routes have to circumvent other barriers before reaching the plasma.

Membranes in the body, whether surrounding individual cells or subcellular structures within those cells, generally consist of a bimolecular lipid layer covered on both sides with a monomolecular layer of protein. Body membranes are about 10 nm thick and are thought to be discontinuous, being interspersed with pores of about 0.4 nm radius. Four mechanisms may be involved in the transport of a drug across a membrane.

Lipid diffusion
Lipid-soluble drugs will dissolve in the lipid portion of a membrane and diffuse down a concentration gradient to the aqueous phase on the other side of the membrane.

Aqueous diffusion
Lipid-soluble hydrophilic substances may cross membranes by passing through the pores in the membrane. Such passage is assisted by a hydrostatic or osmotic pressure difference across the membrane, when water transport may drag dissolved drugs across. This form of passage is limited by the molecular size of the drug. Most drugs have molecular radii considerably in excess of 0.4 nm and cannot cross membranes in this fashion. The vascular endothelium differs from other membranes. Capillary endothelial cells have large channels of up to 4.0 nm radius, and molecules as large as albumin can pass through these pores from plasma to the extracellular fluid or glomerular filtrate.

Active transport
This consists of the movement of a substance against a concentration or electrochemical gradient. Active transport systems, such as the 'sodium pump', are widely distributed in the body. Drugs chemically resembling actively transported substances may be transported by the same mechanisms. Thus α-methyldopa, which resembles phenylalanine, is absorbed from the intestine by an amino acid transporting mechanism.

Phagocytosis and pinocytosis
Drugs of high molecular weight or which exist as molecular aggregates may be transported by being engulfed as small droplets by cells.

Physical properties affecting transfer

Water and lipid solubility
In order to cross a membrane, a drug must first enter into solution in the aqueous phase in contact with that membrane. Thus the rate of absorption of a drug will be a function of its water solubility. Having come into contact with the membrane, the majority of drugs enter into solution in the lipid component of the membrane. Lipid diffusion will depend on the partition coefficient of the drug between aqueous and lipid phases of the membrane. The higher the lipid/water partition coefficient, the more rapidly will a substance be absorbed.

Ionization and absorption
Most drugs are weak electrolytes, containing acidic or basic groups (or both), and are capable of being ionized in aqueous solution. The cell membrane may be considered as being highly impermeable to the ionized form of any drug. The degree of ionization of a drug is a function of its dissociation constant and the prevalent pH. For an acidic drug AH, the ionization constant K_a is given by $[A^-][H^+]/[AH]$. By analogy with pH notation, $pK_a = -\log_{10}K_a$. Although the ionization constant of a basic drug can similarly be expressed in terms of a dissociation constant K_b, by international convention the dissociations of both acidic and basic drugs are expressed on the same K_a scale. The pK_a for a basic drug is equal to $14-pK_b$. The pK_a values of some commonly used drugs are given in *Figure 1.9*.

The degree of ionization of a drug can be calculated from the Henderson–Hasselbalch equation:

$$\text{For a weak acid, pH–pK}_a = \log \frac{\text{(ionized form)}}{\text{(non-ionized form)}}$$

$$\text{For a weak base, pH–pK}_a = \log \frac{\text{(non-ionized form)}}{\text{(ionized form)}}$$

When pH = pK_a, 50 per cent of the substance is present in the ionized form. Small changes in pH can make large changes in the extent of ionization, particularly if the pH and pK_a values are similar. Thiopentone has a pK_a of 7.6. In the stomach it is almost entirely in the non-ionized form and can be rapidly absorbed on ingestion. In blood at a pH of 7.4, about 61 per cent of any thiopentone is non-ionized. Methohexitone has a pK_a value of about 7.9, and 75 per cent of this drug is

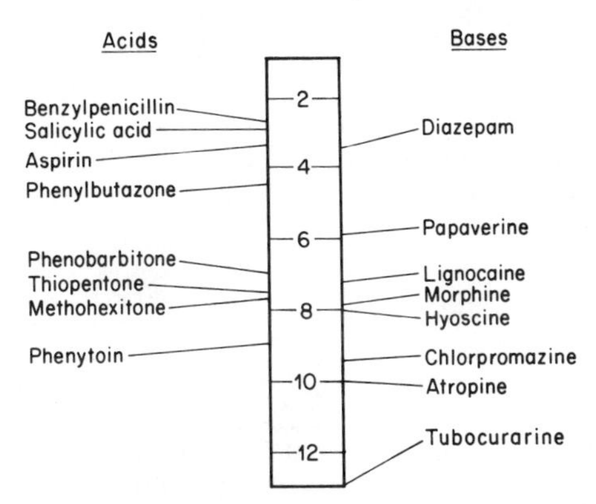

Figure 1.9 The pK_a values of some common drugs

non-ionized at a blood pH of 7.4. This may explain the transiently faster onset of CNS effects with methohexitone compared with thiopentone. As well as being important in determining the absorption of a drug and its passage across cell membranes, the degree of ionization of a substance may greatly affect its excretion by the kidneys.

Transfer across special membranes

Blood–brain barrier

The concept of a blood–brain barrier arose from the observation that many aniline dyes, when given intravenously to animals, stained all tissues except the CSF and brain. The barrier is formed by the close investment of cerebral capillaries by glial cells. These capillaries have permeability characteristics closely resembling those of cellular lipid membranes, and are less permeable than normal capillary endothelial cells. Penetration of the barrier by a drug depends upon the degree of ionization, lipid solubility, and the degree of binding on either side of the barrier. Highly ionized substances such as tubocurarine and hexamethonium cannot cross the boundary. The naturally occurring anticholinesterase, physostigmine, is a tertiary amine which can readily enter the brain; neostigmine closely resembles physostigmine but, being a quaternary compound and highly ionized at plasma pH, is without actions on the CNS.

Brain penetration by non-ionized molecules is a function of lipid solubility. Thiopentone, which is largely non-ionized at plasma pH and very lipid soluble, readily enters the brain. The corresponding oxybarbiturate, pentobarbitone, penetrates the brain slowly because of its low lipid solubility.

Chemotherapeutic agents for the treatment of brain infections must be able to penetrate this barrier. Penicillin penetrates the normal barrier slightly, but passes through more readily in the presence of inflammation. Chloramphenicol, streptomycin, and isoniazid pass into the brain in amounts sufficient to give adequate chemotherapeutic concentrations; tetracyclines and *p*-aminosalicylic acid do not.

Placental barrier

The placenta is best regarded as a modified lipid membrane across which drug passage is chiefly governed by lipid solubility. Besides lipid solubility and ionization, other factors that affect placental transport are the degree of binding of the drug to plasma proteins and the placental blood flow. Highly ionized drugs of low lipid solubility, such as tubocurarine and suxamethonium, penetrate the placenta only slowly. Inhalational anaesthetics and thiopentone rapidly attain equilibrium with fetal blood. Morphine, pethidine, and other narcotic analgesics also readily pass to the fetus. Depressant drugs given to the mother during labour may have untoward effects on the fetus because of the immature drug-metabolizing and excretory systems of the newborn.

Routes of administration

Drugs may be given by various routes. They can be given by mouth in the form of solutions, suspensions, emulsions, or tablets. Tablets are most commonly used for relatively insoluble substances. When made in effervescent form, the solubility is slightly increased and the drug is dispersed more readily. In this form they are known as 'soluble' tablets. The main consideration in the case of a solution for injection is its pH. If the solution is too acidic or too alkaline it may cause irritation and even tissue damage at the site of injection.

Oral route

This is the most common route and normally the best way of giving drugs. Absorption is slow, however, and often irregular. Some drugs may stick in the oesophagus and cause damage to it. Slow-release potassium chloride tablets, doxycycline, and emepronium bromide have been reported to cause oesophageal damage. Other drugs implicated are tetracycline, clindamycin, oral iron preparations, and non-narcotic analgesics such as aspirin. Drugs that are highly acidic (such as doxycycline and tetracycline) or highly basic in solution (such as emepronium bromide) are likely to cause oesophageal damage. Patients at special risk are those who have oesophageal obstruction, for example due to enlargement of the left atrium. Formulation is important; in general, capsules are more likely than tablets to stick or dissolve in the oesophagus. Drugs known to be mucosal irritants should normally be taken with a glass of water to reduce the risk of oesophageal damage. Some substances given orally are absorbed from the stomach, but the majority of drugs administered orally are absorbed from the upper part of the small intestine.

Irritant drugs should be well diluted, cooled if possible, and given after meals to reduce their tendency to cause nausea and vomiting. Drugs that are subject to acid hydrolysis or are highly irritant to the stomach may be given in gelatin capsules which liberate their contents only after reaching the small intestine.

The prevailing pH of the gastrointestinal tract, by affecting the degree of ionization of a drug, will influence absorption. In the stomach the effective pH at the lipid barrier is about 3.5. Acidic substances with pK_a values of less than 2 and bases with pK_a values greater than 5 will be highly ionized and their absorption will be negligible. The higher pH of the small intestine assists in the absorption of bases that may be too highly ionized to be absorbed in the stomach. Rapid absorption from the small intestine occurs with acids with pK_a values above 3 and with bases with pK_a values below 8. It should be noted that contact time is also important. Aspirin (pK_a 3) is less ionized at the pH of the stomach than in the intestine. It is, therefore, more rapidly absorbed in the stomach. However, its transit time in the intestine is normally longer than in the stomach and hence appreciable absorption can occur from the intestine.

Drugs absorbed from the mouth and rectum pass directly into the systemic circulation. Drugs absorbed from elsewhere in the gastrointestinal tract are carried to the liver in the portal vein. Here they may come under the influence of enzymatic detoxicating mechanisms and their activity reduced. The liver may also secrete drugs into the bile. An intestinally absorbed drug may also be secreted in the bile and re-presented to the intestine. Such an enterohepatic shunt tends to prolong the duration of action of a drug.

Some drugs are given by mouth to act locally in the gastrointestinal tract rather than by absorption. In this group are the saline purgatives sodium and magnesium sulphate, which are poorly absorbed and by their osmotic action increase the bulk of the intestinal contents; antacids and absorbents such as aluminium hydroxide and magnesium trisilicate, which neutralize gastric acid to form insoluble salts; and drugs for treating infections of the gastrointestinal tract such as streptomycin, neomycin, and some sulphonamides, which exist in the gastrointestinal tract in a highly ionized form but are not inactivated by intestinal secretions.

Subcutaneous injection

Absorption of drugs given by this route is more rapid than when given by mouth. The rate of absorption is decreased if the drug – or mixture of drugs – causes vasoconstriction, and may be increased by increasing the blood supply to the injection site. Subcutaneous administration may be more painful than other forms of injection because of the rich sensory innervation of the skin. Irritant drugs such as digoxin should not be given subcutaneously as they may cause local sloughing of the skin or abscess formation.

Intramuscular injection

Absorption by this route is faster than by subcutaneous injection, especially when the drug is water soluble. Absorption can be slowed if the drug is in an oily solution or emulsified, when the active drug will be slowly released to pass to the tissues. Water-soluble drugs may be converted into less soluble compounds. The procaine salts of penicillin and the insulin–zinc complexes are examples of the therapeutic advantages of reduced water solubility: prolonged effects can be attained, smoother and more sustained blood levels achieved, and fewer injections needed than if the highly water-soluble parent compounds are used.

Intravenous injection

As the drug in this case is introduced directly into the circulation, its onset of action will be more rapid but its duration of action shorter than when given by any other route (*Figure 1.10*). Substances too irritant for subcutaneous or intramuscular injection can often be given intravenously. The use of this route is not without risk: in cases of overdose or idiosyncrasy the effects are immediate and it may not be possible to antagonize them before serious toxic symptoms or even death have intervened. The effects of a drug given intravenously can be greatly modified by the rate of administration. Mixing of a drug with the circulating blood volume takes several circulation times. With rapid intravenous injection, tissues can be exposed to high concentrations of drug poorly diluted with blood and travelling as a bolus. The rapid onset of sleep when intravenous induction agents are given over a period of 30 seconds or less is related to this 'slug' effect. Subsequent rapid recovery is more dependent upon a fall in effective blood concentration due to mixing than to a rapid initial redistribution to lipid depots.

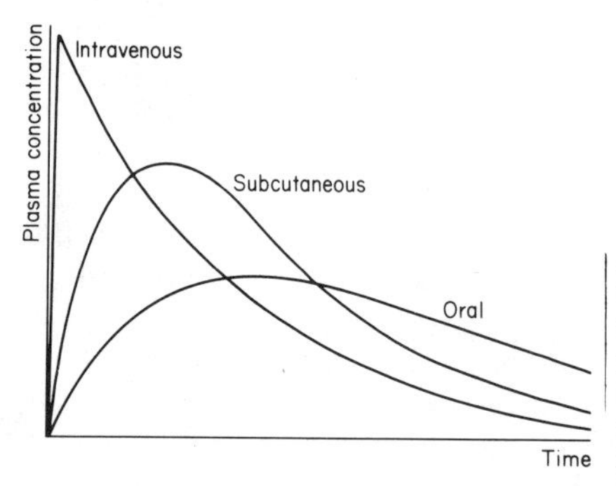

Figure 1.10 Time course of a hypothetical drug given by three different routes. Note the high initial plasma concentration after intravenous injection followed by a rapid fall. After oral administration there is a slow rise and the peak plasma concentration is low. Subcutaneous injection results in a curve with a higher and earlier peak than after the oral route

If a drug is irritant, venous thrombosis can often be avoided by withdrawing blood into the syringe and mixing it with the solution before injection; alternatively, it may be well diluted and given as a slow infusion. A sustained blood level of a drug can also be maintained by giving a continuous intravenous infusion at a controlled rate.

Inhalation

Absorption of drugs through the lungs is rapid as the alveoli have a large surface area and an abundant blood supply. The effect produced by this route is almost as quick as when the drug is given by intravenous injection. The volatile anaesthetics are the most important group of drugs given by inhalation. The factors that govern their absorption are discussed in Chapter 4. Aerosols of sympathomimetic amines are commonly given by inhalation to relieve bronchospasm: untoward and occasionally fatal cardiovascular effects of substances such as isoprenaline may occur due to rapid absorption. A recent hazard in our society is the indiscriminate sniffing of aerosols by people, especially young adolescents, for pleasure. Deaths have occurred due to rapid absorption of toxic substances.

Mucous membranes

Drugs are absorbed through the mucous membranes of the mouth (sublingual), nose, eye, and rectum. The rate of absorption is rapid, being between that of intramuscular and intravenous injection. Sublingual administration is valuable in the case of glyceryl trinitrate in angina. When local analgesics are applied to mucous surfaces they can readily give rise to systemic effects; these can be minimized by the use of a vasoconstrictor such as adrenaline.

Other routes

Drugs are also absorbed through the peritoneum and in small amounts through intact skin. Intrathecal injections of chemotherapeutic agents or local anaesthetics require special care and must be non-irritant.

Factors affecting drug dosage

The required dose of a drug depends mainly on its effect at a given level, on its toxicity, and on the duration of its effect – governed by its rate of inactivation and its mode of excretion. When a new drug is produced, initial animal experiments involving different species can give an approximate idea of its toxicity. If its actions and toxicity do not vary much from one species to another, the chances are that man will behave similarly when exposed to the drug. Initial studies in man are always performed on volunteers to determine by trial what is a reasonable dose to give the desired effect, and the duration of this effect can be studied and correlated with the rate of drug excretion. Gradually information is built up that will enable a reasonable estimate to be made of the dose required. The official dose in the *British Pharmacopoeia* for new drugs is determined in this manner. The dose of the older drugs was determined empirically in a much more haphazard way by trial and error, and it was rare for animal experiments to be employed.

The maximum dose for the majority of drugs depends on the dose level that is effective therapeutically, relative to the toxic effects produced. Some drugs, such as insulin, penicillin, and various antisera, are given in a dose that depends on the severity of the condition, so that a severely ill child may receive more than an adult.

Some drugs are used for one purpose at one dose level and for a completely different purpose at another. Acetylsalicylic acid is an example: it is widely used for certain types of pain in doses of 0.3–1.0 g while in rheumatic fever 10 times the dose may be given for its other actions.

The amount of a drug necessary to produce and maintain a given effect depends on several factors, particularly the rate of clearance. The spacing of dosage is determined by the need to maintain a therapeutic blood level; this is especially important with chemotherapeutic agents or in the use of morphine to maintain prolonged analgesia.

When a drug is given, a peak blood level is reached which subsides as the drug is metabolized and removed from the body. This peak is due to the fact that entry is usually quicker than removal of the drug. It is difficult to determine the end-point when the concentration of a drug in the tissues and the amount being excreted is minimal. For practical purposes it is more convenient to take the half-clearance time.

The frequency and magnitude of doses will obviously vary considerably with different drugs. With benzylpenicillin clearance is very rapid, half being excreted in less than 1 hour; with thyroxine and digitalis half-clearance may take 1 week or more. Between these two extremes are the sulphonamides and salicylates and many of the benzodiazepines, the half-clearance of which takes 2–8 hours.

In many cases the duration of action of a drug and its cumulation follow certain simple general principles related to its clearance curve, which is exponential in type. This type of 'die-away' curve is important because it indicates that the amount of drug removed in unit time is a constant fraction of the amount that still remains. This kind of curve will give a straight line when plotted on semi-logarithmic paper, thus enabling curves similarly constructed to be readily compared. Drugs obeying such laws have a duration of action that varies as the logarithm of the dose, and increasing the dose will therefore have less than the simple arithmetical effect. It is often unwise to give large doses of a drug on a logarithmic scale to increase the duration of action, especially with short-acting drugs quickly excreted or broken down, as the blood concentration necessary may not be tolerated without the occurrence of toxic effects. A longer acting preparation can be substituted if available, smaller doses can be given at more frequent intervals, or the drug may be given by intravenous infusion.

The dose of a drug may have to be decreased after a few days, as in the case of digoxin, because of accumulation. Tolerance or tachyphylaxis may require the dose to be increased. Iodine in thyrotoxicosis and morphine or pethidine given to drug addicts may have to be administered at continually increasing dose levels to evoke the same response.

Paediatric doses

Many equations have been devised for estimating the requirements of children; some are based on age, but the majority on weight. They tend to produce inappropriate doses at the extremes of the scale, and to accommodate this two or three different ranges have to be included.

Many physiological requirements and metabolic processes are more related to surface area than age or weight, and Catzel (1963) has worked out a single schedule covering the range from 1 month to the young adult in which the percentage of the adult dose required is derived from the equation:

$$\text{percentage of adult dose} = \frac{\text{surface area of child}}{\text{surface area of adult}} \times 100$$

It can be seen that even should *Table 1.3* not be available, the four reference points at which the dose is one eighth, one quarter, a half, and three quarters of the adult dose can be simply memorized as approximately 1 month, 1 year, 7 years, and 12 years respectively.

Predicting the requirements of premature infants or normal babies during the first 2 weeks of life, when detoxicating and excretory mechanisms are immature, is much more difficult.

Timing of administration

When a drug is given by mouth it is usually given in divided doses over the day, thus obviating the higher blood concentrations necessary with single doses and reducing the tendency for toxic effects to occur.

The exact time of administration of a drug depends on a number of factors. For example, if a drug is given in order to stimulate appetite, it must be given before food, while gastric irritants should never be given on an empty stomach. Drugs that depress the CNS, such as antihistamines, should as a rule be given at night, while

Table 1.3 Estimation of doses for children as a percentage of the adult dose

Approximate age	*Weight kg*	*lb*	*Percentage of adult dose*	*Fraction of adult dose*
1 month	3.2	7	12.5	1/8
2 months	4.5	10	15	
4 months	6.5	14	20	
12 months	10	22	25*	1/4
18 months	11	24	30	
5 years	18	40	40	
7 years	23	50	50	1/2
10 years	30	66	60	
11 years	36	80	70	
12 years	40	88	75	3/4
14 years	45	100	80	
16 years	54	120	90	
Adult	65	145	100	1

* In the original Table from Butler and Ritchie (1960) an infant weighing 22 lb receives 28 per cent of the adult dose. This has been reduced to 25 per cent for the convenience of remembering that an infant at 1 year requires about ¼ of the adult dose (Catzel, 1963). Reproduced from *Paediatric Prescriber*, by P. Catzel, by courtesy of Blackwell, Oxford.

some CNS stimulants are best given in the early part of the day so as not to interfere with sleep.

The duration of action of a drug governs the spacing of doses. It is essential to maintain adequate drug tissue concentrations if effects are to be maintained in an unbroken manner. This is important to the patient and reduces the tendency for tolerance and addiction to develop.

Binding of drugs

A variable proportion of a drug present in the intravascular compartment is reversibly bound to plasma protein, chiefly albumin. The physicochemical forces involved in the combination of a drug and protein are the same as those involved in the drug–receptor complex (page 5). Only the unbound portion of a drug is pharmacologically active; the bound drug cannot diffuse from the vascular space and is pharmacologically inert, except that the drug–protein complex can act as an antigen.

Binding of a drug, by reducing the concentration in the aqueous phase of plasma, may facilitate absorption, and the degree of binding of a drug may greatly influence its rate of metabolism. Thus when phenylbutazone is present at a plasma level of 100 μg/ml only 2 per cent is unbound. If the plasma level is raised to 250 μg/ml, because the binding sites are approaching saturation, the unbound proportion rises to 12 per cent. Biotransformation now proceeds at six times the former rate, and the level again falls quickly to 100 μg/ml (Brodie, 1965). Binding of tubocurarine to plasma protein slows the distribution of this drug throughout the extracellular fluid and retards the rate of urinary and biliary excretion.

The greater solubility of volatile anaesthetics in plasma and whole blood than can be accounted for by their water or lipid solubility is due to binding of these agents. The binding of anaesthetic agents to protein has been suggested as playing an important part in the mechanisms of anaesthesia at a molecular level.

Other structures besides plasma may bind drugs. Thiobarbiturates, which have a high lipid/water partition coefficient, tend to accumulate in fat. Gallamine has a strong affinity for mucopolysaccharide and is concentrated in connective tissues. Tetracyclines and heavy metals are stored in bone. Carbon monoxide can readily penetrate the red cell membrane and is so firmly bound to haemoglobin that negligible concentrations are present in the plasma. The accumulation of drugs at specific sites may be of great therapeutic significance. The selective affinity of iodine for the thyroid gland is utilized in the diagnosis of thyroid disorders and the treatment of hyperthyroidism with radioactive iodine isotopes. When iodine isotopes are used for investigations not involving the thyroid it is usually necessary to pretreat the patient with a large dose of non-labelled iodine which will saturate thyroid-binding sites and diminish thyroid uptake of the subsequently administered isotope.

Distribution of drugs in the body

At equilibrium the freely diffusible portion of a drug is in equilibrium in all tissues. Because variable fractions of the drug cannot penetrate membranes, due to binding or ionization, different total amounts of drug may be present in different tissues. The total concentration of a drug in a tissue will increase as binding within that tissue increases. Similarly, compartments in which ionization is high will contain a greater amount of a drug than those compartments in which the drug exists mainly in the non-ionized form. This implies that acidic drugs will tend to accumulate in areas of high pH, while basic drugs will accumulate in regions of low pH. As the intracellular pH is lower than the plasma pH, bases thus tend to be concentrated intracellularly.

Drug metabolism

A knowledge of drug metabolism is essential for good therapeutic practice for the following reasons:

1. The metabolite formed may have pharmacological activity; for example, paracetamol, now used extensively as a mild analgesic agent, is in fact the active metabolite of a previously widely used analgesic, phenacetin.
2. The metabolite may have toxic properties: for example, metabolites of methoxyflurane can cause kidney damage.
3. It may be possible to inhibit the metabolism of a drug, thereby prolonging its action; a classic example is the use of an anticholinesterase to prolong the duration of action of acetylcholine.
4. The metabolism of a drug can be increased, thereby shortening its duration of action; for example, barbiturates can decrease the duration of action of oral anticoagulants.

Fish can excrete lipid-soluble drugs through their structured gills into the sea. Frogs can similarly excrete lipid-soluble substances through their skins. Man, however, is devoid of such mechanisms. Lipid-soluble substances may easily pass through the kidney glomeruli into the tubular lumen, but they can be easily reabsorbed back into the circulation through the lipid barrier of the tubular cell. A closed system would therefore exist if there was no mechanism for making such compounds more water soluble (less lipophilic).

Fortunately there are such mechanisms, otherwise the duration of action of lipophilic drugs would be very long. One of the most important is found in the human liver, which contains a system of microsomal enzymes that can modify the chemical structure of such highly lipid-soluble compounds so that the lipid/water partition coefficient of the product is considerably different from that of the original substance. Ontogeny often recapitulates phylogeny. The mammalian embryo undergoes a 'fish-like' stage and therefore it is perhaps not surprising that newborn mammals may be deficient for some time in microsomal enzymes.

Using the technique of electron microscopy, liver cells can be shown to contain a network of lipoprotein tubules diffusing throughout the cytoplasm. Part of this reticulum is studded with ribonucleic acid globules (called ribosomes), and is thus called 'rough endoplasmic reticulum'; the other is smoother in surface and hence is called 'smooth endoplasmic reticulum' (SER). Associated with the SER are a number of enzymes involved in the metabolism of drugs. These are called microsomal enzymes as they can be found on ultracentrifugation in the microsomal fraction. Features of their action are that substances with high lipid solubility usually serve as substrates, and that they are relatively non-specific and will therefore metabolize a wide variety of substances. SER occurs in other cells but many studies have concentrated on hepatic cells.

Liver microsomes (as well as microsomes of other cells) contain a pigment that is important in the metabolism of drugs. The pigment is unusual in that its reduced form has virtually the same spectrum as the oxidized form. The pigmented material is called cytochrome P450. The reduced form forms a complex with carbon monoxide which has an absorption maximum at 450 μ. Microsomal enzyme activity can be modified by pathological processes such as liver damage. Malnutrition can depress it. Drugs may enhance or inhibit microsomal enzyme activity (Conney, 1967).

The majority of drugs undergo some form of metabolism in the body. The metabolic products usually have less pharmacological activity than the unmetabolized drug. Sometimes pharmacologically active metabolites are formed from inactive precursors; such precursors are called pro-drugs. For example, chloral is inactive until converted into trichloroethanol. In other cases the metabolites may have different pharmacological actions to the drugs from which they are derived.

There are four principal pathways of drug metabolism: oxidation, reduction, hydrolysis, and conjugation. Although some drugs are metabolized by a single process, the majority are metabolized by a sequence of at least two processes. Phase 1 consists of transformation by oxidation, reduction, or hydrolysis. In Phase 2 the transformed product is conjugated to produce a pharmacologically inactive, water-soluble, excretory product.

Oxidation

The majority of oxidative transformations involve the microsomal enzymes of the liver and are examples of hydroxylation. Thus aromatic substances such as phenobarbitone and pethidine, and polycyclic compounds such as steroids, undergo aromatic hydroxylation. Thio-ethers such as the phenothiazines undergo sulphoxidation to form sulphoxides. Desulphurization of thiopentone converts it into the parent pentobarbitone.

Not all oxidative transformations involve microsomal enzymes. Caffeine and alcohol utilize non-microsomal enzymes. Alcohols are metabolized by the enzyme, alcohol dehydrogenase. Ethanol is completely converted into water and carbon dioxide:

$$CH_3CH_2OH \rightarrow CH_3CHO \rightarrow CH_3COOH \rightarrow \underset{\text{Acetylcoenzyme A}}{CH_3CO{:}CoA} \rightarrow H_2O + CO_2$$

Monoamine oxidase (MAO) is a mitochondrial enzyme responsible for the conversion of catecholamines into the corresponding aldehydes. MAO is also responsible for the conversion of 5-hydroxytryptamine into 5-hydroxyindoleacetic acid.

Reduction

Reduction is a less common form of drug transformation than oxidation. Again microsomal enzymes of the liver are mainly responsible. Examples of reduction occurring in the liver are the reduction of chloral hydrate to trichloroethanol and the removal of chlorine and bromine from halothane by reductive dehalogenation.

Removal of a radical

Side chains can be removed by oxidative dealkylation or deamination; pethidine to norpethidine is an example of *N*-demethylation; codeine to morphine is an example of oxidative dealkylation.

Splitting a bond

The aromatic ring structure can be opened; for example, the barbiturate ring can be destroyed. Although this can occur, in man it is of minor importance. Oxidation of radicals at the C5 position in the ring is the most important pathway for metabolism of the barbiturates.

Cleavage

A large number of drugs contain the ester linkage $-\overset{\overset{\displaystyle O}{\|}}{C}-O$: examples are esters of choline such as suxamethonium, local anaesthetics such as cocaine, induction agents such as propanidid, and narcotic analgesics such as pethidine. Ester linkages are hydrolysed in the body by specific or non-specific esterases. These are widely distributed in tissues or in the blood.

Hydrolysis is an important mechanism for the metabolism of esters and amides. The best known examples of hydrolysing enzymes are the cholinesterases, which are widely distributed in mammalian tissue and are responsible for the hydrolysis of many ester drugs, including suxamethonium and procaine. Pethidine is similarly hydrolysed by a hepatic microsomal enzyme.

Conjugation

In conjugation reactions, drugs or their metabolic products combine with endogenous substrates. Conjugation plays a major role in the disposition of many products of normal metabolism. Thus the methylation of catecholamines and the glucuronic conjugation of bile salts and steroid hormones are important for normal metabolism.

The endogenous substrate taking part in conjugation reactions is usually a product of carbohydrate or amino acid metabolism. The following conjugation reactions are of importance in man.

Methylation
In these reactions the methyl donor is methionine. A methyl group is transferred from *S*-adenosylmethionine to phenols, amines, and some thiols. *N*-methylation of histamine produces the pharmacologically inactive 4-methylhistamine. Catechol-*O*-methyltransferases are involved in the transfer of methyl groups to the *O*-hydroxyl groups of catechol; these reactions are important in both the synthesis and the degradation of catecholamines.

Acetylation
Acetylcoenzyme A is the acetyl donor. Many alkyl- and arylamines are acetylated by various transferases, including *p*-aminobenzoic acid and sulphonamides.

Glucuronide formation
This occurs with a wide range of compounds. The glucuronyl residue from uridine diphosphate glucuronic acid (UDPGA) is transferred to the acceptor molecule. The UDP glucuronyl transferases which catalyse the reaction are located in the liver microsomes. The general reaction is:

$$\underset{\text{Acceptor drug}}{R-OH}+UDPGA \rightarrow \underset{\text{Glucuronide}}{R-O-C_6H_6O_9}+UDP$$

Among the many drugs that are conjugated with glucuronic acid are morphine, *p*-aminosalicylic acid, and chloramphenicol. Glucuronic acid conjugates are secreted into the bile and enter the small intestine, where they may be hydrolysed by an enzyme, β-glucuronidase. Chloramphenicol and phenolphthalein form glucuronides which are hydrolysed in the intestine by this enzyme; the released active drug is absorbed and carried back to the liver for reconjugation. They thus take part in an enterohepatic shunt.

Amino acid conjugations
Glycine and glutamine form peptide conjugates with acids. The reaction involves the formation of the acetylcoenzyme A derivative of the acceptor molecule, which then reacts with the amino acid:

$$\underset{\text{Acid}}{R-COOH}+CoA+ATP \rightarrow \underset{\text{Coenzyme A complex}}{R{\cdot}CO-CoA} \xrightarrow{\text{Glycine}} \underset{\text{Glycine conjugate}}{R{\cdot}CO-NH-CH_2-COOH}$$

Glycine combines with isoniazid, salicylic acid, and nicotinic acid. Salicylic acids also conjugate with glutamine.

Ethereal sulphate conjugation
Aromatic and aliphatic hydroxyl groups may be converted into a sulphanilic acid, $R{\cdot}OH \rightarrow R{\cdot}OSO_3H$. Sulphate is transferred from the coenzyme adenosine-3-phosphate-5-phosphosulphate. Chloramphenicol can undergo sulphate conjugation. A drug may utilize several metabolic pathways. For example, pethidine can be hydrolysed or, alternatively, *N*-demethylation can occur.

Drug excretion

The kidney and gastrointestinal tract are the major routes of drug elimination. Inhalational anaesthetics are, however, excreted mainly by the lungs, and a few drugs are excreted by the salivary glands. Drugs excreted in milk may have an effect on a breast-fed child.

Drugs may be excreted either in an unchanged form or, after modification, by metabolic processes. Metabolic changes that increase the polarity and reduce the lipid solubility of a substance will facilitate excretion.

Renal excretion

Elimination of drugs in the urine is governed by three factors: glomerular filtration, tubular reabsorption, and tubular secretion. The glomerular filtration of any substance depends on its molecular weight and the plasma concentration of unbound drug. The glomerular capillaries permit the passage of most solutes, but drug bound to plasma protein is retained in the circulation. In the nephron the fate of a drug is largely dependent on its lipid solubility. Molecules that have a high lipid/water partition coefficient and are non-ionized will readily pass back from glomerular filtrates across the tubular epithelium. Ions are unable to traverse this lipid boundary.

The cells of the proximal convoluted tubule possess two separate mechanisms for the active transport of organic acids and bases. These systems transport ionized molecules. Ions compete for these relatively non-specific transport systems. The prolongation of duration of action of penicillin by probenecid is due to a competitive inhibition of renal tubular acid-transporting systems by this acid. Drugs can also reach the urine by passive diffusion across the tubular epithelium. Simple diffusion may be bidirectional. As glomerular filtrate passes down the nephron, water reabsorption increases the concentration of any drugs present and tends to facilitate back-diffusion.

Most drugs are subject to some degree of ionization. The relative proportion of ionized and non-ionized molecules depends upon pK_a and the prevailing pH. The non-ionized portion of a drug tends to come into equilibrium across the tubular epithelium. In alkaline urine, weak acids are more ionized and thus are present in a greater total concentration, and weak bases are similarly excreted more rapidly in acidic urine. Advantage is taken of pH-dependent excretion in the management of salicylate and phenobarbitone overdose. These drugs are weak acids with relatively low pK_a values; alkalinization of the urine by the systemic administration of bicarbonate significantly hastens their rate of renal elimination.

Intestinal excretion

The physicochemical factors involved in the absorption of drugs from the gastrointestinal tract (water solubility and lipid/water partition) also influence the elimination of drugs and their metabolites into the gut and their removal in faeces. The biliary system acts as a specialized transport mechanism for the intestinal excretion of drugs, especially drugs of high molecular weight capable of being metabolically transformed and conjugated. Specialized mechanisms also exist for the active transport of acids and bases from blood to bile. These transport mechanisms closely resemble those of the kidney.

Factors determining biophase concentration

Principle

Size of drug effect (S_E) is a function of the concentration of drug (C) at the site (the biophase) where the effect sequence is initiated:

$$S_E = f(C)$$

Pharmacokinetics is a term used to describe the section of pharmacology that deals with the factors influencing the magnitude of drug effect by determining the amount of drug at various body sites as a function of time. It is usual to divide the time course of drug action into three parts: first, the latency (time for onset of

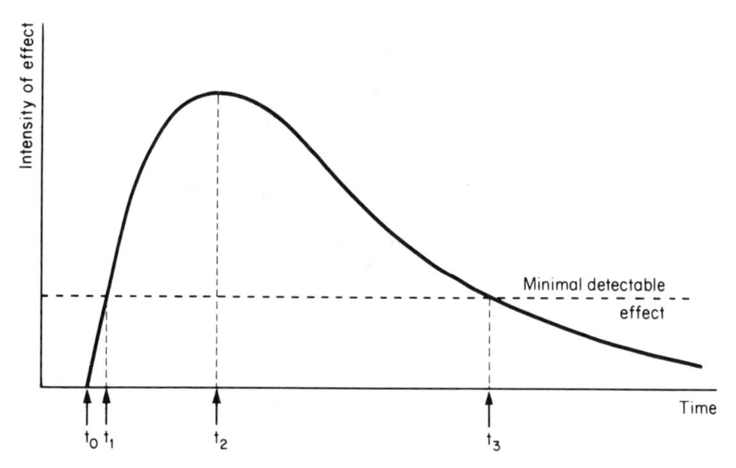

Figure 1.11 Magnitude of drug effect as a function of time. Drug administered at time t_0; latency = $t_1 - t_0$; time to peak effect = $t_2 - t_0$; duration of action = $t_3 - t_0$

action); second, the time to peak effect; and third, the duration of action (*Figure 1.11*). It is often assumed that plasma concentration correlates positively with the intensity of drug effect. This assumption is probably valid if rapid equilibrium occurs between blood and biophase. If the time to equilibrium is long it is unlikely to be true (*Figure 1.12*).

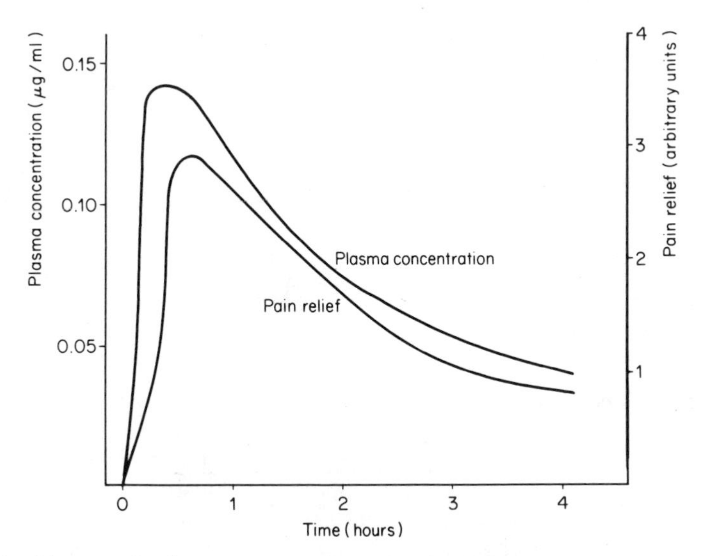

Figure 1.12 In this example plasma concentrations of narcotic analgesic closely follow pain relief obtained by the patient

Rate of drug absorption

In most instances if concentrations are below saturation, first-order kinetics apply. The rate is proportional to the concentration of drug. At higher concentrations zero-order kinetics may apply. Under such conditions rate is constant. Constant rate absorption is important to anaesthetists: if the machines that the anaesthetist uses for administering a volatile anaesthetic replace the anaesthetic removed by the patient during each breath, constant rate absorption occurs. Elimination is the term used to describe the rate at which a drug disappears from the body. More than one process may be involved; for instance, a drug can be metabolized and also excreted in the urine.

Elimination for most drugs follows first-order kinetics: a constant fraction of the total amount of drug in the body is eliminated in equal units of time (*Figure 1.13*). A useful measure is the half-time for elimination, $t_{1/2}$. This is the time required to eliminate 50 per cent of quantity of drug that was present when the measurement was initiated.

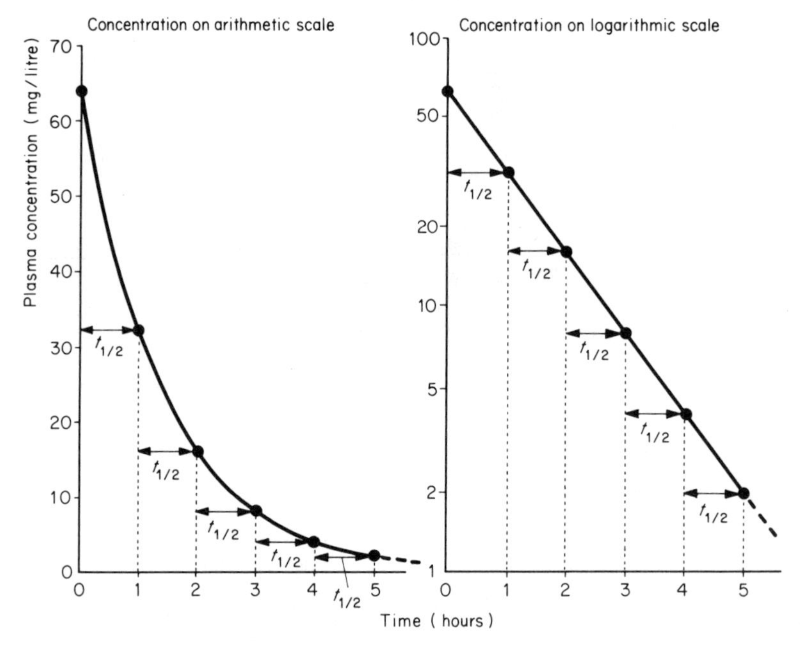

Figure 1.13 Decay of plasma concentration with time for a drug given intravenously whose initial plasma concentration was 64 mg/100 ml; $t_{1/2}$ (indicated by double arrows) is 1 hour. Note: plasma level has fallen to 32 mg/ℓ in first hour; 16, 8, 4, and 2 mg/ℓ respectively in 2, 3, 4, and 5 hours. Conversion of concentration to log concentration will produce a straight line

Since most drugs are metabolized and the metabolism depends on enzymes, the factors determining the velocity of enzyme reaction are important. At low substrate concentration, there will be an abundance of active sites on the enzyme available for occupation, and first-order kinetics will apply. If substrate concentration rises to a level that saturates the active sites, zero-order kinetics will apply. It should be remembered that the 'enzyme complex' contains not only the enzyme but often cofactors. If the demand on these cofactors outruns the supply, zero-order kinetics

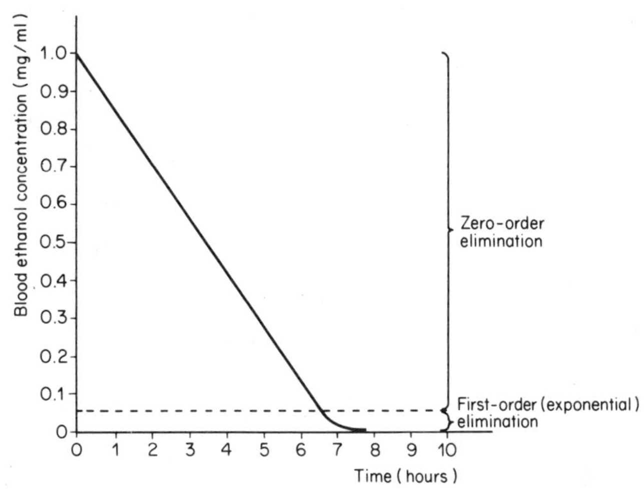

Figure 1.14 Zero-order elimination of ethanol over the concentration range 0.05–1 mg/ml. First-order kinetics apply only at concentrations of ethanol below 0.05 mg/ml

can also occur. Alcohol is a good example of a drug where, at blood levels produced by social drinking, zero-order kinetics apply (*Figure 1.14*).

Compartment models

Pharmacokineticists often use mathematical models to simulate how the body may deal with a drug. The body can be considered to consist of a series of compartments; such compartments are mathematical concepts and need bear no relationship to anatomical or physiological compartments.

The simplest model is a one-compartment model. The body is considered to be one compartment into which a drug, once administered, distributes and equilibrates. Simple though it is, it can adequately model the changes, with time, of plasma concentration of many drugs that rapidly distribute between plasma and tissue after administration. This model does not assume that plasma and tissue concentrations are the same. It does assume that there is a constant relationship between these concentrations, for example that tissue concentrations are always half those of plasma concentrations. Elimination is assumed normally to follow first-order kinetics. Using calculus, the rate of change (dx/dt) in the amount of drug present in the compartment (x) is given by the equation:

$$-\frac{dx}{dt} \propto x \text{ or } \frac{dx}{dt} = -kx \quad (1)$$

where k is a constant, known as the first-order elimination rate constant. Negative sign shows drug is being lost from the compartment.

From equation (1) it is possible to derive by a process of integration and substitution, the following equation:

$$x_t = x_0 e^{-kt} \quad (2)$$

where x_t and x_0 are the amount of drug present at time t and time 0; e is the base e (2.71828), k is the elimination constant.

The amount of drug eliminated in time t is:

$$x_0 - x_t = x_0 - x_0 e^{-kt} \text{ (from equation 2)} = x_0(1 - e^{-kt}) \quad (3)$$

The drug $[x]$ can be considered to be distributed in a certain volume V_d, which is called the volume of distribution:

$$x = V_d C \quad (4)$$

where C is the plasma concentration.

It can be seen that V_d is a proportionality constant. It is important to note that V_d does not represent an actual physiological volume, for example extracellular space. Factors influencing the size of V_d are drug characteristics such as lipid solubility, and patient characteristics such as body size, protein binding, and plasma protein concentration.

Considering now equations (2) and (4):

$$V_d C_t = V_d C_0 e^{-kt} \text{ or } C_t = C_0 e^{-kt} \quad (5)$$

from which may be derived:

$$\log C_t = \frac{-kt}{2.303} \log C_0$$

(logarithms are to the base 10, hence factor 2.303).

If log plasma concentration is plotted against time a straight line is obtained, the slope of which is $-k/2.303$ and the intercept on the y axis is the plasma concentration at time zero C_0.

The half-life of the drug ($t_{1/2}$) can be obtained by substitution in equation:

$$t_{1/2} = e^{-kt_{1/2}} \text{ or } \log(1/2) = -kt_{1/2}$$

$$t_{1/2} = \frac{-\log(0.5)}{k} = \frac{0.693}{k}$$

The clearance of a drug is the fraction of the apparent volume of distribution cleared of drug by the body in unit time

$$Cl = kV_d$$

Clearances are additive and total body clearance is the sum of the clearances by each eliminating organ, that is total body clearance = renal clearance + hepatic clearance + . . .

Two-compartment model

In this model the body is considered to consist of two compartments between which transfer of drug can occur (*Figure 1.15*). Such compartments need have no physiological basis. Injecting a drug into one compartment results in drug level falling in a biphasic fashion. The first phase represents mainly drug transference from one compartment to another; the second slower phase represents mainly elimination after a pseudo-equilibrium between compartments has been reached (*Figure 1.16*). Mathematically the following equations apply to a two-compartment model. The net rate of change of drug concentration x_1 in first compartment A is given by:

$$\frac{dx_1}{dt} = (k_{12} + k_{10})\, x_1 + k_{21}\, x_2$$

(x_2 = drug concentration in second compartment B)

$$x_1 = Ae^{-\alpha t} + Be^{-\beta t}$$

where α is the rate constant of the distributive phase; β is the rate constant of the elimination phase. Both constants can be obtained from the biphasic log drug concentration–time curve.

The distribution half-life ($t_{1/2}^{\alpha}$) is given by:

$$t_{1/2}^{\alpha} = \frac{0.693}{\alpha}$$

and the elimination half-life ($t_{1/2}^{\beta}$) by:

$$t_{1/2}^{\beta} = \frac{0.693}{\beta}$$

$$k_{12} = \frac{AB\,(\beta - \alpha)^2}{(A + B)^2\, k_{21}}$$

$$k_{21} = \frac{A\beta + \beta\alpha}{A + B}$$

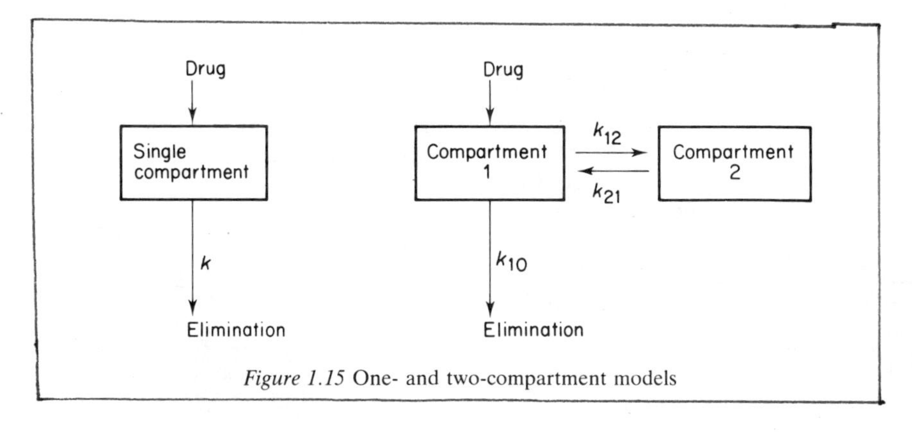

Figure 1.15 One- and two-compartment models

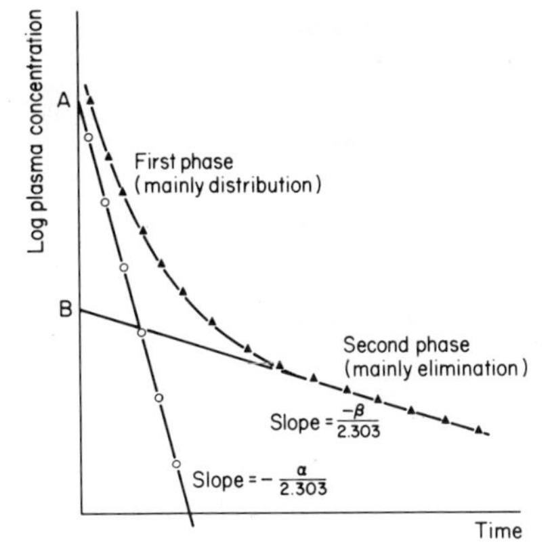

Figure 1.16 Biphasic curve of log plasma concentration–time. Two-compartment analysis can be applied by which A, B and β can be obtained by the method of residuals ('curve peeling'). The line of best fit through the terminal few points of the second phase yields a slope from which β can be calculated. Subtraction of this line from the original data points (▲) yields a series of points (○) to which the 'residual' line can be fitted, giving A and α

Volume of distribution of first compartment:

$$V_1 = \frac{x_0}{A + B} \quad \text{where } x_0 = \text{amount of drug given.}$$

Volume of distribution of second compartment:

$$V_2 = \frac{V_1 k_{12}}{k_{21}}$$

Volume of distribution at steady state:

$$V_{d(ss)} = V_1 + V_2$$

$$= V_1 \left(1 + \frac{k_{12}}{k_{21}}\right)$$

It is possible to construct multicompartment models, for example three-compartment models. It is of interest that the pharmacokinetics of fentanyl is such that a three-compartment model at least is needed to model the experimental data. Readers interested in multicompartment models are referred to the excellent review by Hull (1979).

Multiple dosing

The aim is to maintain plasma concentration of the drug in what has been aptly called 'the therapeutic window', that is between the minimum effective dose and the minimum dose-dependent toxic dose that is allowable in the therapeutic circumstances. To maintain plasma concentrations within the window over a long period of time, for example days, it is necessary to give an initial dose that will quickly establish the desired concentration (called the priming dose). Thereafter maintenance doses need to be given (*Figure 1.17*). The maintenance dose depends on the pharmacokinetics of the drug; the maintenance dose should equal the amount of drug lost from the body in the interval between doses. If it is greater, cumulation can occur and plasma concentration will rise. The rate of elimination of

'loading dose'

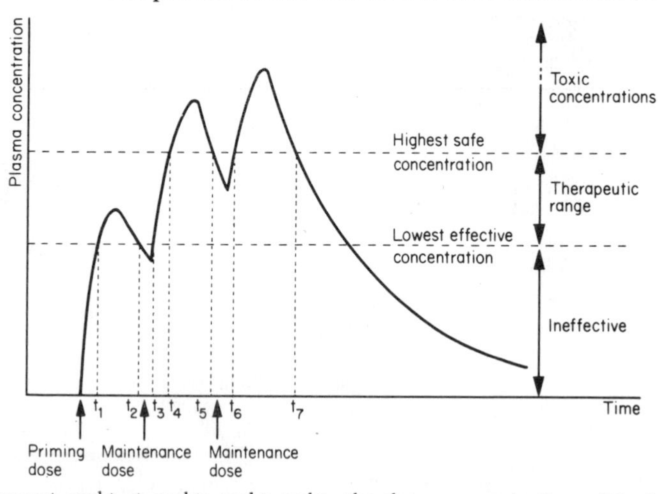

Figure 1.17 Between t_1 and t_2, t_3 and t_4, and t_5 and t_6, the plasma concentrations of the drug falls in the 'therapeutic window'. Because the maintenance dose is too large, between t_4 and t_5, and t_6 and t_7, the plasma concentration is high enough to produce dose-dependent toxicity

most drugs is dependent on first-order kinetics; $t_{½}$ does not change with dose. For such drugs, doubling the dose will not double the duration of action of the drug, but will merely increase it by one biological half-life. If the drug elimination follows zero-order kinetics $t_{½}$ will increase as the dose increases.

Pharmacokinetics of inhalational anaesthetics

For volatile anaesthetics the required pharmacological response is a function of the partial pressure of the anaesthetic (the tension) in the brain. At equilibrium 'brain tension' equals arterial blood tension, which in turn equals the partial pressure of the anaesthetic in alveolar air. In practice this is not obtained. In a gas mixture the fractional concentration of the anaesthetic agent in the mixture is equal to its pressure divided by the total pressure, that is concentration is proportional to partial pressure. To obtain the necessary brain tension quickly, inhalational anaesthetics are given initially at concentrations higher than for maintenance concentration; priming dose followed by a lower maintenance dose is the usual rule.

Four factors determine brain tension. These are the partial pressure of the anaesthetic in the inspired gas mixture; the respiratory rate and depth of respiration; the transfer of anaesthetic through the alveolar wall to the blood flowing through the lung; and the elimination of the anaesthetic from the arterial blood to other tissues.

In the absence of ventilation–perfusion problems, the factors that determine how rapidly anaesthetics pass from the alveolar space into the blood are the anaesthetic's solubility in blood, the rate of blood flow through the lung, and the partial pressures of the anaesthetic in arterial and mixed venous blood. The blood/gas partition coefficient (λ) represents the ratio of anaesthetic concentration in blood to anaesthetic concentration in a gas phase when the two are in equilibrium. Partial pressures will then be equal in both phases. Anaesthetic agents that are very soluble in blood have a high λ (compare methoxyflurane 12.1 with nitrous oxide 0.47). The blood tension rises slowly with soluble agents. The factors that determine the loss of an anaesthetic agent from the blood to the tissues (for example the brain) are the solubility of the agent in the tissue (that is, its tissue/blood partition coefficient), the blood flow to the particular tissue, and the partial pressures of the agent in the tissue and in the blood.

Potency of anaesthetics can be quantitatively compared by determining their minimum alveolar concentration (MAC) values. The MAC of an anaesthetic is defined as the concentration at one atmosphere that produces immobility in 50 per cent of patients or animals exposed to noxious stimuli (Eger, Saidman and Brandstater, 1965). The MAC value for halothane is approximately 0.8 per cent, while that for nitrous oxide is >100 per cent. Halothane is therefore much more potent than nitrous oxide. For further discussion on uptake, distribution, and elimination of anaesthetics *see* Chapter 4.

Bioavailability

While pharmacists have known for many years that the amount of active agent available for absorption depends on its formulation, it is only relatively recently that the therapeutic importance of this phenomenon has become widely appreciated. Two preparations can contain the same weight of active ingredient but produce different therapeutic responses due to their different bioavailabilities.

Bioavailability has been assessed by considering the total amount of drug reaching the circulation following oral dosage. This can be done by measuring the area under a plasma concentration–time curve. If one considers *Figure 1.18* the three dosage forms illustrated have the same biological availability, but only one of these forms will produce the desired therapeutic effect, namely dose form B. Dose form A can produce toxic effects from overdosage, while dose form C would be ineffective. Thus other factors besides total dose absorbed are important. These include absorption rate, peak height and time, and the half-life of the compound.

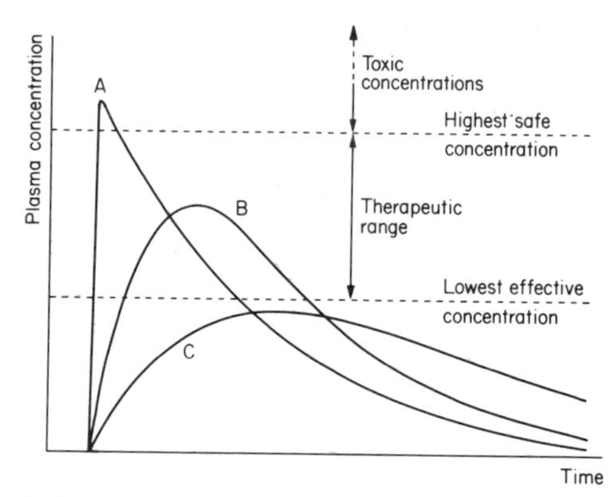

Figure 1.18 Variation of plasma concentration with time for three different dosage forms: A = intravenous; B = subcutaneous; C = oral. These give the same biological availability but are each different therapeutically

Formulation can modify the bioavailability of a drug. Particle size, the tablet disintegration time, and the presence or absence of 'filler' compounds and their composition are important in this regard.

With drugs that have a low therapeutic ratio, slight changes in bioavailability may produce therapeutically important sequelae (Davis, 1973). For instance, different formulations of digoxin containing the same chemical equivalent of digoxin can yield up to seven-fold differences in plasma digoxin levels.

First-pass effect

The majority of drugs when given orally are absorbed through the gastrointestinal tract into the portal circulation and hence pass into the liver. If the liver is very effective in clearing the drug, the amount initially available for systemic distribution will be considerably lower than might have been anticipated. This 'first-pass' effect has been shown to be important for a number of drugs, including salicylates, β-blocking drugs such as propranolol, and tricyclic antidepressants such as nortriptyline. Lignocaine also exhibits a high first-pass effect, as do many of the narcotic analgesics. If a drug is a pro-drug, metabolized to its active metabolite in the liver, first pass will be important in determining initial concentration of the active agent.

Idiosyncrasy

This term is used to describe a qualitatively abnormal reaction to a drug. An example is primaquine anaemia (*see* page 38) which is due to a genetic deficiency.

Allergic reactions (anaphylactic reactions)

These are mediated by an antigen–antibody reaction and involve previous exposure and sensitization to the drug, for example the asthmatic reaction caused by penicillin and haemolytic anaemia caused by methyldopa. The mechanism(s) leading to hypersensitivity are ill understood. The most popular view is that the drug or one of its metabolites acts as a hapten and antibodies are formed which react against the drug. Anaphylactoid reactions have been described previously.

Blood dyscrasia

Many drugs can produce blood dyscrasias; among the most notable is chloramphenicol. The incidence of serious blood dyscrasias following administration of this drug has been variously estimated between 1 in 500 and 1 in 100 000. In the UK the Committee on Safety of Drugs considered that this drug should never be used for the treatment of trivial infections but recognized that it was a highly effective agent in the treatment of *Haemophilus influenzae* meningitis and in typhoid fever. The drug might interfere with the bone marrow by affecting phenylalanine metabolism or, alternatively, by inhibiting the incorporation of iron into the red cell. An allergic basis has also been postulated and genetic factors might influence the sensitivity of patients to chloramphenicol-induced aplastic anaemia. Toxic effects of the drug are more likely to occur in females than males. The phenomenon is usually dose dependent and it is usual to limit treatment to less than 2 weeks. In neonates chloramphenicol can produce the 'grey syndrome'. The child may vomit, there is refusal to suck, and periods of cyanosis. The child becomes flaccid and an ashen colour develops. This is due to a failure of the drug to be conjugated with glucuronic acid, due to glucuronyl transferase not being present in adequate concentrations in the neonate's liver.

There are a number of other drugs that can produce blood dyscrasias. These include phenylbutazone, gold salts, and thiouracil derivatives.

Pharmacogenetics

This term originally covered the study of genetically determined variants that are revealed solely by the effect of drugs. Some investigators now include within the sphere of pharmacogenetics those hereditary disorders which may be revealed spontaneously but are often precipitated or aggravated by drugs. There is a considerable variation in the way different individuals handle and respond to drugs. The population variability can be continuous or discontinuous. Experiments have been done in which a large number of subjects have been given a set dose of a drug. The amount of acetylated product excreted in the urine in a fixed time has then been determined and responses noted graphically. In continuous variation, results form a bell shape or unimodal distribution but in discontinuous variation yield bimodal or trimodal curves. A unimodal distribution implies that metabolism of the drug in question is under the control of many genes (multifactorial) and analysis of genetic factors in such cases is usually not possible.

Genetic variations revealed solely by drugs

ISONIAZID

This drug, which is used in the treatment of tuberculosis, is acetylated (*Figure 1.19*). There are slow, intermediate, and fast inactivators. Slow inactivators are homozygous for an autosomal (non sex-linked) recessive gene. In the USA and Europe about 50 per cent of the population are slow inactivators. Polyneuritis (a toxic effect of isoniazid) is commoner in slow activators. Similarly, there are slow and fast inactivators of hydralazine, phenelzine, and sulphadimidine. Acetylation

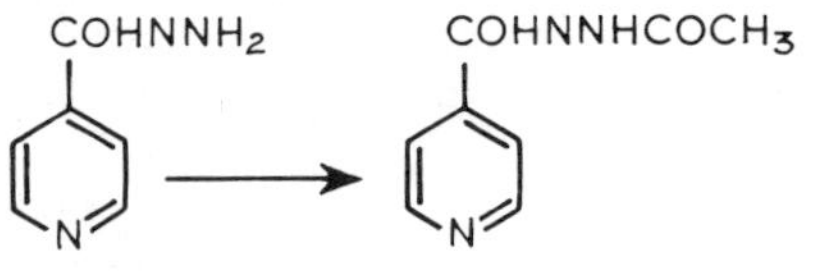

$COHNNH_2$ → $COHNNHCOCH_3$

Isoniazid   Acetylated metabolite

Figure 1.19 Metabolism of isoniazid

is not the only metabolic process whose rate may be genetically determined: for instance phenytoin, which is hydroxylated, also demonstrates fast and slow inactivation.

SUXAMETHONIUM

This drug paralyses all skeletal muscle including the respiratory muscles, thus producing apnoea. Normally it is short acting (2–3 minutes) because it is broken down by plasma cholinesterase. However, about 1 in 3000 patients have apnoea which may last for an hour or more, and this is due to an abnormal form of plasma cholinesterase. Four allelomorphic variants of plasma cholinesterase have been described: the usual, the atypical, the fluoride-resistant, and the 'silent' types (*see* Chapter 10). The atypical variant is the commonest abnormal plasma cholinesterase and is characterized by a relative lack of the inhibition of the hydrolysis of benzoylcholine by the local anaesthetic cinchocaine (dibucaine).

MALIGNANT HYPERPYREXIA

There is a genetic basis for this condition; a dominant gene is responsible. The syndrome occurs during anaesthesia; it is liable to be seen if suxamethonium and/or halothane are used. Muscle rigidity occurs, there is a rapid rise in temperature, and intracellular potassium is released.

PRIMAQUINE

Following administration of this drug some people, after a few days of treatment, began to pass very dark, often black, urine; jaundice developed and the red cell count fell. The cause was found to be a deficiency of an enzyme – glucose-6-phosphate dehydrogenase (G-6-PD). People with G-6-PD deficiency are not only sensitive to primaquine but also to phenacetin, sulphonamides, nitrofurantoin, and salicylates. G-6-PD is inherited as an X-linked recessive trait. Red cell G-6-PD deficiency is much commoner in Negroes than Caucasians, but in affected Negroes activity in *white* cells is normal, whereas it is reduced in most affected Caucasians.

The mechanism of haemolysis is only partially understood. A sufficient quantity of reduced glutathione is necessary for the integrity of the red cell. This substance prevents the damage produced by oxidized products in the red cell such as that produced by oxidizing drugs. A linked process is responsible for maintaining a sufficient supply of reduced glutathione. Lack of G-6-PD diminishes the production of reduced nicotinamide adenine dinucleotide phosphate (NADPH), which is required to ensure that sufficient reduced glutathione can be maintained (*Figure*

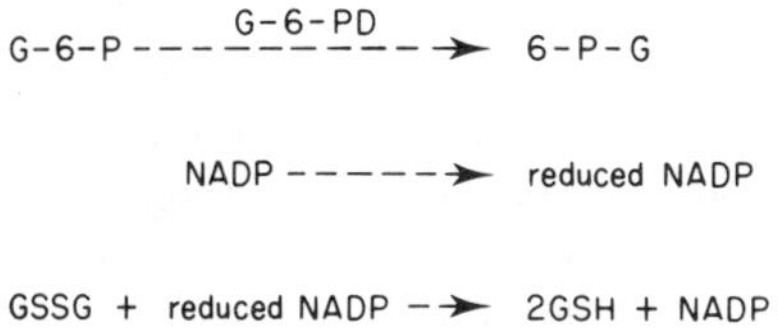

G-6-P --- G-6-PD ---→ 6-P-G

NADP -----→ reduced NADP

GSSG + reduced NADP —→ 2GSH + NADP

Figure 1.20 Linked process: G-6-P = glucose-6-phosphate; 6-P-G = 6-phosphogluconate; NADP = nicotinamide adenine dinucleotide phosphate; GSSG = oxidized glutathione; GSH = reduced glutathione; G-6-PD = glucose-6-phosphate dehydrogenase. Lack of G-6-PD diminishes production of reduced NADP which is necessary for sufficient supply of GSH

1.20). The primaquine-sensitive individual has less reduced glutathione present in his red cells.

Also genetically determined is lack of methaemoglobin reductase (NADH ferrihaemoglobin reductase) in erythrocytes. This causes the persistence of methaemoglobin after intake of nitrites, amidopyrine, or other drugs that cause methaemoglobin formation.

COUMARIN DRUGS

Increased resistance to the effect of coumarin derivatives has been reported, but is very rare. Resistance appears to be transmitted as an autosomal dominant trait. In most instances so-called genetic resistance to these drugs has been proved to be due to other causes. The subject of pharmacogenetics has been reviewed by Watson (1969).

Hereditary disorders with altered drug responses

These are not strictly within the original definition of pharmacogenetics.

ACUTE INTERMITTENT PORPHYRIA

This disease is genetically determined by an autosomal dominant trait. Some individuals have skin lesions, particularly on exposed surfaces. Others may have mental disturbances or severe abdominal pain. An acute attack can be precipitated by barbiturates. In parts of South Africa as many as 1 per cent of the population may have porphyria. There are a number of drugs outside the barbiturate group which can induce porphyria in man. These include griseofulvin, sex steroids, and oral hypoglycaemic agents.

SULPHONAMIDES

These drugs will precipitate haemolysis in patients with certain haemoglobinopathies, for instance haemoglobin H, which consists entirely of β-polypeptide chains.

THIAZIDE DIURETICS

These drugs can precipitate gout in patients genetically predisposed to it (gout is possibly a multifactorial disease). Since thiazides aggravate symptoms of diabetic patients, in the future it may be possible to use chlorothiazide to recognize persons predisposed to diabetes in the population.

Diseases can modify the actions of a drug. For instance, dystrophia myotonica is associated with aberrant reactions to thiopentone and muscle relaxants. In sickle-cell anaemia a slight change in the amino acid structure of the haemoglobin molecule is associated with a marked change in solubility of the reduced form. Precipitation which causes sickling can be induced by hypoxia, acidosis, or infection.

Chemotherapeutic index

It is difficult to compare the therapeutic efficiency of drugs as it involves taking into account both their pharmacological activity and their toxicity. However effective its actions, a drug is of no clinical use if it does not have a sufficient margin of safety. This problem was appreciated by Ehrlich, who took the minimum curative dose as a measure of a drug's efficacy and compared that with the maximum tolerated dose. The therapeutic index of the drug was the ratio of the maximum tolerated dose to the minimum curative dose, and where extremes are concerned, as with penicillin and some of the early arsenicals, it is obvious that with the former the ratio is very high (safe) and with the latter low (unsafe).

Maximum and minimum doses are very difficult to determine, and the minimum lethal dose of a drug was therefore discarded as a measurement in favour of the doses that kill 50 per cent of a group of animals (LD_{50}) and cure 50 per cent (ED_{50}). These are known as the median lethal and median effective doses, respectively. The ratio LD_{50}/ED_{50} has, therefore, replaced the earlier ratio and the index this provides is much more reliable and is now widely used.

Approved names

These are names for drugs selected or devised by the British Pharmacopoeia Commission and published by the Health Ministers, on the recommendation of the Medicines Commission in accordance with the Medicines Act 1968. Trade names are names given by manufacturers to their formulated products. There are advantages besides cost to the patient or health service in prescribing by approved names. Drugs with similar pharmacological actions have similar stems. For instance, propranolol, sotalol, and timolol have the stem -lol, which indicates that they are β-adrenoceptor blocking agents of the propranolol group. The importance of formulation in relation to bioavailability, which can vary between manufacturers as well as by a specific manufacturer, is noted in the section on bioavailability (page 35).

Clinical trials

Many anaesthetists, during the course of their professional lives, will be involved in a clinical trial. It is important, therefore, that they understand the principles and pitfalls. Measurement of the therapeutic efficiency of drugs is more difficult in man than in animals. A carefully planned and executed clinical trial is necessary before the effects of any drug can be assessed. Before administering a new drug to man, the investigator must have good evidence of the lack of toxic effects based upon acute and chronic animal experiments, which may be supported by human pharmacological studies on volunteers. In Great Britain permission has to be obtained from the Committee on Safety of Medicines before a new substance can be used in a clinical trial. Rigorous control over the introduction of new drugs in the USA is exercised by the Food and Drug Administration (FDA).

No firm rules can be laid down for the conduct of a clinical trial. Every trial must be planned in relation to the context in which it is being executed. In planning a trial the investigator should consider the following points.

Ethical considerations

It is important that a patient should not suffer as the result of the administration of a new drug, either by its toxic effects or as a result of being denied orthodox or efficient medication. The investigator performing a clinical trial must ensure that the patient is told that he is to participate in such a trial, that the nature of it is explained to him, and that his informed consent is obtained. He must also be prepared to withdraw a patient from the trial, or even abandon the trial, should it at any time appear that this is in the best interest of the patient.

Detailed planning

It is important to plan as fully as possible every step of a trial before the study begins. A decision on the final form of analysis of experimental data and detailed planning within the limits of this form of analysis should aim at giving maximum utilization of data. The object of the trial should be specified. This will take the form of either testing a hypothesis (that a drug does or does not have a certain action) or more commonly forming an estimate of the quantitative effects of a drug on the body. The population to be tested must also be defined. Clinical trials are commonly carried out on hospital patients or upon volunteers from a hospital population. The eventual aim is to apply the findings of the trial to a much wider population. The investigator must assure himself that the reasons why his patients are in hospital are not such as to influence the result of the trial. The unknown motivation of volunteers may likewise introduce bias in the assessment of, say, psychotropic drugs. It is wise to make the plan of a trial as simple as possible.

The method of collecting the data must be decided. In order to reduce bias, maximum objectivity must be aimed for. A double-blind trial, when neither the subject nor the observer is aware of the nature of the medication given, will tend to reduce bias to a minimum; such trials may be difficult to plan in the context of clinical anaesthetic studies. The use of a piece of apparatus to measure a physiological variable is usually better than reliance upon subjective observation. Machines have random and often measurable degrees of error, while an observer may introduce unconsciously biased and usually unassessable errors.

During intial planning, details of dosage schedules of drugs must be decided. It is also important to decide at this stage upon the management of any untoward complications that may occur during the trial and lay down criteria for the withdrawal of a subject from the trial should he appear likely to suffer harm as a result of continuing.

In performing an estimate of the effects of a drug it is usual to assess drug effects in comparison with those of a standard drug, or an inert drug, that is determine its potency. A new analgesic, for example, may be compared with morphine, while the effects of a mild tranquillizer may be compared with those of inert tablets. Placebo reaction – an apparent therapeutic effect of inert drug – may bedevil a clinical trial, especially one in which subjective effects are being assessed. By the use of inert medications an estimate of the degree of placebo reaction in a population can be obtained.

Potency

The investigator should be aware of the traps associated with the word 'potency'. Consider two drugs used in the relief of pain and their dose–alleviation of pain curves (*Figure 1.21*). The maximum relief of pain that can be achieved with drug B is less than the maximum relief that can be achieved with drug A. Drug A is more

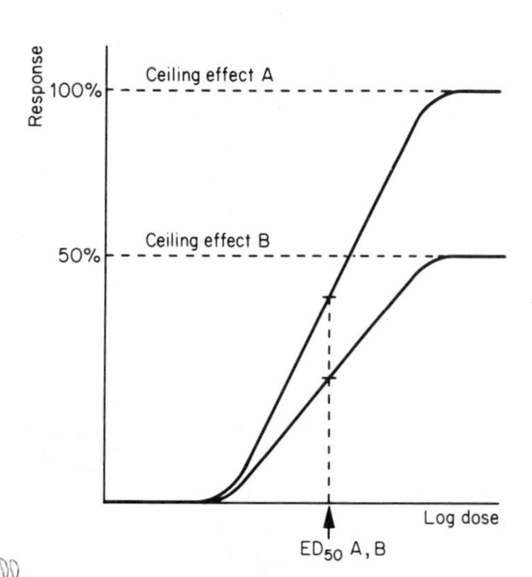

Figure 1.21 Comparison of the ceiling effect of two drugs, A and B

efficacy ~~potent~~ than drug B since it has a higher ceiling effect. Consider two drugs, X and Y, which relax bronchial muscle (*Figure 1.22*). X is more potent than Y but both drugs have the same ceiling effect. Note that there is a parallel shift in the log dose–response curve.

In many clinical trials one dose of the unknown drug (U) under trial is compared with the standard (S), for example in regard to effect on heart rate. Consider *Figure*

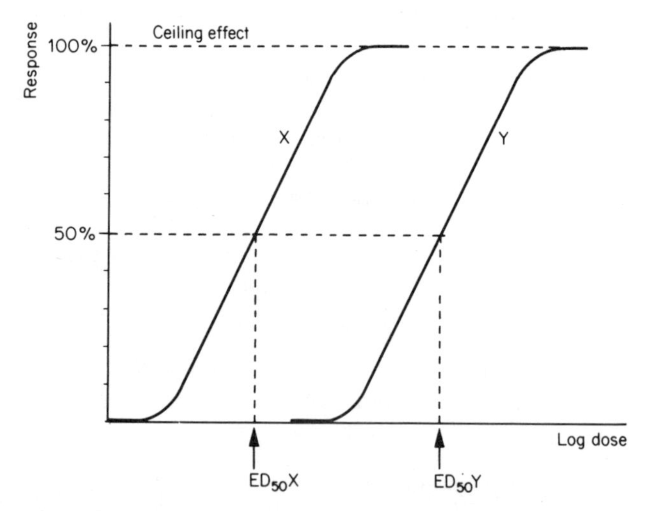

Figure 1.22 Comparison of potencies of two drugs, X and Y. Note the parallel log dose–response curves

1.23; note that if the investigator is interested in comparing the doses of S and U needed to produce a 20 per cent increase in heart rate, U is more potent than S (fewer milligrams of drug U required to produce effect). However, if the investigator is interested in comparing the doses of S and U needed to produce a 70 per cent increase in heart rate, S is more potent than U. In this example the slope of the log dose–response curve for U is not parallel to that for S. The difficulty arises when investigators, having only compared one dose of standard with one dose of unknown, mistakenly infer that the unknown drug is more potent over the whole of the dose–response range.

The form of a clinical trial determines whether the participants will be divided into separate groups receiving separate medication, or whether drug and standard or placebo can be administered in turn to each patient who then acts as his own

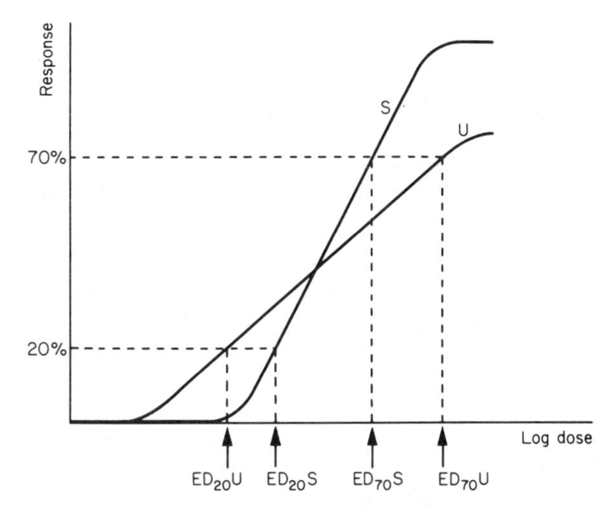

Figure 1.23 Comparison of potencies of two drugs, S and U. Note that the log dose–response curves are not parallel

control. The use of subjects as their own controls simplifies the planning and execution of a trial, but problems of cross-over effects, considered below, may complicate the interpretation of data.

Sampling criteria

In the simplest form of clinical trial two groups of patients are selected from the available population, each given separate drug therapy, and the effects compared. If the comparison is to be valid, no relevant or significant difference must exist between the groups. The analysis also assumes initially that no difference in effect exists between the two medicaments. At the end of the trial this null hypothesis is tested. If the trial supports the null hypothesis, then no discernible drug effect has been found. Failure of the trial to support the null hypothesis will be interpreted as a difference in drug effect, whose magnitude may be calculated.

Sampling – choosing the two groups of subjects – must aim at selecting two groups, both of whom are fully representative of the parent population. It can be shown mathematically that an adequate sample taken at random from a population will tend to be representative of the population, and randomization is the underlying principle in sampling populations for a clinical trial.

Randomization may be achieved in many ways. After the initial decision to admit a patient to a trial, allotment to a group can be determined by coin tossing, the use of previously prepared tables, or the use of tables of random numbers. Apparently random criteria such as alternation of patients on an operating list should be avoided. Such an order may have been decided by events unknown to the investigator which may affect the results of treatment. In more elaborate clinical trials it may be necessary to divide each group into a series of subgroups, depending on such parameters as age, sex, existing disease, or previous treatment. Such sampling demands the use of tables of random numbers.

Carry-over effects

When patients are used as their own controls it is possible that the effects of the first drug administered may modify the responses to subsequent drugs. This modification may be due to pharmacological reasons – the presence of a slowly excreted drug in the body, or an effect on metabolic enzymes – or it may be psychological in origin, for example apprehension when therapy is first administered may be allayed or increased on subsequent occasions. Alternation of the different therapies will usually minimize these carry-over effects.

Sample size

The time taken to complete a clinical trial depends upon the number of subjects who need to be studied in order to provide a valid conclusion. An approximation of the sample size required can be obtained from an initial pilot study. From the analysis of this study one can determine the level of standard deviation that is required to show a statistical difference between groups. Knowledge of the actual standard deviation of the pilot study can then be used to calculate the final sample size. To halve the standard deviation one would have to quadruple the sample size.

A more exact estimate of sample size can be obtained if the experimenter is able to answer the following questions:

1. If no real difference exists between the two drugs being tested, what is the acceptable risk of mistakenly concluding that there is a difference? This is known as a Type I error.
2. If a real difference does exist, what is the acceptable risk of missing it? This is a Type II error.
3. If a real difference does exist, what size difference is important?

The null hypothesis upon which a clinical trial is usually based can never be proved, only disproved. Thus if any difference, no matter how small, is important, the sample required may be infinitely large.

The use of sequential analysis appears at first glance to overcome the problems of determining sample size. Here matched pairs of patients are studied and the comparison between each pair, in terms of greater or lesser effect, is plotted on a graph as a series of vectors. The trial terminates when the line as constructed crosses previously drawn boundaries. However, knowledge of the three factors described above is necessary in order to construct these boundaries. Sequential trials have a very limited application in anaesthetic clinical trials.

Statistical analysis

The wise clinical investigator consults a statistician before commencing a clinical trial to seek his views on whether the design of the trial is appropriate from a statistical point of view. This book is not concerned with statistical methods. There are many good textbooks. Parametric statistics rests on the assumption that the population being considered follows a normal distribution (one of the criteria) before conducting a *t* test. Non-parametric statistics should be used to analyse data from populations that do not conform to a normal distribution. Patients' illnesses may not be normally distributed. If in doubt it is wise to use non-parametric statistics.

Evaluation of reports of clinical trials

To a certain extent the editor and his panel of referees protect the journal reader from conclusions drawn from poor clinical trials. Nevertheless, this is not always so and anaesthetists should be able to make their own judgement as to whether a therapeutic trial has been adequately performed, and if the conclusions drawn are valid. Herxheimer and Lionel (1970) have devised an interesting check-list which covers most points that should be considered. Questions to be answered in relation to the aims of the study include:

Were the subjects suitably selected?
Were the methods of assessment valid?
Was the design appropriate and sufficiently sensitive?
Were enough subjects used?
Are the statistics valid?

It is important to remember, when reading articles in journals, that statistical significance does not necessarily imply therapeutic significance. For instance, a new drug may be shown to be more potent than the one in standard use (probability $P < 0.001$). If the effective therapeutic dose of the new drug is 0.49 mg/day, as compared to 0.5 mg/day for the standard in use, other things being equal, this is not of therapeutic importance.

Legal aspects of drugs

The supply and distribution of drugs that are poisonous or subject to addiction are controlled by law in the UK. The Acts that mainly concern the medical profession are the Medicines Act 1968 and the Misuse of Drugs Act 1971. The Medicines Act 1968 regulates the manufacture, distribution, and importation of medicines for human use. This is controlled by a licensing system. The Act is also concerned with the registration of retail pharmacies. These are concerned with the supply of the majority of medicines to the public. Some medicines may be sold without the supervision of a pharmacist, for example aspirin.

The Medicines Commission is the body appointed to administer the Medicines Act; among the committees appointed by it are the Committee on Safety of Medicines, the Committee on the Review of Medicines, the British Pharmacopoeia Commission, and *ad hoc* committees such as the General Sale List Committee and the Prescription Only Medicines Committee. The licensing authority issues clinical trial certificates. Within the Medicines Act there are powers to control the sale or promotion of medicinal products and the content of data sheets.

Classes or description of medicinal products that can be sold or supplied otherwise than by or under the supervision of a pharmacist are listed in a General Sale List Order; included in the list are antacids such as aluminium hydroxide, purgatives such as cascara, and non-narcotic analgesics such as paracetamol. The majority of medicinal products fall within this list.

When issuing a prescription for a 'prescription only medicine' the prescription must be written in indelible ink (unless it is a carbon copy health prescription, signed in indelible ink by the practitioner giving it). It must contain the following particulars: the name, address, and age (if under 12) of the patient; the total amount of the preparation; the date; signature of the practitioner (note initials or facsimiles are not acceptable) giving it; and the practitioner's address.

Central Midwives Board (CMB) rules

Certified practising midwives may possess certain drugs for use in their work, according to rules promulgated by the CMB. In general, the rules lay down several permissible alternatives, and the local authority makes precise regulations for the midwives employed by them. Midwives working in hospitals are subject to local hospital regulations.

Midwives have access to all medicinal products on a General Sale List and all pharmacy medicines. They can therefore prescribe a mild analgesic such as paracetamol, or a suitable antiseptic. They are entitled to prescribe certain prescription only medicines orally, such as products containing chloral or its active metabolite, pentazocine, and ergometrine maleate. Parenterally they may administer ergometrine maleate, pethidine hydrochloride, pentazocine lactate, naloxone hydrochloride, oxytocin (natural and synthetic), and promazine hydrochloride. For most normal deliveries 200 mg of pethidine should be adequate. Many local authorities insist that a medical practitioner be called if more than this amount is required.

For systemic inhalation analgesia both the drug and apparatus for its administration are covered by the rules. ~~Methoxyflurane may be given using a Cardiff inhaler delivering 0.35 per cent~~; trichloroethylene can be administered from an Emotril or Tecota in concentrations of 0.35 per cent and 0.5 per cent, and pre-mixed 50:50 nitrous oxide and oxygen from an approved demand-valve apparatus. In each case the actual choice rests in the hands of the employing authority. The rules also cover the testing and servicing of such apparatus.

Misuse of Drugs Act 1971

There are four classes of drugs. Those in Schedule 1 are exempt from the most stringent controls and comprise certain commonly used preparations containing codeine, dihydrocodeine, pholcodine, medicinal opium or morphine, cocaine, and diphenoxylate where these substances are present in such small amounts that no serious danger of misuse arises.

Schedule 2 specifies drugs subject to control; the schedule is divided into three parts or classes, partially on the basis of decreasing order of harmfulness. Part A (Class 1) contains morphine. Part B (Class 2) contains amphetamine. Part C (Class 3) contains methaqualone. Cannabis and cannabis resin are found in Part B of Schedule 2, while cannabinol derivatives are found in Part A. These divisions into three classes are solely for the purpose of determining penalties for offences. Included in Schedule 2 are cocaine, dextromoramide, dipipanone, heroin, medicinal opium, levorphanol, methadone, morphine, pethidine, phenazocine, amphetamines, methaqualone, methylphenidate, and phenmetrazine. Dihydrocodeine, codeine, pholcodine, and diphenoxylate are also specified unless they are contained in preparations exempted under Schedule 1. Such drugs are known as Controlled Drugs. A prescription for a drug specified in Schedule 2 to the regulations must:

1. Be in ink or other indelible substance, signed by the prescriber with his usual signature and dated by him;

2. Bear in the practitioner's own handwriting the name and address of the person for whose treatment the drug is prescribed;
3. Specify in the prescriber's handwriting the dose to be taken. When a Controlled Drug is prescribed in the form of a preparation, e.g. tablets, capsules or liquid formulations, the prescription must state the form of the preparation and, if more than one strength of preparation is available, the strength to be dispensed. The prescription must also specify either the total amount of the Controlled Drug to be supplied or the total number of dosage units, e.g. tablets or capsules, to be supplied. Amounts or numbers of dosage units must be stated in *words and figures*;
4. In the case of a prescription for a total amount to be dispensed by instalments a direction must be given specifying the intervals to be observed when dispensing;
5. In the case of a private patient it is also necessary to specify the address of the prescriber;
6. Have written on it the words 'For Dental Treatment Only', or 'For Animal Treatment Only' as appropriate.

It is an offence to *issue or dispense* a prescription for a Controlled Drug which does not comply with the foregoing requirements.

Medical practitioners may not prescribe cocaine and diamorphine for addicts except for the purpose of treating organic disease or injury. All transactions concerning Controlled Drugs must be recorded in a register on the day of the transaction or, if that is impossible, on the following day. Entries must not be cancelled, obliterated, or altered and any corrections must be dated. An entry must be made even when he administers the drugs himself or causes them to be administered under his supervision. Registers must be kept for 2 years after the last entry. Controlled Drugs must be stored in a receptacle that is locked and the key held by the person authorized to hold the drugs. Prescribing arrangements for drugs in Schedule 3 are the same as for Schedule 2, but registers do not have to be kept. The drugs are benzphetamine, chlorphentermine, mephentermine, phenmetrazine, and pipradrol. Schedule 4 includes cannabis and its derivatives and hallucinogens such as lysergide. Nobody is permitted to use drugs specified in this Schedule without a special licence.

There is an Advisory Council on the Misuse of Drugs which keeps under review the situation in the UK with respect to drugs that are or appear likely to be misused. It can advise the appropriate Ministers to take action to restrict the use of such drugs. The Secretary of State has power to direct that a doctor or a pharmacist who has been convicted of an offence under this legislation may not possess, administer, or manufacture Controlled Drugs. The Minister can give such a direction without a conviction if he considers that the practitioner is or has been prescribing in an irresponsible manner. This decision must be ratified subsequently by a tribunal.

Baxter, J. D. and Funder, J. W. (1979) Hormone receptors. *New England Journal of Medicine,* **301,** 1149

Brodie, B. B. (1965) Displacement of one drug by another from carrier or receptor sites. *Proceedings of the Royal Society of Medicine,* **58,** 946

Catzel, P. (1963) The estimation of doses for infants and children. A review and a proposed standardized method. *Medical Proceedings,* **9,** 280

Conney, A. H. (1967) Pharmacological implications of microsomal enzyme induction. *Pharmacological Reviews,* **19,** 317
Davis, S. S. (1973) The biological availability of drugs. *Medicine Today,* **7,** 49
Eger, E. I., Saidman, L. J. and Brandstater, B. (1965) Minimum alveolar anesthetic concentration: a standard of anesthetic potency. *Anesthesiology,* **26,** 756
Gaddum, J. H. (1937) Discussion on the chemical and physical basis of pharmacological action. *Proceedings of the Royal Society (B),* **121,** 598
Grogono, A. W. (1974) Drug interactions in anaesthesia. *British Journal of Anaesthesia,* **46,** 613
Herxheimer, A. and Lionel, N. D. W. (1970) Assessing reports of therapeutic trials. *British Journal of Pharmacology,* **39,** 204P
Hull, C. J. (1979) Pharmacokinetics and pharmacodynamics. *British Journal of Anaesthesia,* **51,** 579
Norman, J. (1979) Drug receptor reactions. *British Journal of Anaesthesia,* **51,** 595
Paton, W. D. M. (1961) A theory of drug action based on the rate of drug–receptor combination. *Proceedings of the Royal Society (B),* **154,** 21
Paton, W. D. M. (1970) Receptors as defined by their pharmacological properties. In *Molecular Properties of Drug Receptors,* p. 3, Ed. Porter, R. and O'Connor, M. London: J. and R. Churchill
Pearson, D. J., Freed, D. L. J. and Taylor, G. (1981) Immunology. In *Essential Sciences for Clinicians,* p. 67, Ed. Tindall, V. R. Oxford: Blackwell Scientific Publications
Schueler, F. W. (1960) *Chemobiodynamics and Drug Design.* New York: McGraw-Hill
Watson, B. M. (1969) Pharmacogenetics: a review of current literature. *Anaesthesia,* **24,** 230

2

Premedicant drugs

Drugs are still widely prescribed prior to surgical operations with the aim of relieving anxiety, aiding induction, and diminishing overall anaesthetic requirements. They are also prescribed for specific purposes related to the agents or techniques that have been selected for anaesthesia. However, certain types of premedication adversely affect the course of anaesthesia with certain agents.

Anxiety

The commonest reason for prescribing premedicant drugs is for the relief of anxiety, and many are still given for this purpose without any knowledge that anxiety is present. Now that modern methods of induction are no longer unpleasant the question is often asked, 'Is the routine employment of sedative drugs really necessary?' The apprehension of the average patient can usually be relieved by a preoperative visit and reassuring talk by the anaesthetist. However, it is not just the induction of anaesthesia which patients fear, but loss of control, and pain or discomfort on waking; there is also an unspoken and often unadmitted fear that consciousness will not return or will return during the surgical procedure. Nevertheless, many of the sedative drugs commonly employed have undesirable side effects, such as nausea and vomiting in the postoperative period and respiratory depression or hypotension during anaesthesia. The only question is how often sedation should be withheld altogether. Much depends on the time available to the busy anaesthetist, the co-operation of the nursing staff and the type of patient to be dealt with. It also depends on the definition of anxiety. Every case must, of course, be judged on its merits, but if there is any doubt it is better to give sedatives than withhold them.

Sedative drugs are not given preoperatively to obstetric patients on account of their depressant effect on the respiration of the infant, and there is no reason to believe that these patients are unduly apprehensive or anxious. They may have previously received analgesics, however, which are still exerting some effect and they receive constant encouragement and reassurance from the midwife and nursing staff.

The sedative drugs most commonly employed prior to operation are papaveretum, morphine and its derivatives, and pethidine. The last drug has only a mild sedative action. The barbiturates are now rarely used in Great Britain. As hypnotics to ensure sleep the night before operation, they have largely been superseded by the benzodiazepines. In the starved patient oral premedication with lipid-soluble drugs appears to be reliable, and many hypnotics and tranquillizers appear to be effective if given 2 hours preoperatively. The phenothiazines are also used, promethazine for its sedative action, and others such as chlorpromazine and trimeprazine for their tranquillizing effect. All of the phenothiazines have an antiemetic action which is particularly important in patients subject to postanaesthetic vomiting. Other tranquillizers such as the butyrophenones and benzodiazepine derivatives are frequently given to anxious patients. One of these, lorazepam, has marked amnesic effects as well as being an anxiolytic. The butyrophenones should not be given alone except in very small doses as they produce dysphoria and extrapyramidal reactions.

When patients are in pain, as is often the case before emergency surgery, powerful analgesics such as morphine and pethidine and their derivatives will be required. Sedatives with only hypnotic activity should then be avoided as they cause restlessness and confusion in the presence of pain.

There have been numerous studies of the efficacy of premedicant drugs in allaying anxiety. Fear is an emotion that cannot be directly measured and such studies have usually been directed at some accompanying autonomic manifestation, such as changes in heart rate or blood pressure, or changes in blood flow in the forearm or fingers. The digital plethysmogram gives a very reasonable quantitative measure of the vasoconstriction that accompanies fear, and its abolition by intravenous sedatives such as haloperidol and lorazepam as well as by anaesthesia has been demonstrated. The fact that this is an effect on the higher CNS can be inferred from the reflex vasoconstriction which still occurs when a cold stimulus is applied to the opposite hand.

Unwanted autonomic responses to anaesthesia

The most common unwanted side effect of many anaesthetics, especially ether, is an increase in bronchial and salivary secretions, which are also stimulated by the presence of an endotracheal tube. This effect is usually prevented by the previous administration of atropine or hyoscine. Many of the phenothiazine derivatives also have some anticholinergic action but it is usually too weak for them to be used alone for this purpose.

Vagal preponderance, which often occurs with halothane and cyclopropane anaesthesia and may cause bradycardia, hypotension, and even cardiact arrest, can also be prevented by atropine. It must be remembered that increased excitability of cardiac muscle occurs with excess of either vagal or sympathetic activity. Hyoscine either slows or has no effect on heart rate in the doses normally given.

Atropine may be given intravenously immediately before induction of anaesthesia instead of 0.5–1 hour before by the intramuscular route. This has the advantage of ensuring that the patient is adequately atropinized during induction and is also relieved of the discomfort of a dry tongue and mouth while waiting for operation.

Other uses of premedication

Premedicant drugs, as well as influencing the drug requirements of anaesthesia, also modify the induction and influence the postoperative behaviour. Induction with intravenous barbiturates may be associated with spontaneous involuntary muscle movements, the incidence of which varies with the drug and is related to the dosage. Methylated barbiturates, such as methohexitone, are particularly prone to exhibit this phenomenon. Premedication with drugs that cause an increase in the sensitivity to somatic pain, such as promethazine, increases the incidence of these muscle movements, whereas analgesic drugs diminish it. Methohexitone induction is also prone to respiratory upsets, such as cough and hiccough. These can be reduced by parasympatholytic premedicant agents, but not by sedative ones. The actual choice of a parasympatholytic agent may also be of importance. For example, the incidence of awareness during anaesthesia for caesarean section is higher after atropine than after hyoscine premedication. This is no doubt related to the amnesic properties of hyoscine.

Many premedicant drugs cause amnesia or potentiate the amnesic effects of anaesthetic agents. They may cause retrograde amnesia for events occurring prior to their administration, or anterograde amnesia for subsequent events. The most potent amnesic drugs of those commonly used as premedicants are lorazepam, hyoscine, and diazepam, particularly if given with opiates. Intravenous administration of premedicants 15–30 minutes before operation markedly potentiates the anterograde amnesic properties of such drugs.

Hypertensive patients are particularly prone to develop dysrhythmias and episodes of severe hypertension associated with ECG evidence of myocardial ischaemia (particularly if antihypertensive therapy has been discontinued) during laryngoscopy and intubation. These adverse autonomic effects can be attenuated by the prior administration of β-blocking agents.

Premedication in children

The avoidance of injections by the use of oral or rectal premedication in children is a widespread practice and many drugs and dose regimens have been tried. None is completely satisfactory; drugs that produce a satisfactory condition in the anaesthetic room may be associated with postoperative restlessness.

Rectal thiopentone, 5 per cent solution in a dose of 40–50 mg/kg, almost always produces narcosis. It is now relatively unpopular, requiring supervision of the patient from the time of administration until the child is handed over to the anaesthetist.

The use of oral trimeprazine syrup (6 mg/ml) is widespread, in doses of 2–4 mg/kg. It has minimal analgesic activity and if given alone may give rise to postoperative restlessness in the presence of pain. It also causes amnesia and pallor if given in doses at the upper end of the range.

Diazepam has been compared with trimeprazine and phenobarbitone in clinical trials. Diazepam (0.22 mg/kg) proved more satisfactory than trimeprazine in the anaesthetic room, but had poor antisialogogic properties. Overall there was little to show that either drug was superior to phenobarbitone (4.4 mg/kg). In another study, triclofos (75 mg/kg; maximum dose 1.6 mg) was found to be satisfactory in 80 per cent of cases. The use of oral sedatives has confirmed that hyoscine is very poor in drying secretions when given by mouth. Adequate drying can be achieved with oral atropine (0.05 mg/kg; maximum dose 1.2 mg).

In unprepared patients, in small babies, in the presence of pain, and where certainty of action is required, standard adult premedicating regimens can be employed with suitable reduction of dose (*see* Chapter 1). It must not be overlooked that equally satisfactory results can be achieved without any sedative premedication, if the anaesthetist has the time and skill to gain the child's confidence on a preoperative visit.

Fuller details of the drugs mentioned in this section are described elsewhere in the book under the appropriate headings.

3

Central nervous system depressants

Narcotics

There are numerous drugs that have the property of producing depression of the CNS. In some, the probable mode of action has been elucidated, particularly those that have been shown to act at dopamine receptors, α-adrenoceptors, or cholinoceptors. However, while animal experiments may reveal differences between drug groups, such differences are often not observed in man, probably because the methodology is not sufficiently sensitive. In practice, therefore, these drugs tend to be used according to convention and convenience rather than on account of any real pharmacological differences that have been shown in man. Conversely, some drugs, such as diazepam, are now used for almost any purpose that involves CNS depression, whether it be as a tranquillizer, sedative, hypnotic, anticonvulsant, or intravenous induction agent. These difficulties should be borne in mind when reading the following paragraphs, in which are discussed the most important general pharmacological actions of drugs that are conventionally classified in one or other of these groups.

Confusion is common concerning the term narcotics as it has both a wide pharmacological meaning and a more restricted one under American Federal and State Laws. In American Federal and State Laws, narcotics are certain specified centrally acting drugs, usually of addiction, and their derivatives which are not themselves necessarily addictive, for example levallorphan. The World Health Organization takes a similar view of drugs of dependence. It is necessary to be aware of this legal use of the term otherwise reference to drugs such as papaverine, marihuana, and cocaine as narcotics may cause confusion.

Pharmacologically, narcotics are those depressants which can produce insensibility. This includes sedatives, hypnotics, analgesics, and general anaesthetics. Thus narcotics are not used to produce only narcosis but all degrees of CNS depression. Narcosis is simply a condition of insensibility, or stupor bordering upon it, from which simple physical stimuli such as noise, shaking, or slapping can achieve at most only partial arousal, and subjects thus roused cannot remain so when such stimuli cease. This state is to be contrasted with true sleep from which rousing by physical stimuli is simple, and can be lasting, except in a few special cases such as sleep after very severe fatigue, or the sleep of the young baby immediately after feeding. Analeptics such as nikethamide will produce some degree of arousal from the effects of narcotics and will stimulate the vital centres in the medulla, but are liable to cause convulsions and other unwanted side effects. The action of the narcotic analgesics is, however, reversed by specific antagonists, such as naloxone.

Deep narcosis is synonymous with general anaesthesia and can be produced by the intravenous narcotics, such as thiopentone.

Various attempts have been made since the turn of the century to produce a sufficient degree of narcosis for the relief of pain and discomfort of minor surgical procedures. 'Twilight sleep' – the administration of full doses of morphine and hyoscine for the relieve of pain in labour – was introduced first, but was soon abandoned because of the respiratory depression it produced in the baby. The technique of basal narcosis followed in the late 1920s.

Drugs first used to produce this state included bromethol, paraldehyde, and barbiturates in comparatively large doses. Hypotension and respiratory depression were common. This technique proved to be too dangerous as at this period modern methods of controlled respiration were not known and doses were adjusted downwards so that a state of deep sleep only was provided. This state was useful in anxious patients, especially those suffering from thyrotoxicosis, who could be brought to the operating theatre unaware of their surroundings and later lightly anaesthetized.

In the early 1940s Laborit and Huguenard introduced their technique of 'artificial hibernation', using the 'lytic cocktail' based on chlorpromazine, promethazine, and pethidine. This produced a state of lethargy, apathy, and tranquillity similar to light basal narcosis with analgesia, but the patient could be readily aroused. This technique and its modifications were used for minor operative procedures, as a form of premedication especially for anxious patients and as a cover for procedures under local anaesthesia. Hypotension accompanied this technique and its popularity gradually waned. It has been adapted into the technique of neuroleptanalgesia in which droperidol or haloperidol replaces chlorpromazine as a neuroleptic agent and phenoperidine or fentanyl provides analgesia. Cardiovascular stability is much greater than with previous techniques although depression of the respiratory centre is common.

Hypnotics

Hypnotics are those depressants of the CNS used to make people go to sleep more easily or more soundly, when wakefulness is not due to cough or severe pain; in other words, they should induce a condition indistinguishable from natural sleep. In fact, even though the physiological state may resemble sleep, the EEG shows characteristic changes with most hypnotics. Optimal results depend largely on giving the right dose of the most suitable drug to the patient which, owing to individual variation, depends on trial and error as much as on experience. They are a class of depressant within the larger category of narcotics and some act mainly upon the reticular activating system. The difference in action between sedatives and hypnotics is mainly one of degree, the same groups of drugs being used to produce either effect, larger doses being necessary to ensure a hypnotic effect. Typical examples occur among the barbiturates, chosen according to the duration of action desired. Some antihistamine drugs, such as promethazine, are now principally employed for their sedative and hypnotic actions, as are many benzodiazepines, particularly nitrazepam, flurazepam, and lorazepam. Other drugs of widely differing chemical composition which are commonly employed as hypnotics include glutethimide, methaqualone, triclofos, and dichloralphenazone. These have largely displaced drugs such as carbromal, bromides, chloral hydrate, and paraldehyde which were either less palatable, less convenient, or potentially more toxic.

Many drugs have various degrees of hypnotic action, but their most powerful effect may be some other type of CNS depression, and this determines their classification. It is then correct to speak of the hypnotic effects of such drugs, but not of the drugs themselves as hypnotics. Morphine, for instance, can produce in a normal pain-free person a feeling of well-being, comfort, and far-awayness of the outside world that tempts sleep. It promotes sleep in a patient kept awake by pain even more so, but its main use is, of course, as an analgesic.

Conversely, true hypnotics given to a patient in slight pain, for example with a mild headache, can induce sleep, and in sleep the pain threshold is always raised. But when severe pain is present, hypnotics cannot induce sleep for they are not analgesics. If the dosage is sufficiently high they may, in the presence of severe pain, produce a state of confusion similar to drunkenness, and if the dosage is pressed indiscriminately a state of total insensibility results. The same is true with regard to wakefulness due to cough, and sleep in the presence of severe pain or cough should therefore be induced by analgesics or cough suppressants primarily, combined with a hypnotic if necessary.

The danger of death from severe overdose lies in depression of the vasomotor and respiratory centres of the medulla. Death may either be rapid, from anoxia and hypotension, or more gradual from pneumonia favoured by a long period of diminished lung movement. However, the benzodiazepines rarely produce deep coma even with gross overdosage. Likewise, ketamine produces a condition in which the patient makes no response to the environment, while medullary centres are relatively undepressed even with large doses. Another compound with a unique ability to produce coma without medullary depression is sodium γ-hydroxybutyrate. This compound is fully metabolized to carbon dioxide and water and would undoubtedly have secured a place in anaesthetic practice if duration of coma had not been long and unpredictable. It is reported that the coma can be terminated with physostigmine.

Distinction should be clear between the pharmacological use of the term hypnosis, meaning drug-induced sleep, and that of hypnosis (originally called neurohypnosis), meaning the sleep-like state inducible in most people by suitable conditions of concentration and suggestion.

Sedatives, tranquillizers and neuroleptics

Sedatives are agents that are given to relieve tension and anxiety, thereby producing calmness and making it easier for the patient to go to sleep, yet they should not make him actually sleepy. They act by causing a mild degree of cortical depression, and the drugs employed consist mainly of the hypnotics in common use, given in small divided doses during the day. Thus the difference is largely one of usage rather than of pharmacological properties.

Tranquillizers are drugs that relieve tension and anxiety without undue sedative action. The difference between these drugs and sedatives is not easy to define; the latter, however, produce sleep more readily in larger doses than do tranquillizing drugs, which in their turn allay anxiety better than sedatives. Some drugs, such as diazepam and benzoctamine, also reduce muscle tension by a peripheral action on internuncial neurones.

In elderly persons, sedatives such as hyoscine or the barbiturates may cause excitement and should be avoided; if barbiturates are used in geriatric cases it is safer to give smaller doses of one of the shorter acting members, at more frequent intervals.

A number of drug groups have tranquillizing properties. These include the phenothiazines (chlorpromazine, promazine, trifluoperazine, and fluphenazine); the butyrophenones (haloperidol and droperidol); and the benzodiazepines (chlordiazepoxide and diazepam). New compounds, such as oxypertine, benzoctamine, and flupenthixol, not chemically related to these groups, continue to be introduced. However, with the more rigorous trials now required by the Committee on Safety of Medicines, the rate of introduction of new drugs is slower. With the introduction of such drugs many of the older ones, such as reserpine and hydroxyzine, are being used less frequently. Meprobamate is still used, often combined in commercial preparations with mild analgesics for the relief of pain associated with muscle tension.

Tranquillizers can be conveniently classified into two groups: the major tranquillizers, often now referred to as neuroleptics, and the minor tranquillizers, which serve as anxiolytics and sedatives. The *neuroleptics* are used to treat psychotic patients with conditions such as schizophrenia and mania, as well as in premedication and in the technique of neuroleptanalgesia. Neuroleptics can be defined in terms of behavioural studies in animals in which such activities as exploration and aggression are diminished while the performance of conditioned responses is preserved. They can also be categorized in psychological terms, as producing a state in which the individual is disinterested in, and indifferent to, his surroundings, readily falls asleep when unstimulated, but can be easily roused to full rational attention. Such drugs also characteristically inhibit agitation and symptoms such as delusions, hallucinations, paranoia, and mania.

It is now well established that the common property shared by the major tranquillizers is the ability to block dopamine-mediated synapses in the CNS. This action is a competitive one on the postsynaptic neurone. Their actions are thus related to effects on those pathways and areas of the brain where dopamine is an important transmitter. These include nigrostriatal and tuberoinfundibular pathways, as well as others (*see* page 231).

As well as their antipsychotic effects, major tranquillizers share other properties which are related to dopaminergic blockade. For example, apomorphine is a powerful agonist of dopamine and this action is blocked by these drugs. More striking in man is the induction of extrapyramidal effects such as pseudoparkinsonism, and in animals, catalepsy. Such drug-induced parkinsonism is not reversed by levodopa because the extra dopamine formed is insufficient to overcome the competitive blockade. The more specific the dopamine-blocking action, the more likely is the drug to produce these effects. Haloperidol and phenothiazines with piperazine side chains are drugs in this category. Many major tranquillizers, however, also have marked anticholinergic properties. As such drugs are useful in the treatment of parkinsonism, tranquillizers with this property have less marked extrapyramidal effects. Chlorpromazine is a drug of this type.

These drugs may also possess antiadrenergic, antihistamine, antiserotonin, or quinidine-like properties and these influence their other actions.

Of the minor tranquillizers, members of the benzodiazepine group are by far the most commonly prescribed drugs. There are currently more than 20 on the market. Many have active metabolites and several have the same metabolite, desmethyldiazepam, in common. This is an interesting compound because it has a very long half-life of 100 hours; in consequence, regular or intermittent doses of a drug that has this metabolite will tend to have a smooth action.

The site of action of the benzodiazepines seems to be predominantly on the limbic system of the brain and particularly on the hippocampi and amygdaloid nuclei. These drugs appear to inhibit selectively discharges from the amygdala and amygdalohippocampal transmission and act on 'benzodiazepine receptors'. These are closely linked to those which respond to the inhibitory neurotransmitter, γ-aminobutyric acid (GABA) – the GABA receptor.

Despite being described as anxiolytic agents, an inhibiting action on a non-specific arousal system clearly accords with the observation that they diminish all excessive emotional responses, whether anger, aggression, or panic.

There are other important reasons why the benzodiazepines have increasingly displaced other drugs, particularly the barbiturates, as the tranquillizers or sedatives of choice, and these are discussed on page 91.

In general, the less sedation a tranquillizing drug produces, the greater is the likelihood of it producing extrapyramidal stimulation with overdosage, and this is often associated with increased wakefulness.

The assessment of the value of tranquillizing drugs is very difficult. The patients to whom these drugs are given all come from a group particularly sensitive to suggestion from their medical attendant who can easily exaggerate unintentionally the effect of a new drug. Such circumstances are optimal for a placebo to produce a beneficial effect, and it is therefore essential for any new drug of this type to be assessed by a double-blind technique if a reliable estimate of its worth is to be made.

Intravenous induction agents

Drugs with various chemical groupings are capable of inducing rapid loss of consciousness when given parenterally, and include thiopentone, methohexitone, Althesin, propanidid, ketamine, etomidate, disoprofol and sodium γ-hydroxybutyrate.

The usefulness of such drugs for this purpose is determined by certain physical properties that they have in common and it is convenient to consider them together rather than scattered throughout the text under their various chemical groupings.

The first group of drugs to be introduced for this purpose were the barbiturates, but experiments to induce anaesthesia by the intravenous route with the earlier members of this series, as exemplified by pentobarbitone, were unsatisfactory: prolonged stupor and drowsiness were common and its action was unpredictable. Hexobarbitone – a methylated compound – was, however, found to be acceptable in spite of excitatory side effects and tendency to prolonged action. The thiobarbiturates then followed, and thiopentone, the most popular member of this group, was the only satisfactory agent for the induction of anaesthesia for nearly 30 years. More recently, further experiments were made with the methylated barbiturates, but only methohexitone was sufficiently free of excitatory side effects to be of value. Further development came with the use of the eugenols, of which propanidid is currently available and is notable for its rapid recovery.

Yet another approach has been what has been termed 'dissociative' anaesthesia. Phencyclidine had an extensive trial, particularly outside the UK, but was associated on occasions with severe psychotic reactions. A related compound, ketamine, appears to have an unusual mode of action. There is a loss of consciousness and an intense analgesia associated with muscle relaxation and yet the pharyngeal and laryngeal reflexes remain brisk. The principal drawback to its use has been the intense dreaming and psychomotor activity which may occur.

A somewhat different approach has been the development of steroids with anaesthetic activity. The first usable compound was hydroxydione; this is pregnanedione (which itself is devoid of anaesthetic activity) with a succinate moiety substituted in the 21 position. This was not a satisfactory compound: onset of anaesthesia was delayed for several minutes, recovery was slow, and it caused an unacceptably high level of venous thrombosis.

Many other steroid compounds have been investigated. C=O groups in the 3 and 20 positions are essential for anaesthetic activity, whereas a double bond between carbon atoms 4 and 5 is essential for hormonal activity. Althesin, which is currently available, is a mixture of two steroids with anaesthetic activity; the problems of solubility have been eased by formulating the drug in a solubilizing agent.

Pharmacokinetics of intravenous induction agents

If a drug is to be of value as an intravenous induction agent there are certain properties that it must possess. Only the non-ionized fraction of the drug is able to penetrate the lipid barrier between blood and brain and the potency of the drug is thus dependent on the degree of ionization at the pH of the extracellular fluid. The rate of penetration is also dependent on the relative solubility of the non-ionized drug in lipid and water. All of the drugs discussed in this section have a high lipid solubility relative to water. Indeed, propanidid, Althesin, and propofol are so insoluble in water that a special formulation in a solubilizing agent is necessary.

They all produce loss of consciousness in one arm/brain circulation time after intravenous injection. Ketamine is unique in that effective narcosis can be produced almost as quickly with the intramuscular as with the intravenous route. Rapid penetration of the brain is accompanied by a rapid redistribution to organs and tissues with a high blood flow, with a rapid fall in the peak blood concentration.

In the case of the barbiturates and thiobarbiturates, this is the principal mechanism leading to the recovery of consciousness. Because of their high lipid solubility, further redistribution then takes place principally into fat depots; 24 hours after administration 67–75 per cent of a dose of thiopentone which is still in the body is in these tissues. However, the role of hepatic metabolism is also significant. The liver removes up to 50 per cent of the thiopentone in the hepatic artery blood, and hepatic dysfunction prolongs its action.

With the non-barbiturates, redistribution also plays a predominant role in the recovery of consciousness after a single injection, but metabolism is of greater importance. Propanidid is broken down by liver and plasma esterases, and cumulation of the drug on repeated administration does not occur. The duration of steroid anaesthesia is significantly affected by hepatic metabolism, and most of a single dose is inactivated by the liver in a few hours. Etomidate and propofol are metabolized rapidly, within an hour or so. These drugs are, therefore, least potentiated by other agents, such as alcohol, if they are given after apparent full recovery of consciousness. Ketamine diffuses from the brain and is broken down more slowly, and is the longest acting of these agents after a single narcotic dose.

Further details about these agents are given in the monographs which follow.

Althesin (This drug has been withdrawn since this edition was prepared because of the high incidence of allergic reactions)

Alphaxalone (*BAN*) mixed with Alphadolone acetate (*BAN*)
Chemical name: 3α-hydroxy-5α-pregnane-11,20-dione (Alphaxalone)
3α,21-dihydroxy-5α-pregnane-11,20-dione 21-acetate (Alphadolone acetate)

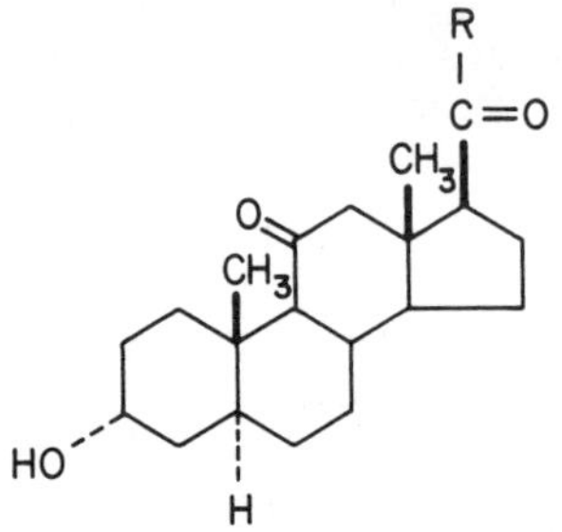

R = CH_3 (Alphaxolone)
R = CH_2 — O — CO — CH_3 (Alphadone)

PHYSICAL CHARACTERISTICS

The drug as supplied contains 3 parts of alphaxalone to 1 part of alphadolone. Final concentrations are 9 mg/ml of alphaxalone and 3 mg/ml of alphadolone. These two steroids differ only in that in the latter R is the acetoxy derivative. Although both steroids have anaesthetic activity, alphadolone is only approximately half as potent as alphaxalone and is included in the formulation because it improves the solubility of the more potent steroid. Both are solubilized in 0.25 per cent saline by the addition of 20 per cent w/v polyoxyethylated castor oil. This can be diluted with an equal amount of isotonic saline before injection.

PHARMACOLOGY

Following intravenous injection, Althesin produces loss of consciousness in about 30 seconds with a duration of approximately 5–10 minutes, depending on the dose. In rats the therapeutic index is approximately four times as great as for the injectable barbiturates. Apart from a weak antioestrogenic action the steroids have no hormonal actions.

Central nervous system The optimal dosage for induction lies between 0.05 and 0.1 ml/kg. Doses lower than this may not lead to loss of consciousness and doses in excess of this range are associated with a higher incidence of excitatory phenomena, such as muscle twitching. The incidence of these is reduced by sedative or analgesic premedication, and is always less than that found with methohexitone and greater than that seen with thiopentone. Surgical anaesthesia persists for approximately half the duration of unconsciousness, or about 2–5 minutes. After the onset of unconsciousness there is good muscle relaxation. Recovery of consciousness is rapid, although there may be some tendency to cumulation on repeat dosage. Nausea and vomiting are infrequent. A mild euphoria on recovery and uncontrollable weeping have both been reported. Althesin produces some retrograde amnesia. The EEG is unlike that seen with intravenous barbiturates in that burst suppression is very commonly seen, even though clinically only a light plane of anaesthesia is present.

Cardiovascular system. Following injection there is peripheral vasodilatation with slight flushing of the skin. There is a fall in central venous pressure and arterial blood pressure of about 10–20 per cent, although cardiac output is maintained or even increased. The heart rate characteristically increases by up to 20 per cent and this is associated with a rise in the threshold to adrenaline-induced arrhythmias. The cardiovascular changes revert to normal rapidly over a period of 2–3 minutes. The timing of the onset of these changes exactly corresponds with those affecting respiration, which suggests a central site of action.

Respiratory system. Following induction there may be some irregularity of ventilation or a short period of apnoea, after which breathing is shallow and rapid. Respiratory rates of approximately 30/min are common in unpremedicated patients. There is a small rise in P_{CO_2} and a fall in P_{O_2} of up to 13 mmHg (1.73 kPa) has been recorded.

Fate in the body. Protein binding is not extensive. The half-life of the drug is 6–8 minutes. Although redistribution is the principal mechanism in the rapid return of consciousness after a single dose, the actions of the drug are terminated by active hepatic metabolism, whose breakdown products are excreted in the bile; 70 per cent appear in the faeces, but enterohepatic recirculation causes the remainder to be excreted in the urine.

Other systems. The drug is painless on intravenous injection, non-irritant to the tissues, and thrombophlebitis has not been a problem. It appears to be compatible with all sedatives and premedicant drugs, with inhalational anaesthetics (with the possible exception of methoxyflurane) and with all muscle relaxants. It can induce anaphylactoid reactions.

INDICATIONS

Althesin is indicated for induction of anaesthesia as an alternative to rapidly acting barbiturates. Its chief merit would appear to be its high therapeutic ratio. It may be of particular value in outpatients because of its rapid metabolism. Althesin may also be used as a sole agent for short procedures since it appears to be more analgesic than the barbiturates. It has been given by slow continuous infusion to maintain light sleep in patients in intensive care units after major surgery and as a sole agent to maintain sleep while analgesia is provided, either by intravenous analgesics or by regional blockade.

DOSAGE AND ADMINISTRATION

Because of the complex formulation it is often convenient to give the dose in terms of millilitres of solution as supplied per kilogram of body weight. Doses below 0.05 ml/kg are ineffective. Doses much in excess of 0.1–0.2 ml/kg may be associated with apnoea or periods of muscle twitching, particularly if combined with hyoscine premedication. Half the dose may be repeated as indicated when used as sole anaesthetic agent for short procedures. To supplement nitrous oxide/oxygen anaesthesia Althesin may be given by continuous infusion which needs to be run to deliver about 17–20 μg/min/kg.

PRECAUTIONS

It is now clear that there is a significantly greater incidence of severe reactions to Althesin than to thiopentone and may exceed 1 in 1000 administrations. Reactions are of two kinds: a skin flush and dermal oedema followed by hypotension and tachycardia, which respond to rapid transfusion of Ringer lactate or plasma substitute; in other cases, histamine release and bronchospasm are predominant. The risk is higher in patients with a personal or family history of atopy and in patients who have recently been exposed to Althesin or other agents formulated in Cremophor EL. Reactions may require treatment with oxygen, plasma volume expanders, and intravenous steroids.

Althesin should also be used with care in the presence of liver disease.

Propofol

Chemical name: 2,6-di-isopropylphenol

PHYSICAL CHARACTERISTICS

Propofol is sparingly soluble in water and was originally presented in Cremophor EL. Because of an unacceptably high incidence of allergic reactions in this preparation, it has been reformulated as a 1 per cent w/v aqueous emulsion in 10 per cent w/v soya bean oil, 1.2 per cent egg phosphatide and 2.5 per cent glycerol.

PHARMACOLOGY

Propofol is a non-barbiturate rapidly acting intravenous induction agent. Of all the non-barbiturate agents, its induction characteristics are most like those of thiopentone. It produces a greater fall in arterial blood pressure than equipotent doses of thiopentone due to a greater fall in systemic vascular resistance. Cardiac output falls slightly, and a compensatory tachycardia does not occur. It is as potent a respiratory depressant as thiopentone.

The duration of sleep is short, broadly comparable to that following an equivalent dose of methohexitone. It has also been used in a continuous infusion to maintain anaesthesia. On cessation of the infusion, the drug decays exponentially and concentrations can be fitted to an open two-compartment model. It is compatible with all premedicant drugs.

INDICATIONS

Propofol is indicated for the rapid induction of anaesthesia; its characteristics suggest that it should be particularly suitable for outpatient anaesthesia. It can be used for the maintenance of anaesthesia by continuous infusion.

DOSAGE AND ADMINISTRATION

For induction of anaesthesia, the ED_{95} in unpremedicated patients is 2.5 mg/kg. Smaller doses need to be given rapidly. To supplement nitrous oxide/oxygen anaesthesia the minimum infusion rate is about 50 μg/kg/min.

PRECAUTIONS

Propofol should be given into an antecubital vein as pain can occur when it is injected into peripheral veins. Muscle movement and respiratory upsets on induction are few and of a minor nature; these are commoner after large doses and in the absence of premedication.

Etomidate

Chemical name: *R*-(+)-ethyl-1-(α-methylbenzyl) imidazole-5-carboxylate

CH_3

C_2H_5O—OC—N—CH—

N

PHYSICAL CHARACTERISTICS

Etomidate is soluble in water and supplied as a 0.15 per cent solution (pH 5.0) in propylene glycol or as an alcohol concentrate for dilution and infusion.

PHARMACOLOGY

Etomidate is an intravenous non-barbiturate narcotic. In doses of 0.2 mg/kg it provides an equal duration of sleep to methohexitone 1.5 mg/kg, but is associated with a more rapid recovery to full ambulation. Even with repeated doses there is little evidence of cumulation. Its other advantage would seem to be greater cardiovascular stability than occurs with other intravenous induction agents. It does not cause histamine release.

Etomidate has been given as a continuous infusion to cover regional analgesia, as a sole anaesthetic agent, and as part of a total intravenous technique with analgesics and relaxants.

Unfortunately, its potential advantages are offset by some practical disadvantages. Moderate or severe involuntary muscle movements occurred in a high proportion of patients given the drug with atropine premedication as an induction agent. The incidence is dose dependent. The frequency is much reduced when analgesic premedicants are given. These movements can persist into the recovery period following infusions of the drug. Other excitatory phenomena such as cough or hiccough occur in 10 per cent of patients. When it is given as a sole agent the occurrence of myoclonus may make conditions quite unsatisfactory. This is largely avoided when potent analgesics and relaxants are used, but this creates some difficulties in ensuring that the patient is unconscious without using large doses.

Nausea and vomiting occur postoperatively in about a third of patients, irrespective of the type of premedication. Pain on injection of the drug occurs in up to 80 per cent of patients when small peripheral veins are used for injection.

Although its extremely rapid recovery makes it seem a very useful agent, on the evidence to date etomidate does not appear to be a satisfactory intravenous narcotic for general use.

DOSAGE AND ADMINISTRATION

The optimum dose for the induction of anaesthesia is 0.3 mg/kg and should be given into the largest available arm vein. Premedication with an analgesic such as pethidine or papaveretum as well as atropine or hyoscine is advisable. For a continuous infusion, used as a sole agent, 0.05 μg/kg/min are needed; when supplemented, doses may be as low as 0.02 μg/kg/min.

PRECAUTIONS

Prolonged continuous administration causes suppression of adrenocortical function and is not recommended for sedation in intensive care.

Ketamine hydrochloride

Ketamine hydrochloride (*BAN* and *USP*)
Chemical name: (±)-2-(2-chlorophenyl)-2-methylaminocyclohexanone hydrochloride

Cl · HCl
NH—CH_3
O

PHYSICAL CHARACTERISTICS
Ketamine is supplied as an acidic solution for intravenous or intramuscular injection as 10, 50, or 100 mg of ketamine base per millilitre. The 50 and 100 mg solutions contain 0.01 per cent benzethonium chloride as a preservative.

PHARMACOLOGY
Central nervous system. Ketamine is a derivative of phencylidine and, like that drug, has been described as a dissociative agent. It produces loss of consciousness in about 30 seconds, given intravenously. A feature of its action is an intense analgesia. Unconsciousness is associated with the maintenance of normal or slightly depressed pharyngeal and laryngeal reflexes. Analgesia may precede the onset of anaesthesia and persists after the return of consciousness. During this state, bizarre hallucinations may occur, associated with the loss of body image and, if stimulated, the patient may react violently and irrationally although remaining amnesic.

A frequently reported feature of ketamine anaesthesia has been the occurrence of vivid and sometimes unpleasant dreams. This response is less common in children. The incidence of these can be reduced by giving sedative drugs during emergence. The drugs most commonly employed hitherto for this purpose have been droperidol, diazepam, or an intravenous barbiturate in small doses. Recently physostigmine has been advocated. Premedication also has marked effects. Opiates with hyoscine, droperidol with nitrazepam, or lorazepam alone are drug regimens that have been found to be the most effective in preventing dreaming and emergence problems.

Amnesia persists for about an hour after apparent recovery of consciousness but the drug does not cause retrograde amnesia. There are persistent marked changes in the EEG with the abolition of alpha rhythm and a dominant theta activity. Increases in cerebral blood flow give rise to acute increases in intracranial pressure. Ketamine differs from other induction agents in that satisfactory induction can be obtained with intramuscular injection of suitable doses.

Cardiovascular system. There is a rise in blood pressure of about 25 per cent and a rise in heart rate of about 15 beats per minute immediately following intravenous injection. These rises occur with all subsequent injections. Cardiac output is unchanged or increased. These responses are blocked or prevented by halothane. Johnstone (1976) believes that these effects of ketamine are due to a veratrine-like facilitation of calcium ion transport across the cell membrane of cardiac muscle and Purkinje fibres, since they can be blocked by verapamil. This would explain the ineffectiveness of β-blockade. The positive inotropic effect of ketamine would, therefore, be akin to that of digitalis. Ketamine sensitizes the heart to small doses of adrenaline and may precipitate dysrhythmias in very anxious patients, in the presence of thyrotoxicosis or phaeochromocytoma, or when adrenaline is used for haemostasis. These can be controlled with β-receptor blocking agents. Ketamine is not vagolytic; the oculocardiac reflex is not obtunded in children.

Ketamine has other important actions on the cardiovascular system; it causes vasodilatation in tissues predominantly innervated by α-adrenoceptors and vasoconstriction in β-adrenergically innervated tissues. This response is comparable to the actions of other powerful sedatives such as haloperidol or lorazepam. However, in the case of ketamine these responses persist even in the presence of severe surgical stimuli. This block of the reflex sympathetic nervous reaction to adrenergic stimuli is not achieved at receptor level, since ergometrine, an α-receptor stimulator, is still effective. Nor can a direct action on the vessels be postulated or β-adrenergically innervated tissues would also be vasodilated. The block may be afferent, associated with intense sensory blockade, or could conceivably be efferent at ganglionic or preganglionic level. This awaits investigation.

Respiratory system. After intravenous injection of 2 mg/kg or more there may be transient apnoea. By comparison with other agents there is preservation of pharyngeal reflexes and a patent upper airway. In fact, obstruction of the airway, laryngeal spasm, and inhalation of vomit have all been reported, although in general these are uncommon.

Other systems. There is a rise in intraocular pressure. Nausea and vomiting are fairly common after sole administration. Adverse effects on the liver or kidney have not been reported.

INDICATIONS

Ketamine may be used as an induction agent prior to general anaesthesia and its positive inotropic effects may be regarded as an indication for its employment in poor-risk patients. It can also be used as a sole agent for surgical procedures that do not require muscular relaxation. Its chief indication would appear to be in situations in which there is difficulty in maintaining an airway, for example severe burns or trauma affecting the face or upper airway. It has also been used for neurodiagnostic procedures, such as pneumoencephalograms and ventriculograms and has also been reported on favourably as a sole agent for cardiac catheterization. It is of value for repeated ocular examination in children and to induce immobility for radiotherapy treatment and other investigations. It may have a place in underdeveloped countries for use by a surgeon working single-handed, particularly if given by the intramuscular route or by continuous intravenous infusion. It is not a suitable sole agent for endoscopies of the pharynx, larynx, or bronchial tree.

DOSAGE AND ADMINISTRATION

An intravenous injection of 2 mg/kg produces surgical anaesthesia within 30 seconds, lasting for 5–10 minutes. Repeated doses may be given if a longer effect is desired, without significant cumulative effects. Intramuscularly, 10 mg/kg produces surgical anaesthesia within 3–4 minutes, with a duration of 15–30 minutes. Continuous administration of 50 μg/kg/min has been recommended for the production of analgesia without loss of consciousness for minor surgery. The concurrent administration of physostigmine antagonizes the distorted perception without reversing the analgesia.

PRECAUTIONS

Ketamine is contraindicated in patients with a history of cerebrovascular accident, with severe cardiac decompensation, severe angina, or sustained hypertension. A severe sustained rise in blood pressure has been reported in a patient receiving thyroid therapy. Ketamine is also contraindicated in the presence of raised intracranial pressure and recent penetrating injury of the eye. The use of ergometrine during ketamine anaesthesia is potentially hazardous. Overstimulation of the patient during the period of emergence should be avoided.

Johnstone, M. (1976) The cardiovascular effects of ketamine in man. *Anaesthesia,* **31,** 873

Methohexitone sodium

Methohexitone injection (*BP*) and Methohexital sodium for injection (*USP*)
Chemical name: sodium α-(±)-5-allyl-1-methyl-5-(1-methylpent-2-ynyl) barbiturate
For structural formula *see Table 3.2*, pp. 100–101

PHYSICAL CHARACTERISTICS

Methohexitone sodium occurs as a white crystalline powder, supplied commercially mixed with anhydrous sodium carbonate, and is readily soluble in water to give solutions of pH 10–11.

PHARMACOLOGY

Methohexitone is a rapidly acting barbiturate and was the product of an intensive search for an intravenous agent with a more rapid recovery than that of thiopentone.

This barbiturate is unusual in having two asymmetric carbon atoms in its structure which allow the formation of four isomers. These have been resolved into two pairs, the α-DL and the β-DL, of which the α-pair produces hypnosis without excessive skeletal muscle activity. The two α-isomers only are present in commercial methohexitone. At body pH more methohexitone is present in the non-ionized state than after a comparable dose of thiopentone. This contributes to its greater potency. It has a lower oil/water partition coefficient, and during the first 12 hours after administration more drug is circulating in the plasma, and this favours more rapid metabolism.

Nervous system. Methohexitone causes loss of consciousness in one arm/brain circulation time. The EEG changes are similar to those seen with thiopentone and propanidid. With doses of approximately 1 mg/kg the immediate recovery of consciousness is rapid and occurs in 2–3 minutes; it is slightly less than with equipotent doses of thiopentone but longer than after equipotent doses of propanidid. There is also a more rapid progression to clinical recovery than with thiopentone. However, blood levels and EEG monitoring during 12–24 hours after the drug has been administered show that the term 'ultra-short-acting' is misleading unless used to describe only the duration of initial unconsciousness, as active drug is circulating for several hours. A tendency to sleepiness is maximal around 4 hours after administration and potentiation of these effects by alcohol can be demonstrated.

Respiratory system. Depending on dosage there is moderate hypoventilation and a rise in arterial P_{CO_2}. Oxygenation is little affected unless respiratory obstruction occurs.

Cardiovascular system. In common with other barbiturates, the evidence concerning the cardiovascular effects of methohexitone is confusing. A single dose causes a fall in the tone of systemic capacitance vessels and a shift of blood from the pulmonary to the systemic circulation. This may be accompanied by a fall in cardiac output. There is vasodilatation of skin vessels. Arterial blood pressure usually shows a moderate fall and there may be a slight tachycardia.

Other systems. Methohexitone is non-irritant and there is little danger of venous thrombosis or damage to tissues following perivenous injection. Intra-arterial injection can cause gangrene in the rabbit's ear and is dependent on dosage, concentration, and volume injected; however, as it is used in a lower concentration, it is proportionately safer than thiopentone.

Compared with thiopentone, induction of anaesthesia with methohexitone is associated with a higher incidence of excitatory phenomena, such as abnormal muscle movements, and cough or hiccough. The incidence of involuntary muscle movements is increased by premedication with antianalgesic drugs, such as promethazine, and diminished by narcotic analgesics. The incidence of cough and hiccough, however, is not affected by analgesic premedication, but is reduced by parasympathetic antagonists. Both types of complication increase with larger doses.

INDICATIONS

Methohexitone can be employed for similar purposes to thiopentone and is especially useful in outpatients when brevity of action is desirable. It has been employed as sole agent in the so-called minimal incremental technique to undertake dental conservation. This usage can no longer be recommended as safer techniques for dental sedation have now been established.

DOSAGE AND ADMINISTRATION

Methohexitone is normally given intravenously in a 1 per cent solution, the dose range being 50–120 mg (1.5 mg/kg) in fit patients.

PRECAUTIONS

Methohexitone should be used with the same precautions as thiopentone. Although the recovery time appears to be short and hangover minimal, effects can be detected electroencephalographically for many hours, and potentiation by alcohol can be shown. It is thus extremely important that patients should be warned against taking alcohol during the subsequent 12 hours. They should be regarded as potential traffic hazards whether as a driver or a pedestrian, and accompanied home by a responsible person. A parasympathetic antagonist is desirable for all patients, and antianalgesic drugs such as promethazine should, in general, not be given alone for premedication, or the incidence of excitatory phenomena will be considerable.

Propanidid (This drug has been withdrawn since this edition was prepared)

Propanidid (*BP*)
Chemical name: propyl-4-diethylcarbamoylmethoxy-3-methoxyphenylacetate

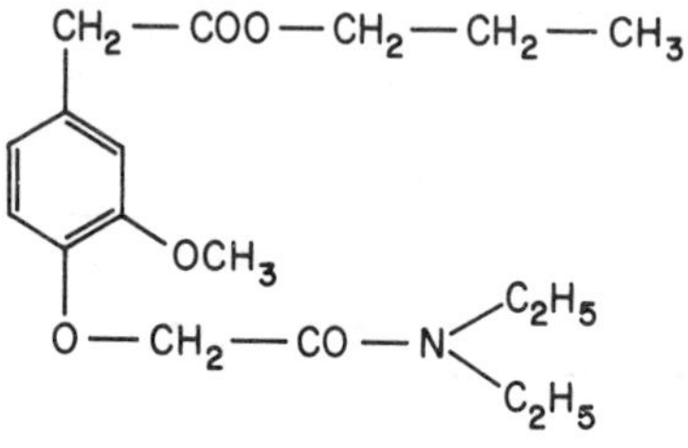

$CH_2—COO—CH_2—CH_2—CH_3$

OCH_3

$O—CH_2—CO—N(C_2H_5)_2$

PHYSICAL CHARACTERISTICS

Propanidid is a colourless or pale yellow oily liquid, insoluble in water; molecular weight 337.4; boiling point 210–212°C; pH 7.8. It is supplied as a 5 per cent solution with a solubilizing agent (Cremophor EL) and can be diluted with an equal amount of isotonic saline.

PHARMACOLOGY

Propanidid is a derivative of eugenol, and produces unconsciousness of short duration when given intravenously. As an induction agent it is approximately half as potent as thiopentone. The drug is redistributed to well-perfused organs, and is rapidly broken down by esterases in the liver and plasma; 90 per cent is eliminated as inert metabolites in the urine within 2 hours. The rate of breakdown is related to the level of plasma cholinesterase: rapid injection, which produces higher blood levels, is associated with a more rapid breakdown. Propanidid is temporarily bound to plasma proteins. Recovery of consciousness takes 3–6 minutes after normal doses.

Central nervous system. Onset of anaesthesia occurs in one arm/brain circulation time. The EEG changes are comparable to those produced by intravenous barbiturates: fast low-voltage activity gives way to progressively slower activity of high voltage (200 µV), which in turn gives way to bursts of low-voltage activity punctuated by periods of electrical silence. In the postanaesthetic period there is a return to a normal pattern within 20 minutes. The potentiating effect of a small amount of alcohol, which can be demonstrated after thiopentone and methohexitone, cannot be demonstrated with propanidid.

Involuntary muscle movements occur in some patients and are more common in the absence of analgesic premedication. Their incidence is similar to those seen with thiopentone but less than after methohexitone.

Respiratory system. The onset of anaesthesia is marked by a period of 15–30 seconds of hyperventilation. This is followed by a variable degree of respiratory depression, or even apnoea. When hyperventilation is marked the hypoventilation may be short, suggesting a biphasic action. No fully satisfactory explanation for these responses exists. In dogs it is unrelated to the solvent or the pH of the solution, and is unaffected by vagotomy. There is either no change or a slight rise in arterial carbon dioxide tension. It is likely that there is an initial stimulation of peripheral chemoreceptors (similar to the effect of lobeline), followed by a slight depression. During the period of hypoventilation there is a demonstrable fall in arterial oxygen tension.

Cardiovascular system. There is a transient fall of about 30 per cent from the resting level of blood pressure with normal doses; this fall is more marked and its recovery slower in hypertensive patients, and is dose related. The principal cause appears to be central depression rather than peripheral vasodilatation. There is also some tachycardia and ECG evidence of a quinidine-like action. Occasional cases of very severe hypotension have been reported.

Musculature. Propanidid may cause a slight rise in resting muscle tension. There is potentiation of the duration of action of suxamethonium, but not of the intensity of the neuromuscular block. This effect is probably due to substrate competition for esterases.

Other effects. Reported instances of accidental and experimental injection into arteries have not been followed by any vascular complications. Extravascular injection induces a painless indurated swelling which resolves without abscess formation. The incidence of venous thrombosis is approximately twice as great as with thiopentone or methohexitone. The drug has a local analgesic action.

There have been a disquieting number of clinical reports of acute hypotension or cardiac arrest shortly after induction with a normal dose of propanidid in fit patients. In many of these cases there has been evidence of a generalized acute hypersensitivity reaction. Skin sensitivity in an anaesthetist has also been reported.

INDICATIONS

Propanidid is chiefly indicated for short surgical procedures when rapid recovery is required. It thus finds its chief application in outpatient procedures. It may also be used as a general induction agent, when the hyperventilation may facilitate blind nasal intubation.

DOSES AND ADMINISTRATION

The usual dose for adults averages 6–7 mg/kg and for children 7–8 mg/kg intravenously. As the drug is rapidly broken down, when it is used as a sole anaesthetic agent any extension of operating time beyond 3–5 minutes will necessitate giving repeated doses at regular intervals of at least half to two thirds of the initial dose.

PRECAUTIONS

When propanidid is used as an induction agent, and immediately followed by suxamethonium, the rapid breakdown of propanidid and the extension of the paralysis can result in the return of consciousness while paralysis persists. The number of clinical reports of anaphylactic reactions suggest that the drug should be given only when positively indicated. Hypotension and the potential fall in arterial oxygen tension make oxygen administration particularly desirable prior to induction in the elderly or unfit.

Thiopentone sodium

Thiopentone sodium (*BP*) and Thiopental sodium (*USP*)
Constitution: a mixture of the monosodium salt of sodium 5-ethyl-5-(1-methylbutyl)-2-thiobarbiturate (100 parts w/w) and exsiccated sodium carbonate (6 parts w/w)
For structural formula *see Table 3.2*, pp. 100–101.

PHYSICAL CHARACTERISTICS

Thiopentone sodium occurs as a yellowish-white hygroscopic powder with a bitter taste and a faint smell of garlic. It is always supplied mixed with anhydrous sodium carbonate, the mixture being readily soluble in water. The sodium carbonate is added because thiopentone is soluble only in strongly alkaline solutions. Thiopentone sodium must be stored in a well-closed container and solutions should be freshly prepared.

Thiopentone is the sulphur analogue of pentobarbitone. It was first used in the USA in 1934 by Lundy and Waters, and was introduced into Great Britain in the following year by Jarman and Abel.

It has been described as an ultra-short-acting barbiturate, but the brevity of its effects is due to redistribution from blood and brain to other tissues rather than to rapid elimination.

PHARMACOLOGY

Nervous system. When given by intravenous injection it rapidly diffuses into the brain and produces its effects within 30 seconds. While having strong hypnotic actions, its analgesic action is poor, and the respiratory centre is readily depressed. These characteristics make it difficult to assess the level of anaesthesia, especially as reactions to stimuli such as surgical incision can occur in the presence of apnoea and apparent deep depression of the CNS. In small doses thiopentone has an antianalgesic action, the pain threshold being actually lowered. The dose that will produce this effect is between 25 and 100 mg in healthy adults, but larger doses when they have become redistributed with the passage of time and reach a corresponding plasma level will have a similar action.

If a given dose is injected rapidly, consciousness returns at a higher plasma level than if the same dose is injected more slowly. This has been attributed by Dundee (1956) to acute tolerance, a concept that is difficult to visualize in either pharmacological or physiological terms. It may be an artifact of the pharmacodynamics of 'slug administration', a mode of administration that results in an exceedingly rapid entry into and exit from the CNS. This causes for some time a distortion of drug distribution between the brain and the peripheral circulation which does not occur with slower rates of administration.

Autonomic system. Vagal tone is not depressed with small doses of thiopentone, but because reflex vagal activity is often marked the impression may be gained that tone is actually increased.

Cardiovascular system. Thiopentone depresses the myocardium and cardiac output decreases as the plasma concentration of the drug rises. Cardiac irritability is unaffected. There is usually a mild initial fall in blood pressure which returns to normal within a few minutes, but when the drug is injected rapidly or in large doses severe hypotension may occur. This is mainly due to peripheral vasodilatation caused by depression of the vasomotor centre, but direct depression of myocardial contractility also plays a part. Such depression of blood pressure is more marked in the presence of cardiovascular disease, especially hypertension.

Respiratory system. Respiration is markedly depressed by thiopentone. Following a few deep breaths a short period of apnoea is common, respiration being resumed with a diminished rate and depth. The degree of respiratory depression depends on the dose of thiopentone administered and the speed of administration, and it is enhanced by the previous administration of other central depressants such as morphine and its derivatives. The sensitivity of the respiratory centre to carbon dioxide is considerably reduced. There is a mild degree of bronchial constriction, but secretions are not increased.

Laryngospasm is not uncommon during light thiopentone anaesthesia. This effect has been attributed to an increased sensitivity of laryngeal reflexes due to parasympathomimetic action, but is more probably caused by the relative absence of depression of this particular nervous arc, as spasm is nearly always associated with some stimulus in the region of the larynx, such as mucus, blood, or the presence of a laryngoscope blade.

Musculature. Skeletal muscle tone is markedly reduced when central depression is at its height. Smooth muscle is unaffected during light anaesthesia but large doses cause depression of activity.

Uterus and placenta. Small doses of thiopentone have little effect on the pregnant uterus, although contractions are depressed by large doses. It rapidly crosses the placental barrier; the fetal blood level is related to maternal blood level but is considerably lower. It is temporarily markedly raised shortly after a 'slug' of drug is administered to the mother.

Fate in the body. After injection, the level of thiopentone in the plasma reaches its maximum rapidly. It is immediately taken up by nervous tissue and other tissues with a high blood flow. It then begins to diffuse more slowly from the plasma to other tissues, mainly liver, kidney and muscles. Most of the thiopentone eventually ends up in fat, but the blood supply of this is so poor that it can play no part in the lowering of brain concentration leading to early awakening. As the plasma level falls, the concentration in the brain falls likewise and consciousness returns. At this time most of the original dose injected is still present unchanged in the body, having merely been redistributed from brain to other tissues.

In the blood, thiopentone is bound to plasma proteins. Decreased binding occurs in malnutrition and other severe wasting illness and this accounts for a large increase in sensitivity to thiopentone. The amount bound depends to a great extent upon the blood pH. Increasing the plasma pH by hyperventilation will increase the plasma concentration of thiopentone, and will therefore increase the effects of a given dose.

Thiopentone is almost entirely metabolized in the liver. Breakdown products are excreted by the kidneys and alimentary tract. Traces are excreted unchanged in the urine. Destruction in the body is slow, 10–15 per cent per hour, and nearly 30 per cent of the original dose may remain after 24 hours. Consequently, if further thiopentone is given there will be a cumulative effect.

Liver and kidney function. No permanent effects have been recorded.

Metabolism.. Oxygen consumption falls in proportion to the depth of anaesthesia. In the absence of surgical stimuli there are no effects on the endocrine system.

ANAESTHETIC PROPERTIES

Thiopentone is a powerful intravenous narcotic. Induction is rapid (15–30 seconds), pleasant, and without excitement. Respiration is quiet, but operating conditions are poor and movement of the patient commonly follows surgical stimulation. Skeletal muscular relaxation is also poor except for a few moments shortly after injection when the drug is exerting its maximum effect. After a moderate dose recovery is rapid, but the patient may be sleepy or confused for some hours. Large or repeated smaller doses may cause severe depression and recovery may be considerably delayed. For this reason thiopentone alone is not a suitable agent for operations lasting more than a few minutes. Postoperative vomiting is rare.

INDICATIONS

Practically all types of operation have at one time been attempted under thiopentone, but respiratory depression and the slow recovery time associated with the use of large doses have led to its abandonment as a sole agent for anaesthesia in favour of more satisfactory methods. Thiopentone is now only used for induction of anaesthesia and in the treatment of status epilepticus. It is used by some anaesthetists for basal narcosis in children by the rectal route. It has largely been superseded by shorter acting agents for examinations under anaesthesia; narcosis to cover spinal, regional, or other forms of local analgesia is better achieved with agents such as diazepam.

DOSAGE AND ADMINISTRATION

Thiopentone is normally given intravenously in a 2.5 per cent solution. It can be given per rectum in a 5 or 10 per cent solution.

The dose of thiopentone required to produce a given depth of narcosis varies considerably according to the age and condition of the patient, and even healthy patients vary in their response. The rate of injection is also important; the faster the injection, the quicker and deeper is the response and the quicker is the recovery. Only the smallest dose necessary to produce the desired effect should be given, and in the judgement of this the experience of the anaesthetist is the important factor.

For the induction of anaesthesia in fit adults a dose of 3–5 mg/kg is usually required; half the dose may be injected over a period of 15 seconds, and after a pause long enough to note the effect the injection is continued until the desired level of narcosis is reached. Respiration must be assisted if unduly depressed.

For basal narcosis by the rectal route, the dose is calculated on the basis of 1 g of thiopentone per 22 kg of body weight. It is given in 5 or 10 per cent solution, and is normally effective within about 15 minutes of administration.

PRECAUTIONS

There are a considerable number of hazards associated with thiopentone anaesthesia; its potency makes it a highly dangerous drug in inexperienced hands. It is very easy to give an overdose, especially to sick and elderly patients.

It should never be given to patients in the sitting position as even a small overdose can cause severe hypotension. It should never be given rapidly to any but fit and robust patients. An apparatus capable of ventilating the lungs should always be readily available when thiopentone is being used.

Outpatients must be allowed to rest for as long as possible after recovering consciousness because confusion and forgetfulness may persist for several hours. They should be accompanied home by a responsible person and told not to take alcohol for 24 hours, drive, or operate machinery.

Atropine or an atropine-like drug should always be given before or with thiopentone to depress vagal reflexes and mucous secretions. Central depressants such as morphine or pethidine are often given before thiopentone to enhance the analgesic effect and to reduce the dose of thiopentone required.

Apart from the absence of suitable veins for its administration, there are few absolute contraindications to the use of thiopentone. It is, however, generally considerd to be contraindicated in the following situations:

1. If the airway is obstructed in conditions such as Ludwig's angina, and where an adequate airway cannot be maintained during operation
2. In uncompensated heart disease, and constrictive pericarditis
3. In severe shock
4. In adrenocortical insufficiency (Addison's disease) following bilateral adrenalectomy, unless adequate cortisone therapy has been previously instituted
5. In status asthmaticus
6. In porphyria.

In some of these conditions, general anaesthesia would, of course, be a hazard in any case.

Relative contraindications, where special care should be exercised both as regards size of dose and the rate of administration, are as follows:

1. Decreased circulating blood volume: severe haemorrhage, burns, dehydration
2. Severe anaemia
3. Cardiovascular disease: conditions affecting the myocardium, severe hypertension
4. Severe liver disease
5. Dystrophia myotonica
6. Myasthenia gravis
7. Adrenocortical insufficiency, even when controlled by cortisone
8. Cachexia and severe toxaemia
9. Raised intracranial pressure
10. Raised blood urea
11. Raised plasma potassium
12. Reduced metabolic rate, as in myxoedema.

Smaller doses than normal will be required in the elderly, and in subjects who have been heavily premedicated with narcotics and other central depressants.

The dose in obstetric cases should be restricted to the minimum necessary for induction.

COMPLICATIONS

Laryngeal spasm. This is uncommon unless the patient is stimulated and even then is likely to be seen only when painful procedures are undertaken under thiopentone alone. Its occurrence in other circumstances suggests the proximity of blood, saliva, or stomach contents to the laryngeal inlet.

Bronchospasm. This may occur in asthmatics whose vagal reflexes are particularly sensitive.

Extravascular injection. This causes pain and swelling which is less severe with the 2.5 per cent than with the 5 per cent solution. Treatment consists of infiltrating the area with lignocaine and hyaluronidase. The arm should be kept at rest.

Intra-arterial injection. This usually causes intense pain shooting down the arm or fingers, blanching of the skin, and disappearance or weakness of the radial pulse. It is not simply due to the alkalinity of the solution and experimentally any spasm is of short duration. Waters (1966) has shown that after mixing thiopentone solutions with blood, precipitation occurs, the pH of the mixture becoming too low for the thiopentone to remain in solution. Crystals thus formed, therefore, are likely to block small arterioles and capillaries. This suggests that stagnation or cessation of the circulation is the initial lesion, and accounts for the rapidity of onset. Its persistence could be due to a sustained release of noradrenaline, provoked by the crystal deposits. The thrombosis is secondary to stagnation.

Serious sequelae may occur, including atrophy of the muscles or gangrene of the fingers, and the operation should be postponed whenever possible. If the needle is still in the artery and there is any flow in the hand, an injection of an α-blocking agent such as phentolamine should be given. Brachial plexus or stellate ganglion block will also improve the blood supply. The latent threat of thrombosis can be counteracted by an immediate injection of heparin and the institution of long-term anticoagulant therapy, unless the operation is to proceed.

Twice as much thiopentone is precipitated from 5 per cent solution as from 2.5 per cent solution. No cases of gangrene have been reported following injection of 2.5 per cent thiopentone into an artery at the elbow, although it has been reported after injection into an artery in the back of the hand. The hazards of this accident can be minimized by using a 2.5 per cent solution and by pausing after injection of 1 ml and asking specifically if there is any pain in the arm or hand.

Thrombophlebitis. This complication sometimes occurs after injection of thiopentone, but is less likely to occur if the 2.5 per cent solution is used. Treatment is symptomatic and may require rest and warmth.

Overdose. An overdose of thiopentone will produce apnoea or serious respiratory depression. Cardiovascular collapse may also occur. Respiratory insufficiency requires controlled respiration with oxygen until normal respiration is resumed. Analeptics should not be given. Thiopentone may cause an anaphylactoid reaction but it is very rare — about 1 in 15 000 administrations.

Dundee, J. W. (1956) *Thiopentone and Other Barbiturates*. Edinburgh and London: Livingstone
Waters, D. J. (1966) Intra-arterial thiopentone. A physico-chemical phenomenon. *Anaesthesia,* **21,** 346

Other injectable barbiturates

Hexobarbitone, which is no longer available, was the first barbiturate to be used safely and effectively for the production of anaesthesia by the intravenous route by Weese and Sharpff in 1932. The principal reason why it lost popularity to thiopentone was a higher incidence of coughing, sneezing, and twitching during induction.

Thiamylal sodium is the thio-derivative of quinalbarbitone, and is slightly more potent than thiopentone. In recent comparisons it has proved indistinguishable from that drug.

Neuroleptics and tranquillizers

Neurolepsis was first described by Delay (1959) as a drug-induced behavioural syndrome in animals and man. Pharmacologically, neuroleptics characteristically block apomorphine-induced vomiting in dogs and antagonize the CNS effects of amphetamine. These actions are due to their general behaviour as competitive antagonists at dopaminergic receptors in the brain (*see* page 231). A neuroleptic state can be induced by various classes of drugs; the butyrophenones are major neuroleptic drugs, as are phenothiazines with a piperazine-type side chain, in that they produce the characteristic syndrome with high specificity. They inevitably also induce extrapyramidal side effects which are also due to dopaminergic blockade.

Many other drugs have significant neuroleptic activity, including many phenothiazines, but also possess anticholinergic or antiadrenergic properties. These modify their side effects: anticholinergic activity counteracts the tendency to extrapyramidal side effects; antiadrenergic activity produces cardiovascular effects. Antihistamine and antiserotonin properties may also be possessed by drugs with significant neuroleptic activity.

Haloperidol · Chlorpromazine · Imipramine · γ-aminobutyric acid (GABA) · Metoclopramide

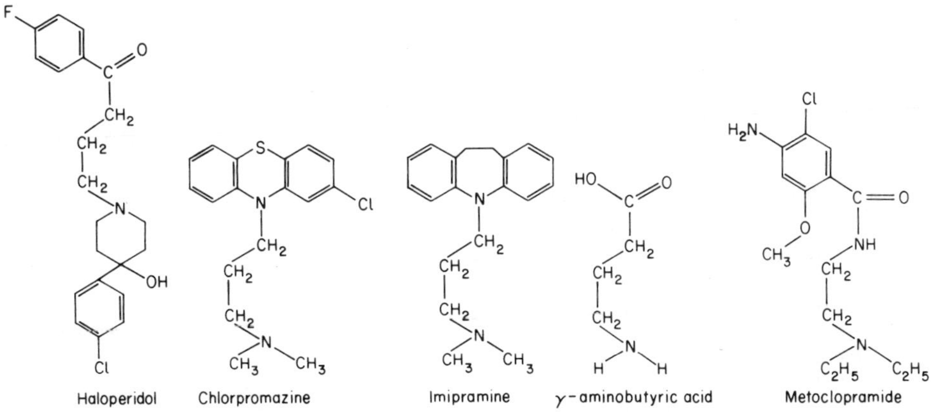

Figure 3.1 Structural formulae of several centrally acting drugs

Although it is not immediately apparent, members of these groups are related structurally. Many contain an S-shaped propylene chain terminating in at least one tertiary nitrogen atom, and often two, with an aromatic ring at one end and sometimes at both. This arrangement is brought out in the structural formulae, together with the significant similarity to the structure of GABA (*Figure 3.1*). At certain synapses, GABA is an inhibitory transmitter and dopamine is the stimulatory transmitter. It is postulated that the neuroleptics compete for the dopaminergic receptors at the postsynaptic membrane and decrease transmission.

They have a predilection for those areas of the brain which are rich in dopaminergic synapses, which include the chemoreceptor trigger zone and extrapyramidal nigrostriatum. Structural relationships to dopamine and other catecholamines are also present. As the structural formulae show, comparable structural groups are found not only in the phenothiazines and butyrophenones, which have marked antiemetic activity, but also in the specific antiemetic, metoclopramide. The dibenzazepine antidepressants also have a similar configuration.

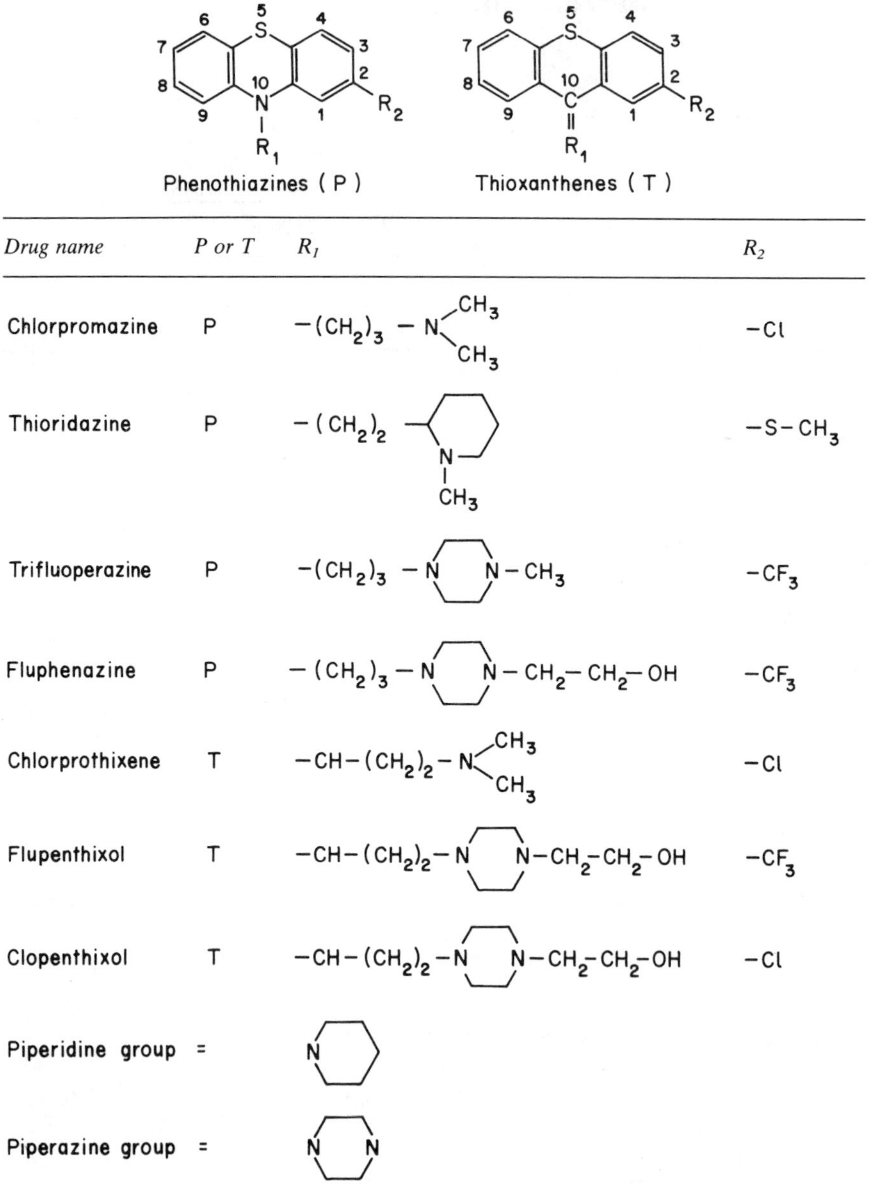

Phenothiazines (P) Thioxanthenes (T)

Drug name	*P or T*	R_1	R_2
Chlorpromazine	P	$-(CH_2)_3-N(CH_3)_2$	$-Cl$
Thioridazine	P	$-(CH_2)_2-$ (piperidine, N–CH_3)	$-S-CH_3$
Trifluoperazine	P	$-(CH_2)_3-N$ (piperazine) $N-CH_3$	$-CF_3$
Fluphenazine	P	$-(CH_2)_3-N$ (piperazine) $N-CH_2-CH_2-OH$	$-CF_3$
Chlorprothixene	T	$-CH-(CH_2)_2-N(CH_3)_2$	$-Cl$
Flupenthixol	T	$-CH-(CH_2)_2-N$ (piperazine) $N-CH_2-CH_2-OH$	$-CF_3$
Clopenthixol	T	$-CH-(CH_2)_2-N$ (piperazine) $N-CH_2-CH_2-OH$	$-Cl$

Piperidine group =

Piperazine group =

Figure 3.2 Structural formulae of some phenothiazines and thioxanthenes

Figure 3.2 shows the structure of phenothiazine. It is a three-ringed structure: two benzene rings are linked by a ring containing nitrogen and sulphur. If the nitrogen in position 10 is replaced by carbon with a double bond to the side chain such compounds are thioxanthenes. The nature of the groups attached to position 10 in the phenothiazine structure modifies its pharmacological activity. If a piperazine ring is present the compound is usually very potent and the compound tends to produce extrapyramidal effects. Such compounds tend to be less likely to sedate or cause a fall in blood pressure which is more easily produced by other substituents. Fluphenazine is a good example. Some piperazine phenothiazines have been esterified with long-chain fatty acids to prolong their duration of action. Fluphenazine enanthate is a good example. Such compounds are used frequently in the outpatient management of schizophrenics.

The phenothiazine groups with the aliphatic side chain, for example chlorpromazine, are less potent than those with the piperazine side chain. Nevertheless, they are clinically effective. They tend as a group to produce sedation and hypotension. Finally, those with the piperidine side chain, for example thioridazine, have potencies usually intermediate between the other two groups. Thioridazine itself has a relatively low incidence of extrapyramidal effects, perhaps due to the atropine-like activity of the compound.

Neuroleptanalgesia and neuroleptanaesthesia

The technique of neuroleptanalgesia was introduced by De Castro and Mundeleer in 1959 and has found a useful place in anaesthetic practice. It is a state produced by combining a potent neuroleptic drug with a potent analgesic. The analgesics commonly used are phenoperidine and fentanyl.

This mixture of drugs has been used in three basically different ways. For minor surgery where the stimulus is not too painful an amount of analgesic can be given which is not enough to depress respiration dangerously. Part of the dose may be given as premedication and the technique is often supplemented with a local analgesic, particularly for ophthalmic surgery.

However, provided that ventilation is controlled, very large doses of analgesic can be given without producing loss of consciousness. This has, therefore, been a popular technique for adult patients undergoing artificial ventilation through an endotracheal tube. It can be extended to the performance of major surgery with the patient in a mentally accessible state.

Nevertheless, most patients prefer to be unconscious, and it has been a short step, therefore, to combining these drugs with nitrous oxide and oxygen to produce what may be termed 'neuroleptanaesthesia'. This has been recommended for cardiopulmonary bypass in which the technique is less depressant to the cardiovascular system than other techniques and in which the analgesia and tranquillity can be extended into the postoperative period. It has also achieved wide popularity for neurological anaesthesia. Unlike halothane, the technique produces no increase in CSF pressure or cerebral blood flow and, indeed, when fentanyl has been used as the analgesic, falls in CSF pressure have been found.

Because of these advantages it is also logically recommendable for the poor-risk and the elderly patients and is regarded by some as the most appropriate form of anaesthesia for any surgical procedure for which general anaesthesia is indicated.

Butyrophenones

By virtue of their inhibition of 'operant' behaviour (that is, purposive movement), these drugs induce a cataleptic immobility in which the patient appears to be tranquil and dissociated from his surroundings. Nevertheless, he is readily accessible if spoken to directly. The apparent tranquillity may mask a state of marked mental restlessness, which has been described on several occasions, particularly by medical patients. This is most noticeable with large doses which can also give rise to hallucinations, loss of body image, and restlessness. Overdose also gives rise to extrapyramidal dyskinesia.

These drugs do not alter the alpha rhythm of the EEG. The reticular activating system is not depressed. These drugs are the most potent inhibitors of vomiting mediated through the chemoreceptor trigger zone, for example that produced by agents such as apomorphine or narcotic analgesics. They also inhibit the CNS effects of amphetamine.

The effects on the cardiovascular system and respiratory system are minimal. The α-adrenergic blocking activity of the butyrophenones appears to have been overemphasized and is inconsistent with the cardiovascular stability, which has been well documented.

De Castro, G. and Mundeleer, P. (1959) Anesthésie sans barbiturates: la neuroleptanalgésie. *Anesthésie, Analgésie, Réanimation,* **16,** 1022

Delay, J. (1959) *Psychopharmacology Frontiers.* Boston: Little Brown

Droperidol

Droperidol (*BAN* and *USP*)

Chemical name: 1-{1-[3-(4-fluorobenzoyl) propyl]-1,2,3,6-tetrahydro-4-pyridyl} benzimidazolin-2-one

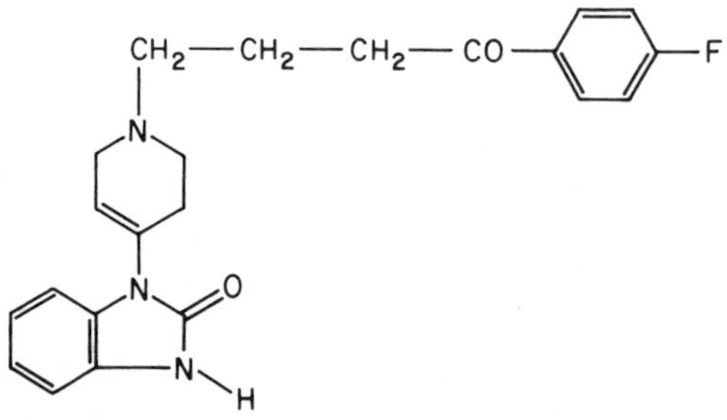

PHARMACOLOGY

Droperidol is a substituted butyrophenone closely resembling haloperidol and certain phenothiazine derivatives. It is described as a neuroleptic and produces a state of mental calm and indifference with little hypnotic effect. Compared with haloperidol it acts faster, has a shorter duration of action and is less toxic. It is a powerful antiemetic, whose action is localized to an area in the chemoreceptor trigger zone, but it does not antagonize motion sickness.

Large doses produce extrapyramidal side effects which may be delayed for some time after administration. Other actions are similar to haloperidol.

On rapid intravenous injection there is a moderate fall in systemic arterial pressure of short duration which is mediated by a direct action on the blood vessels. For a short period this hypotension cannot be reversed by α-adrenergic stimulating drugs, suggesting that the site of action of droperidol is at the α-adrenoceptors.

With oral or intramuscular administration such an effect is not seen, presumably because a high concentration of drug at the receptor is necessary. In ordinary use the marked cardiovascular stability argues against any significant α-blockade. However, it can provide some protection against experimental shock.

Droperidol is metabolized in the liver. The rate of excretion of metabolites is maximal during the first 24 hours.

DOSAGE AND ADMINISTRATION

For premedication 10 mg is given intramuscularly 1 hour before operation. Up to 10 mg may be given intravenously in conjunction with a potent analgesic to initiate neuroleptanalgesia.

PRECAUTIONS

Precautions and side effects are similar to those listed under haloperidol. It is of interest that dystonic reactions have been reported 24 hours or more after administration. These are relieved by diphenhydramine, sedative drugs, and those usually given for the relief of parkinsonism.

Haloperidol

Haloperidol (*BP* and *USP*)
Chemical name: 4-[4-(4-chlorophenyl)-4-hydroxypiperidino]-4′-fluorobutyrophenone
For structural formula *see Figure 3.1*, p. 73

PHARMACOLOGY

Haloperidol is a substituted butyrophenone, its actions resembling those of droperidol. It is classified as a neuroleptic and produces a cataleptic state with little hypnotic action. Its duration of action is longer than that of droperidol, and lasts up to 24 hours. It is a powerful antiemetic, and in its ability to block apomorphine-induced vomiting is 50 times as potent as chlorpromazine.

Haloperidol potentiates both barbiturates and analgesics and blocks the CNS effects of amphetamine in animals. The EEG is not altered by normal doses.

It has virtually no antiadrenergic activity. Blood pressure remains stable and hypotension does not occur, even after intravenous administration. There is no effect on respiration following recommended doses. Although extrapyramidal side effects may occur, toxic effects have not so far been reported.

Haloperidol, like other butyrophenones, is metabolized in the body, probably in the liver. Metabolites have been identified in the urine and also in the faeces.

INDICATIONS

The drug is used in psychiatry for psychomotor manifestations such as delusions, hallucinations, paranoia and mania. It may be used for premedication and for the production of neuroleptanalgesia.

DOSAGE AND ADMINISTRATION

The drug is given orally for psychiatric indications in doses of 1.5–6 mg daily. As a premedicant 5 mg is given intramuscularly 1–8 hours before operation. For neuroleptanalgesia 2.5–5 mg is given intravenously prior to the chosen analgesic, usually phenoperidine or fentanyl.

PRECAUTIONS

The drug should be avoided in patients with lesions in the basal ganglia, including spastic syndromes associated with arteriosclerosis. In such patients, and in normal subjects receiving high doses, extrapyramidal reactions may occur. These may be promptly alleviated by either soporific or antiparkinsonian drugs. High doses may be antisoporific. Solutions should be protected from light.

Phenothiazine derivatives

The term 'phenothiazine derivative', as applied to the drugs used in anaesthesia, refers to those aminated phenothiazine compounds which form a chemical group having the general formula shown in *Table 3.1*, pages 80–81. In this formula, X is either a two- or three-carbon chain, sometimes with an additional methyl substitution at the second carbon atom from the ring, and R_1 and R_2 are alkyl groups or may form part of a heterocyclic ring; furthermore, the benzene rings may be substituted with a halogen, methyl, or methoxy group. It can be seen that the phenothiazine nucleus is attached through its N atom and the divalent hydrocarbon chain to a basic system, which may be either an aliphatic amine, for example the promazines, or a nitrogen-containing heterocyclic system which may be attached through a N atom, for example prochlorperazine, or through a C atom, as in pecazine.

The study of these compounds was commenced simultaneously, but independently, in France and the USA in 1944. The parent substance, phenothiazine, has virtually no depressant action on the CNS and no antihistamine activity, but these pharmacological characteristics are present in the aminated derivatives. Chlorpromazine was synthesized in 1950, and its pharmacological properties became known shortly after. Laborit considered that the effects of these compounds on the CNS could be valuable, especially those of chlorpromazine, promethazine, and diethazine, and together with Huguenard he used the compounds clinically as adjuvants to anaesthesia. Their application to psychiatry followed later. Since these early clinical examinations, the literature on both the pharmacological properties and clinical uses of phenothiazines has become most extensive.

Many of these compounds possess neuroleptic properties. They also lower the metabolic rate and depress the vomiting and temperature regulating centres. Some, such as chlorpromazine, promazine, and trimeprazine, potentiate the actions of anaesthetics, hypnotics, and analgesics; some others have an antianalgesic effect.

Cholestatic jaundice and blood dyscrasias such as agranulocytosis sometimes follow their use. The risk is greatest after prolonged treatment with larger doses. Some members of this group may induce extrapyramidal manifestations. This complication is most likely to occur with phenothiazines containing a piperazine ring in the side chain and/or a trifluoromethyl group in the phenothiazine nucleus. The incidence is high and related to dose. The clinical manifestations may be severe and reports appear from time to time in which an initial diagnosis of tetanus has been made in patients who were subsequently found to have received a relative overdose of a phenothiazine. These side effects can be controlled by antiparkinsonian drugs such as benztropine but not by levodopa.

Their pronounced sedative effects make the phenothiazines unsuitable as routine antihistamines and they are employed mainly for their sedative and neuroleptic properties. Those drugs which have proved useful in connection with anaesthesia include promethazine, chlorpromazine, promazine, prochlorperazine, trimeprazine and methotrimeprazine; they are described more fully under their appropriate headings. Chlorpromazine has become the standard by which all phenothiazine derivatives are judged, mainly on account of the very extensive pharmacological studies that have now been made of it.

Chlorpromazine hydrochloride

Chlorpromazine hydrochloride (*BP* and *USP*)
Chemical name: 3(2-chlorophenothiazin-10-yl)-*NN*-dimethylpropylamine hydrochloride
For structural formula *see Table 3.1*, pp. 80–81

PHARMACOLOGY

Chlorpromazine was first synthesized by Charpentier in France in 1950, following the systematic study of similar phenothiazine derivatives, and was subsequently employed by Laborit and Huguenard in their technique of 'artificial hibernation'. Since then it has been used extensively in general medicine and anaesthesia.

Nervous system. Chlorpromazine is a central depressant with a marked action on the reticular formation, the basal ganglia, and the hypothalamus. It can cause an increase in prolactin secretion by its action on the hypothalamus. Chlorpromazine can also induce a parkinsonian-like syndrome. There is now a considerable body of evidence that chlorpromazine and related drugs antagonize the central effects of dopamine. For instance, they have been shown to antagonize the action of dopamine or dopamine agonists on dopamine-sensitive adenyl cyclase obtained from the limbic or caudate areas and selectively compete with the binding of dopaminergic ligands to membrane fractions from caudate tissues. Neuroleptics increase the turnover of dopamine in the basal ganglia. This may be a secondary response to blockade of the dopamine receptor.

Chlorpromazine produces lethargy, apathy, and tranquillity similar to the state produced by frontal leucotomy. Sleep is induced, but the subject is easily aroused; consciousness is not lost except when very large doses are given. EEG changes are similar to those produced by normal sleep. The stimulant action of the common analeptics is antagonized, but the central action of chlorpromazine is not affected by these drugs and convulsions have followed the use of nikethamide. It has generally been accepted that chlorpromazine potentiates the action of hypnotics, analgesics, and anaesthetics.

There is a marked antiemetic action, which is due to a competitive block at the chemoreceptor trigger zone in the floor of the fourth ventricle. Larger doses of chlorpromazine, however, probably act by direct depression of the vomiting centre. In addition to antagonizing vomiting caused by emetics (apomorphine) it also prevents emesis due to anaesthetic drugs, motion, and radiation.

The temperature-control mechanism is depressed and shivering is thus prevented; although the rectal temperature may fall without active cooling, controlled hypothermia cannot be achieved in the absence of surface or

Table 3.1 Structural formulae of the phenothiazines

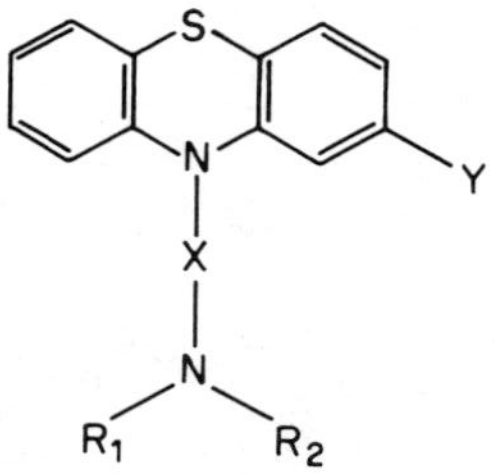

Name	*Y*	*X*	*R_1*	*R_2*
X = 2-carbon chain				
Promethazine	H	$-CH_2-CH(CH_3)-$	CH_3	CH_3
Propiomazine	$CO-CH_2-OCH_3$	$-CH_2-CH(CH_3)-$	CH_3	CH_3
Diethazine	H	$-CH_2-CH_2-$	C_2H_5	C_2H_5

Table 3.1 *cont.*

Name	*Y*	*X*	R_1	R_2
X = 3-carbon chain				
Chlorpromazine	Cl	$-CH_2-CH_2-CH_2-$	CH_3	CH_3
Promazine	H	$-CH_2-CH_2-CH_2-$	CH_3	CH_3
Fluphenazine	CF_3	$-CH_2-CH_2-CH_2-$	$-N\langle\rangle N-CH_2-CH_2-OH$	
Triflupromazine	CF_3	$-CH_2-CH_2-CH_2-$	CH_3	CH_3
Trimeprazine	H	$-CH_2-CH(CH_3)-CH_2-$	CH_3	CH_3
Methotrimeprazine	OCH_3	$-CH_2-C(CH_3)_2-CH_2-$	CH_3	CH_3
Prochlorperazine	Cl	$-CH_2-CH_2-CH_2-$	$-N\langle\rangle N-CH_3$	
Perphenazine	Cl	$-CH_2-CH_2-CH_2-$	$-N\langle\rangle N-CH_2-CH_2-OH$	
Thiopropazate	Cl	$-CH_2-CH_2-CH_2-$	$-N\langle\rangle N-CH_2-CH_2-O-CO-CH_3$	
X = more than 3 carbon atoms in chain				
Pecazine		$-CH_2-$ (piperidine ring, $N-CH_3$)		

bloodstream cooling. There is a marked antiadrenergic action, the effects of which are mostly on the cardiovascular system. A mild anticholinergic action also occurs.

Cardiovascular system. The actions of chlorpromazine on the cardiovascular system are due to its adrenergic blocking effect.

Cardiac output may remain unaltered or slightly increased. The heart rate is increased. Peripheral vasodilatation and a decrease in overall peripheral resistance produce a fall in blood pressure; this is often marked and varies with posture. Systolic pressure falls more than the diastolic pressure with a consequent fall in pulse pressure. There is an increase in peripheral blood flow through the limbs. The response to adrenaline and noradrenaline is reduced, that of the former considerably more than the latter.

The ECG shows little change except in heart rate; an increase in conduction time has, however, been reported in animals following large doses.

Respiratory system. Reports on the effect of chlorpromazine on respiration are conflicting, both depression and stimulation having been recorded. When moderate doses are employed, there is normally little change in rate or depth. It appears to have an antagonistic effect on the respiratory depression due to pethidine. Bronchial secretions are suppressed and dryness of the mucosa of the respiratory tract is marked. Mucous membranes may be congested.

Musculature. Ambulant patients on large doses complain of muscular weakness of the limbs; although it has no neuromuscular blocking action of its own it is said to potentiate the action of muscle relaxants during anaesthesia. Smooth muscle tone is depressed due to a spasmolytic action.

Alimentary system. Salivary and gastric secretions are depressed by the atropine-like action. The bowel is quiet and relaxed, which may lead to constipation during prolonged oral treatment.

Liver function. Jaundice occurs in about 0.5 per cent of patients receiving chlorpromazine, but in those with a previous history of this condition the recurrence rate is about 40 per cent. The reaction is not dependent on the size of the dose or duration of treatment. A case has been recorded after the administration of only 50 mg. Jaundice may also be accompanied by a rash, fever, and eosinophilia.

The liver shows marked cholestasis and a mononuclear and eosinophil reaction in the portal zones. The liver cells show feathery degeneration and occasionally areas of local necrosis. The diagnosis may be confused with acute viral hepatitis and with mechanical obstruction of the bile ducts. Jaundice usually subsides within a few days, although on occasions cholestasis may persist for years and merge into a picture of biliary cirrhosis. The mortality is low.

Metabolism. There is little change in metabolic rate or oxygen uptake. There is increased heat loss, the skin being warm and dry, and there may be a fall in rectal and oesophageal temperatures.

Other effects. These include a mild antihistamine action, the production of local analgesia, and skin rashes following the handling of the drug. A temporary leucopenia may occur, and several cases of agranulocytosis have been recorded. During the first few days of treatment, slight pyrexia may occur and the patient may complain of dizziness and dry mouth.

There is some evidence that chlorpromazine protects the patient against traumatic and haemorrhagic shock. This may be due to its antiadrenergic action, which inhibits the sympathetic vascular response to these conditions.

Fate in the body. The pharmacokinetics of chlorpromazine have been extensively studied. No less than 168 metabolites have been postulated and well over 50 have actually been identified in plasma or urine; most are clinically inactive but 7-hydroxychlorpromazine has biological activity.

The efficacy of chlorpromazine is markedly dependent on the route of administration because the drug is metabolized both in the liver and in the gut wall. This metabolism is highly effective in some individuals with the result that very low blood levels of unchanged chlorpromazine occur. Parenteral administration bypasses this initial metabolism. The metabolic products are of two kinds, those that are psychopharmacologically active and those, such as chlorpromazine sulphoxide, that are inert. There are great individual variations in the way in which the drug is broken down and this is probably genetically determined. The rate of some pathways is also probably affected by enzyme induction produced by other drugs. This may account for the wide variation in response to treatment, those who either metabolize the drug slowly or to active metabolites responding better than those who metabolize the drug quickly to inactive products.

INDICATIONS

Chlorpromazine is used in premedication and to allay anxiety during minor operative procedures and investigations. It was one of the ingredients of the so-called 'lytic cocktail' (*see* page 53). The mental state produced by this mixture is very similar to that of neuroleptanalgesia, although the tendency to sleep is perhaps more pronounced; cardiovascular depression is more evident. It is also used in the treatment of psychiatric conditions, intractable vomiting and hiccough, and together with narcotic analgesics in the treatment of intractable pain.

DOSAGE AND ADMINISTRATION

Chlorpromazine may be given by the oral, intramuscular, and intravenous routes. By mouth its maximal effects appear in about 3 hours; intramuscularly it is effective within 15–30 minutes. A 1 per cent solution may be given intramuscularly, but a more dilute solution is advisable for intravenous injection to avoid thrombosis of the vein. The 1 or 2.5 per cent solution should be diluted with 20 ml of distilled water and injected slowly, either directly into a vein or into the tubing of an intravenous infusion.

Innumerable techniques have been described for the use of chlorpromazine, many of which are exceedingly elaborate and have now fallen into disuse.

For premedication, an intramuscular injection of 25–50 mg may be given about 1 hour before operation, either alone or with a sedative or an analgesic such as pethidine (50–100 mg). Further preoperative sedation in anxious patients may be obtained by giving 50–100 mg of chlorpromazine by mouth the night before operation.

For other purposes the oral dose range is 50–100 mg, and 25–50 mg may be given intravenously or intramuscularly. Considerably larger oral doses are sometimes given in psychiatric conditions.

The 'lytic cocktail' contains chlorpromazine 50 mg, promethazine 50 mg, and pethidine 100 mg in 20 ml of distilled water, and is given slowly intravenously until the desired effect is obtained.

PRECAUTIONS

Chlorpromazine should be used cautiously when combined with sedatives, hypnotics, and anaesthetics as their effects are enhanced.

Special care should also be taken when it is used with other drugs likely to cause a fall in blood pressure, as a dangerous degree of hypotension may ensue. The fall in blood pressure with chlorpromazine is partially due to its α-adrenoceptor blocking activity. Neuroleptics vary in this property. Droperidol is more potent than triflupromazine which is more potent than chlorpromazine. Chlorpromazine in turn is more potent than fluphenazine and haloperidol, and these are more potent than clozapine and pimozide.

The employment of chlorpromazine in anaesthesia for shocked patients is not without risk, and adequate fluid replacement to restore circulating blood volume must be undertaken before anaesthesia is induced.

It should not be given in large doses or over a long period to patients suffering from liver disease or leucopenia or to those receiving drugs known to have a tendency to depress the bone marrow (thiouracil, amidopyrine, and phenylbutazone). If any of these complications develops during treatment, the drug must be withdrawn.

Postural hypotension and drowsiness are likely in the initial stages of treatment in ambulatory patients; they must be advised to limit their activities and avoid the responsibility of controlling vehicles and machinery. They should be kept under observation until they are stabilized and the severity of the side effects are assessed.

Large doses of chlorpromazine when given alone are well tolerated and alarming symptoms due to overdose are rare.

If marked central depression and circulatory collapse occur, especially when other central depressants have also been given, treatment should be symptomatic. Excessive hypotension is best treated with a noradrenaline infusion, preferably in a stronger solution than the 1:250 000 usually given. The pressor amines are, in general, much less effective in restoring the blood pressure in the presence of chlorpromazine, phenylephrine being the most effective single-dose agent.

Fluphenazine hydrochloride

Fluphenazine hydrochloride (*BP* and *USP*)
Chemical name: 2-{4-[3-(2-trifluoromethylphenothiazin-10-yl) propyl] piperazin-1-yl}ethanol dihydrochloride
For structural formula *see Table 3.1*, pp. 80–81.

PHARMACOLOGY

Fluphenazine is a piperazine phenothiazine. It is a more potent antiemetic than chlorpromazine and has a longer duration of action. It exhibits the pharmacological spectrum of the phenothiazines.

INDICATIONS

It is used for the control of postoperative nausea and vomiting and in schizophrenia. Fluphenazine enanthate or decanoate are long-acting preparations especially used in schizophrenia.

DOSAGE AND ADMINISTRATION

Fluphenazine hydrochloride 1 mg once or twice a day orally is the usual dose for control of postoperative nausea. It has been used to prevent postoperative vomiting, in a dose of 5 mg intramuscularly 30–45 minutes before the end of operation. In schizophrenic patients a dose of 0.5 ml of the decanoate or enanthate formulation (12.5–25 mg fluphenazine decanoate or enanthate) can provide adequate maintenance for 2–3 weeks. Some patients require larger doses, up to 4 ml every 2 weeks.

PRECAUTIONS

These are similar to those for other phenothiazines, for example chlorpromazine. Parkinsonian-like states and acute dystonic reactions can occur. With long-term therapy tardive dyskinesias may develop.

Flupenthixol has similar actions to fluphenazine. It is a thioxanthene. It is of interest that the stereoisomers differ in activity. The *cis*-isomer is the more potent in schizophrenia. Depot injections of the decanoate are used in schizophrenia. *Cis*-clopenthixol decanoate is a related compound, also used in maintenance therapy in schizophrenia.

Methotrimeprazine maleate

Methotrimeprazine maleate (*BAN* and *USP*)
Chemical name: 3-(2-methoxyphenothiazin-10-yl)-2-methylpropyldimethylamine
For structural formula *see Table 3.1,* pp. 80–81

Methotrimeprazine has similar pharmacological and clinical effects to chlorpromazine. It has marked hypotensive effects, so that its use in elderly patients or those on the threshold of circulatory failure demands great care. The drug has a strong analgesic action when given alone or with conventional analgesics. Its analgesic action has been compared with that of morphine, 15 mg intramuscularly being equianalgesic with 10 mg of morphine by the same route. It may prove useful in the treatment of severe pain. It is given by mouth or intramuscularly in doses of 10–30 mg and can be given intravenously if required. Larger doses are sometimes given but hypotension is then more likely to be severe. Extrapyramidal manifestations have also been reported.

Perphenazine

Perphenazine (*BP* and *USP*)
Chemical name: 2-{4-[3-2(chlorophenothiazin-10-yl)propyl]piperazin-1-yl} ethanol
For structural formula *see Table 3.1*, pp. 80–81

Perphenazine has similar actions to chlorpromazine but is effective in a considerably smaller dose. Hypotension may occur but is usually less marked. It is a particularly powerful antiemetic.

It is used in psychiatry, in the treatment of vomiting, and in premedication, 4 mg by mouth or 5 mg intramuscularly.

Extrapyramidal side effects are readily produced if doses of 5 mg intramuscularly are repeated too freely.

Prochlorperazine salts

Prochlorperazine maleate (*BP* and *USP*) and Prochlorperazine edisylate (*USP*)
Chemical name: 2-chloro-10[3-(4-methylpiperazin-1-yl)propyl]phenothiazine
For structural formula *see Table 3.1*, pp. 80–81

Prochlorperazine has less potentiating effect on hypnotics than chlorpromazine and does not produce lethargy. It is more effective as an antiemetic, and does not produce hypotension.

It is used in the treatment of migraine, Ménière's syndrome and other labyrinthine disturbances, nausea and vomiting, and in psychiatry.

It is normally given by mouth in a dose of 15–30 mg daily in divided doses; 12.5 mg can be given intramuscularly if tablets cannot be retained in the stomach.

Promazine hydrochloride

Promazine hydrochloride (*BP* and *USP*)
Chemical name: dimethyl (3-phenothiazin-10-yl-propyl)amine
For structural formula *see Table 3.1*, pp. 80–81

Promazine possesses similar properties to chlorpromazine, but weight for weight is less potent. It has been claimed that the absence of the chlorine atom in promazine makes it less toxic. It has less antiadrenergic activity than chlorpromazine and consequently is less likely to cause hypotension.

It is used for similar purposes and in doses approximately the same as those given for chlorpromazine.

Promethazine salts

Promethazine hydrochloride (*BP* and *USP*)
Promethazine theoclate (*BP*)
Chemical name: 1,*N*,*N*,-trimethyl-2-(phenothiazin-10-yl)ethylamine hydrochloride, and 8-chlorotheophyllinate
For structural formula *see Table 3.1*, pp. 80–81

Promethazine hydrochloride

PHARMACOLOGY

Promethazine is a phenothiazine derivative which was first synthesized in France in 1945 in the search for drugs with antihistamine properties. It was first used almost entirely as an antihistamine but is now also employed for its sedative and hypnotic actions.

Nervous system. The action on the CNS is similar although less marked than that of chlorpromazine; the vomiting centre and heat-regulating centres are depressed and the action of other central depressants is potentiated. Its own sedative action, however, is stronger than that of chlorpromazine and sleep is more readily induced. It reduces the analgesic action of pethidine and other analgesics.

It has only a slight antiadrenaline action, but has a more marked anticholinergic effect.

Cardiovascular system. There is no change in cardiac output. Blood pressure normally remains unchanged, although a modest fall is occasionally recorded. Cardiac irritability is decreased, and arrhythmias do not occur. Heart rate may be slightly increased. There is some dilatation of peripheral vessels and capillary permeability is reduced. The action of pressor agents is not affected.

Respiratory system. There is some evidence that promethazine hydrochloride has a mild stimulating action on respiration, both minute volume and rate being increased. Bronchial musculature is relaxed and there is an inhibition of secretions (atropine-like action).

Musculature. There is no action on skeletal muscle, but smooth muscle is relaxed.

Alimentary system. The bowel is quiet due to central depressant and spasmolytic actions. Secretions are diminished.

Liver and kidney function. There is normally little effect on liver and kidney function, but its close chemical relationship to chlorpromazine suggests that its use for prolonged periods may have a similar effect on the liver.

Other effects. It has a marked antihistamine action and is considerably more effective than mepyramine maleate. It also has marked local analgesic properties and is very long acting. Its fate in the body is probably the same as that of chlorpromazine.

INDICATIONS

Promethazine is used in premedication before operation for its sedative, antiemetic, and atropine-like action; any antianalgesic effect that it may possess does not preclude its use for this purpose.

Other uses include the treatment of allergies such as hay fever, urticaria, and anaphylactic reactions, the prevention of motion sickness, and the treatment of intractable vomiting.

DOSAGE AND ADMINISTRATION

Promethazine may be given by mouth, intramuscularly, or intravenously.

For premedication, an intramuscular injection of 25 mg may be given 1 hour before operation with pethidine 100 mg or a similar drug. Atropine may also be given if considered desirable and depending on the anaesthetic to be employed. In anxious patients a similar dose may be given orally, with or without a small dose of a barbiturate the night before operation.

For the prevention of travel sickness and the treatment of allergic conditions 25–50 mg are given by mouth and repeated at 4-hourly intervals if necessary.

PRECAUTIONS

Ambulant patients receiving promethazine hydrochloride must be supervised until its sedative effects have been ascertained. They should not be allowed to drive vehicles or take part in activities requiring full mental alertness.

Overdose will result in central depression which may lead to unconsciousness and circulatory collapse. Treatment should be symptomatic.

Aqueous solutions have an acidic reaction (pH 4.5–5.5) and should be protected from light to prevent discoloration.

Promethazine theoclate has very similar properties to the hydrochloride; its sedative action, however, is said to be less marked.

It is used entirely as an antiemetic in the prevention of motion sickness. For this purpose a dose of 25 mg is given by mouth the night before travelling on long journeys and repeated nightly: for short journeys a similar dose is given 1–2 hours before starting. Treatment of vomiting is not so satisfactory as the tablets are unlikely to be retained in the stomach. It cannot be given intravenously or intramuscularly.

Propiomazine salts

Propiomazine maleate (*BAN*) and Propiomazine hydrochloride (*USP*)
Chemical name: 1-[10-(2-dimethylaminopropyl)phenothiazin-2-yl]propan-1-one hydrogen maleate and hydrochloride
For structural formula *see Table 3.1*, pp. 80–81

Propiomazine is related structurally to promethazine and has similar sedative and antiemetic properties. Its anticholinergic action and antihistamine activity are less marked; it is used as a sedative and in premedication and is given in a dose of 20–40 mg by the intramuscular route.

Trifluoperazine hydrochloride

Trifluoperazine hydrochloride (*BP* and *USP*)
Chemical name: 10-[3-(4-methylpiperazin-1-yl)propyl]-2-trifluoromethyl-phenothiazine dihydrochloride
For structural formula *see Table 3.1,* pp. 80–81

Trifluoperazine is about nine times more potent than chlorpromazine. It is more rapid in onset of action and has a longer duration of effect. It is a powerful antiemetic.

Side effects include parkinsonism, muscular dystonia, torsion spasms, drowsiness, sweating, and increased salivation.

Trifluoperazine is mostly used in psychiatry and is valuable in the control of disturbed behaviour, aggressiveness, hallucinations, and paranoid delusions in acute and chronic psychoses.

Trimeprazine tartrate

Trimeprazine tartrate (*BPC* and *USP*)
Chemical name: *NN*-dimethyl (2-methyl-3-phenothiazine-10-yl)propylamine tartrate
For structural formula *see Table 3.1*, pp. 80–81

Trimeprazine has pharmacological actions intermediate between promethazine and chlorpromazine. It has a greater antihistamine action than promethazine, while its central actions, including antiemetic activity, are similar to those of chlorpromazine. It has some antiadrenergic activity, and blood pressure may be moderately depressed. It also possesses a powerful antispasmodic effect.

It is used as an antipruritic and sedative in dermatology and general medicine, and as a premedicant, especially for children. It is pleasantly formulated as a syrup containing 6 mg/ml.

It is given by mouth in a total daily dose of 10–40 mg in dermatological conditions, and 3–4.5 mg/kg 1–2 hours before operation for full sedation and premedication.

Large doses cause a somewhat flushed appearance with circumoral pallor. On at least two occasions it has been incriminated as a possible trigger of the malignant hyperpyrexia syndrome.

Benzodiazepines

During the past few years, evidence has been obtained that benzodiazepines act at a specific receptor (the so-called benzodiazepine receptor). This interaction increases the affinity of the adjacent GABA receptor for its transmitter. GABA is

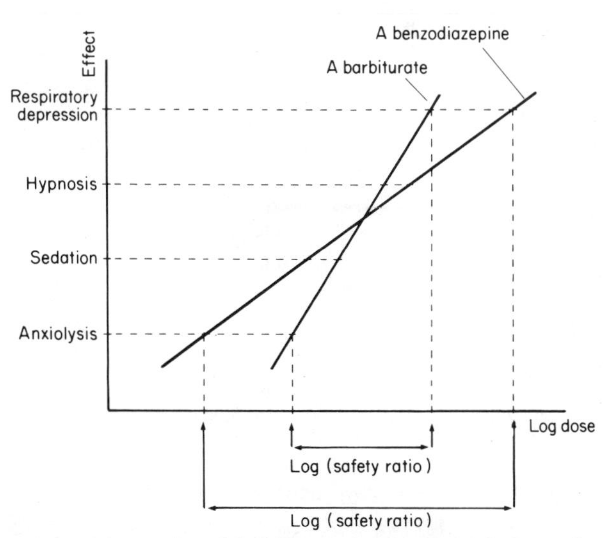

Figure 3.3 Diagrammatic representation of the high margin of safety of the benzodiazepines. Because of the flat dose–effect curves characteristic of the benzodiazepines, the ratio between the lethal dose and the therapeutically useful dose (for example, for anxiolysis) is very high compared with drugs like the barbiturates

an inhibitory transmitter in the CNS and this inhibitory action would fit with the observation that these drugs diminish all excessive emotional responses.

There are now over 20 examples of benzodiazepines on the market. Their site of action is predominantly on the limbic system of the brain, and particularly on the hippocampus and the amygdala. Individual benzodiazepines differ in their duration of action (*see* page 96). They may differ in the amount of sedation produced at anxiolytic doses. Such differences are probably not of therapeutic importance, but are probably more attributable to marketing policy than to pharmacological properties but, as can be seen from *Figure 3.3*, different doses of the same compound can be anxiolytic or sedative, so formulation is important.

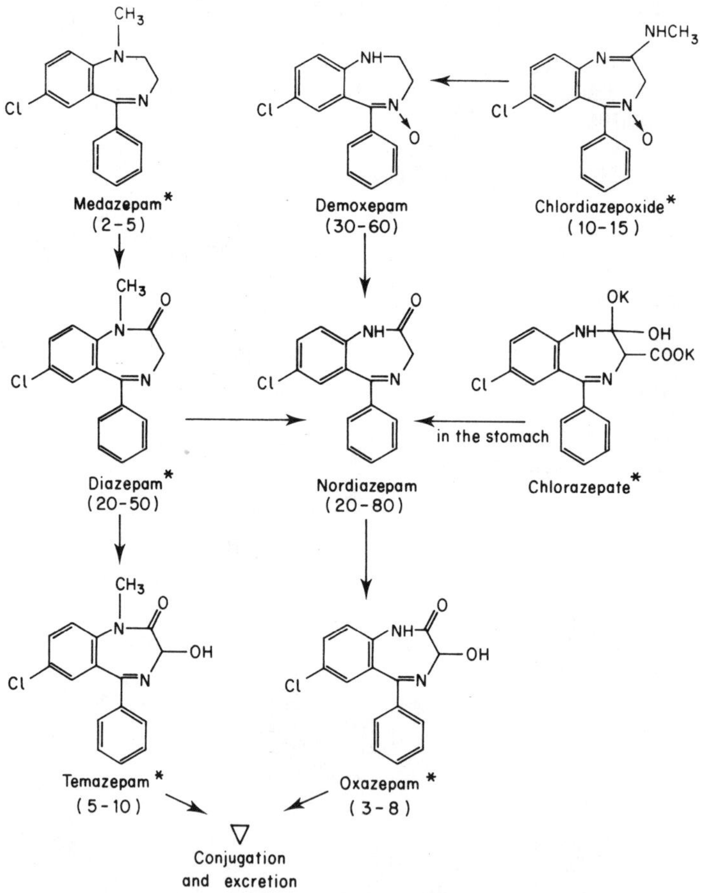

Figure 3.4 Some routes of biotransformation of six commercially available benzodiazepine anxiolytics (*). The figures in brackets indicate half-life in hours. (From Schnieden and Rees, 1980, reproduced by courtesy of the authors and publisher.)

In general, these drugs have a great similarity with one another, the chief difference being potency. Some, such as lorazepam, appear to have a more soporific and amnesic effect than others. However, McKay and Dundee (1980), comparing oral diazepam, flunitrazepam and lorazepam, noted a dose-related amnesic effect produced by all three drugs. This closely paralleled the extent and duration of their sedative action. Most benzodiazepines are metabolized to active compounds and several include nordiazepam (desmethyldiazepam) among them. This metabolite has a very long half-life and this ensures a steady therapeutic effect when intermittent doses of drugs of which this is a metabolite are given (*Figure 3.4*). There may be another mechanism which tends to produce this steady therapeutic effect. A rise in blood diazepam concentration has been observed 4–6 hours after intramuscular injection; an enterohepatic recirculation has been proposed to explain this.

The Committee on the Review of Medicines (1980) has issued guidelines on the use of benzodiazepines in the treatment of anxiety. They suggest that all benzodiazepines are equally effective in the short term for anxiety or insomnia, and to classify specific benzodiazepines as hypnotics or antianxiety agents is invalid. In general, benzodiazepines should be used only for the *short-term* management of anxiety or insomnia, since there is no good evidence to suggest that they are therapeutically of value in the long-term treatment of these conditions.

The great increase in the use of drugs of this group, particularly their displacement of the barbiturates, is based on several favourable pharmacological properties. The slope of their log dose–effect line is much flatter than that of the barbiturates (*see Figure 3.3*). Benzodiazepines have a greater margin of safety than barbiturates and they are freer from serious effects when taken as an overdose. Recovery has followed the consumption of over 100 times the recommended dose. This property accounts for their relative selectivity, that is reduction of anxiety with little sedation.

Benzodiazepines are not analgesic or antidepressants. They may be of value in night terrors or sleep-walking in children, and in the treatment of acute alcohol withdrawal. Their dependence liability is low, although withdrawal symptoms may occur, especially after high doses for a long period of time. These usually manifest themselves 1–10 days after stopping therapy. There may be an impairment of mental function with long-term therapy, and confusional states, tremor, and ataxia may occur, especially in the elderly. Alcohol may interact with benzodiazepines. Driving skills can be impaired, although this is more likely to occur with long-acting benzodiazepines. They have little or no tendency to cause hepatic enzyme induction. Interactions with other agents are therefore less of a problem.

Committee on the Review of Medicines (1980) Systematic review of the benzodiazepines. *British Medical Journal,* **1,** 910

McKay, A. C. and Dundee, J. W. (1980) Effect of oral benzodiazepines on memory. *British Journal of Anaesthesia,* **52,** 1247

Schnieden, H. and Rees, J. M. H. (1980) Psychopharmacological agents and sexual function. Part 1: Anxiolytics. *British Journal of Sexual Medicine,* **7,** 18

Chlordiazepoxide hydrochloride

Chlordiazepoxide hydrochloride (*BP* and *USP*)
Chemical name: 7-chloro-2-methylamino-5-phenyl-3*H*-1,4-benzodiazepine-4-oxide hydrochloride
For structural formula *see Figure 3.5*, p. 92

Chlordiazepoxide was the first member of this group to be studied and used clinically. It has a taming effect on animals and relieves anxiety in human subjects.

Patients become tranquil but remain alert. It also has anticonvulsant and muscle-relaxant properties, the latter effect being due to depression of spinal reflexes. Ataxia can occur after large doses. There is no effect on blood pressure or heart rate in anaesthetized dogs when given intravenously in doses of 1 mg/kg. Respiration is not depressed.

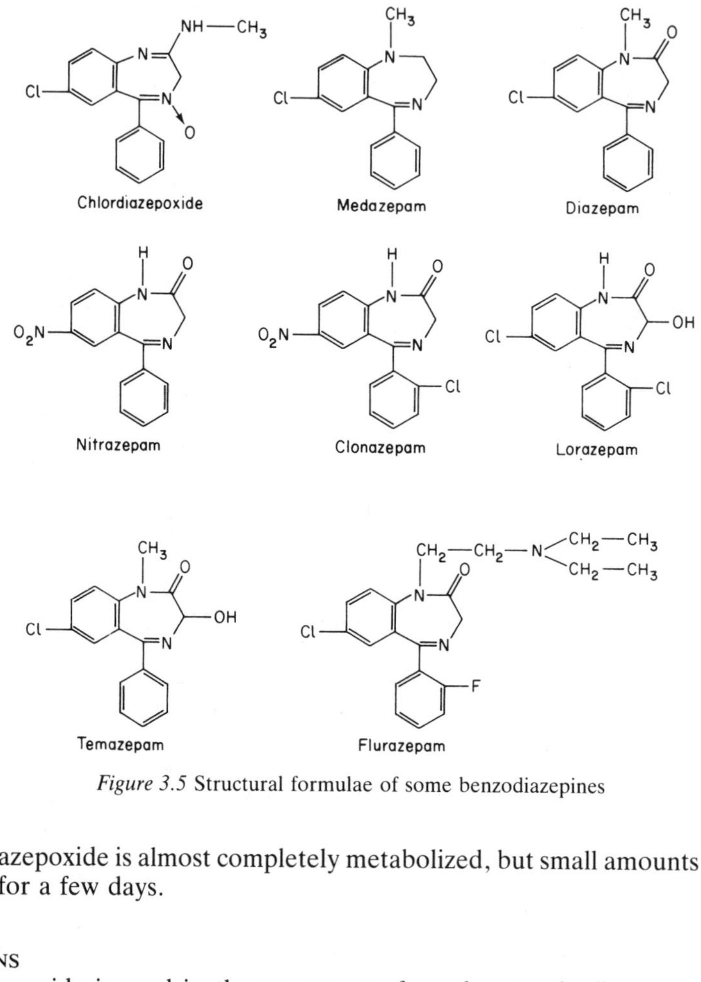

Figure 3.5 Structural formulae of some benzodiazepines

Chlordiazepoxide is almost completely metabolized, but small amounts appear in the urine for a few days.

INDICATIONS

Chlordiazepoxide is used in the treatment of psychosomatic disease and anxiety states and as an alternative to traditional sedatives in preoperative medication.

DOSAGE AND ADMINISTRATION

Chlordiazepoxide may be given by mouth in tablet form or by intramuscular injection. For the relief of anxiety 30–100 mg is given daily in divided doses. Elderly and debilitated patients should be given not more than 10 mg daily initially. For premedication 50–100 mg may be given 1–2 hours before operation intramuscularly or 20–30 mg may be given orally three times a day to surgical patients from the time of admission to hospital until the day of operation.

PRECAUTIONS

The preparation available for intramuscular injection should not be given intravenously. Patients should avoid alcohol while under treatment and should avoid driving or handling machinery.

Clonazepam

Clonazepam (*BAN* and *USP*)
Chemical name: 5-(2-chlorophenyl)-1,3-dihydro-7-nitro-2*H*-1,4-benzodiazepin-2-one
For structural formula *see Figure 3.5*, p. 92

PHARMACOLOGY

Clonazepam is principally of value in epilepsy. It has been shown to suppress seizure activity in animal models of epilepsy, and in epileptic patients clonazepam often limits the spread of discharge from focal lesions without suppressing the primary focus. This may be due to the ability of the compound to enhance polysynaptic inhibitory processes in the CNS. It has been suggested that clonazepam increases the concentration of 5-hydroxytryptamine at synaptic sites or interacts with the neurotransmitter glycine.

Fate in the body. The drug is mainly non-ionized throughout the range of physiological pH and therefore readily crosses the blood–brain barrier as well as the gastrointestinal tract. About 50 per cent is protein bound. Its main metabolite is a 7-amino derivative which has little antiepileptic activity. Less than 5 per cent is excreted unchanged in the urine. Peak serum concentrations occur about 2 hours after administration. The elimination half-life is 20–40 hours in most subjects. The drug does not appear to induce its own metabolism and the addition of clonazepam does not appear to alter significantly the steady-state concentrations of phenobarbitone or phenytoin. However, the addition of phenytoin or phenobarbitone may lower the steady-state concentration of clonazepam. Tolerance may occur.

INDICATIONS

The drug is mainly used for the treatment of petit mal and infantile spasms.

DOSAGE

In children the starting dose is 0.01–0.03 mg/kg/day rising by increments every 3–7 days to a maximum of 0.2 mg/kg/day. In adults the starting dose is 1.5 mg/day or less, rising to 20 mg/day.

PRECAUTIONS

Thrombocytopenia has been reported. It is advisable to withdraw the drug slowly as abrupt withdrawal can precipitate status epilepticus.

Diazepam

Diazepam (*BP* and *USP*)
Chemical name: 7-chloro-1,3-dihydro-1-methyl-5-phenyl-2*H*-1,4-benzodiazepin-2-one
For structural formula *see Figure 3.5*, p. 92

PHYSICAL CHARACTERISTICS
Diazepam is insoluble in water; the solution for injection (5 mg/ml) contains several organic solvents, mainly propylene glycol, ethanol, and sodium benzoate in benzoic acid. The solution is rather viscid and dilution with water or saline causes cloudiness and is not recommended. It should not be mixed with other drugs. These solvents can cause inco-ordination and depression of postsynaptic reflexes.

PHARMACOLOGY
Central nervous system. Diazepam is a benzodiazepine with similar actions to chlordiazepoxide. In animals it is considerably more potent as a tranquillizer, muscle relaxant, and anticonvulsant. These effects are probably due to an additional effect on the ascending reticular activating system and spinal internuncial neurones, as well as the effect on the limbic system. Patients remain alert after small doses but high doses cause drowsiness, and amnesia and unconsciousness can be produced if it is given intravenously. It can be given in doses that cause a state of extreme drowsiness but in which the patient is still accessible and there is marked amnesia. When combined with other drugs as premedicant the incidence of amnesia is increased. A dose of 0.2 mg/kg reduces the MAC (*see* page 130) for halothane by 35 per cent from 0.73 to 0.48 per cent. Doubling this dose brings no further reduction in anaesthetic requirements. The oil/water formulation has a considerably higher LD_{50} in animals. The pharmacokinetics of both formulations are identical.

Respiratory system. Intravenous injection of 0.14 mg/kg depresses the sensitivity of the respiratory centre. The frequency falls and there is a decrease in the slope of the carbon dioxide–ventilation curve.

Cardiovascular system. Following intravenous injection of 0.2 mg/kg at the rate of 10 mg/min, the only significant change is a tachycardia which may persist for some time. There is no effect on cardiac output nor any marked effects on blood pressure.

INDICATIONS
The indications for this drug have multiplied considerably. It has been used as a premedicant both intramuscularly and by mouth, and intravenously to induce anaesthesia. If it is used for the latter purpose, due allowance must be made for the prolonged drowsiness which it causes. It is increasingly employed intravenously in subanaesthetic doses as a sedative for patients with dental phobia, to cover unpleasant procedures in intensive care units, and to accustom patients to artificial ventilators. It has been employed as the sole agent for cardioversion, and has been recommended for cardiac catheterization in children. It is also employed as a sedative during carotid angiography. In fact in almost every conceivable situation in which rapid sedation might be of benefit, diazepam has proved of value and

exhibited a high degree of safety. It is also used orally in the treatment of psychosomatic illness, and has been used in the treatment of tetanus.

It is more effective than pentobarbitone in treating and preventing lignocaine-induced convulsions, and can now be regarded as a drug of first choice in the treatment of convulsive states of all kinds, being associated with a much lower overall mortality.

DOSAGE AND ADMINISTRATION

Diazepam may be given by mouth in tablet form or as a syrup and by intramuscular or intravenous injection. Oral doses for anxiety states vary from 10–30 mg daily in divided doses. For premedication 10–20 mg may be given 1–1.5 hours before operation. When given orally the maximal effect is reached in 60 minutes and there is some suggestion that the oral route is more effective than the intramuscular one. For acute sedation 0.2 mg/kg is usually adequate, but doses up to 0.6 mg/kg may be needed to induce unconsciousness. In the treatment of tetanus doses of about 5 mg/kg/24 h are given by mouth or nasal tube in syrup form. Elderly and debilitated patients require about half the usual dosage, and when the drug is given intravenously it should be injected slowly at a rate not exceeding 10 mg/min.

PRECAUTIONS

Diazepam may potentiate the neuromuscular blocking actions of non-depolarizing muscle relaxants. The consumption of alcohol should be avoided by patients under treatment, or during the day on which an intravenous dose has been given. Diazepam injection cannot be diluted and precipitates when mixed with most other agents. It is painful when injected intramuscularly; there may also be complaints of pain on intravenous administration, particularly if injected into a peripheral vein. It has been reported that the incidence of thrombosis is about 6 per cent if injected into the antecubital vein and up to 23 per cent for a vein in the hand or wrist. Slow injection or dilution with the patient's own blood is said to reduce the incidence.

Diazemuls is a preparation of diazepam in soya bean oil, which has been emulsified in water by means of egg yolk phosphatides and acetylated monoglycerides. Olesen and Huttel (1980) studied about 120 patients who received either diazepam in propylene glycol intravenously or Diazemuls intravenously. In the patients receiving the propylene glycol formulation 78 per cent had pain on injection and there was clinical evidence of thrombophlebitis in 48 per cent. A third preparation of diazepam in Cremophor EL produced anaphylactoid reactions.

Olesen, A. S. and Huttel, M. S. (1980) Local reactions to i.v. diazepam in three different formulations. *British Journal of Anaesthesia*, **52**, 609

Lorazepam

Lorazepam (*BAN* and *USAN*).
Chemical name: 7-chloro-5-(2-chlorophenyl)-1,3-dihydro-3-hydroxy-2*H*-1,4-benzodiazepin-2-one
For structural formula *see Figure 3.5*, p. 92

PHYSICAL CHARACTERISTICS

Lorazepam is insoluble in water. For parenteral use it is dissolved in polyethylene glycol and propylene glycol.

PHARMACOLOGY

Central nervous system. Lorazepam is a benzodiazepine with actions similar to those of diazepam. In the treatment of anxiety neurosis it causes fewer undesirable side effects. It produces anterograde amnesia; an intravenous dose of 5.0 mg invariably produces this effect for up to 24 hours. Lorazepam has no analgesic properties.

Respiratory system. There is an enhanced ventilatory response to carbon dioxide challenge, suggesting that lorazepam may have a stimulant effect upon respiration.

Cardiovascular system. There are no marked changes in blood pressure, pulse rate, or peripheral resistance.

Musculoskeletal system. Lorazepam, like diazepam, has muscle-relaxant properties, probably central in origin.

Fate in the body. Absorption of orally administered lorazepam is rapid, maximum blood concentrations occurring after 2–4 hours and persisting for 24–48 hours. Almost 80 per cent of the administered dose can be recovered in the urine over 5 days, mostly as the glucuronide which is the principal metabolite.

INDICATIONS

Lorazepam is used in a similar manner to diazepam. However, the absence of a depressant effect upon ventilation and its potent amnesic activity may be advantageous in anaesthesia. Most investigations to date have described its value in preanaesthetic medication. Orally, doses from 1–5 mg have generally been found to have similar or superior actions to equipotent doses of diazepam. Sedation, relief of anxiety, and amnesia are produced. Similar doses, given intravenously, have also been used. The relatively long duration of action limits its use when rapid and complete recovery is desired. Postoperatively it virtually abolishes emergence reactions when given intravenously after ketamine anaesthesia.

DOSAGE AND ADMINISTRATION

Lorazepam is approximately five times as potent as diazepam on a weight for weight comparison. Oral doses for the treatment of anxiety range from 1–3 mg two or three times daily. Doses up to 5 mg orally or intravenously are used for preanaesthetic medication. Since it has a long duration of action it may be given simultaneously to all patients on an operating list several hours before the start of the list.

PRECAUTIONS

Lorazepam, like other benzodiazepines, may potentiate the effects of other CNS depressants and may have a prolonged action. It is not recommended for use in children. After intravenous injection of lorazepam thrombosis or thrombophlebitis can be produced. The incidence of thrombophlebitis is less following lorazepam than diazepam.

Other benzodiazepines

The Committee on the Review of Medicines (CRM) divides these drugs into long-acting benzodiazepines whose plasma half-lives (of drug plus active metabolites) exceed 10 hours, and short-acting ones. Long-acting drugs include nitrazepam, medazepam, flurazepam, diazepam, clorazepate, and chlordiazepoxide. The CRM suggests that short-acting benzodiazepines are more suitable than long-acting ones for the treatment of insomnia without anxiety. Lorazepam, temazepam, and oxazepam are in this category.

Nitrazepam is frequently prescribed as a hypnotic, although it is in the long-acting category. It rapidly induces sleep which usually lasts from 6–8 hours. Nitrazepam 5–10 mg before retiring is a common dose for adults, but should be reduced to 2.5–5 mg in elderly patients (Castleden *et al.*, 1977).

Like other long-acting benzodiazepines, it may affect patients' reaction time next morning, so driving performance and operation of machinery can be impaired. Summation with other centrally acting depressants such as alcohol is possible.

Medazepam has a pharmacological profile similar to nitrazepam. It is used in the treatment of anxiety. The initial recommended dose is 5 mg three times a day.

Temazepam is suitable for night sedation, being short acting, and is also used for preoperative sedation. Like diazepam, it depresses the ventilatory response to carbon dioxide (Pleuvry *et al.*, 1980). The dose is 20–60 mg.

Midazolam is a water-soluble benzodiazepine which is stable in solution and non-irritant by intravenous injection. Its general pharmacological profile is typical of the benzodiazepines but it differs from diazepam in being more rapid in onset and having a much quicker recovery. Loss of eyelash reflex or cessation of counting occurs in 0.5–1.5 minutes after a 10-mg dose. Both recovery times and plasma levels show a much shorter duration of action than diazepam, with no evidence of enterohepatic recirculation and no tendency for patients to fall asleep again. The sedative effect lasts for about 2 hours and recovery seems complete in 4 hours (Reves, Corssen and Holcomb, 1978).

Midazolam produces a marked anterograde amnesia significantly more often than does diazepam, lasting between 20 and 40 minutes. Its chief therapeutic application is likely, therefore, to be in situations requiring short periods of intense sedation and amnesia, such as endoscopy of the upper gastrointestinal tract. The drug is administered by slow intravenous injection, the dose being determined by the response of the patient. A dose of 0.07 mg/kg is usually adequate for short procedures, the total dose being between 2.5 and 7.5 mg.

It has been recommended as an intravenous induction agent since it allows a smooth transition to an inhalational anaesthetic even when the patient still retains a lash reflex. Cardiovascular and respiratory effects of normal doses are said to be comparable to those of diazepam and patients will normally retain control of the upper airway. Patients should not drive or operate machinery for 8 hours.

Oxazepam is a metabolite of diazepam and is given as a sedative in doses of 10–30 mg. It has a short duration of action (*see Figure 3.4*).

Castleden, C. M., George, C. F., Marcer, D. and Hallett, C. (1977) Increased sensitivity to nitrazepam in old age. *British Medical Journal,* **1,** 10

Pleuvry, B. J., Maddison, S. E., Oden, R. B. and Dodson, M. E. (1980) Respiratory and physiological effects of oral temazepam in volunteers. *British Journal of Anaesthesia,* **52,** 901

Reves, J. G., Corssen, G. and Holcomb, C. (1978) Comparison of two benzodiazepines for anaesthesia induction: midazolam and diazepam. *Canadian Anaesthetists Society Journal,* **25,** 211

Sedatives and hypnotics

History

Alcohol has been known to man as a sedative since the start of recorded history. Chloral, which yields an alcohol on metabolism, was introduced in 1869. However, the group of sedatives that led modern therapy in this field are the barbiturates which date from 1903 when Fischer and von Mering introduced barbitone, or diethylbarbituric acid. This was followed by phenobarbitone and allobarbitone in 1912, and since that date intensive research has resulted in the production of a very large number of barbiturates, some of which have become established in clinical use.

Chemistry

The combination of urea with organic acids results in the formation of ureides, which, unlike urea, may have hypnotic properties. There are two groups of ureides; monoureides, in which one amino group of urea is condensed with a carboxylic acid, and diureides, in which both amino groups of urea are condensed with a dicarboxylic acid.

The monoureides are weak hypnotics and of little clinical value. An example is carbromal (*see Figure 3.6*).

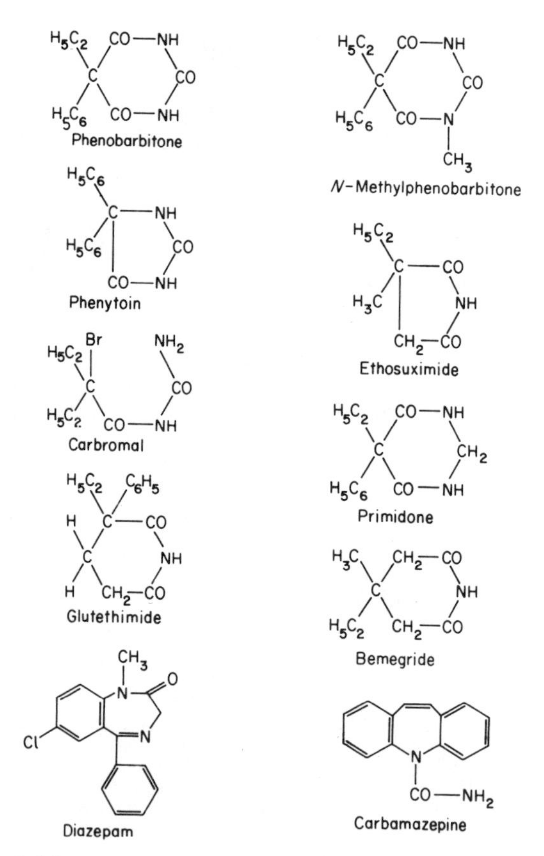

Figure 3.6 Structural formulae of some drugs related to barbituric acid

The diureides are more powerful hypnotics. They include the barbiturates and are of considerable clinical importance.

Barbituric acid is the condensation product of urea and malonic acid, and is malonylurea. Barbituric acid is not itself a hypnotic, but substitution of various organic radicals for both the hydrogen atoms attached to the 5 position results in compounds with hypnotic actions, known as barbiturates, although occasionally barbiturates such as phetharbital are not hypnotically active.

There are a number of substances chemically related to the barbiturates which are interesting from a therapeutic point of view. Efforts have been made by altering the molecule to obtain:

1. Drugs that are better anticonvulsants;
2. Safe hypnotics without the disadvantages of the barbiturates;
3. Specific antagonists to the barbiturate drugs.

The structures of some of these compounds are illustrated in *Figure 3.6*.

There is a specific side chain length for hypnotic effect in the barbiturate series and if the length of the side chains exceeds that of the amyl group (C_5H_{11}) then the sedative property is lost and the drug becomes a stimulant of the CNS instead.

N-Methylation of phenobarbitone produces *N*-methylphenobarbitone, which is equally anticonvulsant, but less sedative. When a C=O group is eliminated from the ring, the 5-membered ring structure phenytoin exerts antiepileptic activity, specifically in grand mal and psychomotor epilepsy, but it is not a general anticonvulsant like phenobarbitone, nor is it such a marked depressant of the CNS.

Further modification of the 5-membered ring of phenytoin gives rise to the oxazolidine derivatives, troxidone and paramethadione. Unlike phenobarbitone, troxidone has no hypnotic effect. It is effective in preventing attacks of petit mal. It is of little use in other types of epilepsy, which may be made worse.

Primidone is another 6-membered ring compound which bears a striking structural resemblance to phenobarbitone although it is not, in fact, a barbiturate. Not surprisingly it is a sedative and anticonvulsant, but is also effective in grand mal epilepsy. Another rearrangement of the ring results in glutarimides which, like the barbiturates, may be either sedative or stimulant. Glutethimide is a hypnotic, whereas bemegride is a stimulant. Seven-membered rings also have sedative and anticonvulsant properties, for example the benzodiazepines and carbamazepine.

Barbiturates

The potentialities of barbiturates in anaesthesia were soon appreciated, and many attempts were made to produce derivatives suitable for intravenous use. In the 1920s and early 1930s intravenous amylobarbitone and pentobarbitone enjoyed a moderate vogue, but their actions by this route were often unpredictable, and their use in this manner was not satisfactory. A notable advance was made in 1932, when Weese and his co-workers introduced hexobarbitone sodium. Two years later Lundy reported the first clinical trials of thiopentone sodium, the first thiobarbiturate to be used clinically (although thiobarbiturates had been synthesized as early as 1911). Since that time numerous thiobarbiturates have been prepared, but only three others–thialbarbitone, thiamylal, and buthalitone–have been found to be of clinical use; thiopentone is now the only one in clinical usage.

Barbiturates are almost insoluble in water, but they possess weak acidic properties because they exist as an equilibrium mixture of keto (—CO—NH—) and enol (—C(OH):N—) forms. The hydrogen of the enol form can be replaced by sodium or other metals to form soluble salts.

A few generalizations can be made on the structure/activity relationship of barbiturates (*Table 3.2*). Alterations in the substitution on the 5 position chiefly affect potency. An increase in potency and a decrease in the duration of action can be produced by increasing the length of the alkyl groups, or by the substitution of alicyclic, branched, or unsaturated side chains for alkyl groups. In practice there is usually a marked dissimilarity between the chains, and one of them is relatively simple. Long or complex alkyl chains may be associated with convulsant properties and gastric and salivary secretion may be increased as the result of central excitation. Specific anticonvulsant properties are associated with the presence of a phenyl group and are more marked in straight-chained alkyl derivatives than in those with branched chains. Substitutions on positions 1 and 2 produce marked changes in properties. A methyl or ethyl substitution in position 1 usually results in

Table 3.2 Classification and chemical structure of the barbiturates

Barbiturate skeleton:

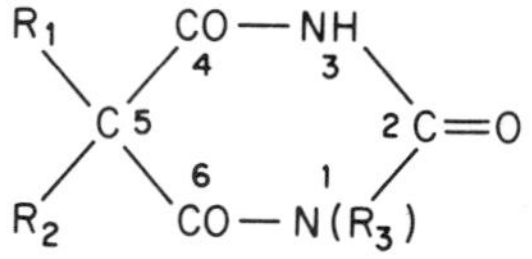

```
R1      CO—NH
  \    /4   3 \
   C 5         2 C=O
  /    \6   1 /
R2      CO—N(R3)
```

	R_1	R_2	R_3
Non-hypnotic			
Phetharbital 5,5-diethyl-1-phenylbarbituric acid	C_6H_5—	C_2H_5—	C_2H_5—
Long acting (8–12 hours or longer)			
Barbitone, 5,5-diethylbarbituric acid	C_2H_5—	C_2H_5—	H—
Methylphenobarbitone, 5-ethyl-1-methyl-5-phenylbarbituric acid	C_2H_5—	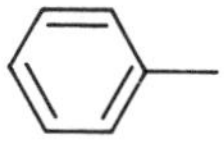	CH_3—
Phenobarbitone, 5-ethyl-5-phenylbarbituric acid	C_2H_5—	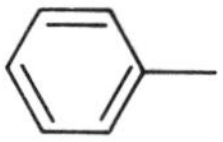	H—
Medium and short acting (2–8 hours)			
Amylobarbitone, 5-ethyl-5-isopentylbarbituric acid	C_2H_5—	$(CH_3)_2CH(CH_2)_2$—	H—
Butobarbitone, 5-butyl-5-ethylbarbituric acid	C_4H_9—	C_2H_5—	H—
Cyclobarbitone, 5-(cyclohex-1-enyl)-5-ethylbarbituric acid	C_2H_5—	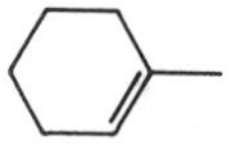	H—
Pentobarbitone sodium, sodium 5-ethyl-5-(1-methylbutyl)bariturate	C_2H_5—	$CH_3(CH_2)_2$ CH— CH_3	H—
Quinalbarbitone sodium, sodium 5-allyl-5-(1-methylbutyl)-barbiturate	CH_2=CH·CH_2—	CH_3 CH— $CH_3(CH_2)_2$	H—

Table 3.2 *cont.*

	R_1	R_2	R_3
Rapidly acting (by intravenous injection) Hexobarbitone sodium, sodium 5-(cyclohex-1-enyl)-1,5-dimethylbarbiturate	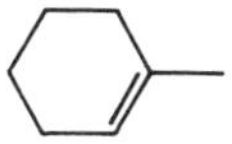	CH_3—	CH_3—
Methohexitone sodium, sodium carbonate and sodium α-(±)-5-allyl-1-methyl-5-(1-methylpent-2-ynyl)barbiturate	CH_2=CH—CH_2—	CH_3 CH— $C_2H_5—C\equiv C$	CH_3—
Thiopentone sodium, 6 parts of sodium carbonate and 100 parts of sodium 5-ethyl-5-(1-methylbutyl)-2-thiobarbiturate	C_2H_5—	$CH_3(CH_2)_2$ CH— CH_3	H—

In Great Britain official names of barbiturates end in -one, e.g. barbitone. In the USA they terminate in -al, e.g. barbital.

a more rapid onset of action and a more rapid recovery, but is also associated with a high incidence of excitatory phenomena during induction, such as tremor and involuntary muscle movements.

The replacement of the oxygen atom in the 2 position with a sulphur atom shortens the duration of action; for example thiopentone is the sulphur analogue of pentobarbitone and thiamylal is the sulphur analogue of quinalbarbitone.

CLASSIFICATION

The barbiturates have traditionally been classified according to the duration of action of a single hypnotic dose into long, medium, short, and ultra-short acting. Long- and medium-acting drugs are used as sedatives. In fact, it may be impossible to distinguish between the hypnotic effects of drugs in each category. In general, the duration reflects the mode of elimination by the body, the more brief the action the greater the amount broken down in the liver prior to renal excretion. When some of the medium- and short-acting drugs are given intravenously they produce anaesthesia after a delay, which is related to their slow rate of penetration into the brain. This is due to the low lipid solubility of the non-ionized part of the drug. The solubility is much increased by thiosubstitution or by methylation in the 1 position. The oil/water partition coefficients of thiopentone and thiamylal at pH 7.4 are 16 and 21 times as high as those of the corresponding barbiturates. A more realistic classification would therefore be:

1. Long acting – preparations used as sedatives or anticonvulsants;
2. Medium and short acting – usually employed as oral sedatives; delayed onset when given intravenously;
3. Rapidly acting – intravenous agents with no delay in onset.

There is little justification for the continued prescription of barbiturates as sedatives and hypnotics, mainly because of the dangers of overdose, their tendency to produce habituation, and the fact that safer alternatives are now available.

Central nervous system. The barbiturates appear to act at all levels of the CNS, but the basis of their clinical usefulness is the greater sensitivity of the cerebral cortex and reticular activating system compared with that of the vital medullary centres. Many attempts have been made to elucidate the biochemical aspects of barbiturate action, but with little success.

Sleep induced by hypnotic doses of barbiturates closely resembles normal sleep but the EEG shows characteristic changes. There is an initial diminution in the proportion of sleep during which rapid eye movements occur, the so-called paradoxical or REM sleep. With continued usage this recovers, and after stopping the administration there is a rebound increase in the proportion of REM sleep. Narcotic doses, however, produce other changes in the EEG which depend on dosage. Initial fast activity gives way progressively to slow-wave high-voltage activity with superimposed bursts of fast activity (the K-complex), and then to periods of electrical silence punctuated by bursts of activity (burst-suppression). With increasing doses the intervals of electrical silence become progressively longer. Hangover effects after hypnotic doses are common with the long-acting members of the group, but rare with those of short duration.

The barbiturates have no significant analgesic action, and in lower concentrations may actually have an antianalgesic effect. Their use in hypnotic doses in the presence of severe pain may produce restlessness and delirium. Even in barbiturate anaesthesia, stimuli which in the conscious state would cause pain may produce marked reflex activity, and this limits the use of barbiturates and of thiobarbiturates as sole anaesthetic agents to only the most minor operations.

In narcotic doses all the clinically employed barbiturates can prevent convulsions, such as occur in epilepsy, strychnine poisoning, or overdosage of local analgesics. Barbiturates with a phenyl group show some specific anticonvulsant action, even in sedative doses, and phenobarbitone and methylphenobarbitone are used in the treatment of epilepsy.

Autonomic nervous system. The barbiturates have only small effects on the autonomic nervous system when given in the usual doses. They may also inhibit synaptic transmission in autonomic ganglia and depress cholinergic receptor mechanisms as, for example, the inhibition of the response of the submaxillary gland to stimulation of the chorda tympani.

Cardiovascular system. Normal hypnotic doses of barbiturates have little effect upon the cardiovascular system, but a slight fall in blood pressure and pulse rate may occur due to the sedative effect. Larger doses cause a fall in blood pressure, due mainly to a direct depressant action on the vasomotor centres, and to a lesser degree to a direct action on the musculature of arterioles. The severe cardiovascular complications of overdose of barbiturates are mainly secondary to respiratory depression.

Respiratory system. The barbiturates are respiratory depressants, the degree of depression being proportional to the dose given. The chief action is a reduction in the sensitivity of the respiratory centre to carbon dioxide. They have no antitussive effect.

Placenta. All the barbiturates cross the placental barrier.

Metabolism. Oxygen uptake is reduced and metabolic rate diminished. Most barbiturates cause increased activity of liver microsomal enzymes. This is particularly the case with phenobarbitone, for which purpose it is a commonly employed research tool. This property is utilized therapeutically in certain cases of hyperbilirubinaemia.

Fate in the body. After absorption, the barbiturates are distributed in all tissues and fluids of the body. In the blood, they are bound to the plasma albumin fraction, the amount varying for different barbiturates from 70–80 per cent in the case of thiopentone to negligible amounts in the case of barbitone.

Except for barbitone and phenobarbitone, equilibrium between the brain and plasma is rapidly attained. With thiopentone, the CSF concentration rapidly reaches the plasma concentration.

The barbiturates are eliminated in two ways: by hepatic metabolism and by excretion by the kidneys. Most members are removed by a combination of these two methods. In general, the shorter acting drugs are metabolized by the liver and the longer acting ones, such as barbitone and phenobarbitone, are removed mainly by renal excretion.

The classic barbiturates are broken down solely by oxidation of their alkyl side chains and give rise to hypnotically inactive compounds. *N*-Methylbarbiturates, such as hexobarbitone, are demethylated to give hypnotically active barbiturates. The latter appear in large amounts in the urine, but are found only in trace amounts or not at all in the plasma.

Thiobarbiturates also undergo desulphuration to yield barbiturates with a hypnotic activity similar to that of the original substances. These metabolic products can always be found in the plasma.

After thiobarbiturate anaesthesia, hypnotically active substances can be detected in the plasma for 3–5 days, but for no longer than 24 hours with pentobarbitone and *N*-methylbarbiturates. The total excretion time of demonstrable metabolic products is 3–7 days with the thiobarbiturates, which is similar to that found with the long-acting barbiturate hypnotics.

Renal clearance of these products, whether free or conjugated with glycuronic acid, is by a combination of glomerular filtration and back-diffusion, similar to that of urea.

INDICATIONS

Barbiturates have been widely used as sedatives, hypnotics, and basal narcotics, but are now mainly used as induction agents and anticonvulsants.

ROUTES OF ADMINISTRATION

The oral route is the commonest method of administration of barbiturates. They are readily absorbed from the gastrointestinal tract, especially the sodium salts.

Rectal administration, in the form of suppositories, solutions or suspensions, may be employed when oral administration is impracticable.

Intravenous administration is now practically confined to thiopentone and methohexitone.

PRECAUTIONS

Barbiturates are contraindicated in porphyria. They should be used with caution in severe liver and kidney disease. They are best avoided during labour, and should not be used in the presence of pain unless combined with a suitable analgesic. Contraindications to the use of thiobarbiturates are discussed under thiopentone.

Natural idiosyncrasy to the barbiturates is rare, but acquired idiosyncrasy or sensitization may occur, particularly in subjects with a tendency to allergy. Reactions disappear rapidly on withdrawal of the drug.

Chronic toxicity may occur due to cumulation, leading to drowsiness, slowness of thought, failing memory, incoherent speech, mental depression, confusion, and disorientation. More serious cases may also develop vertigo, ataxia, nystagmus, diplopia, difficulty of accommodation, dysarthria, paresis of limbs, tremors, paraesthesia, and changes in deep reflexes. There may also be gastrointestinal upset.

Barbiturates are drugs of habituation and withdrawal symptoms occur when their administration is withheld. This complication occurs more frequently with the short-acting compounds given in high dosage.

POISONING

Acute barbiturate poisoning due to overdose, usually taken with suicidal intent, is still common. A number of accidental deaths arise from taking alcohol with barbiturates.

Overdose gives rise to various degrees of central depression and their sequelae. In mild cases, respiratory exchange is usually adequate, and although the patient may be restless or in a deep sleep, bodily functions are within normal limits. Little or no treatment apart from rest is necessary. In more severe cases coma is marked, respiration is depressed and often inadequate, the skin is cold and moist and often cyanotic, the pupils react sluggishly and may become dilated, cardiovascular depression may cause a fall in blood pressure, and reflexes are depressed or absent. Hypostatic pneumonia may develop later. The hypophyseal–hypothalamic mechanism of release of antidiuretic hormone is stimulated and this, together with the lowered blood pressure, decreases the rate of renal excretion of barbiturates.

To aid in differentiation between acute barbiturate poisoning and other forms of coma the presence of barbiturates can be identified in body fluids by ultraviolet spectrophotometry.

Treatment. A conservative method of treatment is now employed comparable to the management of the anaesthetized patient with special attention to his physiological requirements, the use of analeptics being avoided. The general outline of treatment is as follows.

Attention to respiration must be the first consideration: if this is inadequate it should be assisted, or controlled if necessary, by the endotracheal route. Tracheobronchial toilet should be performed frequently to remove secretions as necessary.

Gastric lavage is recommended by some authorities and condemned by others, but it is a worthwhile procedure if the drug has been taken orally within the previous 4 hours and there is a possibility that some is still remaining in the stomach. If pharyngeal reflexes are absent, care must be taken that fluid does not enter the trachea. Preliminary aspiration of the stomach contents is advocated to diminish the danger of forcing them into the duodenum.

A 5 per cent dextrose infusion should be set up as soon as possible as a vehicle for the administration of necessary drugs and to compensate for fluid loss. A fluid input and output chart should be carefully kept and the amount of fluid given adjusted accordingly: in severe cases, repeated estimations of serum electrolytes, pH, and $P\text{aco}_2$ will be necessary to ensure the more accurate control of treatment.

To prevent the onset of pneumonia, the patient's position in bed should be changed frequently and appropriate antibiotic therapy instituted.

Circulatory collapse should be treated by raising the patient's legs to ensure adequate venous return. Lack of response to this procedure requires infusion of a plasma volume expander and the administration of a pressor agent such as mephentermine.

Forced diuresis in the treatment of drug overdosage

If a drug is excreted by the kidneys the rate of its elimination from the body can be increased by inducing a high urine output and, in the case of some drugs, by altering urine pH. The fall in plasma concentration, once equilibrium has been attained, is exponential and the half-life of a drug in plasma is governed by its volume of distribution in body fluids and the rate at which it is cleared by renal excretion:

$$\text{Half-life} = \log_e 2 \times \frac{\text{volume of distribution in ml}}{\text{renal clearance in ml/min}}$$

$(\log_e 2 = 0.69)$

Drugs that pass readily through lipid membranes may have their clearance reduced by back-diffusion from tubular fluid to peritubular blood. During diuresis the concentration of the drug in the distal part of the nephron is kept relatively low and there is, therefore, a relatively small concentration gradient for back-diffusion and a relatively high clearance.

The excretion of acidic or basic drugs may be considerably altered by urine pH. This is because the non-ionized moiety is much more diffusible than the ionized moiety. Raising the urine pH will increase the ionization, and hence the clearance, of acidic drugs; lowering it will do so for basic drugs. These increases of clearance with pH can be very large. For example, salicylate clearance can be increased approximately four-fold for each rise of one unit in urine pH.

Forced diuresis is only of value in certain well-defined instances of drug overdosage and is not without its dangers. Mannitol expands the extracellular fluid and may precipitate left ventricular failure, particularly if the drug is one that is a powerful myocardial depressant, such as methaqualone. It has little to offer in the management of overdosage with short- and medium-acting barbiturates or any of the tranquillizing drugs that have tended to supersede them. It is most applicable to salicylate and phenobarbitone overdosage, when it should be combined with measures designed to render the urine alkaline.

Mannitol in 10 per cent solution (approximately twice isotonic) is the agent most frequently used. Urea has no advantages and its use is no longer justified. Before the method is resorted to, the following points should be borne in mind:

1. An indwelling urinary catheter is essential. It should drain into an accurately calibrated receptacle.
2. There must be no doubt about the ability of the kidneys to excrete the solute load administered.

3. Meticulous attention to the cumulative fluid balance is essential. The method is therefore best confined to intensive care units.

The casual infusion of a bottle of hypertonic mannitol every 4–8 hours resulting in a 24-hour urine volume of 2.5–3 litres is therapeutically ineffective. Before undertaking forced diuresis any fluid deficits judged to be present on admission must be made good. Unless these are unusually great this can be done by giving equal volumes of isotonic saline and 5 per cent dextrose to a total of 40 ml/kg at the rate of 500 ml in 15 minutes. Thereafter:

1. In the first hour infuse 1 litre of 10 per cent mannitol.
2. At the end of the first hour and subsequently at the end of each 2-hour period:
   (a) measure urine volume
   (b) measure urine pH
   (c) calculate the cumulative fluid balance.
3. Fluids are then given as indicated in *Table 3.3*. In phenobarbitone poisoning 1 g of potassium chloride is added to each 500 ml of fluid infused, and in salicylate overdosage 1.5 g of potassium chloride is added to each 500 ml of fluid infused.

Table 3.3 Summary of management of forced diuresis

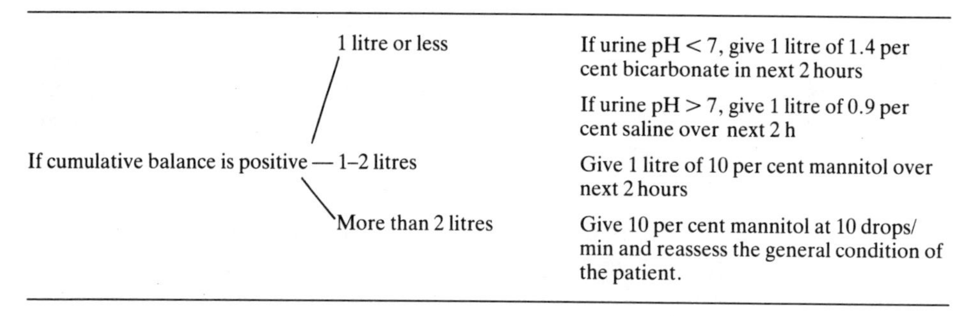

If cumulative balance is positive	1 litre or less	If urine pH < 7, give 1 litre of 1.4 per cent bicarbonate in next 2 hours If urine pH > 7, give 1 litre of 0.9 per cent saline over next 2 h
	1–2 litres	Give 1 litre of 10 per cent mannitol over next 2 hours
	More than 2 litres	Give 10 per cent mannitol at 10 drops/min and reassess the general condition of the patient.

Precautions. It must be stressed that this regimen usually results in progressive accumulation of mannitol and expansion of the extracellular space. If the positive cumulative water balance exceeds 2.5 litres, frusemide should be given. The maximum dose of mannitol infused continuously should not exceed 300 g.

The regimen is continued until the patient is judged to be in a safe state.

Phenobarbitone and phenobarbitone sodium

Phenobarbitone (*BP*) and Phenobarbital (*USP*)
Phenobarbitone sodium (*BP*) and Phenobarbital sodium (*USP*)
Chemical name: 5-ethyl-5-phenylbarbituric acid
For structural formula *see Figure 3.6*, p. 98

PHARMACOLOGY

Phenobarbitone is a long-acting barbiturate; its duration of action may be 8–16 hours. Hangover effects can be marked when other than minimal doses are given.

Besides having a powerful sedative action on the CNS, it specifically depresses the motor cortex and so has an anticonvulsant action. Part is broken down by the liver and other tissues, but the majority is excreted unchanged in the urine, the rate of excretion being increased if the urine is alkaline. Phenobarbitone has proved to be one of the most potent of those agents which induce proliferation of microsomal enzymes in the liver, and thus influence the metabolism of other drugs.

INDICATIONS
Phenobarbitone is used as a sedative in the treatment of neuroses and anxiety states and in the management of epilepsy. It has been used to increase the rate of liver handling of unconjugated bilirubin in Gilbert's disease, but the non-hypnotic analogue phetharbital is now preferred.

DOSAGE AND ADMINISTRATION
Phenobarbitone is given by mouth in tablet form. The sodium salt has the same action as the acid, but being soluble in water can also be given by the intravenous and intramuscular routes. As a sedative, 15–30 mg two to three times a day are generally sufficient. Similar doses are given for the control of epileptic seizures, and may be combined with phenytoin. Larger doses up to 200 mg are sometimes necessary.

In status epilepticus and in the treatment of convulsions due to overdose of analeptics, such as amphetamine, 60–200 mg of the sodium salt may be given intravenously or intramuscularly and repeated if necessary. When given intravenously the solution should be diluted, 200 mg being made up to 10 ml. Solutions for injections should be freshly prepared in CO_2-free water or decomposition with precipitation of phenobarbitone will occur.

PRECAUTIONS
Increased muscular rigidity may occur in patients suffering from parkinsonism and phenobarbitone should not be used in these cases.

Miscellaneous sedatives

Alcohol

Ethanol (96 per cent) (*BP*) and Alcohol (96 per cent) (*USP*)
Chemical name: ethyl alcohol

```
    H   H
    |   |
H—C—C—OH
    |   |
    H   H
```

PHYSICAL CHARACTERISTICS
Alcohol (96 per cent) is a colourless, transparent, mobile and volatile liquid with a characteristic spirituous odour and a burning taste. It boils at 78°C, is readily flammable, and burns with a blue smokeless flame.

Ethyl alcohol is a depressant of the CNS. Inhibitory mechanism and self-criticism are depressed first, and this accounts for the apparent stimulation observed early in its course of action. The subsequent order in which the CNS is depressed is the same as for general anaesthetics, but alcohol is too dangerous for use as such because the safety margin between full anaesthesia and full medullary depression is too narrow and the stage of excitement is too long. It is also an irritant; hence, when strong solutions are given orally they may initiate medullary reflexes by stimulating the pharynx. Solutions of over 12 per cent can cause alcoholic gastritis. Concentrations of alcohol in the blood sufficient to cause respiratory failure have no serious direct toxic effect on the heart, but central vasomotor and respiratory effects are important contributors to the cardiovascular depression by alcohol poisoning. Skin vasodilatation and increased sweating contribute to a loss of body heat, although the subject feels warmer.

The body can metabolize alcohol, like a food, but only at a constant rate (about 10 ml/h) irrespective of the amount present. The liver is the chief organ involved and the metabolic pathway to carbon dioxide and water is via acetaldehyde and acetate. This catabolic process can be speeded up by the injection of soluble insulin which will restore a drunken man to a semblance of normality more quickly. Methyl alcohol, present with ethyl alcohol to the extent of about 4 per cent in methylated spirit, is much more toxic, being oxidized to formic acid which affects the optic nerves, causing blindness.

The oxidation of acetaldehyde can be inhibited by disulfiram, and this has been utilized in the treatment of chronic alcoholism. Alcohol cannot be converted for storage in the body, and when the rate of absorption exceeds 10 ml/h the excess is excreted unchanged by the kidney and in the breath. The concentration in either can be used to make a rough quantitative estimate of the content in the blood. Unfitness to drive a motor vehicle in Great Britain has now been deemed proved by the finding of a blood level of 80 mg/100 ml, although there is no doubt that most people's faculties would be critically impaired by blood levels lower than this, especially when the level is rising. Excretion by the kidney is hastened by a diuresis which is consequent upon a central depression of the release of antidiuretic hormone from the posterior pituitary.

Chronic alcoholics are frequently very resistant to anaesthesia. It is often impossible to anaesthetize these patients with nitrous oxide, and other agents may have to be given in greater than usual quantities. This resistance may be due to several factors. Repeated alcohol ingestion induces proliferation of enzyme systems in the liver which enhances the metabolic breakdown of other drugs. To some degree, however, the apparent resistance may be an example of cross-tolerance, a CNS adaptation found with many other depressants given repeatedly over long periods.

When liver damage occurs from the excessive continued intake of alcohol its progress is slow. It is mainly the result of a deficiency of essential metabolites consequent upon a diminished food intake.

Alcohol is also a protein precipitant, a solvent, and a dehydrating agent; it is germicidal at a concentration of 70 per cent by weight.

The uses of alcohol as an anaesthetic are only of historic interest. Before the introduction of modern anaesthetic agents, wine was often given in sufficient dose to produce a state of stupor to allay the pain of surgical operation. In the early part of this century, a mixture known as A.C.E. (alcohol 1 part, chloroform 2 parts, ether 3 parts) was given on an open mask as an anaesthetic, but alcohol played little or no part in the production of anaesthesia. It has been given as a 10 per cent w/v solution in Ringer lactate but induction is not satisfactory because of complications and side effects.

INDICATIONS

Alcohol may be used for its hypnotic action, which is particularly useful in producing sleep in babies and elderly persons.

In the relief of intractable pain it may be given as a subarachnoid injection. In trigeminal neuralgia the gasserian ganglion or the branches of the fifth nerve may be similarly blocked by alcohol injection.

DRUG INTERACTIONS

Chronic alcohol consumption is associated with a lower blood level of tolbutamide, which may be due to impaired absorption or to more rapid inactivation. Some of the sulphonylureas bloc the enzyme acetaldehyde dehydrogenase and can cause a disuliram-type reaction. Tis has also been reported with the antitrichomonal agent metronidazole.

Alcohol stimulates the metabolism of some other drugs, the most important being phenytoin, isoniazid, and warfarin. It tends to accentuate the gastric irritation produced by salicylates.

There is potentiation of the effects of other CNS depressants, most notably barbiturates, which can give rise to accidental death.

OVERDOSAGE

Alcohol overdose gives rise to excitement followed by general depression leading to coma, respiratory depression, and cardiovascular collapse. Treatment may require gastric lavage and artificial ventilation if respiration is markedly depressed; general supportive therapy should be given, especially if vomiting has been severe and water and electrolyte balance has been disturbed.

Delirium tremens may occur in heavy drinkers upon attempts to withdraw alcohol or after trauma, during an acute infection, after a heavy bout of drinking, or without apparent cause.

Morphine is contraindicated in acute alcohol poisoning because of the raised intracranial pressure.

In an attempt to provide a conscious deterrent to alcohol, patients have been given drugs which, although innocuous in themselves, lead to unpleasant effects if alcohol is taken. Disulfiram and calcium carbimide have been employed in this way.

Chlormethiazole

Chlormethiazole (*BAN*)
Chemical name: 5-(2-chloroethyl)-4-methylthiazole

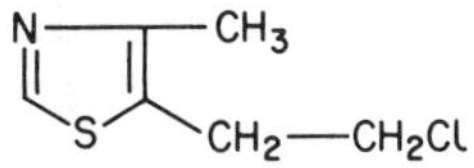

N—CH3 / S — CH2—CH2Cl

Chlormethiazole is a derivative of the thiazole moiety of the vitamin B1 molecule and is available commercially as the edisylate salt, which is a white crystalline powder that is readily soluble in water.

PHARMACOLOGY

Chlormethiazole is basically an anticonvulsant, but is also a powerful sedative and hypnotic with antiemetic properties. It is devoid of action on the autonomic nervous system. Rapid intravenous infusion in healthy volunteers causes little change in cardiac output; blood pressure is little changed or rises but a consistent effect is a marked rise in pulse rate. Respiratory depression and hypotension may follow large doses.

INDICATIONS

It has been widely recommended for the treatment of acute alcoholism during the initial withdrawal phase and during stabilization on an alcohol-free regimen. It is also effective in controlling delirium, tremors, and status epilepticus, and to sedate patients on automatic ventilators and those undergoing uncomfortable manoeuvres in intensive therapy units. It has also been used as a sedative to accompany regional analgesia and in the management of pre-eclamptic toxaemia.

DOSAGE AND ADMINISTRATION

Chlormethiazole may be given intravenously as a 0.8 per cent solution in 5 per cent dextrose for status epilepticus or to severely agitated patients at a rate of 8–20 ml/min, depending on the clinical state of the patient, 40–60 ml usually being adequate. Up to 1 litre may need to be administered in a 12-hour period. Other fluid intake should be restricted if 2 litres need to be given in 24 hours in pre-eclamptic or epileptic patients, to minimize dangers from overhydration.

It may be used orally, commencing with up to 2 g initially followed by 1 g every 3–4 hours. For the treatment of alcohol withdrawal symptoms this dosage is progressively reduced over a period of about 8 days.

PRECAUTIONS AND SIDE EFFECTS

Rapid intravenous injection should be avoided and the strength of the solution should not exceed 0.8 per cent. Gastrointestinal symptoms have been reported after oral treatment and thrombophlebitis after intravenous infusion. A tingling sensation in the nose or sneezing may occur after the first administration.

Glutethimide

Glutethimide (*BP* and *USP*)
Chemical name: 3-ethyl-3-phenyl-piperidine-2,6-dione

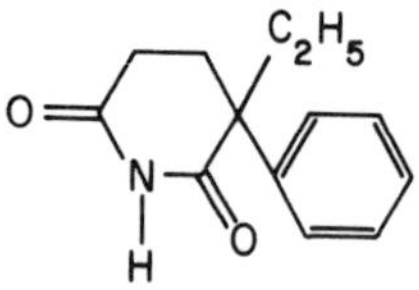

C_2H_5 O N H O

Glutethimide is a CNS depressant with strong hypnotic properties. Its action is rapid – 20 to 30 minutes – and lasts for 6 hours and is comparable to the intermediate-acting barbiturates, to which its potency appears to be similar. Side effects and hangover are stated to be absent. Several cases of withdrawal symptoms following discontinuance of the drug have now been reported and it must be considered to be a drug of dependence.

In normal dosage there is no effect on blood pressure and respiration, but after large doses respiratory depression and a fall in blood pressure may result. Oxygen consumption is not decreased.

Skin rashes sometimes follow the administration of glutethimide. They normally disappear on withdrawal of the drug. Nausea also occurs occasionally.

Liver damage has not been reported. It is broken down in the body, probably to α-phenylglutaric acid imide, as this substance has been found in the urine. It is one of the many hypnotic drugs able to cause liver microsomal enzyme induction.

INDICATIONS

Glutethimide is employed as a hypnotic and is a useful alternative to the barbiturates in elderly subjects, as it is well tolerated.

DOSAGE AND ADMINISTRATION

It is given by mouth in tablet form. The usual dose is 0.25–0.5 g shortly before bedtime. Children may be given 0.125 g at the age of 6 months, increasing to 0.25 g at the age of 6 years and over.

Glutethimide has also been used in premedication – 0.5 g may be given 1 hour before operation.

PRECAUTIONS

Glutethimide, in overdose, is *very* toxic, possibly because of one or more of its metabolites. At all events the death rate from diagnosed cases of poisoning is much higher than for all other hypnotic agents.

Meprobamate

Meprobamate (*BP* and *USP*)
Chemical name: 2-methyl-2-propyltrimethylene dicarbamate

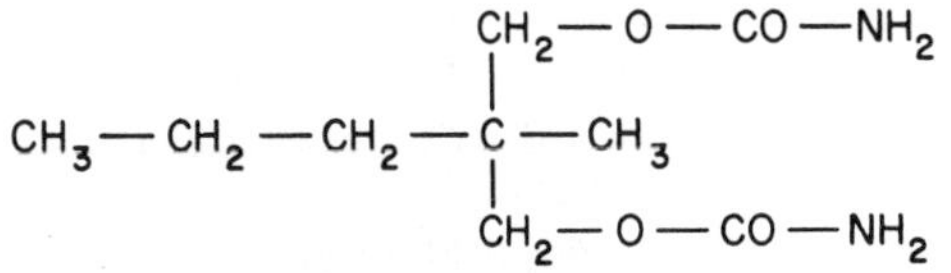

$$\begin{array}{l} \qquad\qquad\qquad\qquad\quad CH_2-O-CO-NH_2 \\ \qquad\qquad\qquad\qquad\quad | \\ CH_3-CH_2-CH_2-C-CH_3 \\ \qquad\qquad\qquad\qquad\quad | \\ \qquad\qquad\qquad\qquad\quad CH_2-O-CO-NH_2 \end{array}$$

Meprobamate is related chemically to mephenesin and has mild muscle-relaxant and anticonvulsant properties. It acts on the internuncial neurones of the spinal cord in a similar manner to mephenesin. It is said to produce a calming effect and induce sleep, but its usefulness is considerably overrated. Although of doubtful therapeutic value it is still used.

Meprobamate has low toxicity but side effects include drowsiness, dizziness, and gastric discomfort and more rarely skin reactions and agranulocytosis.

It is given in tablet form in a dose of 400 mg three times a day, with an additional dose before retiring if necessary. It is combined with an analgesic in some proprietary preparations for the relief of pain associated with muscle tension. It is capable of causing hepatic enzyme induction.

Methaqualone hydrochloride

Methaqualone hydrochloride (*USP*)
Chemical name: 2-methyl-3-*o*-tolylquinazolin-4(3*H*)-one hydrochloride

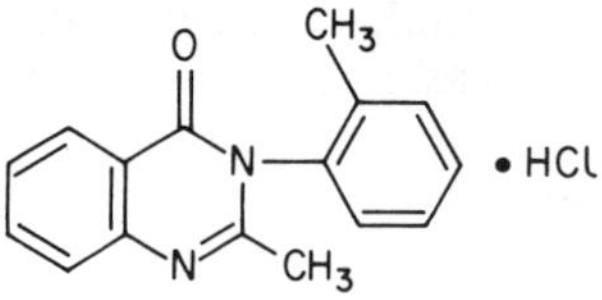

Methaqualone is a quinazolone compound. It has a hypnotic action comparable to that of the barbiturates, and is a suitable alternative particularly in elderly subjects. However, it differs from the barbiturates in not blocking the 'paradoxical' phases of sleep which are associated with dreaming. This may contribute to the absence of hangover which is claimed, and related to the fact that unlike the barbiturates it has not on its own found favour with drug addicts. Side effects are uncommon. Numbness and tingling of the hands have been reported but this complication is rare. It is not teratogenic in rats and rabbits. Methaqualone is given in tablet form and the recommended dose is 150–300 mg.

Methaqualone-diphenhydramine combinations

Methaqualone is notable for the marked potentiation of its hypnotic action which can be induced with the antihistamine diphenhydramine. Indeed, most of the methaqualone that is prescribed is in fact contained in proprietary preparations containing 250 mg of methaqualone with 25 mg of diphenhydramine. The mechanism of this synergism has not been elucidated although competition for binding sites has been suggested. In this connection it is of interest that alcohol markedly interferes with the plasma protein binding of methaqualone, thus increasing its free-water concentration and potentiating its actions.

The addition of diphenhydramine introduces several important differences to the actions of methaqualone. It not only potentiates the hypnotic action, but also markedly shortens the time of onset; patients who have taken toxic overdoses are not only comatose, but also suffer from convulsions; there is frequently a lethal potentiation by alcohol. It is also of interest that although neither drug alone is taken by drug addicts, the combination is very popular; this, of course, may only reflect the relative frequency of prescription. What is undeniable is that while both drugs individually have an enviable record of safety, their combination has figured very frequently in cases of death by self-poisoning, some of which may well have been accidental.

Methyprylone

Methyprylone (*BP*) and Methyprylon (*USP*)
Chemical name: 3,3-diethyl-5-methylpiperidine-2,4-dione

Methyprylone, a piperidine compound, is a CNS depressant with a moderate hypnotic action comparable to that of pentobarbitone. It acts in 30–60 minutes and its effects last about 6 hours. Hangover and side effects are said to be absent.

In normal dosage there is no effect on respiration or blood pressure, but both can be depressed when excessive doses are given.

Its fate in the body has not yet been determined.

Methyprylone is employed as a sedative and mild hypnotic, is given by mouth in tablet form in doses of 50–100 mg three to four times a day for sedation, and 200–400 mg 30 minutes before bedtime as a hypnotic. Children may be given 50 mg at the age of 4 years and up to 200 mg at the age of 10 years.

Metoclopramide hydrochloride

Metoclopramide hydrochloride (*BP* and *USAN*)
Chemical name: 4-amino-5-chloro-*N*-(2-diethylaminoethyl)-2-methoxybenzamide hydrochloride

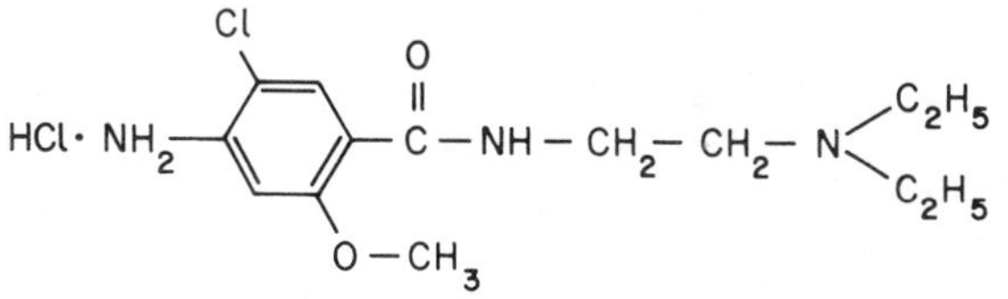

PHARMACOLOGY

Metoclopramide is a specific antiemetic. It is not a phenothiazine, has no antihistamine activity, and in normal therapeutic doses has no narcotic or sedative action. Its mode of action is two-fold; it is effective centrally at the chemoreceptor trigger zone, and also has a peripheral action, diminishing the sensitivity of visceral nerves to local emetics. In addition, it hastens gastric emptying, possibly by a central action on brain stem nuclei controlling gastric motility, and increases the tone of the lower oesophageal sphincter. These peripheral effects are antagonized by atropine.

INDICATIONS

Metoclopramide may be used to control nausea and vomiting associated with peptic ulcer, epidemic vomiting, X-ray therapy, malignant disease, and uraemia. It is as effective as perphenazine in the control of postanaesthetic vomiting and shortens the duration of postoperative ileus. However, the delay in gastric emptying which is caused by narcotic analgesics is not significantly influenced by metoclopramide. It has been employed as an agent for hastening the emptying of the full stomach when general anaesthesia is required after an accident.

DOSAGE AND ADMINISTRATION

Metoclopramide may be given orally or by intramuscular or intravenous injection. The usual dose is 10 mg, which can be repeated three times a day. It is not recommended for children under 5 years, but older children may be given proportionate doses.

PRECAUTIONS

It may produce drowsiness and restlessness; dystonic muscle movements and other extrapyramidal side effects are produced if the dosage exceeds 0.5 mg/kg. Constipation may occur. Atropine antagonizes its action on gastric motility.

Paraldehyde

Paraldehyde (*BP* and *USP*)

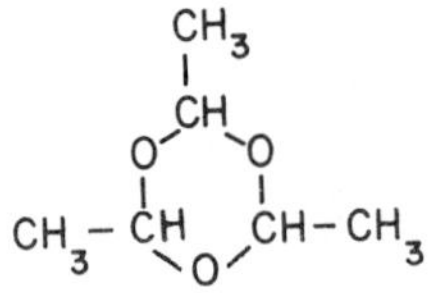

$$\text{Paraldehyde: cyclic trimer } (CH_3CHO)_3 \text{ — 2,4,6-trimethyl-1,3,5-trioxane ring}$$

Paraldehyde is a colourless or very pale yellow liquid with a powerful characteristic odour and unpleasant taste. It solidifies at temperatures below 11°C, and when required the entire contents of the container should be liquefied before use.

PHARMACOLOGY

Paraldehyde is a cerebral depressant with a powerful hypnotic effect. In small doses there is no effect on cardiac or respiratory function, but in larger doses, such as those used to produce basal narcosis, respiration may be moderately depressed. Excitement and restlessness are apt to occur in the presence of fever and pain. Duration of action is about 8 hours and recovery is slow, but after-effects are minimal.

Paraldehyde crosses the placental barrier but does not cause undue depression of respiration in the fetus.

It is quickly absorbed but its fate in the body is not definitely known. The greater part, about 80 per cent, is probably broken down in the liver. The remainder, which is excreted unchanged by the lungs, is responsible for the unpleasant odour in the breath after administration; traces may also be found in the urine.

Paraldehyde is now little used, but has been employed in the control of mania and delirium. Although it may be given by mouth or intramuscular injection, its taste is unpleasant and injections are painful. Thus, if used, it is commonly administered rectally in a dose of 2–10 ml.

PRECAUTIONS

It is contraindicated in liver disease and is incompatible with disposable syringes made of polyethylene.

Triclofos sodium

Triclofos sodium (*BP*)
Chemical name: sodium hydrogen 2,2,2-trichloroethyl phosphate

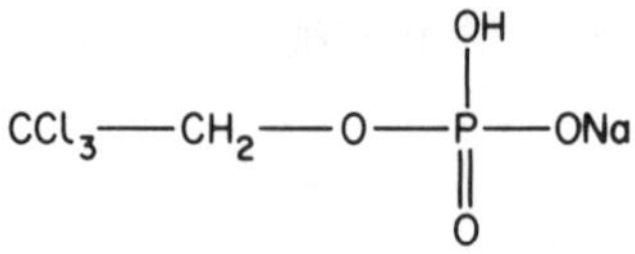

$$CCl_3—CH_2—O—P(=O)(OH)—ONa$$

Triclofos is the phosphoric ester of trichloroethanol. It is rapidly hydrolysed in the body to the organic phosphate and trichloroethanol which is the active principle and responsible for its sedative action. Trichloroethanol is also an active metabolite of chloral hydrate, so the two drugs have similar action. Neither drug is an inducer of liver microsomal enzymes. The main advantages of triclofos are that it can be taken in tablet form or as a pleasant syrup and does not cause gastric irritation. Reports suggest that it is a useful sedative and hypnotic comparable in effect to the medium-acting barbiturates. It is given in doses of 0.5–1 g as a sedative and 1–2 g as a hypnotic; 2–3 g may sometimes be necessary.

Dichoralphenazone is another compound whose action is also due to trichloroethanol, which is produced as a result of hepatic metabolism. Another product of this metabolism is phenazone; this compound is an inducer of microsomal liver enzymes. It also has mild analgesic properties, but as phenazone itself is no longer used on account of its tendency to cause agranulocytosis its presence in this compound cannot be considered an advantage. It is given in a dose of 1–2 g.

Anticonvulsants

Since convulsions may be produced by a number of different metabolic and pathological conditions as well as by convulsant drugs or by electrical stimulation of the CNS, it is not surprising that anticonvulsants in general do not form a well-knit group. The correct antidotes for convulsions due to asphyxia or to hypoglycaemia are obvious and are aimed at their cause, but where convulsions are due to a cause that cannot be rapidly remedied then recourse must be had to substances that prevent the CNS discharges, or sometimes only the peripheral motor function. A large number of CNS depressants will control convulsions but many of these do so only in doses that produce profound sedation or even anaesthesia. For example, this is true of many barbiturates and chlormethiazole. Others produce a useful degree of motor depression in doses that have demonstrable but not incapacitating soporific effects, for example phenobarbitone, methylphenobarbitone, and the benzodiazepines. A few drugs such as carbamazepine and certain hydantoin derivatives, for example phenytoin, exert anticonvulsant actions at dose levels that do not cause drowsiness. Carbamazepine is additionally of interest in that it has also been found to be effective in the control of the paroxysmal pain of trigeminal neuralgia.

Under special circumstances it may not be necessary, or may even be a disadvantage, to quell the nervous discharge of convulsions of central origin. Such would be the case in electroconvulsive therapy for certain mental diseases, and so the problem then is to prevent merely those peripheral motor manifestations of the induced nervous storm that are dangerous. Here the relaxants of striated muscle may be used as anticonvulsants, the choice being from short-acting ones such as suxamethonium.

Convulsions encountered occasionally by the anaesthetist include those caused by drugs. The most common are local anaesthetics and some other antidysrhythmic drugs, particularly those with anticholinergic actions, penicillins, especially benzylpenicillin, psychotropic drugs, particularly chlorpromazine, analeptics, and radiographic contrast media. They are almost always associated with high brain concentrations. These, together with anaesthetic convulsions (so-called ether convulsions), are best treated with diazepam, 10–20 mg given intravenously, or with small doses of thiopentone.

Drug treatment of epilepsy

Not all the manifestations of epilepsy involve overt motor seizures; the most appropriate drug therapy is dependent on the type of epilepsy and a general guide is given in *Table 3.4*.

Table 3.4 Types of epilepsy and drugs of choice

Type of epilepsy	*Drugs*
Grand mal	Phenytoin, phenobarbitone, primidone
Petit mal (3Hz spike and wave)	Sodium valproate, ethosuximide
Focal epilepsy (motor and sensory)	Phenytoin, phenobarbitone
Temporal lobe (psychomotor)	Carbamazepine, pheneturide, sulthiame
Myoclonic and infantile spasms	Clonazepam, sodium valproate
Neonatal fits	Phenytoin, phenobarbitone

Side effects are common with all antiepileptic drugs, particularly when starting treatment. Changes of dosage should be gradual and made under regular supervision. Estimation of plasma drug levels, particularly of phenytoin, can help to avoid toxic effects. Many of these compounds also interfere with folate production and cause megaloblastic anaemia. The incidence of congenital malformation is roughly three times higher than normal in children born to women being treated with anticonvulsants.

The range of drugs with useful anticonvulsant activity is very wide and a brief summary of those in use is given here: monographs are included on phenytoin and sodium valproate which are both widely used and the most effective agents in most cases.

Phenytoin sodium

Phenytoin sodium (*BP* and *USP*)
Chemical name: sodium 5,5-diphenylimidazolidine-2,4-dione

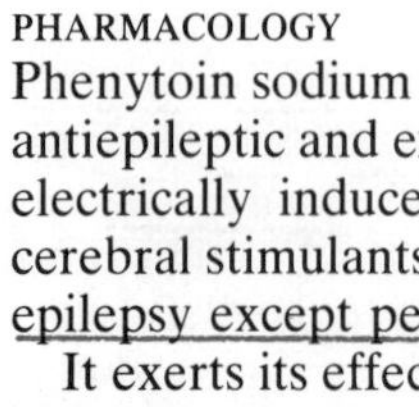

```
H5C6
    \
     C —— NH
    /|      \
H5C6 |       CO•Na
     |      /
     C —— NH
     ||
     O
```

PHARMACOLOGY

Phenytoin sodium does not cause general depression of the CNS, but is powerfully antiepileptic and experimentally is one of the most effective substances in opposing electrically induced convulsions. It is less effective against those produced by cerebral stimulants such as leptazol. Phenytoin is the drug of choice for all forms of epilepsy except petit mal, where it may have an adverse effect.

It exerts its effects by its ability to stabilize excitable cell membranes in the CNS. This effect is also seen in peripheral nerves and in the excitable tissues of the heart.

It is increasingly being used alone rather than in combinations because its metabolism can be influenced by hepatic microsomal enzyme induction caused by other drugs. It is also an enzyme inducer itself. The most effective combination clinically is with phenobarbitone. It often has little effect on the EEG either in the normal person or in grand mal, and the latter condition may be well controlled without any corresponding improvement in the EEG pattern.

Absorption, metabolism, and excretion. The alkalinity of the sodium salt often causes gastric distress, which can be minimized by taking the drug after meals. Phenytoin sodium is absorbed only slowly from the intestine. This is also true of intramuscular administration because of precipitation at the site of injection. The pharmacokinetics of this drug are of special interest and importance for two reasons. First, because of slow absorption and distribution there is a considerable delay in the establishment of a steady-state concentration of the drug. Secondly, the breakdown of the drug does not vary exponentially with the plasma level, as is normally the case with first-order reactions which are usual in drug metabolism. Below 10 μg/ml elimination follows this pattern, but at a higher concentration the metabolic breakdown pathway becomes saturated and any further increase in concentration has no effect on breakdown rate. This rate stays constant, rather like the situation with the metabolism of alcohol. This critical level is close to the therapeutic level and, since the rate of metabolism is determined by genetic influences of a multifactorial nature, normal doses cause continued accumulation in some individuals until toxic blood levels are reached. For this reason, adjustment of dose by reference to plasma concentrations is increasingly employed. Phenytoin is metabolized by hepatic microsomal enzymes and principally undergoes oxidation to a *p*-hydroxyphenyl derivative.

INDICATIONS

Phenytoin is used in all types of epilepsy except petit mal and is the drug of first choice. It may be effectively combined with phenobarbitone. It is particularly useful in the treatment of dysrhythmias due to digitalis for which it is almost specific.

DOSAGE AND ADMINISTRATION

In adults, initial dosage is 100 mg three times a day by mouth. This may be increased if necessary up to 600 mg per 24 hours. Infants and children up to the age of 5 years are given 25–50 mg two to four times a day; children over the age of 6 years may be given 100 mg. The aim is to achieve a plasma level of 10–20 μg/ml (40–80 μmol/ℓ), although seizure control can be achieved at lower plasma levels in some cases. Above 20 μg/ml toxic effects such as ataxia and nystagmus are evident; above 40 μg/ml lethargy becomes apparent. In the control of digitalis-induced dysrhythmias 50–100 mg of phenytoin may be given intravenously every 15 minutes until a satisfactory response is achieved, up to a maximum of 15 mg/kg. Digitalis-induced ventricular dysrhythmias are suppressed at plasma concentrations of 8–16 μg/ml.

PRECAUTIONS

Toxic effects are common and are related to plasma level. The principal effects of overdose, such as nystagmus and ataxia, are manifestations of cerebellar toxicity. Insomnia and gastric disturbances may also occur. A wide variety of hypersensitivity and haematological reactions have been reported and these necessitate stopping the drug. Megaloblastic anaemia is due to altered folate absorption and metabolism and responds to folic acid. After several months of treatment, young patients sometimes develop a hypertrophic condition of the gums, the cause of which is not known.

Administration during pregnancy leads to a typical abnormality, the fetal hydantoin syndrome, which typically includes wide-set eyes, a broad jaw, and finger deformities. There is a three-fold higher incidence of fetal malformations than normal in children born to mothers taking this drug, but the cessation of effective therapy is potentially more dangerous to both mother and child.

Drug interactions can result in both increases and decreases in plasma concentration. Competitive inhibition of metabolic pathways by phenobarbitone, alcohol, chloramphenicol, dicoumarol, and isoniazid has been reported. Conversely, hepatic enzyme induction by phenobarbitone may increase the rate of metabolism and thus lower the plasma concentration for a given dose regimen.

Sodium valproate

Sodium valproate (*BP*)
Chemical name: sodium 2-propylpentanoate

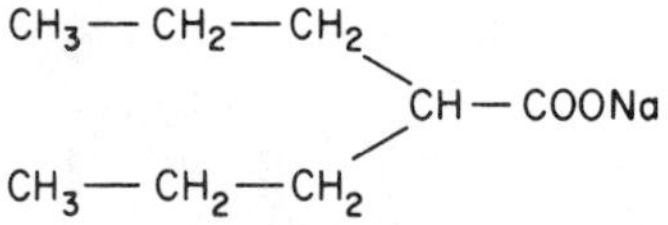

$$\begin{array}{l} CH_3-CH_2-CH_2 \\ \qquad\qquad\qquad\quad \diagdown \\ \qquad\qquad\qquad\quad\ CH-COONa \\ \qquad\qquad\qquad\quad \diagup \\ CH_3-CH_2-CH_2 \end{array}$$

Sodium valproate is an effective anticonvulsant which has been used in the treatment of most forms of epilepsy. It is particularly effective in petit mal, for which it may be the drug of choice.

PHARMACOLOGY

The mechanism of the antiepileptic effect of sodium valproate is not known, although it is probably associated with an increased concentration in the brain of the inhibitory transmitter γ-aminobutyric acid (Whittle and Turner, 1978). The drug is rapidly absorbed from the gut. The plasma elimination half-life is 16–18 hours and this is shortened to 6–8 hours when the drug is used together with an enzyme-inducing anticonvulsant such as phenobarbitone, phenytoin, or carbamazepine. The optimum therapeutic serum concentration has not yet been clearly established, but levels of 200 μg/ml should be exceeded with extreme caution.

The serum concentration of other anticonvulsants may increase when sodium valproate is added. It displaces phenytoin from plasma protein binding sites but also increases phenytoin metabolism. Sodium valproate potentiates the actions of monoamine oxidase inhibitors and tricyclic antidepressants.

DOSAGE

For adults the initial daily dose is 300 mg twice daily, increasing to a maximum of 2600 mg/day. In children and infants the dose must be scaled down.

PRECAUTIONS

After several years of trouble-free usage, there have been reports of serious complications such as fulminant hepatic failure and pancreatitis. Raised transaminases occur in up to 44 per cent of patients, but are usually transient and often are present without clinical manifestations. Children with severe epilepsy associated with mental retardation or structural brain damage are the most at risk of developing severe damage, as well as those who have pre-existing liver disease. The only other drug interactions of which anaesthetists should be particularly aware are reversible haemostatic defects, including decreased platelet adhesiveness, mild hypofibrinogenaemia, and thrombocytopenia.

Whittle, S. R. and Turner, A. J. (1978) Effects of the anticonvulsant sodium valproate on gamma-aminobutyrate and aldehyde metabolism in ox brain. *Journal of Neurochemistry,* **31,** 1453

Benzodiazepines, which are effective as anticonvulsants, include chlordiazepoxide, diazepam, nitrazepam, and clonazepam. Of these, diazepam and clonazepam are of particular value in the management of status epilepticus (*see* pages 93 and 94).

Carbonic anhydrase inhibitors are employed as anticonvulsants. Acetazolamide, which is a diuretic, is effective in many types of epilepsy in some patients, particularly when added to other therapy. A monograph can be found on page 399. Sulthiame is another carbonic anhydrase inhibitor, but it has few obvious advantages over acetazolamide. The adult dose is 200–600 mg daily in divided doses. This dose should be adjusted appropriately in children.

Carbamazepine is chemically and pharmacologically related to the tricyclic antidepressants. It may well prove to be the drug of choice for temporal lobe epilepsy but, strangely, despite clinical improvement, there may be a deterioration in the EEG. It is the drug of choice for the treatment of trigeminal and other neuralgias and has been said to be effective in the control of intractable hiccough. Initially, 100–200 mg may be given once or twice a day, increasing to 600–800 mg daily until an optimal response is obtained. In some instances, 1.6 g daily may be necessary. A wide range of adverse reactions have been reported, ranging from thrombocytopenia to hepatocellular jaundice. It also exhibits toxic effects similar to those of other tricylic antidepressants.

Ethosuximide is the most effective member of the succinimide series. It is used for the control of petit mal, or *absence seizures* which are associated with 3Hz spike and wave discharges in the EEG. It should not be given without such evidence unless an *absence* has been observed. An initial oral dose of 250 mg is given two to three times daily. This may be gradually increased up to 2 g daily as required. The most common side effects involve the gastrointestinal tract (nausea, etc.) and the CNS (drowsiness). Its sole use may unmask tonic–clonic seizures and it is usually combined with phenytoin or primidone.

Phenobarbitone is a safe anticonvulsant for grand mal or focal epilepsy; it is considered in detail on page 106.

Primidone has a similar action, although it is not a barbiturate. In fact, a considerable element of its anticonvulsant activity can be attributed to the formation of phenobarbitone as an active metabolite by oxidation. It does, however, have some anticonvulsant action itself. The commonest side effects are sedation, vertigo, nausea, ataxia, and nystagmus. At the commencement of treatment 125 mg may be given daily in divided doses for 3 days. The dose can then be increased gradually up to 250 mg four times a day as required.

4

General anaesthetics

The word anaesthesia means absence of sensation, and general anaesthesia therefore implies unconsciousness. General anaesthetics include any agents capable of producing total insensibility in a reversible manner. In fact, the term general anaesthetic has come to mean an agent whose actions are qualified in far more detail than this, especially with regard to good relaxation of skeletal muscles and lack of toxicity to tissues so that recovery may be complete.

Stages of anaesthesia

Certain stages are recognized to describe the depth of anaesthesia. These stages were first described for anaesthesia induced with ether given by the semi-open method in unpremedicated patients, and are modified when agents other than ether are used or when premedication is employed. Four stages are described, which can be recognized both during induction of and recovery from anaesthesia.

Stage I: stage of analgesia
This stage lasts from the commencement of induction until loss of consciousness. Respiration is quiet, but often irregular. Reflexes are still present. This stage is utilized during obstetric analgesia, when subanaesthetic concentrations of nitrous oxide, trichlorethylene, or methoxyflurane are administered.

Stage II: stage of excitement or delirium
This stage lasts from the loss of consciousness to the onset of surgical anaesthesia. The patient is unconscious and unco-operative, and may talk, move his limbs, or even become violent. Respiration is irregular and breath-holding may occur; the irregular respiration may result in an irregular rate of absorption of anaesthetic vapour. Reflexes in response to stimuli are active. Retching may occur and if the stomach is not empty, vomiting may result. Premature surgical stimulation may cause excessive release of adrenaline with a danger of ventricular fibrillation. The more quickly and smoothly the patient can be brought through this stage the less likely are these reactions.

Stage III: stage of surgical anaesthesia
This stage extends from the onset of regular respiration, commonly termed 'automatic', until respiratory failure occurs from toxic concentration of anaesthetic agent in the CNS. This stage is divided into the following four planes:

Plane 1. Movements cease and respiration becomes regular and automatic; the eyelid reflex is lost. Eyeball movements are marked. The pharyngeal reflex disappears late in this plane, but the laryngeal and peritoneal reflexes are still present, and so is muscle tone.

Plane 2. The eyes become fixed centrally; muscle tone is decreasing but all muscles of respiration are still functioning. The laryngeal and peritoneal reflexes disappear during this stage.

Plane 3. Onset of paralysis of intercostal muscles, with respiration becoming purely diaphragmatic. Good muscle relaxation.

Plane 4. Respiration becoming gradually depressed with paralysis of diaphragm. A tracheal tug may be present. Muscle relaxation is full.

Stage IV: stage of medullary paralysis, with respiratory arrest and vasomotor collapse

The pupils are widely dilated and the skin is cold and ashen. The blood pressure is very low and the pulse feeble. Respiration is gasping and finally ceases.

These stages are usually well defined with ether or chloroform but are much less clearly marked when halothane is used. If anaesthesia is induced with an intravenous barbiturate the stages become telescoped, the patient passing rapidly into Stage III, Plane 2, or deeper, depending on the dose given, and the intermediate stages are not recognized.

Surgical anaesthesia

Surgical anaesthesia should be a state of harmless and reversible insensibility which allows operations of considerable magnitude to be carried out without hindrance to the surgeon or detriment to the patient. It is convenient to consider this anaesthetic state as consisting of a triad of sleep, analgesia, and muscular relaxation. 'Sleep' in this context differs from natural sleep, where subjects can be awakened by simple and not necessarily painful stimuli, such as touch and noise. By definition, the anaesthetized patient cannot be roused by stimuli of any intensity. Different patients undergoing different surgical procedures will require different degrees of analgesia and muscular relaxation.

It has so far not proved possible to find single drugs that will produce all these effects without causing unpleasant or undesirable side actions. Single anaesthetic agents are rarely used today except for very short and minor operations. The aim now is to attempt to use agents for specific pharmacological actions and in minimal doses so as to produce a state of 'balanced anaesthesia'. A common practice is to use thiopentone to produce initial brief but deep sleep; to maintain sleep and provide analgesia with nitrous oxide supplemented either with low concentrations of a volatile anaesthetic or with incremental doses of a general analgesic; and to use neuromuscular blocking agents to produce the required degree of muscular relaxation. In this way a patient will be enabled to regain his protective reflexes and recover consciousness within a few minutes of the end of an operation and suffer minimal side effects and complications.

Mode of action of anaesthetics

A large number of chemical substances are capable of producing general anaesthesia, and many attempts have been made to produce a single theory of action that would embrace all anaesthetics. These many compounds have no common chemical structure, thus no structure–activity relationships can be defined. They are also chemically unreactive, and unlikely to occupy specific receptors. In most theories, attempts have been made to correlate anaesthetic potency with some physical property of the anaesthetic agents. The majority of these theories infer a major site of action at the cell membrane. The more important theories are considered below.

Lipid solubility theory

The observation by Meyer and Overton that the narcotic potency of members of a chemical series is proportional to their oil/water partition coefficients led to the suggestion that narcotic action is due to drugs becoming dissolved in cell lipids. The relationship between oil/water partition and narcotic activity has been substantiated for many compounds. Better correlation exists between narcotic activity and oil/gas partition, the product of the oil/gas partition coefficient of an anaesthetic agent and its minimum alveolar concentration (MAC, *see* page 130) being approximately constant (Eger *et al.*, 1969). Many exceptions to the lipid solubility theory occur. Chloral hydrate, which has a very low lipid solubility and was held to be the most glaring example, is now thought to be converted into the highly lipid-soluble compound trichloroethanol. The theory does not explain the unequal action of stereoisomers. Nevertheless, the generalizations that may be deduced from the theory that all chemically inert substances that have some lipid solubility will exert a narcotic effect, and that the potency of a narcotic will depend on its affinity for lipid in the presence of body fluid, have been fairly well substantiated.

Thermodynamic activity of narcotics

Ferguson (1939) suggested that chemical potential – the free energy that a substance possesses by virtue of its chemical constitution – would be a more suitable measure of activity than the measurement of partition coefficient or of similar parameters in artificial systems. His method of measuring thermodynamic activity overcame the problems of measuring anaesthetic concentrations within cells or cell membranes. The finding that the chemical or thermodynamic potential so calculated is approximately the same for all compounds showing anaesthetic activity suggests that the action is non-specific in nature. Ferguson's observations explain the several theories that invoke other physical properties of anaesthetics, such as adsorption on surfaces and effects on surface tension. All of these physical properties which have been suggested as causative of narcosis are interrelated molecular properties which, in general, express molecular hydrophobicity.

As a measure of chemical potential, Ferguson used the index 'relative concentration' – the ratio of narcotic tension in a phase to saturated vapour pressure within that phase. In general, the concentration of any anaesthethic required to produce its effect will be directly related to the saturated vapour pressure of that substance, and inversely proportional to its lipid solubility.

Clathrates and gas hydrates

Pauling (1961) and Miller (1961) independently described theories of narcosis involving water. Their theories arose from observations that xenon, which produces anaesthesia in man at a concentration of 71 per cent, can form a hydrate at low temperature or high pressure. Similar hydrates, known as clathrates, occur with some other gases such as argon and nitrogen which can cause narcosis under hyperbaric conditions, as well as with many anaesthetic agents. Owing to their marked hydrogen-bonding properties, water molecules tend to aggregate in clusters, which at low temperatures form stable structures. The formation of a gas hydrate stabilizes the crystal structure. A good correlation exists between the partial pressure of a gas required to produce narcosis and the dissociation pressure of its hydrate at 0 °C. Pauling suggested that gas hydrates, stabilized by amino acid side chains of proteins, could exist as microcrystals and affect ionic mobility or membrane activity. Miller thought that clathrates existed as 'icebergs', which by their presence would affect membrane function. Neither theory defines a locus of action of anaesthetics. Although stable hydrates of anaesthetics can form at 0 °C, high pressures are needed to form such hydrates at body temperature. At 37 °C chloroform hydrate requires a pressure of 63 atm and nitrous oxide hydrate will exist at this temperature only at a pressure of 343 atm. Miller, Paton and Smith (1967) and Eger and colleagues (1969) have shown that narcotic action is more closely correlated to lipid solubility than to clathrate dissociation pressure.

Protein binding

Binding of anaesthetic agents to protein may be involved in their mode of action. Many proteins contain hydrophobic areas to which molecules of anaesthetic drug can become attached by induced dipole bonding. Protein structure has been shown to be reversibly altered in the presence of anaesthetic agents (Halsey, Brown and Richards, 1978).

Membrane permeability

Many theories of narcotic action have invoked an effect on ion transport across cell membranes. The evidence for such an effect is conflicting. There is some suggestion that anaesthetics reversibly inhibit Na^+ and K^+ transport, but much higher concentrations of anaesthetics are required to cause this effect than those used clinically.

Because of the likelihood that anaesthetics act at the cell membrane, it has been suggested that their effects are due to actions on sodium pores. These pores could be blocked by membrane swelling due to anaesthetics or to an action of anaesthetics upon membrane proteins.

Cellular effects of anaesthetics

One of the earliest theories of narcosis was that proposed by Claude Bernard in 1857, who suggested that anaesthesia was due to a reversible coagulation of cell protoplasm. More recently, Allison and Nunn (1968) showed that some anaesthetics (but not diethyl ether) could cause reversible dispersal of labile microtubules. Anaesthetics are well known to cause interruption of mitosis by an arrest in metaphase. The mitotic spindle, composed of microtubules, is dispersed by anaesthetics by a reversible depolymerization. Another effect of anaesthetics, which is probably due to their actions on cytoplasmic structure, is the reduced motility seen with many unicellular organisms and mammalian lymphocytes (Nunn, Sharp and Kimball, 1970). Saubermann and Gallacher (1973) have, however, shown that intact labile microtubules are present in the nerves of animals anaesthetized with halothane. It seems unlikely that microtubule disruption plays an important role in the action of anaesthetics in man.

Pressure reversal of anaesthesia

Many of the effects of inhalational anaesthesia can be reversed by pressures of 50 atm or more. Johnson and Flagler (1950) showed that tadpoles anaesthetized with alcohol awoke if high hydrostatic pressures were applied, and similar reversal of the effects of inhalational anaesthetics has been shown in mammals exposed to high gas pressures (Smith *et al.*, 1975). Halsey and Wardley-Smith (1975) showed that pressure reversal applied not only to inhalational anaesthetics but also to narcotics, tranquillizers, and intravenous induction agents. These effects of raised pressure led to a 'critical volume' hypothesis (Lever *et al.*, 1971; Miller *et al.*, 1973) which proposed a critical hydrophobic molecular site that was expanded by anaesthetics and restored to its normal state by applied pressure. Halsey, Wardley-Smith and Green (1978) have proposed modifications to this theory, suggesting that anaesthesia may be due not to the expansion of a single molecular site but to the expansion of various sites, possibly with differing physical properties.

Uptake and distribution of inhalational agents

After administration via the lungs the rate of entry of general anaesthetics into any tissue depends upon the rate of entry into the circulation, the steepness of the concentration gradient between blood and the tissue concerned, the blood supply of the tissue, and the affinity of that tissue for the anaesthetic. All anaesthetics readily diffuse into the CNS. The attainment of adequate brain tension of an anaesthetic depends upon the balance between the rate of entry of anaesthetic into the blood and its removal into other tissues.

The course of an anaesthetic can in theory be divided into three phases. During induction, the anaesthetic agent is being taken up into body tissues across the concentration gradients that exist. Eventually, tissues come into equilibrium with the inspired tension, and in the maintenance phase there is no net uptake of anaesthetic. During recovery, inspired tension is reduced to zero and elimination of anaesthetic occurs across the reversed tension gradient. In practice, because of the long time constants of some body tissues, equilibrium is rarely achieved during clinical anaesthesia. Uptake of most anaesthetic agents continues for many hours, albeit at a low rate.

The rate of uptake of an anaesthetic agent, and thus the duration of induction, is determined by the rate at which the alveolar anaesthetic tension approaches the inspired anaesthetic tension. Small and negligible differences exist between the tension of an anaesthetic in alveolar gas, arterial blood, and brain, but because of dilution large differences can exist between inspired and alveolar tensions. The important factors that determine alveolar anaesthetic tension are the solubility of the agent in blood, the inspired tension, alveolar ventilation, cardiac output, and venous anaesthetic levels.

Blood solubility

This is best expressed in terms of the partition coefficient of the agent between blood and gas at body temperature (*Table 4.1*). Agents with a high blood/gas

Table 4.1 Chemical structures and physical properties of the inhalational anaesthetics

Drug	*Molecular formula*	*Molecular weight*	*Boiling point at 760 mmHg (101.3 kPa), °C*	*Saturation vapour pressure at 20°C*	*Partition coefficients at 37°C*		*MAC, % v/v*
					Blood/gas	*Oil/gas*	
Chloroform	$CHCl_3$	119.4	61.2	160	8.4	256	*
Cyclopropane	C_3H_6	42.1	−32.86	4800	0.46	11.8	9.2
Diethyl ether	$(C_2H_5)_2O$	74.1	34.6	442	12.1	65	1.92
Enflurane	$CHFClCF_2—O—CF_2H$	184.5	56.5	171.8	1.9	96	1.68
Ethyl chloride	C_2H_5Cl	64.5	13.1	988	3.0	Not known	*
Ethylene	C_2H_4	28.0	−103.7	†	0.41	1.28	*
Fluroxene	$CF_3CH_2—O—C_2H_3$	126.0	43.2	286	1.37	47.7	3.4
Isoflurane	$CF_3CHCl—O—CF_2H$	184.5	48.5	239.5	1.4	91	1.15
Halothane	$CF_3CHClBr$	197.4	50.2	243.3	2.3	224	0.75
Methyoxyflurane	$CHCl_2CF_2—O—CH_3$	165.0	104.8	22.8	12.0	970	0.16
Nitrous oxide	N_2O	44.0	−88.5	38760	0.47	1.4	110.0
Trichloroethylene	C_2HCl_3	131.4	86.7	64.5	9.15	970	*
Vinyl ether	$(C_2H_3)_2O$	70.1	28.3	553	2.8	58	*

* Not yet determined in man.
† Above critical temperature (9.9°C); critical pressure is 50.5 atm. SVP at 20°C is therefore undeterminable.

partition coefficient are removed in large quantities from alveoli by pulmonary capillary blood, reducing the mass and therefore the tension of agent left in the alveoli. As arterial blood is in near tension equilibrium with the alveoli, blood and brain tensions thus rise slowly. In contrast, insoluble agents, such as nitrous oxide and cyclopropane, are removed in only small quantities from the alveoli. Alveolar tension thus rapidly approaches inspired tension and induction of anaesthesia is rapid.

Inspired tension

The prolonged induction phase seen with soluble agents may be shortened to some extent by initially increasing the inspired anaesthetic tension. In this way an

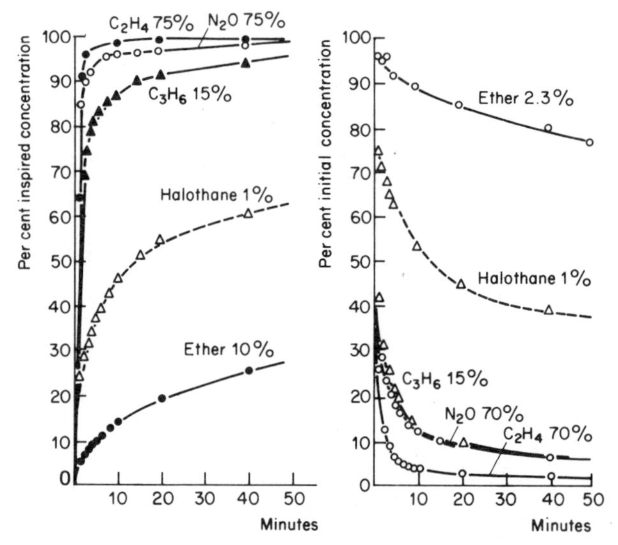

Figure 4.1 Differences between anaesthetics in the rate at which alveolar concentration approaches that inspired. The curves on the left represent induction, and those on the right, recovery. The actual inspired concentration during induction is noted on the respective curves. Alveolar concentrations at the start of recovery are noted on the respective curves. The curves for recovery assume complete tissue equilibration. (From Papper and Kitz, 1963.)

adequate blood tension can be attained long before equilibrium between inspired and alveolar tensions has occurred. Because of the complexities of pulmonary gas exchange, the rate of uptake of an anaesthetic is not a simple function of its inspired tension. This is discussed in the concentration effect below (*Figure 4.1*).

Alveolar ventilation

An increase in alveolar ventilation, by increasing the mass of anaesthetic presented to the lung, will increase the rate of uptake. This factor is of greater importance with soluble agents. Blood is so readily saturated with insoluble agents that the availability of an increased mass of anaesthetic has little effect on the rate of uptake, whereas with soluble agents blood leaving the lungs generally has a largely unsatisfied anaesthetic capacity. Doubling alveolar ventilation during diethyl ether anaesthesia will nearly halve the duration of the induction phase.

Cardiac output

An increase in cardiac output allows more agent to be removed from the alveoli by blood and thus increases the inspired–alveolar tension gradient. When cardiac output is reduced, less anaesthetic is removed from the lungs and alveolar tension approaches inspired tension more rapidly. However, these effects of changes in cardiac output are seen only in the early stages of induction. When cardiac output rises a greater mass of agent is extracted from the alveoli and presented to the tissues, which become saturated more rapidly. The concomitant rise in venous anaesthetic level limits further anaesthetic uptake in the alveoli. During clinical anaesthesia changes in cardiac output are often accompanied by widespread alterations in the distribution of blood, which can have complex and often unforeseeable effects on anaesthetic uptake.

Venous anaesthetic levels

The amount of anaesthetic that is removed from the alveoli is also a function of the arteriovenous anaesthetic tension difference. At equilibrium, arterial and mixed venous tensions are equal and uptake is zero. Arteriovenous difference is due to tissue uptake and depends upon the solubility of an agent in tissues and upon tissue blood flow. Tissue/blood coefficients of anaesthetics vary throughout the body, being highest in lipid tissues. Body tissues can be divided into three compartments. Initially, tissues of the vessel-rich group play a dominant part in uptake. These tissues comprise the brain, heart, kidney, hepatoportal system, and endocrine glands. Uptake by muscle and skin proceeds at a slower rate. The vessel-poor tissues consist predominantly of fat which, because of its poor blood supply and its affinity for anaesthetic agents, often continues to take up anaesthetic for many hours after all other body tissues have reached equilibrium.

Concentration and second gas effects

A relationship exists between the rate at which the alveolar tension of any agent approaches the inspired tension and the actual inspired concentration. In theory, the rate of uptake of all agents is equally rapid when they are administered in 100 per cent concentration; under these circumstances anaesthetic uptake will still leave a 100 per cent anaesthetic mixture within the lung and will not reduce the alveolar tension. With lower inspired tensions, the duration of the uptake phase is progressively increased. When uptake of an agent occurs from the lung, alveolar volume is potentially reduced and additional gaseous inflow occurs in order to maintain intrapulmonary pressure. The effect on the rate of uptake of this additional inspiratory flow is greatest with high inspired anaesthetic concentrations. This ‘concentration effect’ is most marked with agents that can be given over a wide range of inspired concentrations and which can be taken up in large volumes, such as diethyl ether and nitrous oxide.

Closely related to the concentration effect is the ‘second gas effect’. Removal of anaesthetic from the alveoli by the uptake process increases the fractional concentration and therefore the tension of other components of alveolar gas. Uptake of one agent can therefore increase the rate of uptake of a second agent.

A mathematical treatment of many of the factors concerned in anaesthetic uptake can be obtained from the general equation describing the determinants of the alveolar concentration of an inhaled gas. This states that

$$F_{A_x} = F_{I_x} - \frac{\dot{V}_x}{\dot{V}_A}$$

where F_{I_x} *and* F_{A_x} are the fractional concentrations of gax x in inspired and alveolar gas, respectively; $\dot{V}_x$ is the uptake of gas x per unit time; and $\dot{V}_A$ is the alveolar ventilation per unit time. When x represents any anaesthetic, this equation shows that the alveolar concentration will be reduced if uptake increases or if alveolar ventilation falls. Uptake in this equation is a function of blood solubility, cardiac output, and venous anaesthetic levels. This equation does not describe the concentration or second gas effects.

Rubber solubility

Anaesthetic agents are most commonly administered to patients through circuits with rubber conducting pathways. Anaesthetic solubility in rubber may have an important practical influence upon clinical anaesthetic administration. Rubber/gas partition coefficients of the commoner anaesthetic agents are given in *Table 4.2*. During the administration of agents with high rubber solubilities, uptake by the rubber of the circuit may produce large initial differences between the anaesthetic concentration in the inflowing gas and that leaving the circuit and reaching the patient. These differences are maximal at the beginning of administration, and long periods of time may be required for equilibrium within the circuit to occur. The rubber components of a circuit saturated with an agent may give up that agent during a subsequent administration and produce untoward effects. These effects of rubber solubility are minimal with nitrous oxide and cyclopropane, of some significance in the case of halothane, and of considerable importance in the administration of trichloroethylene and methoxyflurane.

Table 4.2 Rubber solubility of some anaesthetics

Anaesthetic	*Rubber/gas partition coefficient at 20°C*
Nitrous oxide	1.2
Cyclopropane	6.6
Diethyl ether	58
Isoflurane	62
Enflurane	74
Halothane	120
Methoxyflurane	530
Trichloroethylene	830

Excretion of volatile anaesthetics

During elimination of volatile anaesthetics by the lung, the factors concerned in uptake operate in a reverse fashion. Alveolar tension is the resultant of the amount of agent released to the alveoli from blood and the amount removed by alveolar ventilation. Insoluble agents are readily released from blood and removed by alveolar ventilation, leading to rapid recovery. Soluble agents, because of their affinity for blood, are removed from the body more slowly.

The duration of the recovery phase is also related to the mass of anaesthetic present in body tissues, and will thus be affected by the duration of anaesthesia and the tissue solubility of the agent. High fat solubility of an agent may lead to the presence during recovery of a large reservoir of anaesthetic which, because it lies in poorly perfused tissues, is released only slowly to the blood. For example, nitrous oxide and cyclopropane have nearly identical blood/gas partition coefficients, and recovery after a brief administration takes a similar time with both agents. If administration is prolonged, the higher lipid solubility of cyclopropane becomes a more dominant factor, and recovery from this agent is then much slower than after nitrous oxide given for a similar period of time.

Metabolism of volatile anaesthetics

General anaesthetics have classically been considered to be inert substances, undergoing no chemical reaction in the body and being excreted in an unchanged form. The lungs are the major route of elimination, small amounts of unchanged agent appearing in the urine, sweat, and other secretions. In the past decade, strong evidence has accumulated to show that many volatile agents undergo biotransformation. By the use of radioactive isotopes of volatile agents and low temperature whole-body autoradiography, volatile and nonvolatile metabolic products of inhaled anaesthetics have been demonstrated in experimental animals.

Biotransformation of drugs in general is a process aimed at reducing the lipid solubility and increasing the water solubility of administered substances. It is not surprising that the inhalational anaesthetics, which have a high lipid affinity and in the main are hydrophobic, should undergo some transformation in the body. As with all drugs, biotransformation of anaesthetics occurs in the liver and is effected by microsomal enzymes, especially cytochrome P450. The commonest transformation is an oxidation resulting in ether cleavage or dehalogenation. Halothane appears to be an exception in undergoing reduction as well as oxidation. Initial transformation is followed by conjugation to form glucuronides. The fraction of anaesthetic transformed varies greatly between agents, ranging from nearly 50 per cent for methoxyflurane to 0.2 per cent for isoflurane, and probably less than 0.01 per cent for nitrous oxide.

Enzyme induction by phenobarbitone increases the rate of breakdown. General anaesthetics themselves induce liver enzymes and repeated exposure to low concentration may lead to an increased degree of metabolism. Metabolic transformation of anaesthetics is reduced by treatment with non-specific enzyme inhibitors such as SKF 525A. There is some evidence to show that high concentrations of anaesthetics inhibit their own biotransformation, and conversely exposure to subanaesthetic concentrations of inhalational agents is associated with a greatly increased rate of metabolism.

Biotransformation of inhalational anaesthetics may have important clinical implications. The formation of chloral hydrate and trichloroethanol during trichloroethylene metabolism may contribute to the prolonged effect of this agent. The nephrotoxicity of methoxyflurane is related to the liberation of inorganic fluoride during metabolism of this compound. The lethal results of prolonged exposure of a variety of experimental animals to fluroxene is due to the production of trifluoroethanol. It has been conjectured that hepatis following halothane may be due to production of a genetically determined reductive toxic metabolite.

Evaluation of anaesthetic potency

The term potency can be used to refer to different attributes of anaesthetic agents. A potent agent may be considered as one that produces its effects in low concentrations. By this definition methoxyflurane and trichloroethylene are the most potent and nitrous oxide the least potent inhalational agents. This use of the term ignores the lengthy period for which these 'potent' agents may have to be administered in order to attain their low effective blood concentrations. In a different sense, potency may refer to the rapidity with which anaesthesia can be produced. Here nitrous oxide and cyclopropane would be considered as agents of high but equal potency, while methoxyflurane and trichloroethylene would be classed as agents of low potency. A third method of comparison is to class as potent those anaesthetics capable of producing deep anaesthesia down to Stage IV of the Guedel classification. By this definition nitrous oxide becomes the least potent of all agents.

Because of the obvious confusion which can arise when the term is used in different ways, any statement of anaesthetic potency should define the criteria by which potency is being evaluated.

Further confusion is possible when attempting to define the concentrations of inhalational agents required to induce and maintain anaesthesia. The inspired concentration, which is easy to measure, often bears a complex and unknown relationship to alveolar and arterial concentrations. The concentration required for induction often depends upon how much time it is considered desirable to spend in going through this phase: induction of anaesthesia with diethyl ether can be achieved with equally effective end-results using inspired concentrations varying from 5 to 50 per cent. Surgical anaesthesia has no sharp end-points, and difficulties arise in determining the concentrations necessary to produce this stage of anaesthesia.

Many of these problems have been simplified by the use of the concept of 'minimum alveolar (anaesthetic) concentration' (MAC). This is defined as the alveolar concentration of an agent which will prevent response to specified stimuli in 50 per cent of subjects. MAC can be converted into a partial pressure (as a percentage of 1 atm) and then represents the tension of anaesthetic at its site of action in the brain. Eger, Saidman and Brandstater (1965) found consistent and reproducible MAC levels for a number of agents in dogs, using skin clamping and electrical stimuli to evoke responses. Lower but equally consistent values were obtained in man when skin incision was used as a stimulus. Average MAC values for most of the commonly used agents are given in *Table 4.1*.

The MAC is unaffected by duration of anaesthesia and changes in $P\text{aco}_2$ or $P\text{ao}_2$ over a wide range. It is affected by age; halothane has an MAC of 1.08 per cent in infants and 0.64 per cent at age 81 years. MAC is affected by drugs that alter CNS catecholamine levels: D-amphetamine raises MAC while catecholamine depleters such as reserpine reduce it. MAC is also affected by temperature. Other inhalational anaesthetics reduce the MAC of any agent in a simple subtractive manner. The addition of 70 per cent nitrous oxide reduces the MAC of halothane and methoxyflurane by about 60 per cent. Narcotic analgesics lower MAC in a non-additive fashion. Premedication with 10 mg of morphine lowers the MAC of halothane by about 7 per cent.

Pharmacology

While the various anaesthetics each have their own pharmacological actions, certain generalizations may be made concerning the physiological changes produced by anaesthesia, whatever the causative agent.

CENTRAL NERVOUS SYSTEM

The paralysis of function of the CNS begins at the cortical level and descends, but fortunately irregularly. The order is cortex, basal ganglia, cerebellum, spinal cord (sensory then motor), medulla. In the medulla the respiratory centre is completely depressed before the vasomotor centre, but only just before with some anaesthetics. It must not be thought that any given level of the CNS is fully depressed before any depression of the next begins; all levels suffer some effect right from the start of anaesthesia, although in some circumstances there may be a phase of reflex stimulation of some areas associated with the depression of other controlling influences. At a neurophysiological level anaesthetics appear to exert most of their influence at the thalamic level, inhibiting transmission from the periphery to the brain (Angel and Knox, 1970). Multisynaptic pathways are no more sensitive to the effects of anaesthetics than those pathways with few synapses. In deep anaesthesia convulsions may occur. This uncommon effect has been reported during the use of all the common anaesthetics with the exception of the barbiturates. The mechanism is not clear, but cerebral cell hypoxia and other systemic biochemical derangements may be important factors.

A point with important practical consequences is the implication of a 'safety margin'. Usually this is stated to be wide if the concentration of anaesthetic required to cause medullary paralysis and cardiac arrest is great compared with the concentration required for surgical anaesthesia, but such a fascination with figures does not take into consideration the relative ease and rapidity with which concentrations may be increased for some anaesthetics without the signs of severely deepening anaesthesia being very obvious (for example, halothane).

AUTONOMIC SYSTEM

Autonomic balance. At first there may be stimulation, later there is normally depression of this system, but the action on the sympathetic and parasympathetic is often unequal; thus the tone of one or the other may predominate and there may appear to be either a parasympathomimetic or sympathomimetic effect. During prolonged light anaesthesia with agents such as halothane and fluroxene recovery occurs from the initial depression of cardiac function, which has been ascribed to a β-stimulant effect of these agents.

Gastrointestinal tract. Nausea and vomiting, much more frequent during recovery than during induction, are mainly of central origin. Irritant vapours of ether or chloroform, for instance, if swallowed may contribute by gastric stimulation. These agents are also particularly potent as depressors of gastrointestinal motility and secretion.

CARDIOVASCULAR EFFECTS

In general, the deeper the anaesthesia the more obvious is the depression of the vasomotor centre, but the precise cardiovascular effects of general anaesthetics vary very much from substance to substance. All anaesthetics cause progressive myocardial depression with increasing dose, but in the intact animal this may be completely masked by sympathetic over-activity, for example during ether anaesthesia or as a response to hypercapnia. Intravenous barbiturates can also cause myocardial depression.

All of the halogenated hydrocarbons and cyclopropane increase cardiac irritability. Cardiac irregularities are not uncommon during their use, and ventricular fibrillation can occur, especially in the presence of an increased carbon dioxide tension, hypoxia, or an increase in circulating adrenaline.

Heart rate. In the first two stages of anaesthesia the rate is increased, but the better the preanaesthetic sedation and the shorter the duration of these early stages, the less marked is the over-activity of the sympathetic nervous system. Even in surgical anaesthesia ether usually causes an increased heart rate by sympathetic stimulation, while halothane generally causes a slow rate, probably by increased vagal tone or sensitivity to the vagus.

Cardiac output and the distribution of blood flow. Cardiac output is decreased during anaesthesia, apart from a temporary rise during induction if accompanied by excitement. Total cardiac output may fall to 3 ℓ/min or less. Local autoregulatory mechanisms ensure that cerebral and coronary blood flows are well maintained. In early and light anaesthesia, in the absence of oligaemia or dehydration, there is a marked increase in skin blood flow and, with most anaesthetics, in muscle flow also. This is probably due to a central depression of vasomotor tone although certain anaesthetics, notably chloroform and halothane, have a direct vasodilator action as well as a central effect. Both liver and kidney suffer considerable reductions in flow in deep anaesthesia, and oliguria or even suppression of urine formation can occur. However, during 'balanced' anaesthesia, urine flow can easily be maintained by adequate parenteral fluid therapy. Since the total peripheral resistance is not markedly reduced, the splanchnic vessels, by inference, are believed to be constricted, and the flow reduced. A major determinant of this is the degree of sympathetic over-activity induced by the anaesthetic agent.

Blood pressure. Light surgical anaesthesia may usually be achieved with blood pressure relatively unaltered or slightly reduced. Occasional increases may be due to carbon dioxide retention or stimulation of the too lightly anaesthetized patient. Falls in pressure during light anaesthesia may be due to unrecognized hypovolaemia. Progressive hypotension during prolonged light anaesthesia is often due to unreplaced fluid loss. Deepening the level of anaesthesia tends to cause a fall in blood pressure, often proportionate to depth, and due to progressive vasomotor paralysis and direct myocardial depression.

RESPIRATION

All anaesthetics depress the medullary respiratory centre when present in sufficient concentration and reduce its sensitivity to carbon dioxide, but there are variations within the pattern of steadily increasing depression, and with some anaesthetics there are even phases of stimulation. Ether increases respiratory minute volume as far as Plane 2 of Stage III, although reflex breath-holding due to irritation from too high a concentration can easily occur in Stages I and II; cyclopropane depresses the thoracic and abdominal components of respiration equally rather than the thoracic first; nitrous oxide may appear to be a respiratory stimulant but stimulation during its administration may be due to asphyxia.

The tendency for respiration to be shallower and more rapid in anaesthesia is often ascribed to effects upon the lung stretch receptors which inhibit inspiration, and upon intrathoracic receptors which initiate inspiration when expiration occurs (deflation reflex). Animal experiments (Whitteridge and Bülbring, 1944) showed that the commonly used volatile and gaseous anaesthetics made the stretch receptors more sensitive, and often stimulated the deflation reflex too. Trichloroethylene was particularly active on both reflexes and this may account for the rapid shallow respiration seen with it. The clinical significance of these observations is debatable, as these reflexes are much less effective in man than in other species.

In light thiopentone or cyclopropane anaesthesia, sudden laryngeal spasm may occur, probably accompanied by bronchoconstriction. This spasm, which relaxes only when asphyxia becomes marked, appears to be due to a grossly increased sensitivity of laryngeal reflex activity, but whether in the afferent or efferent limb of the reflex arc is not known. In contrast, ether, in spite of its irritant property, does not produce the same quality of spasm and, moreover, has a weak sympathomimetic action in dilating the bronchial tree. Excessive salivation and bronchial secretion may occur with irritant anaesthetics, especially during induction.

Some hypoxaemia exists for hours or days after anaesthesia and surgery; the causes are many, and include the site of operation, the degree of pain, and changes in ventilation/perfusion relationships. Although atropine premedication has been alleged to be a factor, there is little evidence that this complex of changes is related to a specific pharmacological effect of any of the drugs used in anaesthesia. It is related to pre-existing disease, age, and the nature of the operation, and probably reflects a continuation after operation of existing impairment of gas exchange in the lungs.

METABOLISM

Metabolism is depressed during anaesthesia, oxygen uptake and carbon dioxide output by tissues falling to basal levels. Biochemical changes which can often be demonstrated during anaesthesia are usually the result of concomitant effects of the agents being administered. Deranged carbohydrate metabolism occurring during administration of diethyl ether is due to stimulation of the sympathetic system by this agent. Non-respiratory acidosis during deep anaesthesia is usually a result of reduced tissue perfusion.

TEMPERATURE

The hypothalamic regulation of heat loss is depressed and body temperature varies with the environment; hypothermia or hyperthermia can result. Serious loss of heat may occur in newborn infants; this may give rise to difficulties in the re-establishment of adequate ventilation after surgery (Calvert, 1962). Hyperthermia is particularly dangerous in older children who are febrile; when such children are atropinized, the use of ether is very liable to cause convulsions.

ELECTROLYTE AND WATER BALANCE

Pituitary and adrenocortical systems appear to be affected in such a way that there is retention of water and sodium in the body and a loss of potassium following anaesthesia. This is mostly due to the stress of surgical trauma.

KIDNEY FUNCTION

There are varying degrees of oliguria resulting from renal vasoconstriction, decreased glomerular filtration, and increased tubular reabsorption. Provided that renal blood flow is unimpaired, glomerular function quickly returns to normal after operation. Increased tubular reabsorption of water usually persists for 36–48 hours but may continue for several days in the elderly. Methoxyflurane causes a high output renal failure, which is due to an effect on the distal tubule of inorganic fluoride released by hepatic metabolism.

LIVER FUNCTION

All anaesthetics depress liver function, especially if anoxia, hypercarbia, or hypotension are allowed to occur during their administration. The halogenated hydrocarbons can cause liver damage, the severity of which depends on the nutritional state of the liver cells. Some agents, for example chloroform, appear more toxic than others, although much of the difference can be attributed to the aggravating effect of physiological disturbances that commonly accompany their administration. Unpredictable liver damage is occasionally reported unrelated to dose or any other factor and this has been ascribed to a sensitivity reaction. This has been most frequently reported after halothane. While some cases have had features consistent with such a view, many have been indistinguishable from random viral hepatitis. Postoperative liver damage has been reported after the use of most anaesthetics, including spinal block. In many cases the cause could be accounted for by other factors, but in some the anaesthetic itself has been held responsible. The production of toxic metabolites, possibly genetically determined, may be the mechanism.

VOLUNTARY MUSCLE

With most anaesthetics the degree of relaxation of voluntary muscle depends entirely on depression of the CNS, but with ether there is a curare-like effect at the myoneural junction and the effects of tubocurarine and other non-depolarizing relaxants are potentiated. Halothane has little effect on myoneural transmission, but potentiates the action of competitive muscle relaxants.

UTERUS

In labour, concentrations of anaesthetics that are merely analgesic do not affect uterine action. Halothane and chloroform cause relaxation of uterine muscle to such an extent as to make their use unsuitable when uterine activity is desirable. Enflurane and trichloroethylene do not appear to relax the uterus in light planes of surgical anaesthesia.

TRANSPLACENTAL PASSAGE

All of the general anaesthetics can cross the placental barrier and reach the fetus, giving degrees of depression proportional to their concentration.

Anaesthetic hazards

The dangers to the patient of drugs used to produce anaesthesia are obvious. While the introduction of agents with fewer side effects and the better understanding of the use of these agents have greatly reduced the hazards of general anaesthesia, constant care must be exercised in the use of these potent and potentially lethal drugs. In recent years increasing interest has been paid to the potential relationships between the metabolism of anaesthetic agents and their toxicity. Several agents – chloroform, methoxyflurane and fluroxene, for example – are known to have toxic effects directly attributable to products of their metabolic transformation. Chloroform is a good example of an agent for which the end-products of metabolism are harmless, but intermediate metabolic products are capable of causing tissue damage. A low level of metabolic transformation is now considered a highly desirable attribute of any new inhalational anaesthetic.

Anaesthetic drugs are potentially hazardous, not to the patient alone but to all who may be exposed to them. Addiction to inhalational anaesthetics is rare but well recognized, and virtually all agents have been implicated in such addiction. Trichloroethylene addiction is commoner among workers in industries where this agent is used as a solvent than in personnel with access to this drug through medical practice.

The atmosphere of operating theatres may contain measurable concentrations of inhalational anaesthetics and these concentrations correlate well with blood levels in staff working in such theatres (Hallén, Ehrner-Samuel and Thomason, 1970). Evidence has been produced which suggests a higher rate of lymphatic, reticuloendothelial, and other malignancies among anaesthetists and anaesthetic nurses than in comparable groups of subjects not exposed to anaesthetic agents (Bruce *et al.*, 1968; Corbett *et al.*, 1973; Cohen *et al.*, 1974). Similarly, there have been several reports suggesting an increased incidence of spontaneous abortion among female anaesthetists and operating theatre nurses (Askrog and Harvold, 1970; Cohen, Bellville and Brown, 1971), and an increased risk of congenital malformations and twin births both in groups of persons occupationally exposed to anaesthetics and in the wives of male anaesthetists. Liver disease (other than serum hepatitis) occurred nearly twice as often among anaesthetists as among paediatricians. Similar findings occurred in a group of dentists chronically exposed to anaesthetics, compared with dentists with limited exposure (Cohen *et al.*, 1975).

Inhalational anaesthetics in small doses would be expected to have deleterious effects on mental performance, and Bruce and Bach (1976) have shown such effects in volunteers with concentrations as low as 50 ppm of nitrous oxide and 1 ppm of halothane. Others (Smith and Shirley, 1976) have failed to show effects on mental performance of these agents in concentrations 10–15 times greater than those used by Bruce and Bach.

Considerable controversy surrounds these findings of potential adverse effects of anaesthetics. No causal relationship has been established between increased morbidity in operating theatre personnel and their spouses and inhalational anaesthetics. Because many of the studies involve low numbers of cases, their statistical evaluation is open to criticism. Vessey (1978), reviewing the epidemiological evidence, concluded that there was reasonable evidence of a moderate increase in the risk of spontaneous abortion among females exposed to anaesthetic atmospheric pollution, but no convincing evidence of any other hazard. However, while many have claimed adverse effects of measurable concentrations of inhalational anaesthetics being present in operating theatres and their environs, no-one has claimed that this is an advantageous or desirable state, and there is some logic in taking steps, such as improved air conditioning and scavenging of waste anaesthetic gases, to reduce their concentrations.

Allison, A. C. and Nunn, J. F. (1968) Effects of general anaesthetics on microtubules. A possible mechanism of anaesthesia. *Lancet,* **2,** 1326

Angel, A. and Knox, G. V. (1970) The effect of anaesthesia on units in the thalamic reticular formation. *Journal of Physiology,* **210,** 167P

Askrog, V. F. and Harvold, B. (1970) Teratogen effekt af inhalationanaestetika. *Nordisk Medicin,* **83,** 498

Bruce, D. L. and Bach, M. J. (1976) Effects of trace anaesthetic gases on behavioural performance of volunteers. *British Journal of Anaesthesia,* **48,** 871

Bruce, D. L., Eide, K. A., Linde, H. W. and Eckenhoff, J. E. (1968) Causes of death among anesthesiologists: a 20-year survey. *Anesthesiology,* **29,** 565

Calvert, D. G. (1962) Inadvertent hypothermia in paediatric surgery and a method for its prevention. *Anaesthesia,* **17,** 29

Cohen, E. N., Bellville, J. W. and Brown, B. W. (1971) Anesthesia, pregnancy and miscarriage: a study of operating room nurses and anesthetists. *Anesthesiology,* **35,** 343

Cohen, E. N., Brown, B. W., Bruce, D. L., Cascorbi, H. F., Corbett, T. H., Jones, T. W. and Whitcher, C. (1974) Occupational disease among operating room personnel: a national study. *Anesthesiology,* **41,** 321

Cohen, E. N., Brown, B.W., Bruce, D. L., Cascorbi, H. F., Corbett, T. H., Jones, T.W. and Whitcher, C. (1975) A survey of anesthetic health hazards among dentists. *Journal of the American Dental Association,* **90,** 1291

Corbett, T. H., Cornell, R. G., Lieding, K. and Endres, J. L. (1973) Incidence of cancer among Michigan nurse anesthetists. *Anesthesiology,* **38,** 260

Eger, E. I., Lundgren, C., Muller, S. L. and Stevens, W. C. (1969) Anesthetic potencies of sulphur hexafluoride, carbon tetrachloride, chloroform and Ethrane in dogs: correlation with the hydrate and lipid theories of anesthetic action. *Anesthesiology,* **30,** 129

Eger, E. I., Saidman, L. J. and Brandstater, B. (1965) Minimum alveolar anesthetic concentration: a standard of anesthetic potency. *Anesthesiology,* **26,** 756

Ferguson, J. (1939) Use of chemical potentials as indices of toxicity. *Proceedings of the Royal Society, B,* **127,** 387

Hallén, B., Ehrner-Samuel, H. and Thomason, M. (1970) Measurements of halothane in the atmosphere of an operating theatre and in expired air and blood of the personnel during routine anaesthetic work. *Acta Anaesthesiologica Scandinavica,* **14,** 17

Halsey, M. J. and Wardley-Smith, B. (1975) Pressure reversal of narcosis produced by anaesthetics, narcotics and tranquillizers. *Nature,* **257,** 811

Halsey, M. J., Brown, F. F. and Richards, R. E. (1978) Perturbations of model protein systems as a basis for the central and peripheral mechanisms of general anaesthesia. In *Molecular Interactions and Activity in Proteins,* Ciba Foundation Symposium 60, p. 123. Amsterdam: Excerpta Medica

Halsey, M. J., Wardley-Smith, B. and Green, C. J. (1978) The pressure reversal of general anaesthesia — a multi-site expansion hypothesis. *British Journal of Anaesthesia,* **50,** 1091

Johnson, F. H. and Flagler, E. A. (1950) Hydrostatic pressure reversal of narcosis in tadpoles. *Science,* **112,** 91

Lever, M. J., Miller, K. W., Paton, W. D. M. and Smith, E. B. (1971) Pressure reversal of anaesthesia. *Nature,* **231,** 368

Miller, K. W., Paton, W. D. and Smith, E. B. (1967) The anaesthetic pressures of fluorine-containing gases. *British Journal of Anaesthesia,* **39,** 910

Miller, K. W., Paton, W. D. M., Smith, R. A. and Smith, E. B. (1973) The pressure reversal of general anaesthesia and the critical volume hypothesis. *Molecular Pharmacology,* **9,** 131

Miller, S. L. (1961) A theory of gaseous anaesthetics. *Proceedings of the National Academy of Sciences,* **47,** 1515

Nunn, J. F., Sharp, J. A. and Kimball, K. L. (1970) Reversible effect of an inhalational anaesthetic on lymphocyte mobility. *Nature,* **226,** 85

Papper, E. M. and Kitz, R. J. (Eds) (1963) *Uptake and Distribution of Anesthetic Agents,* p. 89. New York: McGraw-Hill

Pauling, L. (1961) A molecular theory of general anaesthesia. *Science,* **134,** 15

Saubermann, A. J. and Gallacher, M. L. (1973) Mechanisms of general anesthesia: failure of pentobarbital and halothane to depolymerise microtubules in mouse optic nerve. *Anesthesiology*, **38**, 25
Smith, G. and Shirley, A. W. (1976) Failure to demonstrate effects of low concentrations of nitrous oxide and halothane on psychomotor performance. *British Journal of Anaesthesia*, **48**, 274
Smith, R. A., Winter, P. M., Halsey, M. J. and Eger, E. I. (1975) Helium pressure produces a non-linear antagonism of argon or nitrogen anesthesia in mice. *American Society of Anesthesiologists Annual Meeting Scientific Abstracts*, 217
Vessey, M. P. (1978) Epidemiological studies of the occupational hazards of anaesthesia — a review. *Anaesthesia*, **33**, 430
Whitteridge, D. and Bülbring, E. (1944) Changes in activity of pulmonary receptors in anaesthesia and their influences on respiratory behaviour. *Journal of Pharmacology and Experimental Therapeutics*, **81**, 340

Halogenated hydrocarbon anaesthetics

The discovery of the anaesthetic properties of chloroform has been followed by the production of many halogenated hydrocarbons with useful anaesthetic properties. Chief among these are halothane and trichloroethylene. Ethyl chloride and chloroform itself are nowadays rarely used.

The substitution of halogen atoms for the alkyl hydrogen atoms in hydrocarbons usually leads to the production of compounds with enhanced narcotic activity. Increasing halogen substitution leads to increasing narcotic action, but when halogen substitution is continued to the total exclusion of hydrogen, narcotic activity declines. Thus, in the methane series, methyl chloride is a more potent narcotic than methane, and activity increases with increasing chlorine substitution to reach a maximum with chloroform. Carbon tetrachloride, however, is less potent than chloroform.

Increasing narcotic potency due to halogenation is accompanied by increased side effects, especially cardiac irritant and hepatotoxic effects. This again is well exemplified by the methane series, protoplasmic toxic effects increasing with increasing chlorine substitution to reach a maximum with carbon tetrachloride.

The pure bromo- and iodo-derivatives of hydrocarbons tend to be rapidly hydrolysed into the corresponding alcohol or re-converted into the parent hydrocarbon and are therefore of little clinical use. In the past, halogenation has been largely confined to the insertion of chlorine into hydrocarbon molecules. Most of the recently introduced anaesthetic agents have been produced by fluorine substitution, either alone or together with other halogens.

Chloroform

Chloroform (*BP*)
Chemical name: trichloromethane

```
      Cl
      |
H  —  C  —  Cl
      |
      Cl
```

PHYSICAL CHARACTERISTICS

Chloroform is a colourless volatile liquid with a specific gravity of 1.48; the vapour density is 4.12. While not flammable it is broken down by heat and light to form phosgene.

The anaesthetic properties of chloroform were discovered by Flourens in 1847 and in the same year it was used clinically by Simpson of Edinburgh and by his colleagues, Duncan and Keith. It enjoyed considerable popularity in the latter part of the nineteenth century, but increasing awareness of its toxic effects led, by the early part of this century, to its largely being supplanted by diethyl ether.

PHARMACOLOGY

Chloroform has acquired a fearsome reputation as a highly potent and highly dangerous anaesthetic, with a liability to cause death either from vagal cardiac arrest during induction or from ventricular fibrillation during maintenance. Much of this reputation could be ascribed to the uncontrolled administration of excessive inspired concentrations of chloroform to unprepared, hypoxic, and hypercapnic subjects. In most of its anaesthetic properties chloroform resembles halothane. Its higher blood solubility leads to a longer induction period than for halothane, and at equilibrium, concentrations of about the same levels for both agents are needed for maintenance. Chloroform has more cardiac irritant properties than most other inhalational agents. Waters (1951) recorded ventricular dysrhythmias in 20 out of 52 patients and also reported four cases of temporary cardiac arrest. Less dramatic cardiac effects were seen by Payne and Conway (1963), when chloroform was given from calibrated vaporizers, and three out of 25 patients developed ventricular dysrhythmias. Like most anaesthetic agents chloroform is a respiratory depressant.

The major disadvantage of chloroform is its effect on the liver, as severe liver damage can follow short exposures. In so-called delayed chloroform poisoning the effects of chloroform administration appear 24–48 hours after administration. There is centrilobular necrosis which, in severe cases, may extend to be mid-zonal or even massive. This form of liver damage is said to be more likely to occur in starved, dehydrated, and toxic patients or in those repeatedly exposed to chloroform. Liver damage due to chloroform differs from the rare non-specific liver damage due to halothane and other agents in being specific. In experimental animals this damage is greatly potentiated by enzyme-inducing agents and this suggests the presence of a toxic metabolite. Marked inhibition of liver microsomal enzymes has been found to occur (Hallén and Johansson, 1975), and stimulation of lipid peroxidation has been suggested as a major factor in chloroform toxicity (Slater and Sawyer, 1971). During chloroform breakdown the free radicals $:CCl_2$ and $\cdot CCl_3$ are formed, and it is these highly reactive intermediate products of metabolism which are responsible for tissue damage. Because of the danger of liver damage, and in spite of its cheapness, acceptable odour, non-flammability, and useful anaesthetic properties, there appear to be no indications for the use of chloroform when safer and equally effective agents are available.

Hallén, B. and Johansson, G. (1975) Inhalation anesthetics and cytochrome P-450-dependent reactions in rat liver microsomes. *Anesthesiology,* **43,** 35

Payne, J. P. and Conway, C. M. (1963) Cardiovascular, respiratory and metabolic changes during chloroform anaesthesia. *British Journal of Anaesthesia,* **35,** 588

Slater, T. F. and Sawyer, B. C. (1971) The stimulatory effects of carbon tetrachloride and other halogenoalkanes on peroxidative reactions in rat liver fractions *in vitro. Biochemical Journal,* **123,** 805

Waters, R. M. (Ed.) (1951) *Chloroform: A Study After 100 Years.* University of Wisconsin Press

Trichloroethylene

Trichloroethylene (*BP* and *USP*)

```
H   Cl
|   |
C═══C
|   |
Cl  Cl
```

PHYSICAL CHARACTERISTICS

Trichloroethylene is a colourless liquid with low volatility and an odour not unlike chloroform. The liquid has a specific gravity of 1.47 and a vapour density of 4.35. Trichloroethylene vapour is not flammable in the presence of air, but under certain conditions will ignite in the presence of oxygen in concentrations of 10–65 per cent. It is decomposed by alkalis and heat and breaks down to form a toxic and flammable substance, dichloroacetylene. This may break down further to phosgene and carbon monoxide, and therefore cannot be used with soda lime in closed circuits. It is supplied commercially with the addition of 1:10 000 of thymol as a stabilizing agent and coloured with Waxoline blue (1:200 000) for identification purposes.

Trichloroethylene, although described in 1864 and used as an anaesthetic in the USA by Jackson in 1934 and Striker in 1935, did not come into general use until 1941 following the work of Langton Hewer, since when it has been widely used. Recent fears as to the potential mutagenic effects of this agent have resulted in its being withdrawn as an anaesthetic in the USA.

PHARMACOLOGY

Nervous system. Its action on the CNS is the same as that of all general anaesthetics. Paralysis of the respiratory and vasomotor centres does not readily occur, and is extremely rare with the vapour concentrations normally employed in anaesthesia. There is some increase in vagal tone. It was at one time thought to have a specific paralysing action on the sensory fibres of the trigeminal nerve, but this has since been shown to be due to impurities in the vapour. Apart from its anaesthetic properties is is a powerful analgesic, used in midwifery and often effective in relieving the pain of trigeminal neuralgia. The utility of trichloroethylene as an analgesic is due to the high blood solubility of the agent. For this reason (and possibly also because of rapid metabolism) the first stage of anaesthesia can be maintained for long periods without consciousness or the ability to co-operate being lost.

Cardiovascular system. Depression of cardiac muscle is minimal and blood pressure is usually unchanged. The pulse rate is usually slower but cardiac irritability is increased. The sensitivity of the heart to adrenaline is increased. Dysrhythmias are rare during controlled ventilation but not uncommon during spontaneous ventilation when carbon dioxide accumulation is more common.

Respiratory system. Respiratory effects of trichloroethylene become prominent at any but the lightest planes of surgical anaesthesia. Tidal volume is decreased and respiratory rate increased. Tachypnoea with a rate of 40 breaths/min is common. Following the animal studies of Whitteridge and Bülbring (1944) it has become common to ascribe these respiratory effects to an increased sensitivity of the Hering–Breuer reflex mediated through stretch receptors in the alveoli and possibly deflation receptors in the small pulmonary arterioles. This reflex is weak in man. The respiratory effects of trichloroethylene are more likely to be central in origin, and represent in an exaggerated form the respiratory response evoked by the majority of inhalational anaesthetics. It has been fairly common practice to control the tachypnoea with small doses of pethidine. On the face of it, it seems unsound to treat respiratory inadequacy with a respiratory depressant, and an already raised P_{CO_2} may rise still further if this treatment is employed.

Alimentary system. There is no marked change in intestinal tone or salivary secretions.

Muscular system. Skeletal muscle tone is depressed, but to a much lesser extent than by ether and other general anaesthetics. There is little effect on plain muscle.

Liver and kidney function. There is some depression in function of these organs, but considerably less than that caused by ether or chloroform. Liver damage has been reported, but is rare.

Metabolism. There is little effect on normal metabolic processes, but acidosis following carbon dioxide retention is not uncommon. Nausea and vomiting are frequent, especially after prolonged administration.

Uterus and placenta. Trichloroethylene depresses uterine muscle during anaesthesia, but there is little effect when it is used in analgesic concentrations for short periods. It rapidly passes from the mother into the fetal circulation.

Fate in the body. Trichloroethylene differs from other inhalational anaesthetics in being chemically reactive and it is not surprising that it undergoes a significant degree of metabolic transformation. It is first oxidized to chloral hydrate and this is then either further oxidized to trichloroacetic acid or reduced to trichloroethanol (Kelley and Brown, 1974). Both chloral hydrate and trichloroethanol have hypnotic properties. Detectable concentrations of trichloroacetic acid are found in the urine up to 10 days after exposure. The transformation of trichloroethylene involves a rearrangement of its three chlorine atoms without release of chlorine. The degree of biotransformation of this compound is greater than with any other inhalational anaesthetic. Mapleson (1963) suggested that hepatic metabolism clears blood of 25 per cent of its trichloroethylene content.

ANAESTHETIC PROPERTIES

Although a powerful analgesic, trichloroethylene is a relatively weak anaesthetic and suitable only for the production of light anaesthesia. The vapour is non-irritant and induction with this agent is not unpleasant. It is usual, however, to induce anaesthesia with an intravenous induction agent or nitrous oxide.

No significant degree of muscular relaxation can be obtained with trichloroethylene. Normal doses of muscle relaxants may be used.

INDICATIONS

Trichloroethylene can be used for all operations where light anaesthesia is required. It is also used for the production of analgesia in obstetrics. The main advantages of this agent are freedom from explosion risk, marked analgesic properties, lack of irritation to the respiratory tract, and low cost. The overriding disadvantages are its respiratory effects and its failure to produce muscular relaxation. These disadvantages become less important when it is used to supplement light nitrous oxide–oxygen relaxant anaesthesia.

In the past trichloroethylene has also been used in the treatment of trigeminal neuralgia and angina pectoris.

DOSAGE AND ADMINISTRATION

On account of its low volatility the administration of trichloroethylene by the open mask method is unsatisfactory. It can, however, be used alone in the 'draw over' apparatus designed by Marrett, and as a supplement to nitrous oxide and oxygen in the Boyle's and similar anaesthetic machines. Vapour strengths of 0.2–1.5 per cent are required to produce light anaesthesia. The Tritec is a calibrated vaporizer delivering concentrations between 0.17 and 1.5 per cent of trichloroethylene.

Vaporizers used for obstetric analgesia, such as the Emotril and Tecota Mark VI, deliver accurate concentrations of either 0.35 or 0.5 per cent trichloroethylene in air.

PRECAUTIONS

Soda lime at a temperature above 60°C converts trichloroethylene into a toxic compound, dichloroacetylene, which may cause paralysis of cranial nerves; this agent must not, therefore, be used in a closed circuit with an absorber.

Tachypnoea, which will lead to carbon dioxide retention and possible hypoxia, must not be allowed to persist. If reducing the concentration of the vapour does not have the desired effect, ventilation must be controlled or the agent withdrawn and another one substituted.

Occasional extrasystoles are usually of no significance. Marked dysrhythmias are usually a sign of carbon dioxide retention and should be treated by a reduction of inspired concentration and if necessary institution of controlled ventilation. The use of a β-blocking agent, such as propranolol or practolol, is effective in controlling dysrhythmias, but usually unnecessary.

Prolonged trichloroethylene administration leads to a slow recovery from anaesthesia. This may be minimized by using low vapour concentrations and ceasing administration some time before the end of the surgical procedure.

Users of trichloroethylene may become addicted to the vapour. The incidence is probably not great, but it has occurred among industrial workers and even anaesthetists.

Overdose of trichloroethylene is characterized by cardiac dysrhythmias and tachypnoea. Adrenaline should not be administered to patients receiving trichloroethylene unless special precautions are taken (*see* page 324).

Kelley, J. M. and Brown, B. R. (1974) Biotransformation of trichloroethylene. *International Anesthesiology Clinics,* **12,** 85

Mapleson, W. W. (1963) Quantitative prediction of anesthetic concentrations. In *Uptake and Distribution of Anesthetic Agents,* Ch. 9, p. 104, Ed. Papper, E. M. and Kitz, R. J. New York: McGraw-Hill

Whitteridge, D. and Bulbring, E. (1944) Changes in activity of pulmonary receptors in anaesthesia and their influence on respiratory behaviour. *Journal of Pharmacology and Experimental Therapeutics,* **81,** 340

Halothane

Halothane (*BP* and *USP*)
Chemical name: 1-bromo-1-chloro-2, 2-trifluoroethane

```
     F    H
     |    |
F—C—C—Br
     |    |
     F   Cl
```

PHYSICAL CHARACTERISTICS

Halothane is a colourless liquid with a sweet, non-irritant odour. It has a specific gravity of 1.87 and a vapour density of 6.8. Halothane is non-flammable and non-explosive. Some decomposition occurs on exposure to light, but it is more stable in the presence of thymol 0.01 per cent w/w and when stored in amber glass bottles. It is unaffected by soda lime and can be used in a closed circuit. It is absorbed by rubber.

Stephen and Little (1961), Sadove and Wallace (1962), and Greene (1968) deal very fully with all aspects of the pharmacology and clinical use of halothane.

PHARMACOLOGY

Central nervous system. CNS depression follows the pattern of all general anaesthetics, but the stage of excitement is minimal and often absent. Paralysis of the vasomotor centre follows that of the respiratory centre much less rapidly than with chloroform, but more readily than with ether. Halothane is much less soluble in the phospholipids of brain cells than in the neutral fats of adipose tissue: this, together with its low blood/gas partition coefficient, accounts for the relatively rapid recovery of consciousness. A characteristic feature of the use of halothane in neurosurgical anaesthesia is an increase in cerebral blood flow (McDowall, 1967) and in intracranial pressure (Jennett *et al.*, 1969). This is more marked in the presence of an intracranial space-occupying lesion, and in association with hypoventilation.

Autonomic system. The sympathetic system is depressed more than the parasympathetic system; the tone of the latter therefore preponderates. Sympathetic ganglia are mildly blocked, and the block produced by hexamethonium and trimetaphan is potentiated. Mild β-stimulant effects of halothane have been demonstrated on the cardiovascular system.

Cardiovascular system. The outstanding effect of halothane on the cardiovascular system is a reduction in blood pressure proportional to the depth of anaesthesia. This hypotension reflects the myocardial depressant action of halothane. Eger and colleagues (1970) showed that during controlled ventilation halothane caused a reduction in cardiac output, stroke volume, and myocardial contractility, while right atrial pressure rose. Prolonged anaesthesia was associated with a recovery of cardiovascular function, due to a sympathetic stimulant action of halothane. Bahlman and colleagues (1972) found that during spontaneous ventilation there was much less cardiovascular depression than during controlled ventilation. This difference reflects the rise in carbon dioxide levels associated with spontaneous ventilation during halothane anaesthesia and a consequent β-adrenergic stimulation. During spontaneous ventilation, recovery of cardiovascular function with prolonged anaesthesia still occurred.

Bradycardia is not uncommon during induction and may be associated with hypotension; both may be reversed with small doses of atropine (0.2–0.3 mg). The most common dysrhythmias seen during halothane anaesthesia are nodal rhythm and ventricular extrasystoles. These often occur under deep anaesthesia with spontaneous ventilation and are related to the concomitant hypercapnia. Like other hydrocarbon anaesthetics halothane sensitizes the myocardium to the dysrhythmic effects of catecholamines.

Respiratory system. The usual respiratory response is a reduced tidal volume associated with an increased respiratory rate, resulting in a diminished alveolar ventilation. During light anaesthesia there may be no change or even a fall in the rate of breathing and the response is variable from patient to patient. Halothane does not provoke salivary or bronchial secretions, and coughing is less easily provoked and more quickly suppressed than is the case with diethyl ether or trichloroethylene.

Muscular system. There is no myoneural block in the cat: the effect of tubocurarine is potentiated, but that of suxamethonium is diminished. These actions are also clinically apparent in man. The potentiation of non-depolarizing relaxants by halothane is less than that produced by isoflurane and enflurane.

Renal function. Halothane has no particular effect on renal function as distinct from that of other anaesthetic agents.

Liver function. Since the introduction of halothane in 1956 there have been many reports alleging a causal relationship between the administration of this agent and postoperative hepatitis. Multiple exposures to halothane have been a common feature of many of these reports. It is well recognized that many factors may be involved when a patient develops postoperative jaundice, and in the past all the commonly used anaesthetics, including local anaesthetics, have been incriminated.

Concern as to the possible hepatotoxic effects of halothane led to a number of retrospective surveys, the largest of which was the United States National Halothane Study (Bunker, 1966), which analysed over 850 000 anaesthetics administered in 34 institutions. Eighty-two cases of fatal massive hepatic necrosis occurred, of which all but nine could be attributed to a recognizable cause: seven of these nine cases had halothane. Although the report gave a guarded conclusion, Dykes and Bunker (1970) commented that 'there was not a single patient in the National Halothane Study who was jaundiced after the administration of halothane, who died after a second administration, and who was found at autopsy to have suffered massive or intermediate hepatic necrosis'.

Since this large study a considerable amount of work has been carried out on the possible hepatotoxic effects of halothane, especially in relation to the metabolic products of halothane. Little advance has been made in the identification of a form of liver damage specific to halothane. Many studies have concentrated on enzyme changes following halothane administration. Thus Fee and his colleagues (1979), in a 3-year prospective study on patients exposed to halothane or enflurane, showed a greater incidence of increased liver enzyme activity following repeated halothane administration. Greater changes were seen in obese subjects, the suggestion being that relative tissue hypoxia in the obese may increase halothane toxicity. McLain, Sipes and Brown (1979) have produced an animal model of halothane hepatotoxicity, and demonstrated that hypoxia increases the rate of reductive metabolism of halothane with the production of reactive intermediates. The weight of evidence lends cautious support to the view that halothane hepatitis is a rare but reasonably well-proven clinical entity (Brown, 1979).

Uterus and placenta. The contractility of the uterus is inhibited rapidly by inspired concentrations of 2–3 per cent; the myometrium is presumably directly affected and regains its normal tone soon after withdrawal of halothane (Embrey, Garrett and Pryer, 1958).

Fate in the body. Compared with other common anaesthetic agents, halothane is relatively insoluble in blood. Even so, the arterial tension takes a considerable time to approach the inspired tension; it is only due to the fact that a sufficiently high vapour pressure exists at room temperature, relative to its potency, that induction can be made rapid by giving much higher concentrations during induction than are necessary for maintenance (over-pressure technique). The concentration in organs with a very rich blood supply, such as the heart and brain, closely follows arterial tensions. Areas with a poor blood supply and high solubility, such as adipose tissue, however, take up the anaesthetic for a considerable time, and it has been estimated that it would take 20–30 hours at a constant inspired tension for the whole body to come to equilibrium.

Halothane is metabolized in the body by hepatic microsomal enzymes. Both oxidative and reductive metabolic pathways exist. Dechlorination and debromination appear to be the initial steps in its breakdown. Cohen and colleagues (1975) isolated trifluoracetic acid, *N*-trifluoracetyl-2-aminoethanol and *N*-acetyl-L-cysteine from the urine of patients given halothane. Bromide has also been shown to be released, but negligible amounts of inorganic fluoride are formed. Enzyme induction and a consequent greater breakdown of halothane have been shown to occur after pretreatment with phenobarbitone, and followed repeated or chronic exposure to halothane. Metabolic pathways for halothane are rapidly saturated and its metabolism is depressed by high concentrations.

ANAESTHETIC PROPERTIES

Halothane is a potent inhalational anaesthetic. The deeper the level of anaesthesia, the greater the degree of respiratory depression and hypotension.

Induction is smooth and not unpleasant for the patient as the vapour is non-irritant, consciousness is quickly lost, and surgical anaesthesia can be produced in 2–5 minutes with little excitement; intubation is normally possible at this stage. Induction with a small dose of thiopentone followed by suxamethonium if intubation is necessary, however, is a more common practice, and it is more pleasant for the patient.

Maintenance of anaesthesia with vapour strengths of the order of 0.5–2 per cent provides good operative conditions. Respiration is usually quiet; a rapid respiratory rate is often a sign of overdose. Muscle relaxation is usually good, but the deep anaesthesia required to produce adequate relaxation for upper abdominal surgery is often accompanied by marked cardiovascular depression. The hypotension associated with halothane anaesthesia reduces capillary bleeding and gives a relatively bloodless field. The degree of hypotension will be dependent on the depth of anaesthesia and will also be affected by the patient's posture.

Other advantages claimed for halothane anaesthesia are suppression of salivary and bronchial secretions, suppression of sympathetic activity, and rapid recovery when the anaesthetic is withdrawn. The speed of recovery, however, is dependent on the concentration of the vapour employed and the length of administration, and can be considerably delayed if deep anaesthesia is maintained for long periods. Shivering may occur during recovery, and restlessness is not uncommon in the immediate postoperative period due to the poor analgesic action of the drug.

INDICATIONS

Since its introduction, halothane has been widely used for every type of operation. Until recently it was the most widely used volatile anaesthetic. Its use has now started to decline, due mainly to medicolegal fears. It is most useful in operations where considerable but not full muscular relaxation is required. Uraemia resulting from intrinsic renal disease is not a contraindication to its use.

DOSAGE AND ADMINISTRATION

Inspired concentrations of 2–3.5 per cent are necessary for induction and anaesthesia can be maintained with inspired concentrations of 0.5–2.5 per cent. The concentrations required will depend to a considerable extent on the degree of previous sedation, and whether nitrous oxide is used in the vaporizing gases. It may be given by the open drop method, by the OMV inhaler (with air), and by most of the anaesthetic machines in common use, the halothane fluid being placed in vaporizing bottles already fitted to the machine or special bottles designed for its use.

Calibrated vaporizers such as the Fluotec are recommended as they give accurate vapour concentrations under normal working conditions irrespective of temperature, flow-rate, and the amount of fluid in the vaporizer. Halothane can be used in a closed circuit, the vaporizer being either outside or inside the circuit; if the vaporizer is outside the circuit it must be capable of evolving 40–80 ml/min of halothane vapour with a fresh gas flow of 500 ml/min or less. For this purpose a Fluotec vaporizer calibrated to give 10 per cent halothane vapour has been used in the past. If the vaporizer is inside the circuit it will only be safe if it is relatively inefficient and has a small capacity; halothane concentration in the circuit is a function of the patient's minute volume. Dangerously high concentrations will be attained if ventilation is assisted or controlled.

PRECAUTIONS

Although, on rare occasions, halothane may cause liver damage, its use should not be prejudiced on this account. It is contraindicated in obstetrics when uterine tone must be preserved, for example caesarean section.

There is no evidence that liver damage is more likely in the presence of existing liver disease. In the present climate of opinion, however, an unexplained pyrexial illness, unexpected liver damage after halothane anaesthesia or a recent exposure to the drug would counsel against a second exposure.

It is recommended that the patient should be well atropinized before induction with halothane to decrease vagal tone; this will prevent bradycardia and a serious fall in blood pressure. Atropine 0.6–0.9 mg may be given in the normal way 30 minutes before operation, or 0.6 mg intravenously just before induction. Hyoscine is not effective in depressing the cardiac vagus in normal doses. Heavy sedation with morphine or its derivatives is inadvisable as they tend to cause an increase in respiratory depression and hypotension. Pethidine in a dose of 50–100 mg does not appear to have this effect. If hypotension associated with bradycardia occurs during anaesthesia, atropine 0.3 mg should be given intravenously. If the pulse rate is within normal limits and blood pressure falls unduly the inspired concentration of halothane should be reduced.

Should controlled ventilation be necessary, care must be taken that high concentrations of vapour are not forced into the patient's lungs. If the vaporizer is within the circuit it must be turned off before controlled ventilation is started.

Hypotensive agents, such as hexamethonium and trimetaphan, have been used with halothane, but it must be remembered that halothane potentiates their action and they must therefore be given cautiously. Adrenaline should not be given to patients during halothane anaesthesia, unless special precautions are taken (*see* page 324).

Bahlman, S. H., Eger, E. I., Halsey, M. J., Stevens, W. C., Shakespeare, T. F., Smith, N.T., Cromwell, T. H. and Fourcade, H. (1972) The cardiovascular effects of halothane in man during spontaneous ventilation. *Anesthesiology,* **36,** 494

Brown, B. R. (1979) Halothane hepatitis is a reasonably well-proved clinical entity. In *Controversy in Anesthesiology,* p. 31, Ed. Eckenoff, J. Philadelphia: W. B. Saunders

Bunker, J. P. (Chairman) (1966) Sub-committee on the National Halothane Study of the Committee on Anesthesia, NAS-NRC. Summary of the National Halothane Study. Possible association between halothane and postoperative hepatic necrosis. *Journal of the American Medical Association,* **197,** 775

Cohen, E. N., Trudell, J. R., Edmunds, H. N. and Watson, E. (1975) Urinary metabolites of halothane in man. *Anesthesiology,* **43,** 392

Dykes, M. H. M. and Bunker, J. P. (1970) Hepatotoxicity and anesthetics. *Pharmacology for Physicians,* **4,** 15

Eger, E. I., Smith, N. T., Stoelting, R. K., Cullen, D. J., Kadis, L.B. and Whitcher, C. E. (1970) Cardiovascular effects of halothane in man. *Anesthesiology,* **32,** 396

Embrey, M. P., Garrett, W. J. and Pryer, D. L. (1958) Inhibitory action of halothane on contractility of human pregnant uterus. *Lancet,* **2,** 1093

Fee, J. P. H. *et al.* (1979) A prospective study of liver enzyme and other changes following repeat administration of halothane and enflurane. *British Journal of Anaesthesia,* **51,** 1133

Greene, N. M. (1968) Halothane. *Clinical Anaesthesia,* **1,** 1

Jennett, W. B., Barker, J., Fitch, W. and McDowall, D. G. (1969) Effect of anaesthesia on intracranial pressure in patients with space-occupying lesions. *Lancet,* **1,** 61

McDowall, D. G. (1967) The effects of clinical concentrations of halothane on the blood flow and oxygen uptake of the cerebral cortex. *British Journal of Anaesthesia,* **39,** 186

McLain, G. E., Sipes, I. G. and Brown, B. R. (1979) An animal model of halothane hepatotoxicity: roles of enzyme induction and hypoxia. *Anesthesiology,* **51,** 321

Sadove, M. S. and Wallace, V. E. (1962) *Halothane.* Oxford: Blackwell

Stephen, C. R. and Little, D. M. (1961) *Halothane.* Baltimore: Williams and Wilkins

Ethyl chloride

Ethyl chloride (*BP* and *USP*)

```
   H   H
   |   |
H—C—C—Cl
   |   |
   H   H
```

PHYSICAL CHARACTERISTICS

Ethyl chloride is a gas at room temperature but is usually stored under slight pressure as a liquid in glass containers. The liquid has a specific gravity of 0.92 and the vapour a density of 2.23. It forms flammable mixtures with air (4–15 per cent), oxygen (4–67 per cent), and nitrous oxide (2–33 per cent). When the liquid is sprayed on to the skin the latent heat of vaporization is sufficient to cause refrigeration and local analgesia.

PHARMACOLOGY

The effects of ethyl chloride resemble those of chloroform. Its lower blood solubility allows for more rapid induction and recovery. The major problem in its administration is the difficulty in controlling inspired concentration. It is too volatile to be used in a conventional vaporizer and has commonly been given on an open mask. As excessively deep levels of anaesthesia may be attained very rapidly and uncontrollably this agent has no place in current anaesthetic practice.

Anaesthetic ethers

Since the introduction of diethyl ether as an anaesthetic in 1846, a large number of ethers have been found which have anaesthetic properties, although few have been clinically useful. Divinyl ether, methyl n-propyl ether, and ethyl vinyl ether all bear a close chemical resemblance to diethyl ether. Methoxyflurane, fluroxene, enflurane, and isoflurane are all fluorinated ethers. The search for new anaesthetic agents has in recent years concentrated on the methyl-ethyl ethers. Many clinically used ethers are flammable. As a class most ethers do not potentiate the arrhythmic effects of catecholamines. There is a tendency among the ethers to flammable properties, but this has been overcome in newer members of the class.

Diethyl ether

Anaesthetic ether (*BP*) and Ether (*USP*)

```
    H   H       H   H
    |   |       |   |
H — C — C — O — C — C — H
    |   |       |   |
    H   H       H   H
```

PHYSICAL CHARACTERISTICS

Diethyl ether is a colourless, highly volatile liquid with a not unpleasant pungent odour. Unlike most inhalational anaesthetics it is significantly soluble in water, its water/gas partition coefficient being 13.1. It has a specific gravity of 0.714 and a vapour density of 2.6. Diethyl ether is highly flammable and ignites at 154°C. Its vapour forms flammable mixtures with air (1.85–36.5 per cent), oxygen (2–82 per cent), and nitrous oxide (1.5–24 per cent). It is decomposed by air, light, and heat, the most important decomposition products being acetaldehyde and ether peroxide. Decomposition is retarded in the presence of copper or hydroquinone. It should be stored in a cool place in sealed opaque containers.

With the exception of nitrous oxide, ether is the oldest inhalational anaesthetic still in use. It was first used by Crawford Long in 1842 and by Morton in 1846, since when it has enjoyed considerable popularity, and for many years was the anaesthetic of choice for major surgery.

Nervous system. During induction of anaesthesia there is depression of the cortex, resulting in loss of many higher inhibitions, and the medulla and spinal cord, where both two-neurone arc (stretch) reflexes and multineurone arc (nociceptor) reflexes are depressed. Paralysis of the respiratory centre precedes that of the vasomotor centre by a considerable margin. There is stimulation of the sympathetic system, with an increase in circulating catecholamines.

Cardiovascular system. During light planes of diethyl ether anaesthesia there are usually only minor changes in blood pressure, cardiac output, and peripheral resistance. During deeper anaesthesia, myocardial depression and paralysis of the vasomotor and other vital centres may lead to circulatory failure. In Plane 3 of Stage II, 15 minutes of diethyl ether anaesthesia may cause as great a depression of blood pressure as 2 hours in Plane 2. Diethyl ether predisposes to early and extensive deterioration of the peripheral vascular compensatory mechanisms and a decrease in the tolerance to haemorrhage. Thus this agent does not afford the patient in shock or with haemorrhage a wide margin of safety.

The innocuous effects of light diethyl ether anaesthesia are due to the sympathetic stimulation produced by this agent. In the absence of a sympathetic response diethyl ether anaesthesia is associated with evidence of marked myocardial depression.

Respiratory system. Unlike other inhalational agents, diethyl ether produces respiratory stimulation until the deepest planes of surgical anaesthesia are reached. The cause of this stimulation is unknown; it does not appear to be related to the irritant effects of the agent or to catecholamine release. Arterial $P\text{CO}_2$ levels of 30 mmHg (4kPa) are commonly met during clinical diethyl ether anaesthesia. When the alveolar concentration of diethyl ether rises above 6 per cent respiratory depression usually ensues.

The vapour of diethyl ether is irritant to the respiratory tract. Laryngeal spasm is not uncommon during induction. Bronchial secretions are increased, but are prevented by the previous administration of adequate doses of atropine. Diethyl ether may be useful in some cases of asthma and bronchitis because of its property of producing bronchial muscle relaxation.

Alimentary system. Salivary and gastric secretions are increased at first, but are decreased during deep anaesthesia. Bowel movement is decreased, due in part to stimulation of dilator fibres and also to depression of plain muscle. The degree of handling of the viscera during operations is as important a factor, or more so, than the anaesthetic. Nausea and vomiting are common with diethyl ether, their incidence varying with the length of operation and the depth of anaesthesia.

Muscular system. Skeletal muscle tone is markedly reduced, especially during the deeper levels of anaesthesia. This is due mainly to depression of transmission at the neuromuscular junction by an action similar to that of curare. Tremors are sometimes noticed during light diethyl ether anaesthesia, but are unrelated to convulsions (*see* below). Plain muscle is also depressed.

Liver and kidney function. Liver function is depressed, and some impairment may persist for several days. Irreversible damage does not occur.

Renal vasoconstriction causes a reduction in renal plasma flow and therefore of glomerular filtration rate. A further tendency to oliguria is due to tubular reabsorption of water caused by raised levels of antidiuretic hormone.

Metabolism. Glycogen is mobilized by the liver, and hyperglycaemia follows. This effect is mediated by increased sympathetic activity. Some degree of metabolic acidosis may occur due to decreased tissue perfusion produced by increased sympathetic activity. Many of the changes in blood chemistry observed after diethyl ether, such as decreased serum bicarbonate, increased lactate, rise in lactate/pyruvate ratio, and decreased serum potassium, are qualitatively similar to those produced by physiological amounts of adrenaline.

Uterus and placenta. The pregnant uterus is not affected during light anaesthesia, but is relaxed during deep anaesthesia. Diethyl ether passes rapidly from mother to child and may cause depression of respiration in the infant.

Fate in the body. About 15 per cent of an inhaled dose of diethyl ether is metabolized in the liver, via acetaldehyde and ethanol, to carbon dioxide and water. There are no indications that the metabolites of diethyl ether exert any untoward toxic effects.

ANAESTHETIC PROPERTIES

Diethyl ether is a potent inhalational anaesthetic. Because of the high solubility of this agent in blood, induction is slow and may be further prolonged by breath-holding and coughing due to the irritant effect of the vapour. Muscular relaxation is good during deep anaesthesia. When light anaesthesia is used in association with muscle relaxants, smaller doses of non-depolarizing agents than usual are required because of the curare-like action of diethyl ether.

Respiration is often of a blowing or tugging nature during deep anaesthesia and is sometimes an embarrassment to the surgeon during upper abdominal surgery. This may be avoided by lightening anaesthesia, using a muscle relaxant, and controlling respiration. In the inadequately atropinized patient bronchial and salivary secretions are troublesome, but they can be inhibited by a further dose of atropine.

Capillary bleeding is more prominent during diethyl ether anaesthesia than in more modern forms of balanced anaesthesia. Coagulation time may be shortened by diethyl ether anaesthesia but the bleeding time is unchanged; the prothrombin time is somewhat prolonged. As with other general anaesthetic agents, there is a polymorphonuclear leucocytosis.

Recovery is slow after prolonged administration.

INDICATIONS

Since the introduction of the muscle relaxants, the popularity of ether has waned. It is, however, a very safe and reliable anaesthetic and may be used for operations in all branches of surgery and obstetrics, especially where good muscle relaxation is required. Although now only occasionally employed as a sole or main anaesthetic in major surgery, it is still used in some short operations, such as tonsillectomy. It is a particularly useful agent for those working in remote parts of the world where elaborate apparatus is not available.

DOSAGE AND ADMINISTRATION

Diethyl ether may be given on an open mask or by means of the vaporizer of any of the anaesthetic machines in common use. Vapour strengths of up to 20 per cent are required for induction; light anaesthesia can be maintained on strengths in the region of 3–5 per cent, but deep anaesthesia may require concentrations up to 10 per cent or more in resistant subjects. There is a tendency to cross-tolerance between alcohol and the volatile hydrocarbon anaesthetics. This is especially noticeable during the induction period, when, as is common knowledge, it is difficult to anaesthetize addicts to alcohol or morphine.

Accurate administration of known vapour concentrations is not possible with the Boyle type of vaporizer owing to the number of variables, such as the rate of flow of gases, position of the plunger, and changes in temperature. The EMO inhaler, however, will deliver known concentrations between 0 and 25 per cent under all normal conditions and when relaxants are used it has been found that 3 per cent diethyl ether vapour in air will maintain unconsciousness. This combination has wide applicability in all circumstances in which cylinders of nitrous oxide are not readily available. Patients anaesthetized with 3 per cent diethyl ether vapour regain consciousness very quickly and the incidence of nausea and vomiting is no greater than with the conventional nitrous oxide–oxygen–relaxant technique. Diethyl ether may safely be used in closed circuits with soda-lime absorption. It has been administered intravenously (5 per cent solution in isotonic saline), and per rectum (65 per cent solution in olive oil); these methods, however, are unreliable and not without danger, and should not be employed.

PRECAUTIONS

Diethyl ether should not be used in cases of diabetes mellitus and severe liver disease, and its use is inadvisable in patients with fever under hot and humid operating conditions. This particularly applies to children and those who have been atropinized: such patients are liable to have convulsions. If these occur the anaesthetic should be withdrawn, the patient should be cooled by sponging with cold water if hyperthermia is present, and small doses of thiopentone or diazepam should be given intravenously until convulsions cease. Small doses of a muscle relaxant may also be employed in resistant cases. Convulsions occurring during anaesthesia are not confined to diethyl ether. Although the majority of cases reported have occurred with this agent, convulsions have followed chloroform, trichloroethylene, and other anaesthetics. Hypoxia, often occult, may be an important factor in the production of this condition.

When used on an open mask or with air, the large mass of diethyl ether in the inspired atmosphere inevitably leads to hypoxaemia. To prevent this a small flow of oxygen should be added under an open mask or to air draw-over vaporizers.

The flammability of diethyl ether contraindicates its use in the presence of diathermy, and care to avoid static discharge must be taken in hot dry climates.

As with trichloroethylene, addiction to diethyl ether vapour can occur.

An overdose of diethyl ether is characterized by respiratory failure and later cardiac arrest. Normal respiration will usually be resumed following controlled respiration with oxygen.

Enflurane

Enflurane (*BP* and *USP*)
Chemical name: 2-chloro-1,1,2-trifluoroethyl difluoromethyl ether

```
     F    F        F
     |    |        |
H----C----C---O----C----H
     |    |        |
     Cl   F        F
```

PHYSICAL CHARACTERISTICS

Enflurane is a halogenated ethyl-methyl ether and an isomer of isoflurane. Early clinical evaluations of this drug were made by Virtue and his colleagues (1966) and Dobkin and his colleagues (1968). Numerous reports of the clinical use of enflurane have appeared and this agent is now widely used and regarded as a satisfactory anaesthetic agent for a great variety of surgical procedures.

Enflurane is a colourless liquid of specific gravity 1.5. It is a stable compound, not affected by ultraviolet light, and may safely be stored in clear glass bottles. The vapour has an ethereal odour, and vapour concentrations above 6 per cent are flammable. Because of its low blood/gas partition coefficient (1.9) induction of anaesthesia is rapid, depth of anaesthesia may readily be controlled, and prompt recovery follows withdrawal.

PHARMACOLOGY

Central nervous system. Although it is a potent anaesthetic, enflurane can also produce marked central stimulant actions, and therein differs from other inhalational anaesthetics. During enflurane adminstration the EEG commonly shows episodes of paroxysmal activity and periods of burst suppression. Neigh, Garman and Harp (1971) have shown that these EEG responses are a function of anaesthetic depth and that they are exacerbated by a reduction in $P\text{CO}_2$. Episodes of tonic or clonic twitching of the jaws have been observed in many patients. The EEG effects of enflurane may persist for up to 30 days after its administration (Burchiel *et al.*, 1977). Seizures have been reported by Ohm and his colleagues (1975) up to 1 week after enflurane anaesthesia. Abnormal EEG activity during the use of enflurane is seen more commonly in children than in adults. Under conditions of normocapnia enflurane does not exacerbate pre-existing epileptic activity (Opitz and Oberwetter, 1979). These EEG abnormalities should be regarded as signs of overdosage, possibly associated with hypocapnia.

Cardiovascular system. Light enflurane anaesthesia is usually accompanied by a slight decrease in arterial pressure and increase in heart rate. Cardiac output, stroke volume, peripheral resistance, and myocardial contractility have been shown by Calverley and his colleagues (1978) to be reduced during light (1.0 MAC) enflurane anaesthesia in man. While the cardiovascular effects of this level of enflurane anaesthesia were similar to those of halothane, these workers found that deepening anaesthesia often produced profound cardiovascular depression with little evidence of adaptation with time. More marked circulatory changes were seen during controlled ventilation than in spontaneously breathing subjects.

The spontaneous appearance of cardiac dysrhythmias is uncommon during enflurane anaesthesia. Johnston, Eger and Wilson (1976) showed in man that the amount of adrenaline needed to produce ectopic ventricular contractions during enflurane anaesthesia was some five times that needed during halothane anaesthesia.

Respiratory system. Enflurane commonly causes respiratory depression. This is usually the result of a reduced tidal volume associated with a slight increase in rate. Royston and Snowdon (1979) showed that during enflurane anaesthesia respiratory rate is slower and tidal volume greater than during halothane administration. Enflurane is a more powerful respiratory depressant than either halothane or isoflurane. Respiratory depression is dose related and some recovery occurs over a period of time. The respiratory depressant effects of enflurane are partly antagonized by the stimulus of surgery.

Neuromuscular transmission. Enflurane can produce a marked degree of muscular relaxation and can be used alone to provide adequate operating conditions for abdominal surgery. The concentration of enflurane needed for this may, however, produce severe cardiovascular depression. Smaller amounts of neuromuscular blocking agents are needed during enflurane anaesthesia. Fogdall and Miller (1975) have shown that during 1.25 MAC enflurane anaesthesia the dose of tubocurarine needed to produce a 50 per cent depression of twitch height was 1.6 mg/m^2, while the same degree of block during comparable halothane anaesthesia required a dose of 5.6 mg/m^2.

Liver and kidneys. Extensive studies in both animals and man have failed to reveal any significant hepatic effects of enflurane. A few clinical reports of impaired liver function after enflurane anaesthesia have appeared, but the influence in these cases of other factors such as blood transfusion and viral hepatitis cannot be excluded.

Renal blood flow and glomerular filtration rate are reduced by enflurane, the changes being of the same order as with other volatile anaesthetics. Inorganic fluoride is produced during enflurane metabolism, although the concentrations are far less than with methoxyflurane. A few cases of renal failure have been reported after enflurane anaesthesia and it may be wise to avoid using this agent in patients with pre-existing renal disease.

Metabolism. Enflurane undergoes much less metabolic degradation than halothane. As with methoxyflurane, inorganic fluoride is the most important product of its metabolism, fluoride levels being related to the inspired enflurane level and the duration of exposure. Maximal serum fluoride levels are in the order of 25 µmol/ℓ and they decline more rapidly than after methoxyflurane. Cousins and Mazze (1973) showed that serum fluoride levels of 50 µmol/ℓ were needed to produce nephrotoxicity, but more recently Mazze, Calverley and Smith (1977) have demonstrated significant reductions in the maximum urine-concentrating ability when serum fluoride levels were in the order of 20 µmol/ℓ. These effects of enflurane should not be of great clinical importance in well-hydrated patients with normal renal function.

INDICATIONS

Inspired enflurane concentrations of 3–4 per cent are required for induction of anaesthesia and of 1–3 per cent for maintenance, lesser concentrations being needed in the presence of nitrous oxide. Both induction and recovery from anaesthesia are more rapid than with halothane. The central stimulant effects of enflurane have not caused major problems. The relative lack of myocardial sensitization to catecholamines and the rarity of cardiac dysrhythmias during enflurane anaesthesia make this agent suitable for use when catecholamines are being used for haemostatic purposes or when high catecholamine levels are anticipated, as in patients with phaeochromocytomas. Although in unstimulated subjects severe cardiovascular and respiratory depression are seen at only moderate levels of enflurane anaesthesia, surgical stimulation usually counters these effects. Because of potential nephrotoxicity, enflurane should be avoided in subjects with pre-existing renal disease or during procedures in which renal function may be compromised.

Burchiel, K. J., Stockard, J. J., Calverley, R. K. and Smith, N.T. (1977) Relationship of pre- and post-anesthetic EEG abnormalities to enflurane-induced seizure activity. *Anesthesia and Analgesia,* **56,** 509

Calverley, R. K., Prys-Roberts, C., Eger, E.I. and Jones, C.W. (1978) Cardiovascular effects of enflurane anesthesia during controlled ventilation in man. *Anesthesia and Analgesia,* **57,** 619

Cousins, M. J. and Mazze, R. I. (1973) Methoxyflurane nephrotoxicity — a study of dose response in man. *Journal of the American Medical Association,* **225,** 1611

Dobkin, A. B., Heinrick, R. G., Israel, J. S., Levy, A. A., Neville, J. F. and Ounkasem, K. (1968) Clinical and laboratory evaluation of a new inhalation agent: compound 347. *Anesthesiology,* **29**, 275

Fogdall, R. P. and Miller, R. D. (1975) Neuromuscular effects of enflurane alone and combined with d-tubocurarine, pancuronium and succinylcholine in man. *Anesthesiology,* **42,** 173

Johnston, R. R., Eger, E. I. and Wilson, C. (1976) A comparative interaction of epinephrine with enflurane, isoflurane and halothane in man. *Anesthesia and Analgesia,* **55,** 709

Mazze, R. I., Calverley R. K. and Smith, N. T. (1977) Inorganic fluoride nephrotoxicity: prolonged enflurane and halothane anesthesia in volunteers. *Anesthesiology,* **46,** 265

Neigh, J. C., Garman, J. K. and Harp, J. R. (1971) The electroencephalographic pattern during anesthesia with Ethrane: effects of depth of anesthesia, $Pa\text{CO}_2$, and nitrous oxide. *Anesthesiology,* **35,** 482

Ohm, W. W., Cullen, B., Amory, D. W. and Kennedy, R. D. (1975) Delayed seizure activity following enflurane anesthesia. *Anesthesiology,* **42,** 367

Opitz, A. and Oberwetter, W. D. (1979) Enflurane or halothane anaesthesia for patients with cerebral convulsive disorders? *Acta Anaesthesiologica Scandinavica* (Suppl.), **71,** 43

Royston, D. and Snowdon, S. (1979) Comparison of respiratory characteristics during enflurane and halothane anaesthesia. *British Journal of Anaesthesia,* **51,** 567P

Virtue, R. W., Lund, L. O., Phelps, M., Vogel, J. H. K., Beckwitt, H. and Heron, M. (1966) Difluoromethyl 1,1,2-trifluoro-2-chloroethyl ether as an anaesthetic agent: results with dogs and a preliminary note on observations in man. *Canadian Anaesthetists' Society Journal,* **13,** 233

Fluroxene is a colourless liquid with a not unpleasant smell. Its vapour is heavier than air (specific gravity 1.13). The vapour is both flammable and explosive, the lower limits of flammability being 4 per cent in air and 4.5 per cent in oxygen.

Introduced clinically in 1954 under the name of Fluoromar, it was the first of the group of fluorine-substituted hydrocarbons and ethers. Although overshadowed by halothane in Great Britain it did enjoy wide popularity in North America, but has been withdrawn owing to its toxic effects on laboratory animals.

Central nervous depression resembles that with other inhalational agents. The analgesic state is marked, both during induction and recovery. Excitement is minimal. Like diethyl ether, fluroxene stimulates the sympathetic nervous system.

Fluroxene has direct myocardial depressant effects which are usually masked by concomitant sympathetic stimulation. Deep fluoroxene anaesthesia is associated with significant falls in arterial pressure. Fluroxene does not sensitize the myocardium to catecholamines. Clinical concentrations of fluroxene vapour are not irritant to the respiratory tract. Fluroxene anaesthesia is often associated with tachypnoea accompanied by a reduced tidal volume and alveolar hypoventilation. Postanaesthetic derangement of hepatic and renal function has not been demonstrated in man or experimental animals. Prolonged deep anaesthesia, especially if associated with hypercapnia, causes immediate postoperative nausea and vomiting.

Significant metabolic transformation of fluroxene occurs. Repeated exposures of experimental animals to fluroxene invariably led to death following one to three exposures. The animals developed bloody diarrhoea, ataxia, hypotension and seizures. Blood coagulation changes were seen in dogs. These effects seem to be due to the production of trifluoroethanol by metabolic transformation. In man no occult blood or blood coagulation changes have been detected after clinical fluroxene anaesthesia. Biotransformation of fluroxene does not seem to lead to significant trifluoroethanol production in man.

A further disadvantage of fluroxene is its potential mutagenic action which has been shown in the Ames Salmonella microsome assay system.

Isoflurane

Isoflurane (*BP* and *USAN*)

Chemical name: 1-chloro-2,2,2-trifluoroethyl difluoromethyl ether

```
    F   H       F
    |   |       |
F — C — C — O — C — H
    |   |       |
    F   Cl      F
```

PHYSICAL CHARACTERISTICS

Isoflurane is the latest ethyl-methyl ether to be introduced into clinical practice. Although it was first synthesized in 1965, only 2 years after its isomer enflurane, problems in its purification have delayed its introduction. A suggestion that this agent might be carcinogenic (Corbett, 1976) further delayed clinical use of isoflurane.

The physical properties of isoflurane resemble those of enflurane, but it has a lower boiling point and a higher vapour pressure, and is less soluble in blood (partition coefficient 1.4). Like enflurane, isoflurane is stable in the presence of ultraviolet light.

PHARMACOLOGY

Central nervous system. The CNS effects of isoflurane are similar to those of other volatile anaesthetic agents. Unlike enflurane it does not have any convulsant actions, even at deep levels of anaesthesia with hypocapnia. Cerebral blood flow is increased during moderate to deep isoflurane anaesthesia. While the rise in cerebral blood flow is less with isoflurane than with halothane or enflurane, large rises of intracranial pressure can occur with all three agents in the presence of a space-occupying lesion.

Respiratory system. Isoflurane is capable of producing profund respiratory depression in the spontaneously breathing subject. This is evidenced by a dose-related increase in $P\text{CO}_2$ and a reduced ability to respond to an imposed carbon dioxide load. Isoflurane-induced respiratory depression is seen in its most marked form in unstimulated volunteers (Cromwell *et al.*, 1971; Flemming *et al.*, 1975). The degree of respiratory depression is more than that seen with halothane, but less than that produced by enflurane. France and his co-workers (1974) showed that this respiratory depression was countered by surgical stimulation, and during routine clinical use only moderate rises in $P\text{CO}_2$ occur when isoflurane is given to spontaneously breathing subjects.

Circulatory system. Light and moderate levels of isoflurane anaesthesia are associated with a small degree of cardiovascular depression. Arterial pressure, stroke volume, and total peripheral resistance fall but cardiac output is usually maintained by a rise in heart rate (Stevens *et al.*, 1971). The cardiovascular effects of isoflurane are greatest in unstimulated and ventilated volunteers. Surgical stimulation reduces the degree of cardiovascular depression (Graves, McDermott and Bidwai, 1974), and during spontaneous ventilation carbon dioxide retention may lead to an increased cardiac output, although an increase in systemic arterial pressure rarely occurs.

Isoflurane does not increase the sensitivity of the heart to the dysrhythmic effects of catecholamines. Joas and Stevens (1971) showed that in dogs under isoflurane the same order of dose of adrenaline needed to be administered to produce dysrhythmias as in the awake state, and a similar lack of effect of isoflurane on catecholamine sensitivity in man has been demonstrated by Johnston and his co-workers (1976).

Muscular effects. Isoflurane alone can produce a good degree of muscular relaxation, and has been used without muscle relaxants during upper abdominal surgery. Miller and his colleagues (1971a) have shown that isoflurane produces a dose-related decrease in the ability of skeletal muscle to sustain a contraction in response to tetanic stimulation. Isoflurane also potentiates the effects of muscle relaxants. Miller and his colleagues (1971b) showed that the dose of tubocurarine needed to produce a 50 per cent depression of twitch response was 1.7 mg/m^2 during isoflurane anaesthesia and 5.6 mg/m^2 during comparable levels of halothane anaesthesia. Similar although less marked differences were seen with pancuronium.

Liver and kidneys. Isoflurane produces negligible changes in liver function as evidenced by studies of changes in liver function tests and enzymes during and following administration of this agent. Similarly, the effects of isoflurane on the kidney resemble those of other inhalational agents and include a reduction in renal blood flow and glomerular filtration, with a full recovery of renal function after anaesthesia.

Metabolism. Early studies by Halsey and his co-workers (1971) suggested that isoflurane did not undergo metabolic degradation in experimental animals. Later studies by Holaday and his colleagues (1975) showed that about 0.17 per cent of administered isoflurane was metabolized. Serum fluoride levels rise slightly after isoflurane administration. The plasma inorganic fluoride levels seen after isoflurane are greater than those seen after halothane, but in the order of 10 per cent of those occurring after enflurane. The minimal biodegradation seen with isoflurane can be related both to the stability of its molecule and to its rapid elimination from the body after its administration.

The minimal level of isoflurane metabolism is of importance in relation to its potential toxic effects. Corbett (1976) in a pilot study suggested that isoflurane could induce liver tumours in mice. A later and more detailed study by Eger and his co-workers (1978) did not substantiate these findings. No evidence has yet been adduced to show any carcinogenic or mutagenic effects of isoflurane.

INDICATIONS

Isoflurane has been used to anaesthetize without incident a wide range of patients for a large variety of procedures. Eger (1981) has claimed that isoflurane approaches the ideal inhalational agent more closely than any other agent. The marked muscular relaxation and stable cardiovascular system are particular advantages of isoflurane. Because of its lower blood solubility induction with isoflurane can be more rapid than with halothane, although the pungent odour of isoflurane leads to a greater incidence of breath-holding and coughing and may limit the rate of induction.

A further advantage of isoflurane over halothane and enflurane is its lack of deleterious side effects, especially those relating to hepatic and renal function. The lack of toxicity of isoflurane has been related to the low level of metabolic breakdown of this agent that occurs. This aspect of the safety of isoflurane should be considered with some caution. Methoxyflurane was administered to some 12 million patients before its harmful renal effects were noted. Isoflurane has not been used as extensively as other inhalational agents, and time alone will prove or disprove how safe an agent it is.

DOSAGE AND ADMINISTRATION

Isoflurane has a MAC of 1.15. Concentrations of 1.5 per cent – that is, 1.3 times the MAC – can be used to maintain light anaesthesia. Higher concentrations are needed if any significant level of relaxation is desired. The inspired concentration of isoflurane can be greatly reduced if the agent is given together with 60–70 per cent nitrous oxide. Under these circumstances isoflurane MAC falls to about 0.5.

Isoflurane should be administered from a calibrated vaporizer. Halothane and isoflurane have nearly identical vaporizers, and Steffey (1980) has shown that a calibrated halothane vaporizer can be used to deliver nearly accurate concentrations of isoflurane. However, hazards can arise if a vaporizer specifically designed for one agent is filled with a different agent and this practice is not recommended.

Corbett, T. H. (1976) Cancer and congenital anomalies associated with anesthetics. *Annals of the New York Academy of Science,* **271,** 58

Cromwell, T. H., Stevens, W. C., Eger, E. I., Shakespeare, T. F., Halsey, M. J., Bahlman, S. H. and Fourcade, H. E. (1971) The cardiovascular effects of Compound 469 (Forane) during spontaneous ventilation and CO_2 challenge in man. *Anesthesiology,* **35,** 17

Eger, E. I. (1981) *Isoflurane (Forane). A compendium and reference.* Wisconsin, USA: Airco Inc.

Eger, E. I., White, A. E., Brown, C. L., Brava, C. G., Corbett, T. H. and Stevens, W. C. (1978) A test of the carcinogenicity of enflurane, isoflurane, halothane, methoxyflurane and nitrous oxide in mice. *Anesthesia and Analgesia,* **57,** 678

Flemming, D. C., Kallos, T., Mull, T. and Smith, T. C. (1975) Ventilatory and cardiovascular effects of isoflurane and halothane in combination with oxymorphone and naloxone. *Isoflurane New Drug Application,* p. 2367

France, C. J., Plumer, M. H., Eger, E. I. and Wahrenbrock, E. A. (1974) Ventilatory effects of isoflurane (Forane) or halothane when combined with morphine, nitrous oxide and surgery. *British Journal of Anaesthesia,* **46,** 117

Graves, C. L., McDermott, R. W. and Bidwai, A. (1974) Cardiovascular effects of isoflurane in surgical patients. *Anesthesiology,* **41,** 486

Halsey, M. J., Sawyer, D. C., Eger, E. I., Bahlman, S. H. and Impelman, D. M. (1971) Hepatic metabolism of halothane, methoxyflurane, cyclopropane, Ethrane and Forane in miniature swine. *Anesthesiology,* **35,** 43

Holaday, D. A., Fiserova-Bergerova, V., Latto, I. P. and Zumbiel, M. A. (1975) Resistance of isoflurane to biotransformation in man. *Anesthesiology,* **43,** 325

Joas, T. A. and Stevens, W. C. (1971) Comparison of the arrhythmic doses of epinephrine during Forane, halothane and fluroxene anesthesia in dogs. *Anesthesiology,* **35,** 48

Johnston, R. R., Eger, E. I. and Wilson, C. (1976) A comparative interaction of epinephrine with enflurane, isoflurane and halothane in man. *Anesthesia and Analgesia,* **55,** 709

Miller, R. D., Eger, E. I., Way, W. L., Stevens, W. C. and Dolan, W. M. (1971a) Comparative neuromuscular effects of Forane and halothane alone and in combination with d-tubocurarine in man. *Anesthesiology,* **35,** 38

Miller, R. D., Way, W. L., Dolan, W. M., Stevens, W. C. and Eger, E. I. (1971b) Comparative neuromuscular effects of pancuronium, gallamine and succinylcholine during Forane and halothane anesthesia in man. *Anesthesiology,* **35,** 509
Steffey, E. P. (1980) Isoflurane concentrations delivered by isoflurane and halothane specific vaporizers. *Anesthesiology,* **53,** 519
Stevens, W. C., Cromwell, T. H., Halsey, M. J., Eger, E. I., Shakespeare, T. F. and Bahlman, S. H. (1971) The cardiovascular effects of a new inhalation anesthetic, Forane, in human volunteers at constant arterial carbon dioxide tension. *Anesthesiology,* **35,** 8

Methoxyflurane (This drug has been withdrawn since this edition was prepared)

Methoxyflurane (*BP* and *USP*)
Chemical name: 2,2-dichloro-1,1-difluoroethyl methyl ether

```
      Cl   F         H
      |    |         |
H  —  C  — C — O  —  C  — H
      |    |         |
      Cl   F         H
```

PHYSICAL PROPERTIES

Methoxyflurane is a clear colourless liquid with a fruity odour. It has a specific gravity of 1.43 and the vapour has a density of 7.36.

Under normal working conditions it is non-explosive and non-flammable, but concentrations exceeding 4 per cent may ignite above 75°C. It is stable in the presence of oxygen, air, light, moisture, and soda-lime. Prolonged exposure to light causes a brown colour to develop which is of no significance. Its vapour accelerates the deterioration of rubber, in which it is highly soluble.

The saturated vapour pressure of methoxyflurane at room temperature is only 20 mmHg (2.7 kPa) and this corresponds to a concentration of 3 per cent methoxyflurane which it is not possible to exceed under normal working conditions. The latent heat of vaporization of methoxyflurane is 49 cal/g, thus the temperature of the liquid changes little during prolonged use.

Methoxyflurane was investigated by Artusio and colleagues (1960) and they first reported its use in man. Since then it has been widely used in the USA and in Canada. Its popularity has greatly diminished since its nephrotoxic actions were demonstrated.

PHARMACOLOGY

Nervous system. Both induction of anaesthesia and recovery are prolonged. This can be attributed to the high solubility of methoxyflurane in blood. There is no specific effect on the autonomic system and atropine is not necessary in premedication. Deep levels of anaesthesia produce direct depression of the respiratory and vasomotor centres. Low concentrations of methoxyflurane have a powerful analgesic action.

Cardiovascular system. Methoxyflurane resembles halothane in its cardiac effects. Blood pressure tends to fall to a degree proportional to the depth of anaesthesia. This fall is accompanied by a fall in cardiac output. Peripheral resistance is unchanged and muscle blood flow is not increased. Marked pallor of the face and extremities can occur with deep anaesthesia. Methoxyflurane does not cause an increase in the level of circulating catecholamines (Romagnoli and Kornan, 1962). Methoxyflurane does not sensitize the heart to the dysrhythmic effects of adrenaline.

Respiratory system. During the lighter levels of anaesthesia there is a slight increase in respiratory rate associated with a fall in tidal volume. This is marked in the absence of opiate premedication, but in any case the rise in rate fails to compensate for the fall in tidal volume and the $P\text{CO}_2$ tends to rise to levels comparable to those produced by halothane. Deep anaesthesia is associated with inadequate ventilation and assisted or controlled respiration is then essential.

Skeletal muscle. The skeletal muscle tone is reduced as anaesthesia is deepened. There is no evidence of any action at the myoneural junction.

Liver. Although a few cases of hepatic necrosis have been recorded following methoxyflurane administration, there is no evidence of a specific toxic effect of this agent on the liver.

Kidney. Following methoxyflurane anaesthesia a syndrome of high output renal failure has been recorded by many authors, characterized by an increased output of dilute urine, dehydration, and uraemia. Mazze, Shue and Jackson (1971) consistently found evidence of impaired renal function in man after relatively deep methoxyflurane anaesthesia. Oxaluria is a prominent feature, and this is believed to be derived from the metabolic transformation of methoxyflurane. The toxic picture, however, is almost certainly due to an effect of the fluoride ion on the distal renal tubule, rendering it unresponsive to antidiuretic hormone (Jones, 1972). Inorganic fluoride can be demonstrated in blood and urine after administration of other fluoride-containing anaesthetics, especially enflurane. However, the concentration of fluoride present after methoxyflurane administration is much greater than with these other agents. The high solubility of methoxyflurane in tissues (which may be associated with covalent binding of the drug to tissues) exposes methoxyflurane to metabolic actions for a much longer time than other agents.

ANAESTHETIC PROPERTIES

Induction is slow and it is essential to administer 2–3 per cent methoxyflurane vapour for several minutes before consciousness is lost. Induction with thiopentone is therefore advisable, and the administration of a muscle relaxant if intubation is necessary. Even with this form of induction the patient is unlikely to be ready for operation in under 10 minutes. Muscular relaxation is variable and unpredictable, and depends on the depth of anaesthesia: if this is pressed, serious respiratory depression and hypotension will result. It is safer, therefore, to employ light levels of anaesthesia with a muscle relaxant if full relaxation is required. One of the main disadvantages of methoxyflurane is its slow recovery time, which is often associated with amnesia, analgesia, and dizziness which may last for many hours. Reports as to the incidence of postoperative vomiting vary considerably. Hudon (1961) has reported nausea 13 per cent and vomiting 4.5 per cent in the recovery room, while Denton and Torda (1963) have reported a high incidence of this complication, often delayed for at least 2 hours after the return of consciousness. Only 40 per cent of their series were entirely free from nausea or vomiting.

INDICATIONS

Methoxyflurane can be used for operations in all branches of surgery. It is especially useful as an adjuvant to nitrous oxide–oxygen–relaxant anaesthesia, prolonged postoperative analgesia being a useful attribute in this technique. Much lower concentrations of the vapour are necessary than those previously used, and provide adequate anaesthesia with little alteration in cardiac or respiratory function. Subanaesthetic concentrations are used to provide awake analgesia in obstetrics and for minor painful surgery. The very real danger of renal failure after moderate periods of methoxyflurane administration, especially in patients with pre-existent renal disease, has greatly reduced the application of this agent.

DOSAGE AND ADMINISTRATION

High concentrations (2–3 per cent) are desirable during induction. Methoxyflurane administration is hampered by the severe limitation of vapour strength that can be obtained: because of its low saturated vapour pressure it is not possible at room temperature to attain concentrations much greater than 3 per cent. Significant absorption of methoxyflurane by the rubber of anaesthetic circuits further reduces the concentration of vapour reaching the patient. During maintenance, concentrations of 0.2–0.5 per cent are needed. Because of its prolonged effects, methoxyflurane administration can be discontinued 15–20 minutes before the end of surgery. Concentrations of 0.35 per cent are used for analgesia; special pre-set vaporizers are available for this purpose.

Artusio, J. F., Van Poznack, A., Hunt, R. E., Tiers, F. M. and Alexander, M. (1960) A clinical evaluation of methoxyflurane in man. *Anesthesiology,* **21,** 512

Denton, M. H. V. and Torda, T. A. G. (1963) Methoxyflurane. Clinical experiences in fifty orthopaedic cases. *Anaesthesia,* **18,** 279

Hudon, F. (1961) Methoxyflurane. *Canadian Anaesthetists' Society Journal,* **8,** 544

Jones, N. O. (1972) Methoxyflurane nephrotoxicity — a review and case report. *Canadian Anaesthetists' Society Journal,* **19,** 152

Mazze, R. I., Shue, G. L. and Jackson, S. H. (1971) Renal dysfunction associated with methoxyflurane anesthesia. A randomized, prospective clinical evaluation. *Journal of the American Medical Association,* **216,** 278

Romagnoli, A. and Korman, D. (1962) Methoxyflurane in obstetrical anaesthesia and analgesia. *Canadian Anaesthetists' Society Journal,* **9,** 414

Vinyl ether is a highly volatile liquid, lighter than water. The vapour is highly flammable and explosive when mixed with air (1.7–27 per cent) or oxygen (1.8–85 per cent). Vinyl ether is highly unstable. Available preparations contain 3.5 per cent of absolute alcohol to lower its volatility and reduce its freezing point and 0.01 per cent of phenyl-α-naphthylamine as an antoxidant.

Many of the actions of vinyl ether resemble those of diethyl ether. Induction, as would be expected with a low blood/gas partition coefficient, is more rapid, respiration is not stimulated, and the vapour is less irritant. Many cases of centrilobular hepatic necrosis have been reported following prolonged administration of vinyl ether.

Vinyl ether has been mainly used in the past as an induction agent, especially in children. Because of its flammability, potency, and the great difficulty in controlling inspired concentrations, it has virtually passed from current use.

Anaesthetic gases

The most widely used anaesthetic gas is nitrous oxide. Cyclopropane, ethylene, and acetylene have been used in the past. Xenon has anaesthetic properties very similar to those of nitrous oxide, but its prohibitive cost has precluded its clinical use.

By definition, the anaesthetic gases have a vapour pressure above ambient pressure at room temperature and there are no limitations upon the concentrations that may be administered. These gases are stored in cylinders, usually compressed to a liquid form at moderate pressure.

Nitrous oxide and cyclopropane differ in many of their anaesthetic properties. They have in common the property of low blood solubility. Because of this, induction with these agents is more rapid than with any of the volatile anaesthetic liquids. They also share the property of being resistant to metabolic transformation in the body.

Nitrous oxide

Nitrous oxide (*BP* and *USP*)
Chemical formula: N_2O

Nitrous oxide is a colourless gas with a slightly sweetish odour. It has a density compared to air of 1.5 and a critical temperature of 36.5°C. It is neither flammable nor explosive, but will support combustion. It is supplied in blue cylinders, compressed to a liquid at a pressure of 650 lb/in^2 (4481 kPa).

Nitrous oxide, or laughing gas, was first used as an anaesthetic agent at the beginning of the nineteenth century, and is still in universal use. It was prepared by Priestley in 1772. Humphry Davy tried it on himself in 1799, noticed the anaesthetic properties and suggested it be used to allay pain. It was first used in clinical practice in 1844 by Colton and Wells in the USA.

PHARMACOLOGY

Many of the effects that have been ascribed to nitrous oxide are the direct result of hypoxia rather than those due to the agent itself. In the presence of adequate oxygen the effect on the body systems is not great. Hypoxia has been used in the past to prolong anaesthesia for dental and other operations. The combination of nitrous oxide and hypoxia is most dangerous and has led to pulmonary oedema, atelectasis, and to heart failure. Death from acute oxygen want, and organic brain damage with early or late neurological and psychiatric manifestations, have also occurred.

Nervous system. CNS depression is similar to that caused by all general anaesthetics, but paralysis of the respiratory and vasomotor centres does not occur if normal oxygen requirements are satisfied.

Cardiovascular system. Because of the difficulties of measuring the effects of nitrous oxide alone, uncomplicated by other factors, evidence of its effects on the circulation must be interpreted with caution. Eisele and colleagues (1969) gave 60 per cent nitrous oxide to conscious, trained, instrumented dogs and found a small fall in maximum aortic blood flow acceleration (indicative of reduced ventricular contractility), together with a small fall in cardiac output. In contrast, substantial evidence of both α- and β-adrenergic stimulant effects of nitrous oxide when added during stable halothane anaesthesia has been demonstrated by Smith and colleagues (1970). Kawamura and his co-workers (1980) have shown that within the first 15 minutes of administration of 60 per cent nitrous oxide to spontaneously breathing man heart rate and cardiac output rise, but these variables have returned to normal levels after 2 hours of nitrous oxide administration. These effects were associated with a rise in $P\text{CO}_2$, and this rather than nitrous oxide *per se* was probably responsible for the cardiovascular effects seen.

Respiratory system. Although psychic factors operate during induction of nitrous oxide anaesthesia, ventilation usually increases. Hypoxia, painful stimuli, or relief of pain may mask the slight respiratory effects of nitrous oxide. Hornbein and colleagues (1969) showed mild depressant effects of nitrous oxide on alveolar ventilation and the ventilatory response to added carbon dioxide.

Muscular system. Depression of skeletal muscle tone is minimal and plain muscle is unaffected.

Haemopoietic system. Bone marrow depression follows prolonged nitrous oxide administration. This was first reported by Lassen and his colleagues (1956), who were using nitrous oxide in the management of tetanus. Nitrous oxide has been shown to react chemically with vitamin B_{12} (Banks, Henderson and Pratt, 1968) and Amess and his colleagues (1978) showed that megaloblastic bone marrow depression could follow inhalation of 60 per cent nitrous oxide for 6 hours. Minty and her colleagues (1979) have shown that nitrous oxide affects the B_{12} coenzyme, methylcobalamin, interfering with the activation of methyl synthetase which is required to convert homocysteine to methionine.

Other effects. There is no effect on kidney or liver function. Nausea and vomiting are likely to occur if anaesthesia is associated with hypoxia. Nitrous oxide crosses the placental barrier but does not cause respiratory depression in the fetus.

Fate in the body. Nitrous oxide is rapidly excreted by the lungs. A small amount diffuses through the skin. Hong and his colleagues (1980) have shown that intestinal bacteria can break nitrous oxide down, eventually to nitrogen, and suggest that some 0.004 per cent of administered nitrous oxide is metabolized in man.

ANAESTHETIC PROPERTIES

Nitrous oxide is a weak anaesthetic, as can be deduced from its indirectly determined MAC of 110 per cent. When used with air it is impossible to produce anaesthesia without some degree of hypoxia. With oxygen at near atmospheric concentration the first plane of surgical anaesthesia can be reached in average subjects, although difficulties can occur with alcoholics, habitual takers of narcotics, and fit, powerfully built adults. Induction is rapid and not unpleasant, but hallucinations and some violence in the second stage are not uncommon. Arterial blood reaches approximately 90 per cent saturation in 10 minutes, there being a net gas uptake of about 1 ℓ/min during induction. Full equilibrium does not occur for several hours, and uptake continues at a greatly diminished rate for the entire course of most clinical administrations. Recovery is rapid (1–4 minutes) even after prolonged administration.

Because of the limited depth of anaesthesia attainable with nitrous oxide, relaxation is poor and insufficient for major surgery. Limb movements are apt to occur following painful stimuli.

INDICATIONS

Nitrous oxide is still occasionally used with oxygen as a sole agent for short minor procedures, such as dental extractions, although there is an increasing tendency to supplement its actions with low concentrations of more powerful volatile agents. With supplementary agents it is widely used for all branches of major surgery. Two advantages accrue from using potent agents with nitrous oxide: 60–70 per cent nitrous oxide will reduce by approximately two thirds the alveolar concentration of other agents needed to maintain light anaesthesia; because of the marked initial net uptake of nitrous oxide there is a noticeable 'second gas effect' which initially hastens the uptake of other agents.

Subanaesthetic concentrations of nitrous oxide are widely used to produce analgesia. Employed mainly in obstetrics, this practice is spreading to other situations that require controllable and easily administered pain relief, such as trauma and for the relief of pain associated with chest physiotherapy postoperatively.

DOSAGE AND ADMINISTRATION

In the past, nitrous oxide was widely used with air as an analgesic. This practice has been replaced by the use of 1:1 nitrous oxide–oxygen mixtures, delivered either from pre-set intermittent-flow machines, such as the Lucy Baldwin, or from pre-mixed cylinders attached to an Entonox demand flow head.

Nitrous oxide and oxygen can be given by many different types of apparatus. When used for minor surgery, intermittent-flow machines are still widely employed. Many techniques have been described for inducing and maintaining this form of anaesthesia; most, unfortunately, allow varying degrees of hypoxia, but if patience is exercised light anaesthesia can usually be maintained on mixtures containing 20 per cent oxygen. Indeed, Vickers and Pask (1966) showed that less than 20 per cent oxygen is of no benefit once the technique ceases to rely on hypoxia. Inhalation of 100 per cent oxygen for 3–5 minutes is advantageous before nitrous oxide administration. Smith (1971) has pointed out that removal of nitrogen from the lungs does not in itself hasten nitrous oxide induction. The main advantage of pre-oxygenation is to allow the initial use of high inspired nitrous oxide concentrations without danger of hypoxia.

Although anaesthesia for major surgery may be maintained with nitrous oxide, oxygen, and muscle relaxants alone, it is more usual to supplement such anaesthesia with a low concentration of a volatile agent, or to administer an analgesic.

PRECAUTIONS

The most obvious problem arising with nitrous oxide administration is hypoxia. An inspired oxygen concentration of 20 per cent or even slightly less is usually safe for induction, especially if 3–5 minutes pre-oxygenation is performed. The 'second gas effect' due to nitrous oxide uptake effectively increases arterial oxygen tension during the first few minutes of administration. Such oxygen concentrations are inadequate during prolonged administration; because of the inevitable impairment of oxygen transport across the lungs during general anaesthesia, inspired oxygen concentrations of at least 30 per cent should be given. During upper abdominal and thoracic surgery, especially in patients with pre-existing cardiac or respiratory disease, an inspired oxygen concentration of at least 50 per cent may be needed to ensure adequate arterial oxygenation. These considerations of necessity limit the concentration of nitrous oxide that can be administered.

Hypoxia can occur during recovery from nitrous oxide administration if patients breathe air. 'Diffusion anoxia' was first described by Fink (1955) and is due to the rapid elimination into the alveoli of large volumes of nitrous oxide and a consequent diminution in alveolar oxygen concentration. Although usually mild, diffusion hypoxia may present a risk to the patient with depressed or impaired cardiac or respiratory function. Diffusion hypoxia is only important when an appreciable volume of nitrous oxide has been taken up. It can easily be prevented by oxygen administration during the initial phase of nitrous oxide elimination.

During nitrous oxide anaesthesia any closed gas-filled cavity in the body will expand, due to the exchange of small volumes of nitrogen from the cavity for large volumes of nitrous oxide from blood. Expansion of a pneumothorax, pneumopericardium, or pneumoperitoneum may have serious consequences. Gas-filled obstructed intestine will also expand, although a poor blood supply will limit the rate, and therefore the significance, of nitrous oxide passage into the intestine. Air accidentally entering the circulation during nitrous oxide anaesthesia will greatly increase in volume. Air injected during pneumoencephalography will also expand and may raise the CSF pressure. Nitrous oxide diffusing into the middle ear may interfere with middle ear mechanics.

Prolonged nitrous oxide administration depresses bone marrow function. Animal studies have indeed shown a minimal teratogenic effect of prolonged nitrous oxide administration.

Although vigilant care is taken during the preparation of nitrous oxide to ensure its purity, fatalities have been caused in the past due to cylinders contaminated with higher oxides of nitrogen, principally nitric oxide and nitrogen peroxide. A syndrome of chemical pneumonitis, severe hypoxaemia, methaemoglobinaemia, metabolic acidosis, and hypotension is caused by the inhalation of these impurities.

Pre-mixed cylinders. Although nitrous oxide readily liquefies under pressure, mixtures of nitrous oxide and oxygen can be prepared that will remain gaseous when pressurized. Under these circumstances nitrous oxide may be considered as being dissolved in oxygen. A constant composition mixture is released from such pre-mixed cylinders. The stability of these mixtures decreases as the nitrous oxide fraction is increased. Pre-mixed cylinders containing 50 per cent nitrous oxide are now in widespread use. If cooled below −8°C, the contents separate into liquid nitrous oxide and gaseous oxygen. The cylinders will then initially deliver a high oxygen-containing mixture, but eventually nearly pure nitrous oxide will emerge. Ideally, these cylinders should not be stored in the open. If accidentally exposed to low temperatures, they should be brought indoors to warm up, and inverted several times to re-establish the stable mixture.

Amess, J. A. L., Burman, J. F., Rees, G. M., Nancekievill, D. G. and Mollen, D. L. (1978) Megaloblastic haemopoiesis in patients receiving nitrous oxide. *Lancet,* **2,** 339

Banks, R. G. S., Henderson, R. J. and Pratt, J. M. (1968) Reactions of gases in solution. Part III: some reactions of nitrous oxide with transition-metal compounds. *Journal of the Chemical Society (A),* **12,** 2886

Eisele, J. H., Trenchard, D., Stubbs, J. and Guz, A. (1969) The immediate cardiac depression by anaesthetics in conscious dogs. *British Journal of Anaesthesia,* **41,** 86

Fink, B. R. (1955) Diffusion anoxia. *Anesthesiology,* **16,** 511
Hong, K., Trudell, R. S., O'Neill, J. R. and Cohen, E. N. (1980) Metabolism of nitrous oxide by human and rat intestinal contents. *Anesthesiology,* **52,** 16
Hornbein, T. F., Martin, W. E., Bonica, J. J., Freund, F. G. and Parmentier, P. (1969) Nitrous oxide effects on the circulatory and ventilatory responses to halothane. *Anesthesiology,* **31,** 250
Kawamura, R., Stanley, T. H., English, J. B., Hill, G. E., Liu, W-S. and Webster, L. R. (1980) Cardiovascular responses to nitrous oxide exposure for two hours in man. *Anesthesia and Analgesia,* **59,** 93
Lassen, H. C. A., Hendrikson, E., Neukirch, F. and Kristensen, H. S. (1956) Treatment of tetanus. Severe bone marrow depression after prolonged nitrous oxide anaesthesia. *Lancet,* **1,** 527
Minty, B., Deacon, R., Lumb, M., Perry, J., Halsey, M. J., Nunn, J. F. and Chanarm, I. (1979) Effect of nitrous oxide on B-12 requiring enzymes. *British Journal of Anaesthesia,* **51,** 65P
Smith, N. T., Eger, E. I., Stoelting, R. K., Whayne, T. F., Cullen, D. and Kadis, L. B. (1970) The cardiovascular and sympathomimetic responses to the addition of nitrous oxide to halothane in man. *Anesthesiology,* **32,** 410
Smith, W. D. A. (1971) Pharmacology of nitrous oxide. *International Anesthesiology Clinics,* **9,** 91
Vickers, M. D. and Pask, E. A. (1966) Less than 20% oxygen or not? *Anaesthesia,* **21,** 261

Cyclopropane

Cyclopropane (*BP* and *USP*)
Chemical name: trimethylene

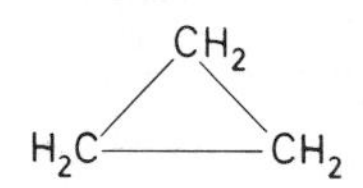

PHYSICAL CHARACTERISTICS

Cyclopropane is a colourless gas with a characteristic odour resembling that of solvent naphtha, and has a pungent taste. The vapour has a density of 1.45. It is manufactured by heating trimethylene dibromide with zinc. It also occurs in natural gas in the USA. Cyclopropane is highly flammable and forms explosive mixtures with air (2.4–10.4 per cent) and oxygen (2.5–60 per cent). It is supplied compressed to a liquid at a pressure of 75 lb/in^2 (517 kPa) in orange-coloured cylinders. These cylinders should be kept in a cool place and away from material of a flammable nature. It diffuses through rubber, which it attacks. In the theatre, precautions against static discharge should be taken. The addition of 30 per cent or more helium to the cyclopropane–oxygen mixture aids in preventing explosions.

The anaesthetic properties of cyclopropane have been known for many years but, on account of its high cost, it was not until Waters perfected closed-circuit anaesthesia during the 1930s that it was used to any great extent. It rapidly became popular, but since the introduction of balanced anaesthesia it has been used much less frequently.

PHARMACOLOGY

Nervous system. The CNS is depressed, as with all general anaesthetics. Paralysis of the respiratory centre readily occurs, but precedes that of the vasomotor centre by a safe margin unless anaesthesia is deepened rapidly. There is a preponderance of vagal tone. Postoperative headache is more common than with other anaesthetics.

Cardiovascular system. Cardiac output may be initially increased, but falls as anaesthesia is deepened. Blood pressure is slightly increased. Severe hypotension may occur when the anaesthetic is withdrawn (so-called 'cyclopropane shock'). This was investigated by Dripps (1947), who showed that the degree of hypotension was directly related to the severity of the respiratory acidosis which had occurred. Cyclopropane anaesthesia is associated with marked increases in the levels of circulating adrenaline and noradrenaline, and withdrawal of cyclopropane is accompanied by an abrupt fall in these levels.

Pulse rate is slowed but atropine will usually restore the rate to normal. There is an increase in cardiac dysrhythmias if the $P\text{CO}_2$ is allowed to rise.

Cullen, Eger and Gregory (1969), in a controlled study of the effects of cyclopropane in volunteers when the effects of other drugs or surgical stimulation could be avoided, found little change in cardiac output, heart rate or stroke volume. Mean arterial pressure and total peripheral resistance were raised. Mean right atrial pressure rose considerably and skin blood flow was increased six-fold. There was peripheral vasoconstriction with a marked reduction in venous compliance. During prolonged administration only a minor degree of recovery occurred with time. The cardiac index–carbon dioxide response curve was depressed by cyclopropane, but less so than by halothane or a thiopentone–narcotic–relaxant sequence.

Respiration. Cyclopropane is a marked respiratory depressant. Respiration is slow and shallow and minute volume is decreased. During spontaneous ventilation severe respiratory depression may limit the achievement of adequate depth of anaesthesia. There is constriction of bronchial musculature and bronchospasm, and laryngospasm may occur during light anaesthesia. Bronchial secretions are increased during light anaesthesia and decreased during deep anaesthesia.

Muscular system. Depression of skeletal muscle tone is not marked; smooth muscle is unaffected.

Liver and kidney functions. There is only a transient and slight depression of the function of these organs. In the absence of hypoxia, permanent liver damage does not occur.

Alimentary system. The bowel is constricted at first, but becomes relaxed as anaesthesia is deepened. Salivary secretion increases during light anaesthesia.

Metabolism. There is a slight increase in blood sugar; other metabolic processes are little affected. Respiratory acidosis will occur if ventilation is depressed. Nausea and vomiting are common.

Uterus and placenta. Cyclopropane passes the placental barrier and can cause respiratory depression in the fetus.

Fate in the body. It is excreted by the lungs unchanged; a small amount diffuses through the skin. Although Van Dyke and Chenoweth (1965) suggested that [^{14}C]cyclopropane was converted into $^{14}CO_2$ in rats, Sawyer and colleagues (1971) were unable to demonstrate biotransformation of cyclopropane following liver perfusion in miniature swine.

ANAESTHETIC PROPERTIES

Cyclopropane is a rapidly acting anaesthetic, full surgical anaesthesia being obtainable within 5 minutes. Induction is not unpleasant. Respiration is quiet, but muscular relaxation is insufficient for abdominal surgery. Capillary oozing from cut surfaces is more pronounced than with other anaesthetic agents.

Because of the low blood solubility of cyclopropane it is easy to achieve deep levels of anaesthesia quickly. For the same reason recovery is rapid, normally within a few minutes of terminating the administration, but owing to its higher oil solubility recovery is relatively slow after long administration.

INDICATIONS

Cyclopropane can be used in all branches of surgical practice when diathermy is not necessary and has been recommended for 'bad-risk' patients on the grounds that it allows good oxygenation and is rapidly eliminated without metabolic or visceral damage. However, it is not without interest that one of the incidental findings of the National Halothane Study (Bunker, 1966) was that cyclopropane was associated with a higher mortality than any other agent or technique, and this was true even when allowance was made for the preoperative status of the patient and the nature of the operation. In the UK almost the only usage of cyclopropane is for inducing babies and small children as it does not cause breath-holding and coughing and unconsciousness can be achieved with only a very few breaths. The very real explosion risk suggests that cyclopropane should be used only when there is a positive indication.

DOSAGE AND ADMINISTRATION

On account of its high cost, cyclopropane is normally administered in a closed circuit with carbon dioxide absorption.

Concentrations of 3–5 per cent produce analgesia, 7–10 per cent light anaesthesia, 20–30 per cent moderate to deep anaesthesia, and respiratory paralysis will occur in the region of 40 per cent.

PRECAUTIONS

An adequate dose of atropine should be given before anaesthesia to prevent the effects of increased vagal tone.

If respiration is controlled an overdose may easily be given.

Ventricular dysrhythmias are most commonly provoked by a raised level of carbon dioxide in the arterial blood, and increasing the ventilation and reducing the concentration of the anaesthetic will correct many dysrhythmias without resort to β-receptor blockade. Adrenaline must not be given during cyclopropane anaesthesia.

Bunker, J. P. (Chairman) (1966) Subcommittee on the National Halothane Study of the Committee on Anesthesia. NAS–NRC. Summary of the National Halothane Study. Possible association between halothane and postoperative hepatic necrosis. *Journal of the American Medical Association,* **197,** 775

Cullen, D. J., Eger, E. I. and Gregory, G. A. (1969) The cardiovascular effects of cyclopropane in man. *Anesthesiology,* **31,** 398

Dripps, R. D. (1947) The immediate decrease in blood pressure seen at the conclusion of cyclopropane anesthesia: "cyclopropane shock". *Anesthesiology,* **8,** 15

Sawyer, D. C., Eger, E. I., Bahlman, S. H., Cullen, B. F. and Impelman, D. (1971) Concentration dependence of hepatic halothane metabolism. *Anesthesiology,* **34,** 230

Van Dyke, R. A. and Chenoweth, M. B. (1965) Metabolism of volatile anesthetics. *Anesthesiology,* **26,** 348

5

Systemic analgesics

Pain

Following the stimulation of pain nerve endings, impulses can travel by two routes to reach the CNS: one via the myelinated delta group of A fibres and the other by a slower passage through non-myelinated C fibres. Both groups of fibres end in the dorsal horn of the spinal cord where they synapse.

According to the 'gate' theory, normal sensory input inhibits further transmission of the nerve impulse. However, excessive activity from pain fibre stimulation allows the gate to open and pain impulses pass through. It is postulated that there is a central control modulating the threshold of the 'gate' and this accounts for the variation in response to pain from patient to patient and from situation to situation.

The postsynaptic secondary nerve fibres cross the cord and ascend in the spinothalamic tract. Impulses are recognized as crude pain in the thalamus and the localization of the pain takes place in the cortex.

An alternative pathway exists consisting of collaterals which relay in the reticular formation. Again impulses reach the cortex but this time through the reticulocortical pathways.

Rapid impulse conduction results in a sharp stinging pain being appreciated at cortical level; slow impulse conduction results in dull constant pain.

For almost a century the choice of an analgesic has been between a narcotic analgesic of the morphine type and a mild agent, related to salicylic acid, pyrazolone, or *p*-aminophenol. The former are centrally acting powerful analgesics which will relieve pain associated with surgery, trauma, and cancer; the latter have mild central actions which are supplemented by a mechanism that relieves pain by modifying inflammatory processes peripherally.

In recent years, intensive research has been devoted to finding non-addictive powerful analgesics. One line has been the development of narcotic analgesics that are predominantly antagonist such as buprenorphine. Cannabinoids have analgesic effects and one, levonantradol, is now on trial. It tends to cause sedation and psychotropic effects. Nefopam is another interesting compound which is sufficiently powerful to be used for moderate to severe pain. Despite the fact that there has been some loss of distinction between various kinds of analgesics, it is still convenient to consider them under two broad headings, the narcotic analgesics and the non-narcotic analgesics, the latter being divided into mild analgesics and non-steroidal anti-inflammatory drugs (NSAIDs).

Morphine skeleton

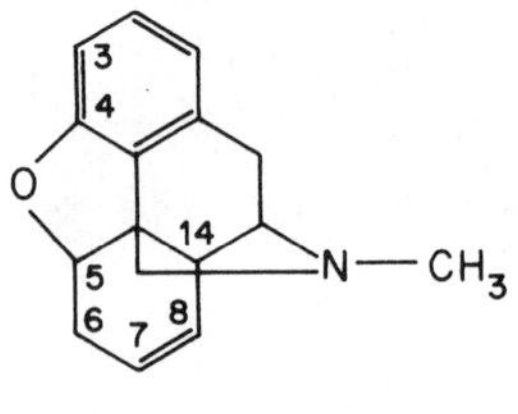

Official and/or common name	*Substituents on morphine skeleton*						
	3	*4–5*	*6*	*14*	N	*7*	*8*
Morphine	HO	O	HO	—	CH_3	—	—
Codeine	CH_3O	O	HO	—	CH_3	—	—
Dihydrocodeine	CH_3O	O	HO	—	CH_3	H	H
Diamorphine (heroin)	CH_3COO	O	CH_3COO	—	CH_3	—	—
Dihydromorphinone	HO	O	O	—	CH_3	H	H
Oxymorphone	HO	O	O	HO	CH_3	H	H
Naloxone	HO	O	O	HO	C_3H_5	H	H
Nalorphine	HO	O	HO	—	C_3H_5	—	—
Levorphanol	HO	—	H	—	CH_3	H	H
Levallorphan	HO	—	H	—	C_3H_5	H	H

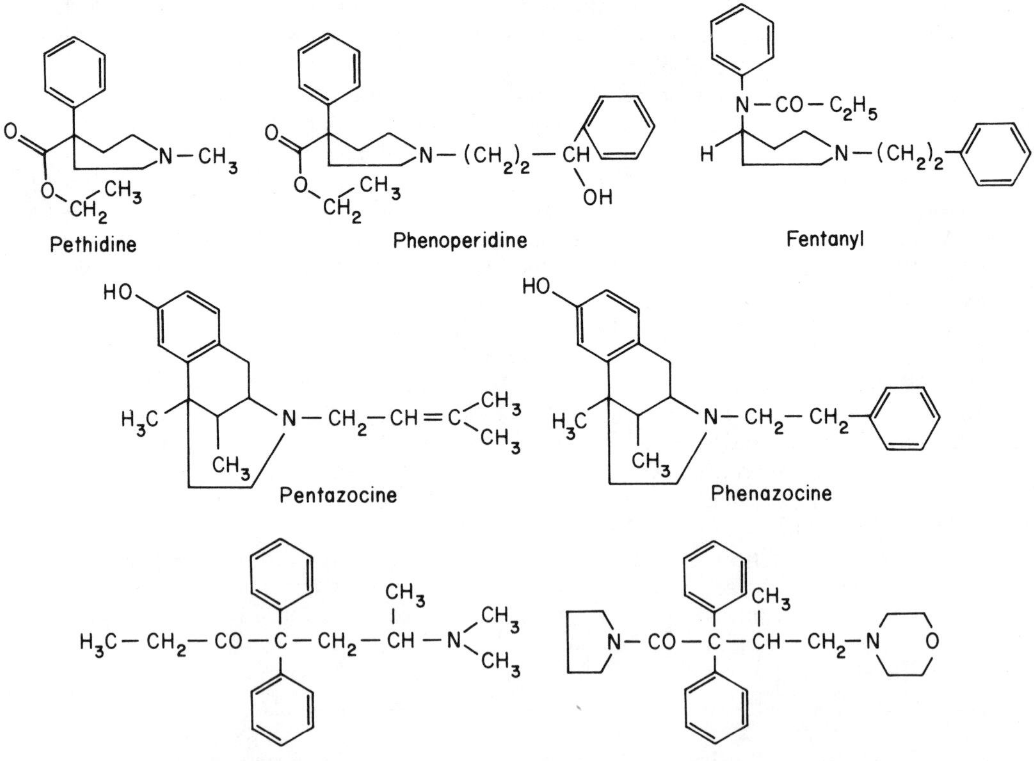

Pethidine

Phenoperidine

Fentanyl

Pentazocine

Phenazocine

Methadone

Dextromoramide

Figure 5.1 The chemical structures of morphine derivatives and some other narcotic analgesics

Narcotic analgesics

All the members of this group are complex chemical compounds; some occur naturally while others are prepared synthetically. They include the alkaloids of opium, especially morphine and its derivatives – codeine, dihydrocodeine, diamorphine, dihydromorphinone, levorphanol, and oxymorphone; pethidine and its derivatives – phenoperidine and fentanyl; and methadone and its derivatives – phenadoxone, dipipanone, and dextromoramide. Other powerful analgesics unrelated chemically to the above groups are piritramide, phenazocine, and pentazocine. The chemical structures of some of these compounds are shown in *Figure 5.1*.

Drugs of this type can possess two types of activity. They can have agonist actions like morphine and cause respiratory depression and analgesia. Alternatively, they can possess antagonist activity and reverse the active effects of morphine. The ratio of agonist to antagonist activity differs from compound to compound (*Figure 5.2*); those that have both agonist and antagonist activity are often referred to as partial agonists. Thus these drugs are on a spectrum of activity ranging from those with pure agonist actions (for example diamorphine) to those with pure antagonist actions (for example naloxone). Between these extremes are a large number of drugs which are partial agonists. Agonist actions include analgesia, euphoria, stimulation of the chemoreceptor trigger zone, and respiratory depression; those with only partial agonist activity also exhibit dysphoria and hallucinations.

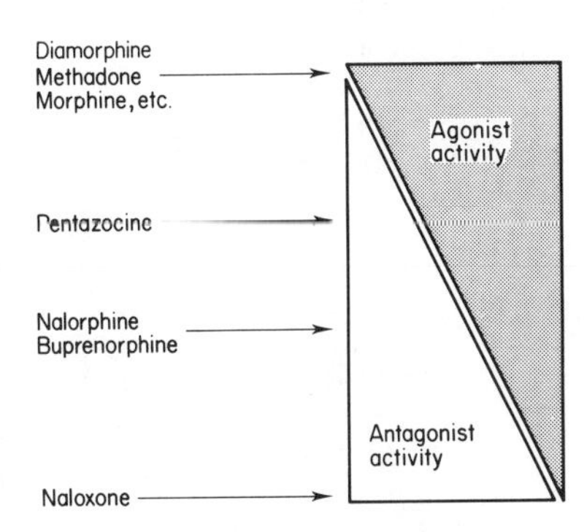

Figure 5.2 Agonist/antagonist activity of some opioids

As can be seen from *Figure 5.2*, pentazocine has both agonist and antagonist activity. Drugs such as nalorphine and pentazocine, which have some antagonist activity, will antagonize drugs nearer the agonist end. The antagonism, however, is unreliable because of the partial agonist activity. Naloxone, with no agonist activity, is the only drug that will safely antagonize all the agonist actions.

Addiction potential is an agonist action; drugs that are well towards the antagonist end of the spectrum produce such additional unpleasant symptoms that they could never be addictive.

The mechanism of action of morphine has been a subject of speculation for many years. Most hypotheses have tried to link the actions with changes in brain amines or brain acetylcholine levels. Morphine inhibits the release of acetylcholine from nerve endings and this almost certainly accounts for the gastrointestinal paralysis that it produces. There is reasonable evidence that this mechanism indirectly accounts for many of the central effects also. Analgesia is associated with changes in central cholinergic activity in certain critical areas. In addition, all these compounds are partial dopamine agonists. The most powerful agonist is apomorphine and this is a powerful stimulator of dopamine receptors in the chemoreceptor trigger zone. Dopamine antagonists, such as neuroleptics, are therefore the most logical and effective antiemetics to counteract this action of these drugs.

Our modern views on the subject date from the mid 1970s when Snyder and Pert (1975) showed specific binding of labelled opiates to parts of the CNS. Selective binding was noted in the limbic system (amygdaloid and septal nuclei), in the cortex (frontal and temporal lobes), and in parts of the pain pathway (thalamic nuclei, aqueductal grey matter, and substantia gelatinosa). Other sites that bound labelled opiates in high concentrations were the area postrema of the fourth ventricle and the locus coeruleus. These structures have been implicated in vomiting, sleep, emotional response, and the pain pathways. Hence the distribution of binding sites correlated well with the actions of opiate-like drugs which cause vomiting, produce sedation and euphoria, and diminish pain.

In 1975 Hughes reported that certain brain extracts could mimic the actions of morphine on tissue preparations. Later that year Hughes and co-workers identified two pentapeptides from brain which had morphine-like activity. These were methionine and leucine enkephalin (*Figure 5.3*). Shortly after this it was noted that

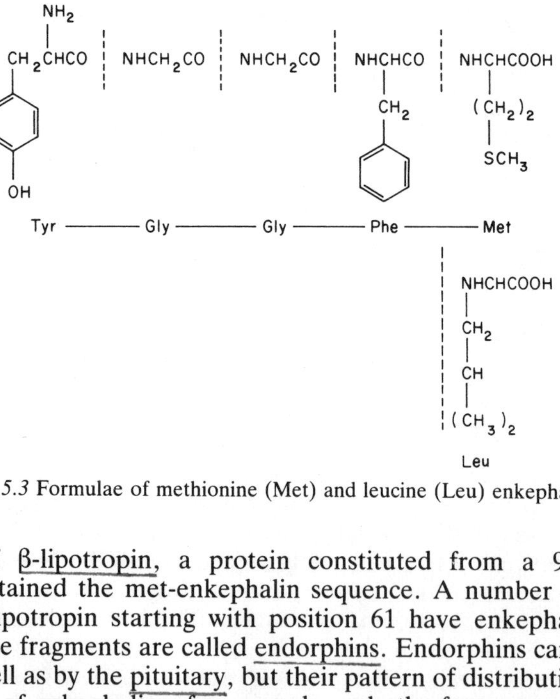

Figure 5.3 Formulae of methionine (Met) and leucine (Leu) enkephalin

the structure of β-lipotropin, a protein constituted from a 91 amino acid polypeptide, contained the met-enkephalin sequence. A number of polypeptide fragments of β-lipotropin starting with position 61 have enkephalin-like action (*Table 5.1*). These fragments are called endorphins. Endorphins can be formed by brain tissue as well as by the pituitary, but their pattern of distribution in the brain differs from that of enkephalins; for example, only the former are present in the hypothalamus. Pharmacologically both endorphins and enkephalins have morphine-like actions; however, enkephalins have a very short duration of action while β-endorphin has a duration of action similar to morphine.

It is now thought that corticotrophin, intermediate lobe peptides, and related lipotropins are derived from a common glycoprotein called pro-opiocortin (molecular weight approximately 30 000).

It seems likely that there are separate synthetic pathways for the synthesis of endorphins and enkephalins, the latter being synthesized from pro-enkephalin. It is possible that growth hormone and the enkephalins share a common precursor. A third enkephalin has also been isolated (Hughes, 1979).

This is a rapidly developing field and it is possible that within the next few years other endorphins or enkephalins will be discovered and also their functions better understood. At present there is evidence, based on the fact that naloxone will antagonize the effects of endorphins and enkephalins, that the effects of acupuncture may be mediated via opiate receptors (Chung and Dickenson, 1980), that patients with high pain thresholds are being stimulated by physiological opiate-like substances, and that the placebo response to pain may be mediated by an enkephalin or endorphin mechanism (Anon, 1980).

Table 5.1 The endorphins and the amino acids in β-lipotropin which constitute them

Endorphin	*Part of B-lipotropin*
α	61–76
β*	61–91
	61–77
γ	61–86

* Also called fragment c. This is a potent analgesic.

The concept that a drug can act at more than one receptor site is not novel. Martin (1979) suggested that there were three types of opioid receptor which he called μ (mu), κ (kappa), and σ (sigma) receptors (*Table 5.2*). Another type of receptor, δ (delta), has also been postulated (Lord *et al.*, 1977). Morphine has a low affinity for such receptors, enkephalins a high affinity. It is suggested that opioids produce their spectrum of activity by their interactions with such receptors. For instance, pentazocine is a weak competitive μ-receptor agonist, a σ-receptor agonist, and a more potent κ-receptor agonist.

Table 5.2 The opioid receptors and the effects produced by opiate agonists on them

Receptor	*Effects produced by agonists*
μ (mu)	Supraspinal analgesia, physical dependence (morphine type), euphoria
σ (sigma)	Dysphoria, mydriasis, respiratory stimulation
κ (kappa)	Sedation, spinal analgesia, cyclazocine-type dependence

Drugs with predominantly agonist activity produce coma or stupor when used in high doses. Respiratory depression is then the greatest immediate danger. Addiction is a bar to their indiscriminate and continued use. Nausea, vomiting, and constipation are potentially troublesome side effects, especially when treatment is prolonged. Combining treatment with partial antagonists, such as levallorphan, to prevent respiratory depression or other side effects is of doubtful value; the concurrent administration of non-specific arousal agents such as amiphenazole enjoyed a vogue in the treatment of severe terminal pain but has not been widely adopted.

It is not easy to compare the relative potency and effectiveness of different analgesics; pain is difficult to assess, and drugs that will relieve experimentally produced pain are not necessarily equally effective in pain of pathological origin, and vice versa. Morrison, Loan and Dundee (1971) have compared the efficacy of 14 preparations in the relief of postoperative pain.

Anon (1980) Opiate peptides, analgesia and the neuroendocrine system. *British Medical Journal*, **1**, 741

Chung, S. and Dickenson, A. (1980) Pain, enkephalin and acupuncture. *Nature*, **283**, 243

Hughes, J., Smith, T. W., Kosterlitz, H. W., Fothergill, L. A., Morgan, B. A. and Morris, H. R. (1975) Identification of two related pentapeptides from the brain with potent opiate agonist activity. *Nature*, **258**, 577

Hughes, J. (1979) Opioid peptides and their relatives. *Nature*, **278**, 394

Lord, J. A. H., Waterfield, A. A., Hughes, J. and Kosterlitz, H. W. (1977) Endogenous opioid peptides, multiple agonists and receptors. *Nature*, **267**, 495

Martin, W. R. (1979) History and development of mixed opioid agonists, partial agonists and antagonists. *British Journal of Clinical Pharmacology*, **7**, 273

Morrison, J. D., Loan, W. B. and Dundee, J. W. (1971) Controlled comparison of the efficacy of fourteen preparations in the relief of postoperative pain. *British Medical Journal*, **3**, 287

Snyder, S. H. and Pert, C. B. (1975) Regional distribution of the opiate receptor. In *Opiate Receptor Mechanisms*, p. 34, Ed. Snyder, S. H. and Matthysse, S. Cambridge (Mass): MIT Press

Intrathecal and extradural opiates

Following animal trials, the practice of applying opiates directly to the spinal cord has spread rapidly into clinical practice. Opioid receptors have been identified, particularly in the substantia gelatinosa. Both intrathecal and extradural routes have been used, doses tending to be lower in the former.

When injected intrathecally, the onset of analgesia takes only 2–3 minutes and lasts up to 24 hours; there is virtually no motor blockade and no sympathetic blockade. Despite these tremendous advantages, the method is not without drawbacks, the principal one being the occasional development of severe respiratory depression many hours after administration. This is principally found after intrathecal administration but has been reported after extradural administration. It is due to direct spread rostrally to the respiratory centre. In fact, changes in the sensitivity of the respiratory centre can be detected in most subjects. It has been reported that it can be reversed by naloxone, and that this has no effect on spinal analgesia. Further complications are the development of itching and of urinary retention.

A variety of opiates can be used in this way; given intrathecally, the rate of onset is dependent on physical properties such as lipid solubility.

The technique is generally unsatisfactory for the pain of the first stage of labour, as might be expected. It has been enthusiastically reported on in the relief of postoperative pain. Mixing the narcotic with a conventional local anaesthetic before surgery has been recommended as a technique that meets the needs of both surgery and postoperative pain relief, but it is too early to be sure of the best way to exploit this new mode of therapy. The technique has also been used to treat chronic pain conditions and in one series (Magora *et al.*, 1980) 56 per cent of a heterogenous group of patients had good pain relief. The authors suggest that opiate drugs have a direct antinociceptive effect on the spinal cord.

In the case of morphine, the intrathecal dose is 2–4 mg; extradurally the dose may need to be increased to 8 mg. Other narcotics can be given in appropriate equipotent doses. Solutions must be preservative-free for intrathecal use.

Magora, F., Olshwang, D., Eimerl, D., Shorr, J., Kulznelson, R., Cotev, S. and Davidson, J. T. (1980) Observations on extradural morphine analgesia in various pain conditions. *British Journal of Anaesthesia,* **52,** 247

Addiction to narcotic analgesics

Those members of this group of drugs in which agonist actions predominate induce a compulsive desire and continuous need for their influence, and this is accompanied by the development of a psychological and often physical dependence upon them. The effect is detrimental to the individual and to society and the craving is so great that the former will go to criminal extremes, if necessary, to procure supplies. A tolerance is acquired, and a cross-tolerance will then exist for drugs of related function.

Physical dependence is perhaps more correctly described as a chemical dependence, in that the drug has entered into the functioning of the body, probably into some enzyme systems, in such a way that the individual is used to its presence and without it rapidly becomes ill. Withdrawal symptoms are often severe and always unpleasant, and consist of nervousness, restlessness, and anxiety followed by sweating, twitching of muscles, and painful cramps in the legs and abdomen; vomiting and diarrhoea occur frequently. Objective signs of abstinence disappear in about 7–10 days, but the addict may complain of insomnia, nervousness, and muscle aches and pains for several weeks. The use of a morphine antagonist, such as naloxone, can rapidly precipitate such a state and can be dangerous. Used with care, it may be helpful in diagnosing addiction to morphine and related drugs, such as heroin, pethidine, and methadone.

A committee of the World Health Organization has defined drug addiction as a state of periodic or chronic intoxication produced by the repeated consumption of a drug (natural or synthetic). Its characteristics include:

1. An overpowering desire or need (compulsion) to continue taking the drug and to obtain it by any means;
2. A tendency to increase the dose;
3. A psychic (psychological) and generally a physical dependence on the effects of the drug;
4. An effect detrimental to the individual and to society.

The danger of addiction to drugs in the absence of pain is probably not great in mentally stable individuals, but the euphoria they produce is usually irresistible to neurotic and psychotic personalities.

The treatment of drug addiction is unsatisfactory and relapses are common. When the drug has been withdrawn, total abstinence offers the only hope of permanent cure. In addiction, as distinct from habituation, the dose of the drug must be reduced slowly and sedation may be necessary to control the abstinence syndrome. Chemically related drugs, such as methadone or pethidine for the heroin or morphine addict and, later, even codeine, are often helpful in these circumstances during the 'weaning period'; cyclazocine, a morphine-like analgesic, has been used in a similar way to methadone. Tranquillizers or chlorpromazine, initially parenterally, or orally later, may be of help. Two of the most important aspects of therapy, after recovery from the initial stages, are attention to general health and social rehabilitation.

Buprenorphine hydrochloride

Chemical name: (2*S*)-2-[(−)-(5*R*,6*R*,7*R*,14*S*)-9a-cyclopropylmethyl-4,5-epoxy-3-hydroxy-6-methoxy-6,14-ethanomorphinan-7-yl]-3,3-dimethylbutan-2-ol hydrochloride

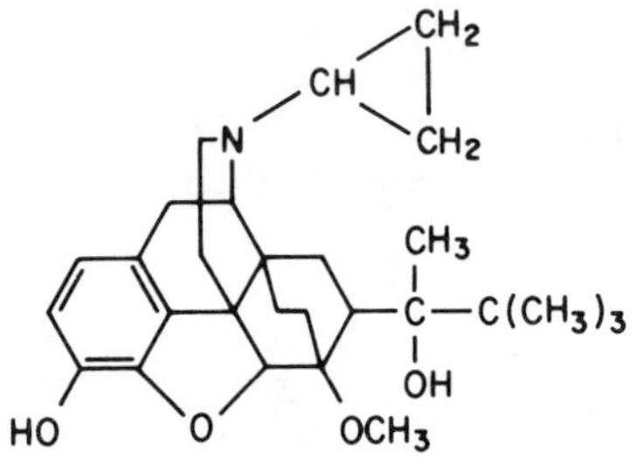

PHARMACOLOGY

Based on animal studies, buprenorphine appears to be a partial μ-receptor agonist. It might, therefore, be expected to produce supraspinal analgesia but cause less physical dependence than morphine. Tests in animals show it to have a low physical dependence potential and this has been confirmed in man (Jasinski, Pevnick, and Griffiths, 1978).

Buprenorphine dissociates very slowly from opiate receptor sites. Such a slow dissociation may give time for homeostatic mechanisms to come into play following abrupt withdrawal. Its respiratory effects suggest a slow rate of association also. When given intravenously the peak effect was not seen for over 25 minutes (Slattery *et al.*, 1982). Naloxone had little antagonistic effect.

It is about 20–50 times as potent as morphine as an analgesic. Its duration of action has generally been found to be longer than that of morphine. Unlike morphine, it does not necessarily produce constipation. The main side effect is drowsiness; less frequently, nausea and vomiting may occur. In single doses it can produce euphoria and constrict the pupils. Naloxone is unable to precipitate an abstinence syndrome during chronic treatment. Coltart and Malcolm (1979) used the drug in patients following coronary artery grafting or valve replacement. Apart from a small fall in heart rate, it had no effect on ECG, cardiac output, and arterial blood pressure.

Fate in the body. The drug is metabolized in the liver by *N*-dealkylation and glucuronide conjugation and the metabolites are excreted in the bile.

INDICATIONS

It has been found to give satisfactory analgesia after surgery and was virtually indistinguishable from morphine when given either intravenously or intramuscularly by an 'on demand' self-administration system. Robbie (1979) found it a useful analgesic when given sublingually to patients with cancer pain.

DOSAGE AND ADMINISTRATION

Buprenorphine is given by intramuscular or slow intravenous injection 0.3–0.6 mg three to four times per day. The duration of action of a single dose is 6–8 hours. It may also be given sublingually 0.4–0.8 mg every 6–8 hours.

PRECAUTIONS

As with other opiate-like compounds, liver dysfunction can prolong its duration of action. Buprenorphine can cause drowsiness which may be potentiated by other central depressants, including alcohol. It may cause vomiting and an interaction with monoamine oxidase inhibitors (MAOIs) is possible. Overdosage leading to respiratory depression is not easily reversed by naloxone and doxapram may need to be administered as well. General supportive measures to maintain adequate oxygenation and ventilation may also be necessary.

Coltart, D. J. and Malcolm, A. D. (1979) Pharmacological and clinical importance of narcotic antagonists and mixed agonists — use in cardiology. *British Journal of Clinical Pharmacology,* **7,** 309

Jasinski, D. T., Pevnick, J. S. and Griffiths, J. D. (1978) Human pharmacology and abuse potential of the analgesic buprenorphine. *Archives of General Psychiatry,* **35,** 501

Robbie, D. S. (1979) A trial of sublingual buprenorphine in cancer pain. *British Journal of Clinical Pharmacology,* **7,** 315

Slattery, P. J., Harmer, M., Rosen, M. and Vickers, M. D. (1982) Respiratory depression with buprenorphine: onset time and reversal. In *Proceedings of the European Academy of Anaesthesiology,* p. 68, Ed. Prys-Roberts, C. and Vickers, M. D. Heidelberg: Springer-Verlag

Butorphanol tartrate

Butorphanol tartrate (*USP*)
Chemical name: (−)-17-(cyclobutylmethyl)morphinan-3,14-diol tartrate

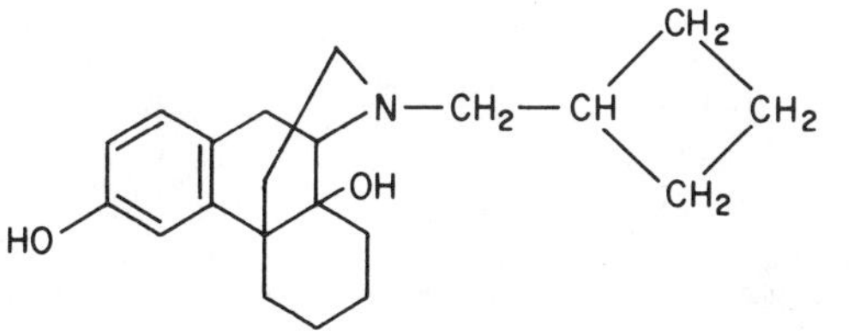

PHARMACOLOGY

Butorphanol is a potent partial agonist analgesic which is approximately seven times as potent as morphine when given intramuscularly for the relief of postoperative pain. It appears as effective as other opioids for premedication or when used as part of balanced anaesthesia. Compared with equianalgesic doses of morphine, the drug produces similar respiratory depression at low doses. However, there are reports that as the dosage of butorphanol is raised, further depression of respiration is less than that produced by equianalgesic doses of morphine. This ceiling effect has been suggested as an advantage. Whether a true ceiling exists is difficult to determine in man, but the drug certainly produces changes in respiratory pattern at lower doses. Butorphanol's actions are reversed by naloxone, but the dose required is higher than for reversal of a pure agonist such as morphine.

Fate in the body. The drug is well absorbed when given orally, but there is a marked first-pass effect and availability of the oral dose is only about 20 per cent of the intravenous dose. Peak levels in man occurred 1.5 hours after oral administration and 30 minutes after intramuscular administration. The drug is mainly metabolized to inactive hydroxybutorphanol but about 10 per cent of a parenteral dose is excreted in the bile. *O*-Dealkylation and conjugation of the drug also occurs. The elimination half-life in healthy subjects is about 3 hours.

INDICATIONS

The drug is used for the relief of moderate or severe pain. It is effective in postoperative pain, cancer pain, and labour pain. For the latter, 1–2 mg butorphanol is equivalent to 40–50 mg pethidine.

DOSAGE AND ADMINISTRATION

As a partial agonist it can reverse the actions of morphine and can be expected to produce withdrawal symptoms in patients dependent on morphine. Since it can produce miosis and it has a respiratory depressant effect, its use is contraindicated in head injury. The drug has been reported to increase pulmonary arterial pressure and therefore is not recommended in acute myocardial infarction. It can produce physical dependence, although it appears to have a lower liability than morphine.

Codeine phosphate

Codeine phosphate (*BP* and *USP*)
Chemical name: phosphate of 3-*O*-methylmorphine
For structural formula *see Figure 5.1*, p. 168

PHARMACOLOGY

Codeine is one of the chief alkaloids found in natural opium. Its actions are all much weaker than those of morphine and it is less constipating and less liable to produce nausea and vomiting. Its analgesic action is considerably weaker and its sedative action is poor but it is a useful suppressor of the cough reflex. If the dose is increased too much it may cause excitement rather than sedation. Even in large doses, however, it does not produce severe respiratory depression.

Fate in the body. Codeine is partly demethylated and partly conjugated in the body; some remains unchanged and this is excreted by the kidneys. The demethylation can produce either morphine or norcodeine according to which methyl groups are attacked, so that the urine will contain free and conjugated forms of codeine, norcodeine, and morphine. It has been suggested that its analgesic action is entirely due to the morphine which is produced by its degradation in the liver.

INDICATIONS

Codeine phosphate is used in the treatment of minor degrees of pain, often in combination with other analgesics such as acetylsalicylic acid and paracetamol. Its main use, however, is as an antitussive and in the treatment of diarrhoea.

DOSAGE AND ADMINISTRATION

Codeine phosphate is given by mouth in a dose of 10–60 mg but doses up to 100 mg are sometimes employed. Higher dosage does not achieve a greater degree of analgesia. A common formulation is 250 mg each of aspirin and paracetamol and 8 mg of codeine phosphate.

PRECAUTIONS

Precautions are basically the same as for morphine; side effects in the doses normally employed are rare and addiction is uncommon.

Diamorphine hydrochloride

Diamorphine hydrochloride (*BP*)
Synonym: heroin hydrochloride
Chemical name: 3,6-*O*-diacetylmorphine hydrochloride
For structural formula *see Figure 5.1,* p. 168

PHARMACOLOGY

Diamorphine is the diacetyl analogue of morphine. It is a more powerful analgesic, but its main disadvantage is that it is extremely likely to cause addiction. In the USA and other countries its manufacture and use are forbidden by law.

In optimal doses, about half those required with morphine, it produces more profound analgesia, and it is less depressing on the respiratory centre. Nausea, vomiting, and constipation are less common. Diamorphine has always been noted for its euphoric effect but there is little difference between the two drugs in their ability to relieve anxiety or produce euphoria. Its duration of action is less than half that of morphine. Diamorphine is hydrolysed to morphine.

INDICATIONS

Although diamorphine is now rarely used as a routine analgesic, it is of value in really severe pain. However, without some specific indication it should be used with caution because of the readiness with which addiction can develop. It is normally given subcutaneously in doses of 5–10 mg but is also included in Brompton Hospital mixtures. Precautions and treatment of overdose are as for morphine.

Dihydrocodeine tartrate

Dihydrocodeine tartrate (*BP*)
Chemical name: 7,8-dihydro-3-*O*-methylmorphine hydrogen tartrate
For structural formula *see Figure 5.1*, p. 168

PHARMACOLOGY

Dihydrocodeine tartrate must be stored away from light in well-closed containers. It is closely related chemically to codeine and its analgesic potency lies between that of codeine and pethidine. A dose of 30 mg gives similar analgesia to 10 mg of morphine. Compared with morphine, its sedative effect is less, and its duration of action is slightly shorter. Side effects such as respiratory depression, nausea, and vomiting are minimal, although constipation may be troublesome after prolonged treatment. Even when given intravenously, respiration is scarcely affected and there is little change in minute volume, the slight reduction in rate being almost compensated by an increase in depth. There is little or no effect on blood pressure when given in recommended doses.

INDICATIONS

Dihydrocodeine may be used as a substitute for morphine or its derivatives in the treatment of postoperative and chronic pain.

DOSAGE AND ADMINISTRATION

Dihydrocodeine is effective by mouth and may be given in a dose of 30–60 mg; similar doses may be given subcutaneously, or 20–30 mg intravenously. Side effects are less troublesome than with morphine but similar precautions should be taken regarding its use.

Fentanyl citrate

Fentanyl citrate (*BP* and *USP*)
Chemical name: *N*-(1-phenylethyl-4-piperidyl)propionanilide dihydrogen citrate
For structural formula *see Figure 5.1*, p. 168

Fentanyl, like phenoperidine, is chemically related to pethidine but weight for weight is even more potent. Its action is similar and respiratory depression will occur if doses exceeding 200 µg are given intravenously. Its duration of action is considerably shorter than that of phenoperidine and repeat doses need to be given every 10–20 minutes during major surgery. The cardiovascular system usually remains stable but high doses can cause hypotension; 200 µg is equianalgesic with 10 mg of morphine but this dose when given as a premedicant has more marked unwanted side effects.

INDICATIONS

Fentanyl is given as an analgesic supplement during light nitrous oxide anaesthesia and in neuroleptanalgesia.

DOSAGE AND ADMINISTRATION

Fentanyl may be administered orally or intramuscularly but is usually given intravenously; 100–200 µg usually allows adequate respiration, and 200–600 µg may be given when respiration can be controlled. It is one component of a commercial mixture with droperidol in a proportion of 50:1 (2.5 mg of droperidol and 50 µg of fentanyl in 1 ml). As these drugs have half-lives of approximately 4 hours and 20 minutes respectively, the logic of this fixed-ratio mixture cannot be well founded.

PRECAUTIONS

Respiratory depression if present at the end of operation should be treated by the administration of naloxone. Large doses have a prolonged effect.

Alfentanil. This is a derivative of fentanyl which has all its pharmacological characteristics but is about one-third as potent, more rapid in onset and of much shorter duration of action.

Levorphanol tartrate

Levorphanol tartrate (*BP* and *USP*)
Chemical name: (−)-9a-methylmorphinan-3-ol hydrogen tartrate
For structural formula *see Figure 5.1,* p. 168

PHARMACOLOGY

Levorphanol is a morphine-like agent in which the oxygen bridge, the double bond, and the alcoholic hydroxyl group are absent. Its actions are similar to those of morphine. It is more powerful as an analgesic, but has little hypnotic effect and anxiety is not relieved. Its duration of effect is longer, and side effects are said to be less marked, vomiting being less common. In postoperative abdominal pain, it is particularly effective, chiefly because pain relief is associated with minimal depression of consciousness.

It is broken down in the liver and only small amounts are found unchanged in the urine.

INDICATIONS

Levorphanol is used in the relief of severe pain; its lack of sedative action is an advantage in the treatment of ambulant patients. A striking characteristic is that it produces cheerfulness in pain-depressed patients the morning after an evening dose.

DOSAGE AND ADMINISTRATION

Levorphanol may be given by mouth or by subcutaneous, intramuscular, or intravenous injection. When given by mouth the average duration of analgesia with 1.3 mg is 8 hours, with 2 mg it is 10 hours and with 4 mg it is 14 hours. Orally, it need be given only once or twice a day.

Precautions and antagonists are as for morphine.

Methadone hydrochloride

Methadone hydrochloride (*BP* and *USP*)
Chemical name: (±)-6-dimethylamino-4,4-diphenylheptan-3-one hydrochloride
For structural formula *see Figure 5.1,* p. 168

PHARMACOLOGY

Methadone is a synthetic heptanone; the *laevo* isomer is many times more powerful than the *dextro* isomer and is the active constituent of the racemic compound. In general its actions are similar to, although less marked than, those of morphine.

It is a powerful analgesic of similar potency to morphine, but has only about a quarter of its sedative action and euphoria is minimal. In equianalgesic doses there is less depression of respiration, spasmogenic effect on smooth muscle, and stimulation of the vomiting centre. There is effective depression of the cough reflex. Marked tolerance to the analgesic, sedative, and respiratory depressant actions of methadone have been observed in man; methadone-induced miosis is less prominent than that caused by morphine, and the addict develops complete tolerance to this action.

Fate in the body. The ultimate fate of methadone in the body is unknown. It is probably metabolized in the liver, 20–30 per cent being excreted unchanged in the urine. The rate of degradation is similar to that of morphine.

INDICATIONS

Methadone is used in the treatment of severe pain, morphine addiction, and in premedication. In morphine addiction it may be substituted for morphine and withdrawn more readily than the latter drug.

As a premedicant it is less effective than morphine as it has little sedative or tranquillizing action, but it is satisfactory in the presence of severe pain.

DOSAGE AND ADMINISTRATION

Methadone may be given by mouth, subcutaneously, or intramuscularly.

The official dose is 5–10 mg by any of the above routes and may be repeated at 4-hourly intervals if necessary. Doses up to 200 mg may be required if pain is very severe, or as tolerance develops; 10–15 mg may be given for premedication 1–1.5 hours before operation; 2.5 mg by mouth will depress the cough reflex.

PRECAUTIONS

Precautions are the same as for morphine. Side effects, however, are less marked. Respiration is likely to be seriously depressed if methadone is given intravenously. Overdose is treated similarly; nalorphine, naloxone, and levallorphan are antagonists.

Methadone derivatives

Dextromoramide is a synthetic potent analgesic which is fully effective by mouth. It can be used whenever a morphine-like drug would be used but is most suitable for chronic intractable pain as in inoperable carcinoma. The oral dose is 5 mg initially. Suppositories and solution for injection are also available.

Dextropropoxyphene is only one of four stereoisomers to possess analgesic activity and it is also structurally related to methadone. It produces analgesia by CNS actions which are qualitatively similar to those of codeine. It is often combined with aspirin or paracetamol for the relief of mild and moderate pain. A common formulation is dextropropoxyphene hydrochloride 32.5 mg and paracetamol 325 mg.

A dose of 65 mg of the hydrochloride (100 mg of the napsylate) is generally regarded as equianalgesic with 325–500 mg of aspirin. At a dose of 32.5 mg there is little evidence that a therapeutically significant analgesic effect occurs after oral administration. It has an abuse potential and chronic consumption of over 800 mg daily has been associated with psychosis and convulsions. An acute overdose produces respiratory depression which can be reversed with naloxone or nalorphine in appropriate doses.

Dipipanone is another methadone derivative. Its actions are similar to those of methadone and it does not appear to have any particular advantage.

Morphine salts

Morphine hydrochloride (*BP*)
Morphine sulphate (*BP*) and Morphine sulfate (*USP*)
For structural formula *see Figure 5.1*, p. 168

PHARMACOLOGY

Morphine is the oldest analgesic known to man; it is obtained from opium, which is the dried juice from the unripe poppy heads of *Papaver somniferum*. It is the most active constituent of opium and has been used at least since biblical times. The first undisputed reference to poppy juice is found in the writings of Theophrastus (200–300 BC). A phenanthrene derivative, it was first isolated by Serturner in 1803, but its synthesis was achieved only comparatively recently and was a considerable chemical feat. There is no commercial production except by extraction from opium. It acts mainly upon the CNS and involuntary muscle. Its name derives from the Greek, *Morpheus,* God of Dreams, while opium is the Greek for juice.

Central nervous system. The greatest effects of morphine are on the CNS throughout its various levels and result from a mixture of stimulant and depressant actions. Although the latter usually predominate, morphine is not an anticonvulsant and often acts synergistically with convulsant drugs. Its depressant action on the cerebrum reduces the ability to concentrate and deal with complex thought processes. Mental and physical performances are impaired, especially for newly acquired skills, yet motor function is unimpaired. Normal fears and apprehension are diminished and this gives rise to the condition known as euphoria. This elevation of mood normally occurs in the presence of pain, discomfort, fear, and anxiety, but occasionally is displaced by dysphoria in normal individuals or when morphine is followed by nalorphine.

Analgesia and the relief of anxiety are the most powerful effects of morphine, and hunger is allayed. Other sensations include nausea and sometimes vomiting, a feeling of body warmth, heaviness of the extremities, dryness of the mouth, sweating, and itching, especially of the nose.

The effect on the cerebellum is mainly depressant, causing an ataxic gait by inhibiting motor co-ordination. All morphine alkaloids have a strychnine-like action and spinal reflexes are stimulated. Thus it depresses the CNS from above downwards, and stimulates from below upwards. In clinical doses this mixture of excitement and depression is of no significance, except in rare cases when morphine given postoperatively, for example, may excite rather than sedate a patient.

Various medullary areas are affected. The respiratory centre is depressed and becomes less sensitive to the stimulant effects of carbon dioxide. This effect is detectable even after the smallest effective analgesic doses of morphine and after overdosage it is the cause of death. The cough centre is also depressed, but various morphine derivatives (for example, codeine and diamorphine) do this relatively more in proportion to their other actions.

In contrast, the chemoreceptor emetic trigger zone and the parasympathetic portion of the oculomotor nucleus are stimulated. Nausea therefore occurs, and nearly 50 per cent of ambulant patients may be affected and 16 per cent may vomit. Nausea and vomiting are less common in patients who are at rest and receive morphine when pain is already present. In either case any preliminary stimulation of vomiting may be followed by depression, so that morphine can also have an antiemetic action; other emetics are usually ineffective after morphine. Nausea and vomiting are therefore commoner with the first dose, or when doses are spaced at too great intervals.

The pupils are constricted by the effect on the oculomotor nucleus, which is probably due to the removal of an inhibitor tone to this nucleus from a higher level, and in morphine poisoning the pupils may be pin-point in size. This stimulant effect is not followed by depression, and such pin-point pupils dilate again only when the effect of the morphine wears off or when asphyxia supervenes. Mydriatics such as atropine or hyoscine or others with the same mode of action can counteract morphine miosis. Morphine has no local effect in causing pupillary constriction.

The vagal and vasomotor centres are not significantly affected by morphine in man. The effect on heart rate and blood pressure is discussed below.

Analgesia. The analgesic effect reaches its peak about 20 minutes after intravenous injection and about 1.5 hours after intramuscular or subcutaneous injection. The duration of action is about 4 hours. The best effects are obtained when dosage precedes the onset of painful stimuli, in which case the pain threshold is demonstrably raised. When the drug is given after pain is established, relief is mainly due to alteration in the pattern of reaction to pain, which is still recognized by the subject but appears distant and does not give rise to anxiety. Under favourable circumstances sleep may ensue and dreams may be prominent. On the other hand, in the absence of pain small doses of morphine (5–10 mg), in contrast to the larger doses normally given, may actually increase anxiety and general discomfort. Continuous dull pain is relieved more effectively than sharp intermittent pain. The lightning pain of tabes dorsalis is one of the few types that resists morphine analgesia. In sharp contrast to the salicylates and related analgesics, morphine is effective against pain arising from viscera as well as from muscles, joints, and integumental structures.

Morphine appears to relieve pain in at least four ways: by raising the threshold for pain; by altering the pattern of reaction to pain; by inducing sleep, which in itself raises the pain threshold to an appreciable extent; and by inducing hypercapnia, which produces a similar effect. Reduction in body temperature may also be a contributory factor.

Cardiovascular system. Therapeutic doses have negligible effects upon heart rate and blood pressure but larger doses slow the heart by depressing conduction; a stimulant action on the vagal nucleus may contribute to this effect. With anoxia and central vasomotor depression added, a fall in blood pressure will occur. In man the peripheral blood vessels are dilated by therapeutic doses, producing a feeling of warmth in the skin. Peripheral vasodilatation becomes more marked when morphine is injected rapidly intravenously and will cause a fall in blood pressure. All the alkaloids of opium produce a histamine-like weal when injected intradermally and histamine release may well be a factor in producing vasodilatation and hypotension, as can be shown in the cat.

Respiratory system. All phases of respiratory activity are depressed by therapeutic doses of morphine. The rate, minute volume, and tidal exchange are decreased. The diminished minute volume is primarily due to the slower rate of breathing. After intravenous injection, morphine produces a reduction in amplitude of respiration in nearly all subjects; when given by other routes the depth of breathing may be increased or decreased, but is usually unaltered. With overdose, Cheyne-Stokes type of periodic breathing may be seen. From work in dogs it is thought that morphine causes 'pharmacological decerebration' by inactivating cortical and subcortical suppression mechanisms which modify the activity of more caudally located respiratory centres.

Although respiration is decreased by morphine it is important to note that its analgesic effect vastly improves respiration where this has been fast, shallow, and inefficient, due to pleuritic pain. Similarly, where the lungs are oedematous, as in left ventricular failure, central depression by morphine prevents the Hering–Breuer reflex from initiating expiration before a useful inspiratory volume is reached. Bronchial constriction by a central vagal action is normally too slight to matter, but it can be dangerous in bronchial asthma.

Gastrointestinal tract and biliary tract. Morphine is constipating yet stimulant to the gastrointestinal muscle. The tone of the visceral muscle is raised, especially that of the pyloric, ileocolic, and anal sphincters. Segmenting contractions increase and truly propulsive activity diminishes. The delay of intestinal contents in the colon allows an increased absorption of water to take place and, finally, the normal defaecation reflex is inhibited more easily than usual because the distended rectum no longer produces the usual discomfort. In addition to the alleviation of pain, hunger and thirst are relieved or abolished, and vomiting if it occurs is not necessarily associated with the usual unpleasant emotional reactions even when it is violent and repeated.

The tone of the biliary musculature is raised and spasm may result, including that of the sphincter of Oddi. This extra spasm may increase pain originating in biliary colic already present and is unrelieved by the belladonna alkaloids.

Urinary tract. Ureteric tone is increased as markedly as is that of the biliary tract, but it can be completely relaxed by the belladonna alkaloids. The detrusor musculature of the bladder is stimulated, but so is the sphincter, so that urgency may be created and difficulty also, but the central analgesic effect prevails. Catheterization may become necessary. Morphine, experimentally in dogs, can be shown to cause antidiuresis due to release of antidiuretic hormone and a reduction in the number of nephrons functioning, but whether this effect occurs in patients receiving therapeutic doses is uncertain.

Uterus. The natural contractions during labour are not affected by analgesic doses although the stimulant effect of oxytocic agents may be slightly diminished.

Placenta and fetus. The placenta is permeable to morphine which can thus reach the fetus and depress the respiratory centre, making the initiation of respiration after birth difficult. Intrauterine addiction can occur when the mother is addicted.

Metabolism. Any fall in body temperature is usually the result of large doses and is due to lowered muscular activity, increased heat loss through cutaneous vasodilatation and sweating, and decreased metabolic rate. The last named is of the order of 10–20 per cent and is due to a decrease in oxygen consumption, which is of considerable benefit in cardiac disease. Hyperglycaemia and even glycosuria may be seen from adrenaline release, and when there is respiratory depression acidosis occurs with increased bicarbonate and lactic acid levels.

Fate in the body. Although the most profound actions of the drug are on the CNS, only small traces are detectable there. About 90 per cent of a dose is eliminated, mainly by the kidneys, and mostly in a conjugated form. The fate of the remainder is unknown. The liver is the chief organ for the conjugation, and severe liver damage decreases the proportion of conjugated to free morphine detectable in the urine. Both codeine and pethidine are converted into the nor- form by *N*-demethylation in man, and this is probably the case with morphine, but it has been demonstrated only in rats. About 75 per cent of a dose appears in the urine within 24 hours and most of it appears within the first 6 hours. A small amount is excreted into the stomach and bile and appears in the faeces. Traces are found in sweat and milk.

Tolerance. Tolerance occurs to morphine, as detected by the need to increase the dose to obtain the same degree of effect. Such tolerance is called acquired tolerance and usually takes 2–3 weeks to develop on moderate therapeutic doses, but will occur more rapidly if the dosage is raised. On discontinuing the use of morphine the tolerance goes within 2 weeks, but probably not completely, at least for the analgesic effect. Acquired tolerance exists only towards the depressant actions of the drug and never becomes absolute. Thus, the miotic and constipating actions of morphine persist unabated, whereas tolerance to the respiratory depression is great but never a total safeguard. By the time addiction occurs tolerance is usually demonstrable, but the presence of tolerance does not mean that addiction is necessarily present. A cross-tolerance occurs to drugs of closely related chemical structure, for example other phenanthrene derivatives. Tolerance is not due to enzyme induction and no increase in metabolic turnover can be shown. It is an adaptive process within the CNS. It has been postulated that if the mechanism of action involves the inhibition of acetylcholine release, this may lead to receptor induction, and that withdrawal symptoms are like other examples of denervation hypersensitivity. In animals made tolerant there is a rise in brain enkephalin levels, which fall when an abstinence syndrome is induced. Thus acetylcholine and enkephalins may be involved in opioid tolerance and in the abstinence syndrome.

Addiction. Subjects receiving morphine regularly are in danger of becoming powerfully addicted to it. In the more emotionally unstable it may become apparent after about 10 days on the drug, but in more stable people it is likely to take about 25 days. When addiction is established, denial of the drug produces a typical abstinence syndrome within 15–20 hours with a peak in 2–3 days, and remission in 10–14 days. The antagonist nalorphine can produce the abstinence syndrome within 30 minutes, and the use of this drug has shown that some degree of physical dependence to morphine can be demonstrated after only 48 hours on continuous medication, that is at least a week earlier than psychological dependence can be shown to be developing.

Abstinence syndrome. When the addict is suddenly deprived of his supply of morphine, the well-known withdrawal symptoms occur. They usually commence about 10–12 hours after the last dose with yawning, sweating, and running of the eyes and nose. Then follows a restless irregular sleep for 18–24 hours. The previous signs and symptoms then return, accompanied by mydriasis, 'gooseflesh', and cramps and later by insomnia, nausea, vomiting and diarrhoea. Signs and symptoms reach their peak in 72 hours and they decline over the next 7–10 days.

During the withdrawal period tolerance to morphine is rapidly lost, and the syndrome may be terminated at any time by a suitable dose of morphine or related drugs. The longer the period of abstinence, the smaller will be the dose required.

INDICATIONS

Morphine is used in the treatment of acute pain which may follow trauma, cardiac ischaemia, acute abdominal conditions, and operations, and in severe chronic pain such as that which may occur in the terminal stages of cancer. It is also useful in the treatment of severe pleuritic pain and left ventricular failure. It was the first drug to be used as a sedative before anaesthesia and is still used extensively in premedication.

DOSAGE AND ADMINISTRATION

Morphine may be given by mouth, but since absorption is slow and the effect variable, it is normally given by subcutaneous or intramuscular injection. The intravenous route can also be employed.

Acute pain. In the treatment of acute pain the official dose is 8–20 mg, but larger doses up to 30 mg may sometimes be required. In acute pain associated with shock it should be given intravenously, as when given by the other routes its action is delayed owing to the poor circulation in peripheral tissues.

Chronic pain. In chronic pain, such as that associated with cancer, an initial dose of 15 mg may be given subcutaneously and repeated at 4-hourly intervals as required, but as tolerance develops the dose and frequency of administration may have to be increased and doses of 20–30 mg may become necessary.

In premedication. A dose of 10–15 mg according to the condition of the patient is usually given by subcutaneous or intramuscular injection 1–1.5 hours before operation. It is normally better to avoid the use of morphine in the elderly.

PRECAUTIONS

As morphine causes marked respiratory depression, it should not be given when there is increased intracranial pressure, and in conditions where respiration is already depressed or ineffective as in bronchial asthama and emphysema. It is also contraindicated in adrenocortical insufficiency, severe liver disease, hypothyroidism, diverticulitis and other spastic conditions of the colon, biliary colic, in patients who are being treated with MAOIs, in cachetic or elderly patients, and during labour.

As morphine is a drug of addiction, it should be used with due circumspection when repeated doses are likely to be required. This, of course, does not apply to the terminal stages of painful disease such as cancer, when duration of life can be only a matter of months.

Apart from respiratory depression, other side effects of morphine include drowsiness, confusion, nausea, vomiting, and constipation. They are more marked when the patient is ambulant. Overdose causes respiratory failure, cardiovascular collapse, and coma. Treatment consists of supportive therapy and the administration of an antagonist such as naloxone 0.2–0.4 mg or nalorphine 3–5 mg intravenously.

Artificial ventilation may be necessary and hypotension requires the administration of a pressor drug and fluids to increase the circulating blood volume.

Other morphine derivatives include dihydromorphinone hydrochloride and oxymorphone hydrochloride. Their actions are similar to those of morphine and they have no particular advantages.

Naloxone hydrochloride

Naloxone hydrochloride (*BAN* and *USP*)
Chemical name: (−)-(5*R*,14*S*)-9a-allyl-4,5-epoxy-3,14-dihydroxymorphinan-6-one hydrochloride
For structural formula *see Figure 5.1,* p. 168

PHARMACOLOGY

Naloxone is the *N*-allyl derivative of oxymorphone. It is a specific narcotic antagonist and possesses no agonist activity. If administered alone it produces no detectable effects or symptoms unless a gross overdose is given (200 times the therapeutic dose). If given in adequate dosage it will reverse opiate-induced analgesia, euphoria, respiratory depression, pupillary constriction, delayed gastric emptying, coma, and convulsions. It can also antagonize the dysphoria and depressant effects of pentazocine. It is also effective in dextropropoxyphene overdose. However, it has little or no effect on the actions of buprenorphine. It is unable to antagonize CNS depression produced by any other group of drugs.

Pharmacokinetics. The blocking effect is apparent 1–2 minutes after intravenous injection. The plasma half-life is between 1 and 1.5 hours, so that the effect is apparent for about 45–60 minutes.

INDICATIONS

Naloxone is used to antagonize the respiratory depression or other effects of morphine, pethidine, methadone, or any of their derivatives. It is of particular value as an antagonist for overdose by pentazocine for which there is no other reliable antagonist. It can be used partially to antagonize overdose by phenoperidine or fentanyl after neuroleptanalgesia. It is of particular value in the immediate treatment of neonatal asphyxia when due to narcotic analgesics. It may also be used as a diagnostic aid in suspected acute narcotic overdose and in the diagnosis of narcotic addiction. It has also been used to block endogenous endorphins in alcohol poisoning, obesity, and septic shock, but these uses are still experimental.

DOSAGE AND ADMINISTRATION

Naloxone may be given subcutaneously, intramuscularly, or intravenously; it is normally given intravenously in doses of 0.2–0.4 mg when a rapid action is required. In children the initial dose is 10–20 µg/kg. It can be given intramuscularly in a dose of 20–70 µg/kg for a more prolonged effect. This may be of particular value in the neonate depressed by pethidine transferred from the mother.

PRECAUTIONS

The duration of action after intravenous administration may be shorter than that of some of the agents whose effects it is required to antagonize. It will rapidly induce withdrawal symptoms if given to patients addicted to one of the narcotics.

Nalorphine is a morphine-like derivative. It is a partial agonist and hence acts as a competitive antagonist to the actions of morphine and some other narcotic analgesics.

In established respiratory depression due to these drugs respiration is stimulated, and the minute volume may be increased by as much as 200–300 per cent. There may also be some improvement in blood pressure, and deep sleep may be lightened. Nalorphine passes the placental barrier and is effective in neonatal asphyxia.

Its duration of action is similar to that of morphine.

Nalorphine can be used to antagonize the effects of morphine, pethidine, methadone, and their derivatives, but this usage is likely to be superseded wherever naloxone is available. The dose is 3–5 mg by the intravenous route.

As nalorphine causes respiratory depression when used alone, it must not be given to patients whose respiration is depressed by drugs other than those known to be antagonized by it.

Levallorphan is a morphine-like compound bearing the same relationship to levorphanol as nalorphine does to morphine. It has a greater analgesic effect than nalorphine but antagonizes the effects of morphine and other narcotic analgesics. It will not cause withdrawal symptoms in morphine addicts. The drug has fallen into disuse now that naloxone is available.

Nefopam hydrochloride

Nefopam hydrochloride
Chemical name: 3,4,5,6-tetrahydro-5-methyl-1-phenyl-1*H*-2,5-benzoxazocine hydrochloride

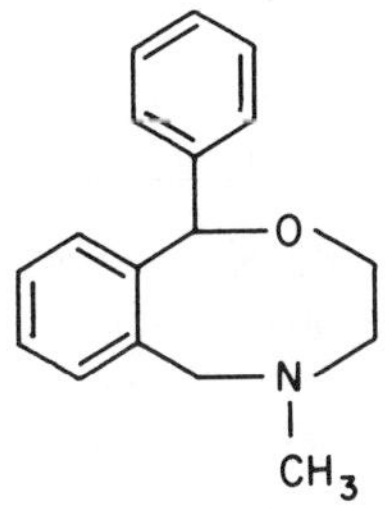

PHARMACOLOGY

It is an analgesic which has been reported to be approximately eight times as potent as aspirin. Its potency as compared to morphine has been estimated in patients. In one trial 20 mg nefopam has been rated as almost as effective as 12 mg morphine (Sunshine and Laska, 1975). After parenteral intramuscular injection the peak effect is reached after 1 hour.

DOSAGE AND ADMINISTRATION

The oral dose is 30 mg three times a day which can be increased up to 90 mg three times a day. By intramuscular or slow intravenous injection the dose is 20 mg, followed by further similar doses at 6-hourly intervals if necessary.

PRECAUTIONS

The drug can produce atropine-like effects – blurred vision, dry mouth, tachycardia. It should probably be avoided in patients with glaucoma or urinary retention. Convulsive disorders and myocardial infarctions are other contraindications. After injection it can produce fainting and it is best administered to patients who are lying down and who remain so for about 20 minutes after injection. It can produce insomnia and nausea.

Sunshine, A. and Laska, E. (1975) Nefopam and morphine in man. *Clinical Pharmacology and Therapeutics,* **18,** 530

Opium

Constitution: the dried latex obtained from the unripe capsules of *Papaver somniferum*

Official preparations: powdered opium (*BP* and *USP*) (cont. 10 per cent anhydrous morphine); opium tincture (*BP*) (cont. 1 per cent anhydrous morphine) *synonym:* laudanum; camphorated opium tincture (*BP*) (cont. 0.05 per cent anhydrous morphine); paregoric (*USP*) (cont. 0.04 per cent anhydrous morphine); ipecacuanha and opium powder (*BPC*) (cont. 1 per cent anhydrous morphine) *synonym:* Dover's powder; ipecacuanha and opium tablets (*BPC*) (cont. 1 per cent anhydrous morphine) *synonym:* Dover's powder tablets

Raw opium varies in consistency from being firm and plastic to brittle. It occurs as irregular masses of a chocolate or dark brown colour, having a strong characteristic odour and bitter taste. Powdered opium (*BP*) is a fine or moderately fine light brown powder.

Papaveretum (*see* below) and the proprietary product Nepenthe are standardized preparations of opium alkaloids which may be given by injection as well as by mouth.

Opium contains about 25 different alkaloids which occur in combination with meconic acid (of which about 5 per cent is present) and with sulphuric acid. The alkaloidal contents may vary with different types of poppy, and where these are grown. The most important alkaloids are morphine (9–20 per cent), codeine (methylmorphine) (0.3–4 per cent), narcotine (2–8 per cent) and thebaine (0.2–0.5 per cent). The remaining alkaloids, including narceine and papaverine, together constitute only just over 1 per cent of the drug.

Opium is a valuable drug. It is still unexcelled for many purposes as a narcotic and analgesic, being used extensively in various forms to relieve pain and anxiety. It is used as an astringent in diarrhoea and dysentery and as a sedative in certain forms of cough and dyspnoea. Its action is substantially that of morphine, being rather more excitant owing to the presence of the other alkaloids, some of which, such as narcotine, potentiate the analgesic action of morphine, while papaverine reduces its tendency to cause nausea and vomiting; also, depression of respiration by morphine is less when papaverine is present. Papaverine is the most important of the benzylisoquinoline group of alkaloids found in opium, and is distinct from morphine chemically and in its pharmacological actions.

The alkaloids of opium can be divided into those which resemble morphine and stimulate plain muscle and those, such as papaverine, which relax plain muscle. The muscle sites affected are not identical, as papaverine affects, among others, arteriolar muscle, which is not affected by morphine. Like morphine, papaverine is a histamine liberator. Papaverine has been used to control spasm of blood vessels due to emboli or local damage and to relax smooth muscle in spastic conditions of the intestinal tract. All the important alkaloids have narcotic and strychnine-like actions. The former effect decreases and the latter increases in the order morphine, papaverine, codeine, narcotine, thebaine. Thebaine has virtually only strychnine-like and no narcotic actions. Codeine can be extracted from opium, but is usually made by methylating morphine.

Papaveretum is the most commonly used preparation in anaesthetic practice; its actions and uses are more fully discussed below. Nepenthe (0.91 per cent total alkaloids of opium and 0.84 per cent anhydrous morphine) is sometimes used as a premedicant in children in a dose of 0.06 ml intramuscularly for each year of age. Precautions are the same as for morphine.

Papaveretum

Papaveretum (*BPC*)
Constitution: the hydrochlorides of the alkaloids of opium

PHARMACOLOGY

Papaveretum is a preparation containing the water-soluble alkaloids of opium, standardized to contain 50 per cent anhydrous morphine. The other 50 per cent consists of the hydrochlorides of the remaining opium alkaloids (mainly papaverine, codeine, narcotine, thebaine). It should be stored in dry dark conditions.

Milligram for milligram, its sedative and analgesic actions are less powerful than those of morphine. It should be noted that morphine, when prescribed as such, is given as a salt (the sulphate, hydrochloride, or tartrate) and includes five molecules of water of crystallization. Papaveretum, containing 50 per cent of *anhydrous* morphine, therefore contains more than 50 per cent of its weight as effective morphine when compared with that drug as normally prescribed. Twenty milligrams of papaveretum are therefore more effective than 10 mg of morphine even though the other alkaloids do not exert much sedative or analgesic effect.

INDICATIONS

Papaveretum is used for the relief of severe pain and in premedication before operation. It has been advocated for the treatment of colic, but the amount of papaverine in the preparation has little effect on plain muscle spasm.

DOSAGE AND ADMINISTRATION

Papaveretum may be given by mouth in tablet form or by subcutaneous injection. The official dose is 10–20 mg. In the treatment of severe pain 20 mg is the usual adult dose given by the appropriate route under the circumstances. As with morphine, larger doses are sometimes necessary. A similar dose range is employed in premedication.

The dose should be reduced to 15 mg in patients over the age of 55 years, and to 10 mg in those over 65 years. It is best avoided in those over the age of 70 years.

Papaveretum is often combined with hyoscine (scopolamine). This combination is very satisfactory in children and fit adults, but may cause severe depression in the elderly, and atropine should normally be substituted in those over the age of 60 years.

PRECAUTIONS

Precautions in the use of papaveretum are as for morphine.

Pentazocine and salts

Pentazocine (*BP* and *USP*)
Pentazocine hydrochloride (*BP* and *USP*)
Pentazocine lactate injection (*BP*)
Chemical name: (2*R**,6*R**,11*R**)-1,2,3,4,5,6-hexahydro-6,11-dimethyl-3-(3-methylbut-2-enyl)-2,6-methano-3-benzazocin-8-ol
For structural formula *see Figure 5.1,* p. 168

PHARMACOLOGY

Pentazocine is a benzmorphan derivative related to phenazocine. It is a powerful analgesic, 20–30 mg having an effect equivalent to that of 10 mg of morphine. As can be seen from *Figure 5.2,* it has both agonist and antagonist activity. In consequence, it is only midly sedative and in large doses it tends to produce dysphoria rather than euphoria. It is also, therefore, able to antagonize the effects of drugs, such as morphine and heroin, with almost exclusively agonist activity but cannot itself be antagonized by other drugs with some agonist action such as nalorphine and levallorphan. It can, however, be antagonized by the 'pure' antagonist naloxone. Because of its tendency to produce dysphoria there is little liability to addiction and it is not subject to the Controlled Drugs regulations. Its respiratory and cardiovascular effects are similar to those produced by morphine, but there is no effect on the pupil. Nausea, vomiting, and constipation are said to occur less frequently, but dizziness has been reported after larger doses. It produces less pupillary constriction than equianalgesic doses of morphine and reaction to light is preserved. In the absence of a rise in $Pa{CO_2}$, it causes a small fall in intracranial pressure.

Between 5 and 25 per cent of an administered dose is excreted unchanged in the urine, the proportion being dependent on the blood level achieved. Less than 2 per cent appears in the faeces, and the remainder appears as metabolites in the urine.

INDICATIONS

Pentazocine can be used in the relief of all types of pain for which a narcotic analgesic is usually necessary. It may prove particularly useful for the management of chronic pain where habituation or addiction might otherwise be a problem; 25–100 mg may be given by mouth or intramuscularly. The Central Midwives Board has approved its use by midwives.

A somewhat novel use for pentazocine has been its employment in the techniques of 'anesthesie analgesique sequentielle'. In this technique, the short-acting analgesic fentanyl is used throughout the operation, and its respiratory depressing action is then terminated by a suitable dose of pentazocine. Excellent postoperative analgesia for an average of 10 hours has been claimed for this technique.

PRECAUTIONS

Similar precautions should be observed as for morphine; overdosage can be reversed with naloxone. It is important to remember that levallorphan and nalorphine are ineffective.

Decozine is structurally related to pentazocine. It has been reported to have a potency similar to morphine although other workers have reported it to be about half as potent. The latency of onset and duration of action therapeutically are similar to morphine. In one trial no psychotomimetic effects were reported. It may be an alternative to pethidine or morphine. In monkeys it has less abuse potential than morphine.

Phenazocine is a benzmorphan derivative and has powerful analgesic properties. It has little sedative action. Although it is claimed that it causes less respiratory depression than morphine, reports are conflicting and there is probably little difference between the two drugs. Other side effects such as nausea, vomiting, and constipation are possibly less prominent.

It may be used for the same purposes as morphine and is given intramuscularly in a dose of 1–3 mg.

Pethidine hydrochloride

Pethidine hydrochloride (*BP*) and Meperidine hydrochloride (*USP*)
Chemical name: ethyl-1-methyl-4-phenylpiperidine-4-carboxylate hydrochloride
For structural formula *see Figure 5.1,* p. 168

Pethidine, a piperidino compound, shares many properties with morphine and atropine; structurally it is similar to atropine, but its relationship to morphine is less apparent.

PHARMACOLOGY

Nervous system. Pethidine is a central depressant with strong analgesic action, its potency lying between those of morphine and codeine. Its hypnotic effect is mild, but medullary depression of the respiratory centre is proportional to the dose administered. Overdose causes depression of the vasomotor centre. Euphoria and elevation of mood often follow its administration, although depression sometimes occurs in the absence of pain. Large doses may cause cerebral irritation, and convulsions can occur. Summation effects are noted when it is given with barbiturates and other central depressants. After parenteral administration pethidine may produce corneal analgesia and abolish the corneal reflex. Pupillary size and accommodation are unaltered.

For clinical purposes, equianalgesia would require a dose 8–10 times that of morphine. Duration of analgesia is only about three quarters of that of morphine, and the more severe the pain the shorter is the duration of analgesic action. All types of pain are relieved, but the drug is more effective in pain of visceral origin, probably because of its atropine-like action.

The drug is of value in the relief of intractable pruritus which may be aggravated by giving morphine. It is sometimes effective although dangerous to administer it in bronchial asthma as it may lead to addiction. Morphine addicts will use pethidine, but prefer morphine. Tolerance is not as complete as with morphine and with high daily doses of 3–4 g, the amount which some addicts take, convulsions may occur.

The pethidine addict is usually less able to work than the morphine addict, but withdrawal symptoms are less severe and appear more rapidly. They commence about 3 hours after the last dose, reach 50 per cent of maximum in 4–5 hours and are maximal within 8–12 hours, after which the syndrome rapidly subsides. They resemble those of morphine (*see* page 184), twitching of skeletal muscle and extreme restlessness being particularly prominent.

Autonomic system. There is a mild anticholinergic action, which produces an atropine-like effect.

Cardiovascular system. Pethidine has a quinidine-like action which reduces cardiac irritability, and ventricular dysrhythmias may often be prevented or controlled if already present. Blood pressure is normally unaffected, but sometimes falls; this may be due to relaxation of the muscle of vessel walls, histamine release or, in the case of overdose, vasomotor depression. The heart rate may be slightly increased, but in the presence of cardiovascular collapse it may be slowed.

Respiratory system. Respiration is depressed in proportion to the dose given, but less than with an equianalgesic dose of morphine. The main effect is on the rate which may be markedly slowed; apnoea will follow large intravenous doses. The cough reflex is unaffected, but laryngeal reflexes are depressed. Bronchi are not affected, but if in spasm will relax. Secretions are moderately reduced.

Musculature. There is no effect on skeletal muscle. Minor effects are exerted on smooth muscles which cause spasm in some – for example, the sphincter of Oddi – and relaxation in others. Spasm, with the exception of biliary colic, is usually relieved. The atropine-like effect of the drug probably plays some part in this process.

Alimentary system. There is little action on the bowel, but when in spasm it is relaxed. Unlike morphine, it has little constipating effect, but nausea and vomiting are not uncommon. However, in analgesic doses, pethidine virtually suppresses gastric emptying in pregnant women in labour.

Liver and kidney function. Pethidine has no adverse action on the liver. Urinary output and peristaltic movements of the ureter are decreased.

Uterus and placenta. Uterine contractions are unaffected. Pethidine passes the placental barrier and will cause depression of respiration in the infant at birth.

Histamine release. The action of liberation of histamine is a local one, a weal often being noticed along the course of the vein used for injection. General effects are rare.

Fate in the body. Pethidine is absorbed in 20–60 minutes when given by mouth, 15 minutes by intramuscular injection, and its effects are noticeable within 2–4 minutes when given intravenously. It is mainly detoxicated by hepatic metabolism, either by demethylation to norpethidine or by hydrolysis to meperidinic acid. Only about 5 per cent is excreted unchanged in the urine. Pregnant women, neonates, and women on oral contraceptives excrete a higher proportion of unchanged drug.

In severe liver disease and in patients under treatment with MAOIs the degradation of the drug is inhibited.

The urinary excretion of pethidine is pH dependent; if the pH is reduced below 5.0, as much as 25 per cent is excreted unchanged. Whereas only 1 per cent per hour is excreted in urine at normal pH, the rate is increased to 4 per cent per hour if it is highly acidic.

INDICATIONS

Pethidine is used for the following:

1. The treatment of acute pain in the preoperative and postoperative periods, and the intractable pain associated with carcinoma;
2. Premedication before operation;
3. As a supplement to nitrous oxide and oxygen anaesthesia, with or without muscle relaxants;
4. The early stages of labour;
5. Minor procedures, such as painful dressings, which do not require full anaesthesia;
6. To allay anxiety and apprehension during operations performed under spinal and other forms of local analgesia;
7. To produce basal narcosis with such drugs as chlorpromazine and promethazine.

Pethidine is also used to prevent tachypnoea which may occur during trichlorethylene or halothane anaesthesia.

It has proved particularly useful in pulmonary and cardiac surgery as cardiac and bronchial reflexes are depressed.

DOSAGE AND ADMINISTRATION

Pethidine may be given by mouth, intramuscularly, or intravenously. Intravenous solutions employed vary from 1–5 per cent.

For analgesia. A dose of 50–100 mg is given orally or intramuscularly and repeated every 3–4 hours as necessary. The intravenous route may be used in emergency.

For premedication. An intramuscular injection of 100 mg is given 1 hour before operation; 50 mg is usually sufficient for frail or elderly subjects. Children aged 2–12 years may be given 25–75 mg (2.0 mg/kg, maximum 100 mg). It is often combined with promethazine 25–50 mg intramuscularly.

As a supplement to nitrous oxide and oxygen anaesthesia. The initial intravenous dose after induction is 10–25 mg, according to the age and condition of the patient. Supplementary doses are normally necessary every 20–30 minutes. Healthy and robust subjects, however, may require supplementary doses at shorter intervals. It is advisable to wait for respiration to return following induction with thiopentone and muscle relaxants before giving the initial dose as otherwise it may be difficult to determine which drug is responsible should apnoea be unduly prolonged.

In the treatment of tachypnoea, up to 25 mg may be given intravenously.

In obstetrics. When pains have become regular and intense, an initial dose of 100 mg, or up to 150 mg in large and obese subjects, is given intramuscularly. These doses may be repeated every 2–3 hours as required. If delivery occurs while the drug could still be affecting the fetus, respiratory depression can be reversed by naloxone. While this may be given to the mother before delivery, it is generally kinder to administer the drug to the infant after delivery. There is some evidence that the intramuscular administration of a relatively large dose to the baby is more beneficial than administration by intravenous injection. Behavioural improvements extend over several days and may be related to the earlier establishment of feeding and quicker urinary clearance of pethidine. Although there is no evidence that the giving of pethidine and levallorphan together will prevent respiratory depression without affecting analgesia, this mixture (as well as pethidine alone) is approved by the Central Midwives Board for use by midwives.

PRECAUTIONS

Pethidine is contraindicated in severe liver disease and in patients who are under treatment with MAOIs, as inability to metabolize the drug at the normal rate will cause them to go into coma.

It is usually advisable to give atropine with pethidine when it is used in premedication before operation, as its antimuscarinic action is rarely sufficient when used alone.

Pethidine is a drug likely to cause addiction, and should be used in repeated doses for the relief of chronic pain only in exceptional circumstances.

Side effects such as nausea and vomiting, excitement or depression, and confusion are not uncommon, and ambulant patients must be warned to adjust their activities accordingly.

When given intravenously, pethidine is liable to cause respiratory depression or even apnoea. This can be adequately dealt with by assisted or controlled respiration during anaesthesia, otherwise naloxone may be necessary to restore adequate ventilation.

Apart from respiratory depression, overdose of pethidine may cause convulsions, cardiovascular collapse, and coma. Treatment is symptomatic: respiration requires assistance, small doses of suxamethonium may be necessary to control convulsions, and naloxone (0.2–0.4 mg) should be given as an antagonist. Hypotension can occur without other symptoms and following even relatively small doses; if severe a small dose of a pressor agent should be given.

If coma and other signs of overdose are associated with liver disease or the administration of MAOIs the urine should be acidified as soon as possible. This may be accomplished by the intravenous infusion of 10 g of L-arginine hydrochloride dissolved in 500 ml of 5 per cent dextrose and given over 30 minutes. Ammonium chloride 1 per cent (187 mEq/ℓ) can be given for the same purpose provided that there is no impairment of liver function. Not more than 1 mEq/kg should be given, that is, about 250–300 ml in an average adult. Arginine is safer and preferable.

Pethidine derivatives

Anileridine and **alphaprodine** are closely related to pethidine and have similar actions. The dose range of both these compounds is 30–60 mg given by mouth or intramuscular injection.

Phenoperidine hydrochloride

Phenoperidine hydrochloride (*BAN*)
Chemical name: ethyl 1-(3-hydroxy-3-phenylpropyl)-4-phenylpiperidine-4-carboxylate hydrochloride
For structural formula *see Figure 5.1*, p. 168

PHARMACOLOGY

Phenoperidine is chemically related to pethidine and on a weight-for-weight basis is considerably more potent as an analgesic. It acts within 2–3 minutes when given intravenously and its effect lasts for 0.5–1 hour. Some degree of analgesia persists for 4–6 hours. In recommended doses the cardiovascular system remains stable but respiration is readily depressed; 2–5 mg given intravenously will cause apnoea. Other actions are similar to those of pethidine. Its emetic effect is similar to that of pethidine and can be counteracted by any antiemetic drug effective at the chemoreceptor trigger area.

Phenoperidine is mainly excreted by the kidneys, about 50 per cent being found in the urine. The remainder is broken down in the liver to pethidine and then pethidinic acid, most of which also appears in the urine.

INDICATIONS

It is used as an analgesic supplement to light nitrous oxide and oxygen anaesthesia, in neuroleptanalgesia, and as a respiratory depressant to assist conscious patients to acclimatize to mechanical ventilation. It can also be used in place of other analgesics in the relief of severe pain.

DOSAGE AND ADMINISTRATION

For the relief of pain without undue respiratory depression 0.5–1 mg may be given intravenously. As a supplement to nitrous oxide and oxygen anaesthesia, 0.5–1 mg is usually sufficient if spontaneous respiration is being maintained. When respiration can be controlled 2–5 mg may be given. Phenoperidine may also be given orally and intramuscularly.

PRECAUTIONS

Respiratory depression may persist at the end of operation, and should be antagonized by the administration of naloxone or another narcotic antagonist. Respiration should also be observed carefully even when small doses are given. Other precautions are similar to those described for pethidine.

Piritramide is a tertiary amine of the diphenylpropylamine series. It is a powerful narcotic analgesic but has little structural similarity to other drugs of this class.

Its duration of action is about 6 hours. Equianalgesic doses depress ventilation to a lesser extent than morphine. Compared with morphine, vomiting is comparatively rare. A dose of 15 mg is approximately equivalent to 10 mg of morphine. The chief side effect appears to be drowsiness which may be an advantage in the postoperative period.

Mild analgesics

These drugs include the salicylates, of which acetylsalicylic acid is the most commonly used; aniline derivatives, phenacetin, paracetamol, and acetanilide; and pyrazolones such as amidopyrine and phenazone. Of these, amidopyrine and phenazone have proved too toxic to the bone marrow for general use, although other closely related pyrazolones such as phenylbutazone and oxyphenbutazone have established a place as anti-inflammatory agents (*see* below). Acetanilide has been abandoned for similar reasons, and phenacetin has been prohibited in commercial mixtures in the UK and dropped as an official drug in the USA because of toxic effects on the kidney. Another widely prescribed mild analgesic is dextropropoxyphene. It is a common ingredient of oral compound analgesic preparations. It is, however, a methadone derivative and in sufficiently high dosage can produce morphine-like effects. It is considered on page 180.

Many of these drugs, particularly the salicylates, also exhibit anti-inflammatory properties but at a higher dose level than that needed for mild analgesia. It seems likely that the mild analgesic effect is a central one whereas the anti-inflammatory effects are due to one or more actions on peripheral mechanisms. Another important property often found in this group of drugs is an antipyretic action in the presence of pyrexia, which is mediated via the hypothalamus and leads to increased sweating and skin vasodilatation.

Because of their ready availability they are often taken in overdose in suicide attempts: it is somewhat ironic that these drugs, which in the recommended doses are safe enough to be freely available, when taken in overdose produce toxic effects that are difficult to treat effectively and are often fatal.

Acetylsalicylic acid

Aspirin (*BP* and *USP*)
Chemical name: 2-acetoxybenzoic acid

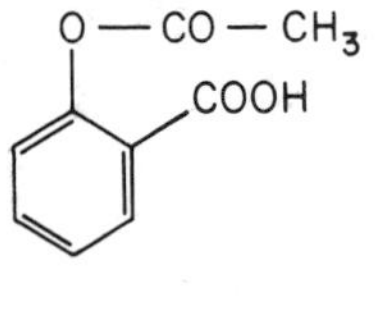

O — CO — CH_3
COOH

PHARMACOLOGY

Acetylsalicyclic acid is one of the most potent of the salicylate drugs as an analgesic. It is about 50 per cent more effective and toxic than sodium salicylate in doses containing equal amounts of salicylate. Analgesia is usually adequate for pain from integumental structures, for example bones, joints, muscles, and teeth, but poor for visceral pain.

The analgesic action is confined to a small dose range below which there is little effect, and above which an increase in dose produces toxic effects with little increase in analgesia. There is no graded response as with the morphine group. It seems likely that the analgesia achieved by small doses (up to 1 g) is a central effect, whereas bigger doses may additionaly relieve pain by a peripheral anti-inflammatory effect.

Acetylsalicylic acid, like the other salicylates, has an antipyretic action and a slight hypnotic effect. The former, which occurs only in pyrexia, is mediated via the hypothalamus, and invokes increased heat loss by sweating and hyperaemia of the skin. It is also a primary metabolic stimulant, but the rapid fall in temperature due to profuse sweating normally overcomes the stimulant effect. If sweating fails to occur, as in the case of electrolyte depletion, hyperpyrexia will result.

In addition to these effects the drug has an anti-inflammatory action. The possible mechanisms by which drugs such as acetylsalicylic acid exert this action are discussed on page 202.

Salicylates have important effects on carbohydrate metabolism. Large doses may reduce glycosuria in diabetic patients; in normal subjects hyperglycaemia and glycosuria occur. They also inhibit the action of many enzymes including succinate dehydrogenase, α-ketoglutaric dehydrogenase, and hyaluronidase, and uncouple oxidative phosphorylation.

Acetylsalicylic acid has a paradoxical dose-dependent action on the excretion of uric acid. At daily doses of 1–2 g, net excretion is diminished because the drug depresses active tubular excretion more than reabsorption. Above 4–5 g per day, however, the effect on tubular reabsorption dominates, and the net effect is enhanced excretion. The side effects of such doses make it an unsuitable drug for this purpose. Salicylates inhibit the uricosuric action of probenecid (but not its capacity to inhibit tubular excretion of penicillin) and the activity of other uricosuric drugs such as sulfinpyrazone. No entirely satisfactory explanation for this has been advanced. Further details on the interaction of uricosuric drugs are provided by Gutman (1966).

Acetylsalicylic acid is a common cause of bleeding from gastric erosions. Patients in whom there is strong circumstantial evidence that the drug precipitated the bleeding subsequently show a normal susceptibility. Acetylsalicylic acid also inhibits platelet aggregation and there is now some evidence that the rare severe gastric bleeding episodes that are associated with this drug are a manifestation of an abnormally increased susceptibility of the platelets to this inhibiting action. Chronic bleeding occurs in about 80 per cent of all patients who take 4 g or more of acetylsalicylic acid per day. The loss is usually between 3 and 10 ml/day, although in some there is sufficient bleeding to cause an iron deficiency anaemia. Most of the available preparations, including the soluble ones, are equally responsible, but effervescent aspirin and aloxiprin cause significantly less bleeding. In large and repeated doses salicylates tend to cause haemorrhages by prolonging the prothrombin time, an effect antagonized by vitamin K. Doses of 3–4 g/day also shorten erythrocyte survival time.

Absorption, distribution, and fate. Absorption is mainly from the upper part of the small intestine, although some is absorbed from the stomach when the contents are particularly acid. Sodium bicarbonate has often been given with salicylates to prevent the tendency for free salicylic acid to cause gastric irritation, but although it may help in this respect, it increases urinary excretion and therefore to obtain the same blood level, with bicarbonate, a larger dose is necessary.

After absorption, salicylate is rapidly distributed throughout all the body tissues; it is secreted in saliva, milk, and bile and crosses the placental barrier. Acetylsalicylic acid is detectable for only a short time in the plasma after absorption, as the ester is rapidly hydrolysed to salicylic acid. Salicylate is found in the urine; between 60 and 90 per cent is in the free form when the urine is alkaline and it is almost entirely conjugated with glycine as salicyluric acid and with glycuronic acid when the urine is acidic. Ferric chloride will give a reddish-violet colour in a urine containing excreted salicylate, even after boiling, which distinguishes it from the colour obtained in ketonuria.

INDICATIONS

Acetylsalicylic acid may be used for the relief of minor degrees of pain such as that of rheumatism, fibrositis, headache, and toothache. It is the drug of choice in the treatment of acute rheumatic fever.

It may be employed alone or with barbiturates when pain prevents these agents being effective, and it is often combined with codeine to produce a slightly greater analgesic effect.

DOSAGE AND ADMINISTRATION

The official dose of acetylsalicylic acid is 0.3–1 g. In adults 0.6 g is usually given in tablet form when required and repeated at 4-hourly intervals if necessary. A plasma level of 30 mg/100 ml is necessary for an adequate therapeutic effect.

In acute rheumatic fever, as much as 12 g may be given in the first 24 hours, after which the dose is reduced to about 5 g/day.

PRECAUTIONS

Acetylsalicylic acid, especially when given in large or repeated doses, may cause tinnitus and dizziness, gastric irritation and bleeding. The latter complication can be minimized by use of the aluminium preparation aloxiprin; acetylsalicylic acid is best avoided altogether in the presence of known gastric or duodenal ulceration.

Aspirin sensitivity, so-called, is manifest as wheezing, sometimes accompanied by urticaria and rhinorrhoea. It occurs in up to 2 per cent of all asthmatics. It seems likely that this is in fact a consequence of prostaglandin synthetase inhibition: antibodies to aspirin are not involved and cross-reaction to all other prostaglandin synthetase inhibitors occurs. PGE_2 is a bronchodilator and $PGF_{2\alpha}$ is a bronchoconstrictor; the synthesis of the former is preferentially blocked by these drugs, thus allowing bronchoconstriction to preponderate. Because of this effect, caution should be exercised in prescribing acetylsalicylic acid to known asthmatics, particularly children.

Gutman, A. B. (1966) Uricosuric drugs, with special reference to probenecid and sulfinpyrazone. *Advances in Pharmacology,* **4,** 91

Salicylate poisoning

Salicylates are the commonest cause of death by poisoning in children under the age of 4 years, and many cases follow therapeutic use. Two clinical phases can be described which depend on the speed of development of three different toxic mechanisms.

In the first phase there is an initial direct stimulation of the respiratory centre, with the development of a respiratory alkalosis. This induces renal compensation in which hydrogen ion is conserved, and bicarbonate, sodium, and potassium are excreted. As a consequence, serum bicarbonate levels fall and the pH is shifted back towards normal at the expense of buffering capacity. At the same time, tissue metabolism is stimulated directly and the increase in carbon dioxide production maintains the hyperpnoea. Oxygen consumption can go up by 100 per cent.

Hyperpyrexia will develop if sweating is limited by dehydration, and tetany may also be induced.

The second clinical phase is dominated by the effects of salicylates on carbohydrate and lipid metabolism. The general stimulation of metabolism increases the demand for glucose. However, at least two essential enzymes of the Krebs cycle, succinic dehydrogenase and α-ketoglutaric dehydrogenase, are inhibited by salicylates. This blocks normal glucose metabolism and metabolic requirements become increasingly dependent on fatty acid catabolism, with consequent overproduction of keto acids. This metabolic acidosis now comes to dominate the clinical picture and, as a result of the previous cation loss and dehydration, can be neither buffered nor effectively compensated for by the kidney.

In young children, and in cases of severe poisoning, the first phase of alkalaemia may have passed before the patient reaches hospital, but in adults and older children this phase lasts 12–24 hours.

Acute renal failure, possibly due to tubular necrosis, has been reported, and a review of the literature suggests that renal damage in salicylate poisoning may be commoner than is generally appreciated.

Treatment. Treatment should include gastric aspiration, lavage, and full supportive therapy. As salicylate poisoning gives rise to complex changes in acid base balance, it can be best treated if pH and $Paco_2$ or standard bicarbonate estimations are repeatedly made. Rapid alkalinization of the urine accompanied by a forced diuresis with osmotic diuretics increases the rate of excretion of salicylates to values comparable to exchange transfusion or dialysis. The regimen of forced diuresis combined with alkalinization of the urine, as described for barbiturate poisoning on pages 105–106, is suitable for older children and adults. Small children aged 1–4 years (the commonest age-group in which salicylate poisoning occurs accidentally) are usually in a state of metabolic acidosis on admission. Their relatively high rate of water loss, often exaggerated by hyperpyrexia, makes osmotic diuretics unsuitable. Initial rehydration may be with 80–100 ml/kg of 5 per cent dextrose plus 3 mmol/kg of sodium bicarbonate (6 ml/kg of 4.2 per cent solution) in the first 2–3 hours, followed by a similar volume of fluid containing a further 1 mmol/kg of bicarbonate during the rest of the 24 hours; 2–4 g of potassium chloride should also be given during this period.

Adults characteristically exhibit respiratory alkalosis and virtually never develop metabolic acidosis regardless of the severity of the poisoning. Although the danger of tetany if sodium bicarbonate is given in such cases has probably been overemphasized, little may be gained by doing so if the urine is already alkaline. Tubular excretion of bicarbonate is the normal renal response to overbreathing and sodium bicarbonate should not be given unless arterial blood pH is less than 7.5 and urinary pH less than 7.6. Paper indicating strips of the appropriate range are sufficiently accurate for monitoring urinary pH. In adults, the arterial pH tends to rise with increasing blood salicylate levels. In severely alkalotic patients (arterial pH > 7.6) intravenous calcium may be given to reduce the risk of tetany.

Curarization and mechanical ventilation are extremely valuable in severe salicylate intoxication in children. This should be considered if coma, hyperpyrexia ($> 40°C$), and tetany occur.

In severe cases in which a diuresis cannot be obtained because of renal failure, dialysis will be necessary.

Benorylate

Benorylate (*BAN*)
Chemical name: 4-acetamidophenyl *O*-acetylsalicylate

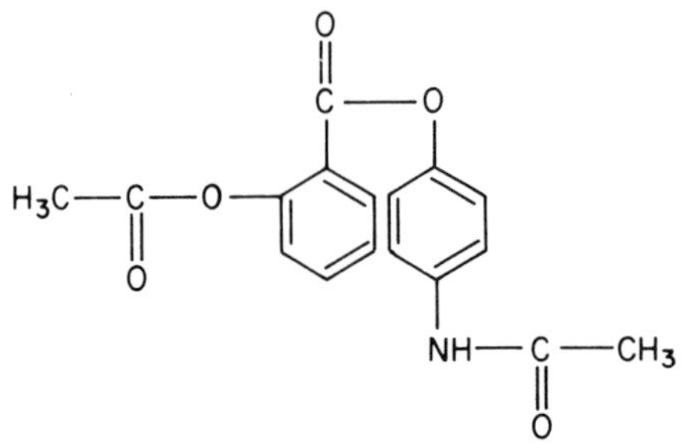

This compound illustrates an interesting pharmaceutical development by which normal metabolism is deliberately employed to deliver as active metabolites drugs that give rise to problems when given directly.

As can be seen from the chemical formula, the drug is a combination of aspirin with paracetamol, by a simple ester linkage. The compound is tasteless and readily absorbed unchanged from the gastrointestinal tract and does not cause gastric bleeding. Following absorption it is hydrolysed to produce acetylsalicylic acid and paracetamol. The compound, therefore, has the properties of these drugs and is analgesic, antipyretic, and anti-inflammatory. Effects on the kidney are not yet known, but it seems likely that nephrotoxicity could occur with big doses. There is evidence that some unmetabolized benorylate is stored in fat and slowly released. Accordingly, it need only be given twice daily in doses of 6–8 g daily; 2 g is equivalent to 1.2 g of acetylsalicylic acid.

Paracetamol

Paracetamol (*BP*) and Acetaminophen (*USP*)
Chemical name: *N*-(4-hydroxyphenyl) acetamide

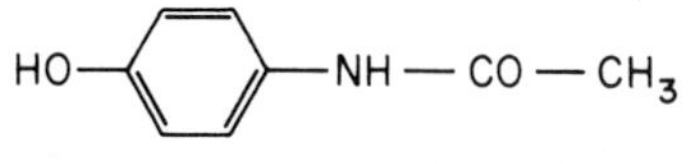

PHARMACOLOGY AND METABOLISM

Paracetamol is the metabolite of phenacetin responsible for its analgesic and antipyretic action. It is of similar potency as an analgesic and few adverse side effects have been reported. Its excretion is rapid, over 85 per cent being excreted in the urine in conjugated form. In contrast to phenacetin, it does not cause methaemoglobinaemia.

INDICATIONS, DOSAGE, AND ADMINISTRATION

It may be used for the relief of minor degrees of pain as a substitute for acetylsalicylic acid or phenacetin. It is given by mouth in tablet form in a dose of

0.5–1 g and may be repeated at 4-hourly intervals. As will be seen from the larger dose, it is a weaker analgesic than aspirin and phenacetin, but is less irritant to the stomach in those who cannot tolerate aspirin, and is generally less toxic in normal doses than any in this group.

PRECAUTIONS

Overdose with paracetamol gives rise to hepatic necrosis.

Paracetamol poisoning

This takes the form of a dose-dependent hepatic necrosis and may follow the ingestion of 10–15 g. A single intake of over 25 g is potentially fatal. It is caused by a toxic metabolite (the *N*-hydroxy derivative) which is inactivated by glutathione; toxicity results when the amount of this metabolite exceeds the stores of glutathione available for its inactivation. Regular consumers of alcohol or other drugs that induce liver microsomal enzymes produce metabolites at a greater rate and have an increased risk of developing hepatic damage.

All intensive care units who may have to treat paracetamol overdose should be able to obtain blood level estimations. A special kit is available which is accurate to the nearest 50 μg/ml in amateur hands. Such estimations are of value within the first 10 hours after ingestion as a guide to therapy. Hepatic damage is likely if the blood level is over 200 μg/ml at 2 hours after ingestion or 120 μg/ml at 10 hours after ingestion, and active therapy is indicated. Any compound rich in sulphydryl groups can be given: cysteamine is effective but causes unpleasant side effects; methionine and acetylcysteine are also effective and the latter has the advantage of being available for intravenous use. The initial dose should be 150 mg/kg in 200 ml of 5 per cent dextrose over 15 minutes followed by 50 mg/kg over 4 hours and 100 mg/kg over the next 6 hours. To be effective, treatment must be started within 10 hours of ingestion of the overdose of paracetamol.

Phenacetin

Phenacetin (*BP*)
Chemical name: *N*-(4-ethoxyphenyl) acetamide

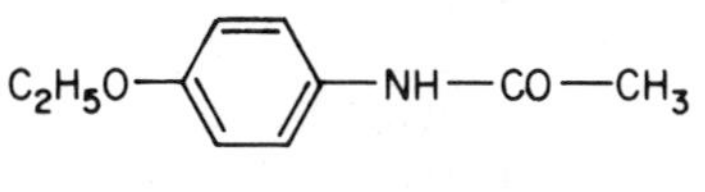

$C_2H_5O—C_6H_4—NH—CO—CH_3$

Phenacetin (acetophenetidin) is an aniline derivative which has analgesic and antipyretic action of a similar potency to that of acetylsalicylic acid and is believed to act in a like manner. Compared with acetylsalicylic acid it is less soluble, more slowly absorbed, and causes less gastric irritation. Its action is due to a metabolite, *N*-acetyl-*p*-aminophenol. Another metabolite, *p*-aminophenol, is therapeutically inactive, but may produce methaemoglobinaemia. These metabolites are excreted in the urine in conjugated form.

During the past decade there have been a number of reports of renal damage following the administration of phenacetin. This takes the form of necrosis of the renal papillae and chronic interstitial nephritis. Anaemia, probably due to haemolysis, has also been reported. Because of these toxic effects the drug has now been withdrawn from all proprietary analgesic preparations in the UK.

Analgesic nephropathy

There is a clear lack of correlation on this subject between experimental work in animals and clinical experience. In acute experiments in rats a large number of aspirin and phenacetin derivatives cause renal damage which, however, is confined to the proximal convoluted tubule. Phenacetin alone in animals has only rarely induced papillary necrosis but aspirin does so readily. In man, the evidence is the reverse. Numerous cases of analgesic nephropathy have been reported in patients taking mixtures containing phenacetin; by contrast, considering the enormous consumption, less than half a dozen cases have been reported in patients taking aspirin alone. The chief metabolite of phenacetin is *N*-acetyl-*p*-aminophenol (paracetamol). But again, despite widespread consumption, there is little evidence that ingestion of this compound alone causes nephropathy.

Anaesthestists should be alert for possible analgesic nephropathy in patients undergoing major surgery, particularly gastric surgery for ulceration. Dehydration and renal ischaemia are both capable of exacerbating experimental nephropathy and they may occur in surgical patients for a variety of reasons. There have been clinical reports of a high mortality in surgical patients with known analgesic nephropathy, and agents that are less likely to cause renal vasoconstriction are therefore indicated, combined with adequate fluid therapy.

Non-steroidal anti-inflammatory drugs (NSAIDs)

As well as some of the mild analgesics given in larger doses (particularly the salicylates) there are an increasing number of compounds available in which anti-inflammatory action is predominant, and which may have little or no analgesic effect in the absence of inflammation. These fall into several chemical groups: substituted acetic acids such as indomethacin, sulindac, and tolmetin; other pyrazolones such as phenylbutazone and oxyphenbutazone; propionic acid derivatives such as ibuprofen, fenoprofen, ketoprofen, flurbiprofen, and naproxen; and phenylacetic acids such as fenclofenac. Diflunisal can be regarded as a derivative of aspirin but is claimed to be better tolerated and without effect on platelets. There are a few others which do not fall into these groups such as azapropazone and flufenamic acid, but which exhibit very comparable pharmacological actions. Yet another drug is zomepirac which is not only anti-inflammatory but has marked central actions and is claimed to have an analgesic effect comparable to that of morphine.

Mechanisms of anti-inflammatory action

Many actions can be identified experimentally, but have been demonstrated only at dose levels above the clinically effective range. It seems likely that the major effects are mediated peripherally at the site of inflammation. The inflammatory process in rheumatic disorders involves the combination of an antigen with an antibody (rheumatoid factor) and complement. This releases local chemotactic factors which attract leucocytes; these not only phagocytize these complexes but release lysosomal enzymes which cause local injury. Local prostaglandin synthesis is also initiated by the leucocytes because of the release of phospholipases from lysosomes. These hydrolyse lipids to yield precursors of prostaglandins. These substances markedly potentiate the effects of chemical mediators of inflammation such as 5-hydroxytryptamine and bradykinin.

A property of most drugs in this category is inhibition of cyclo-oxygenase (prostaglandin synthetase), essential to the production of prostaglandins. These compounds, particularly those of the E series, are not only mediators of inflammatory responses, but also protectors of the gastric mucosa. Their effects must in part be due to this common property. However, there are other parts to the pathway and one drug (benoxaprofen) has little activity as a prostaglandin synthetase inhibitor (and little ulcerogenic potential) but inhibits monocyte migration.

In addition, there are systemic effects which may be important. The corticosteroids are transported in the plasma by binding to a globulin for which the binding affinity constant is very high. Many anti-inflammatory drugs have been shown to displace the steroid, and their ability to do so is similar to their potency as anti-inflammatory drugs. The binding of antirheumatic drugs to protein also displaces small molecules such as L-tryptophan and anti-inflammatory peptides; the proportion of unbound L-tryptophan is also increased in jaundice and pregnancy, conditions in which remission of rheumatoid arthritis often occurs. It has therefore been suggested on this indirect evidence that the displaced compounds exert a protective effect. This theory still requires further confirmation.

Clinical properties of NSAIDs

The different NSAIDs have been compared in numerous clinical trials, often with conflicting results. They seem, overall, remarkably similar in efficacy and (with some exceptions) in toxicity. However, this disguises the fact that there may be striking differences between these drugs, in both efficacy and toxicity, in individual patients.

They are the drugs of first choice in the active stages of rheumatoid arthritis and arthritides such as ankylosing spondylitis, and are more effective than simple analgesics in relieving symptoms in osteoarthritis where there is secondary inflammation. They relieve pain and stiffness and may reduce the swelling of inflammation. They do nothing to treat the underlying disease process. NSAIDs act within 48 hours and have their maximal effect within 1–2 weeks.

Their principal side effect, which is common to all NSAIDs to a greater or lesser degree, is gastrointestinal ulceration and bleeding. This is most noticeable with phenylbutazone, aspirin, and indomethacin. This is said to be because, as weak acids, they accumulate in the parietal cells of the stomach where they inhibit prostaglandins which are normally protective. However, benoxaprofen (which has now been withdrawn from the market) has no prostaglandin synthetase inhibitory activity, but is equally prone to produce gastric symptoms. To avoid this common problem some pro-drugs such as benorylate (*see* page 200) and sulindac have been developed which rely on hepatic metabolism to produce the active principle from an inert compound.

NSAIDs are also prone to effects on coagulation: aspirin inhibits platelet aggregation while many of the others, being highly protein bound, are able to displace anticoagulants. Other less common but well-substantiated side effects include tinnitus (particularly in the elderly), onycholysis, and photosensitivity. Aspirin can cause renal damage (*see* above) and an asthma-like sensitivity. Relatively uncommon effects include bone marrow suppression, hepatic toxicity, and the Stevens–Johnson syndrome.

Included below are monographs on one compound from each group and short notes on the principal differences claimed for other members of the group.

Ibuprofen

Ibuprofen (*BP* and *USP*)
Chemical name: 2-(4-isobutylphenyl)propionic acid

$$(H_3C)_2CH-CH_2-C_6H_4-CH(CH_3)-COOH$$

Ibuprofen is a mild analgesic, antipyretic, and anti-inflammatory agent whose actions compare favourably with those of acetylsalicylic acid. It is related to ibufenic acid which was withdrawn in 1968 because of its tendency to cause jaundice. Ibuprofen has no effect on liver function, no glucocorticoid activity, and no teratogenic effects in rabbits or mice. It is comparatively free from side effects, but occasional cases of dyspepsia, malaise, and rashes have been reported. On rare occasions gastrointestinal haemorrhages have followed its use.

Ibuprofen is rapidly absorbed when given by mouth. It is mainly excreted as two metabolites in the urine, but some re-enters the intestine by excretion in the bile. It is cleared from the serum within 24 hours. About 90 per cent is bound to serum albumin.

Ibuprofen is used in the treatment of rheumatoid arthritis and other similar conditions, and is useful in the treatment of patients intolerant to acetylsalicylic acid. At the start of treatment 1.2 g may be given daily in divided doses. This is then followed by a maintenance dose of 200 mg three to four times a day. Because of its good safety record, it can now be bought without prescription in the UK.

Other propionic acid derivatives

Fenoprofen is a pro-drug without anti-inflammatory activity in the stomach, which is converted by the liver to active metabolites with long half-lives. It can be given as a once daily dose of 600 mg in the evening.

Flurbiprofen has marked prostaglandin synthetase inhibition but does not seem to be unusually effective clinically. It must be taken three times daily in a dose of 150 mg–300 mg per day.

Ketoprofen is well tolerated and can be given twice or three times a day; it is also available as a suppository. The dose is 150 mg daily.

Naproxen has a low incidence of side effects and a long half-life (10–17 hours). It can be given by suppository. The dose is 500 mg–1 g daily.

Indomethacin

Indomethacin (*BP* and *USP*)
Chemical name: [1-(4-chlorobenzoyl)-5-methoxy-2-methylindol-3-yl]acetic acid

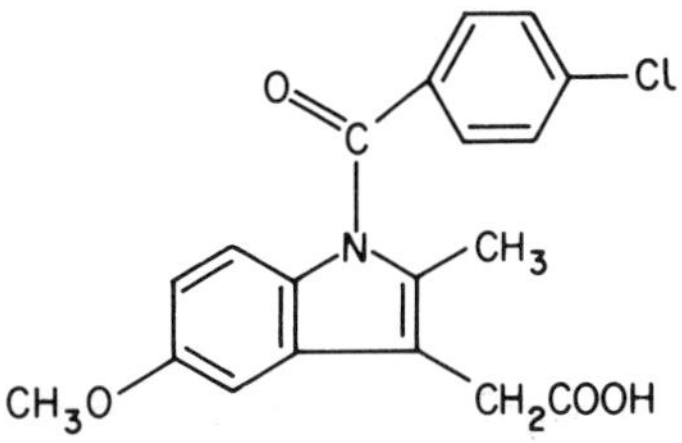

PHARMACOLOGY

Indomethacin is a mild analgesic and antipyretic, somewhat more effective than acetylsalicylic acid. It also has anti-inflammatory activity not dependent on the integrity of the pituitary–adrenal axis. Combination with steroids is more effective in inhibiting oedema formation than either agent alone. Gastrointestinal disturbances are a relatively common side effect and headache often occurs during the early stages of treatment. Other side effects that have been reported include drowsiness, mental confusion, blurred vision, pruritus, and skin rashes. It may also cause silent giant peptic ulcers, similar to those produced by corticosteroids. Both perforation and haemorrhage have been reported. The incidence of this complication appears to be related to the daily dose. Since recommended doses have been reduced to those suggested below, the incidence of all side effects has fallen considerably.

Indomethacin is insoluble in acid, and is absorbed only when it reaches the small intestine. Absorption, therefore, depends on gastric emptying, and peak levels occur about 2 hours after administration. It is well absorbed from the rectum. Two thirds of the drug are excreted as the glucuronide in the urine, while the remainder is excreted mostly unchanged in the faeces.

INDICATIONS

Indomethacin is used in the treatment of rheumatoid arthritis and osteoarthritis, gout, and other musculoskeletal disorders.

DOSAGE AND ADMINISTRATION

The initial dose is 25 mg three times a day, which is then gradually increased up to about 100 mg per day. It should be given with meals. Smaller doses may be combined with a corticosteroid. Alternatively, the drug may be given as a suppository containing 100 mg.

PRECAUTIONS

Indomethacin shold not be given to patients with active peptic ulceration, and should be used with caution if there is a history of peptic ulcer.

Sulindac is a fluorinated pro-drug which undergoes hepatic metabolism to the sulphide metabolite. It is claimed to have fewer side effects than indomethacin but clinical experience has shown that, nevertheless, side effects do occur in some patients. The dose is 100 mg–200 mg twice daily.

Tolmetin is closely structurally related to indomethacin and must be given three or four times per day. The dose is 800 mg–1600 mg daily.

Mefenamic acid

Mefenamic acid (*BP* and *USAN*)
Chemical name: *N*-(2,3-xylyl)anthranilic acid

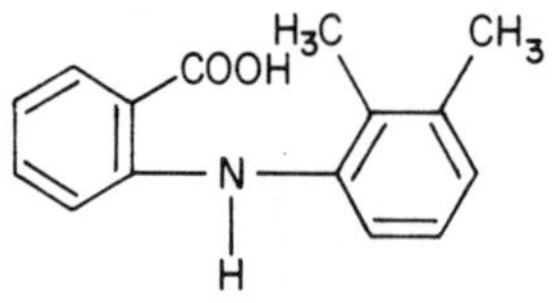

Mefenamic acid is a mild analgesic with anti-inflammatory properties. Its analgesic action is similar to that of codeine and its anti-inflammatory effect is greater than that of acetylsalicylic acid. It relieves the pain of rheumatism and has a uricosuric action in gout. Side effects have been increasingly reported. Diarrhoea is common and sometimes severe gastrointestinal haemorrhage and ulceration have been reported, as have exacerbations of allergies. Many blood dyscrasias have also been noted. It enhances the effects of oral anticoagulants. It is excreted in the urine, both in the free form and combined with glycuronic acid.

Mefanamic acid may be used for similar purposes as acetylsalicylic acid. It is given by mouth in capsule form, the dose being 750 mg–1500 mg daily in three divided doses.

Flufenamic acid is also an anthranilic acid derivative and has similar properties. It is given three times a day up to a maximum of 600 mg daily.

Phenylbutazone

Phenylbutazone (*BP* and *USP*)
Chemical name: 4-butyl-1,2-diphenylpyrazolidine-3,5-dione

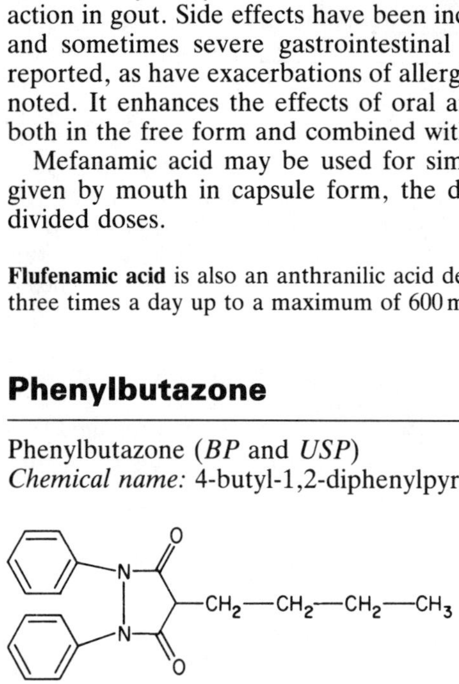

PHARMACOLOGY

Phenylbutazone, which is closely related chemically to amidopyrine, is an effective, long-acting, anti-inflammatory analgesic; it suppresses the inflammatory effects on the skin of ultraviolet light and other irritants, and has some antihistamine action. It is an inhibitor of prostaglandin synthetase and can thus inhibit many aspects of inflammation such as oedema.

In rheumatoid arthritis, it reduces the pain and tenderness in joints better than either amidopyrine or salicylates. Judging these cases subjectively, the drug will produce improvement in 70–90 per cent of cases, which is of the same order as that produced by cortisone or corticotrophin. Phenylbutazone does not, however, equal cortisone in its effectiveness in reducing joint swelling, there being little change except in a small percentage of patients treated.

Despite their effectiveness, drugs of this type have serious side effects: in addition to the expected peptic ulceration they can cause bone marrow aplasia, and a less toxic NSAID should be used for long-term therapy.

Certain metabolic effects are seen after administration of phenylbutazone which affects the transport mechanism of the renal tubules. In the case of uric acid, by depression of tubular reabsorption, there is increased excretion, while in the case of sodium chloride, by increasing the tubular absorption of both ions, there will be water retention to the extent of 1–3 litres. This may not be enough to cause oedema of the tissues, but it may increase the load on the heart and induce failure in patients with a diminished cardiac reserve.

Absorption and fate in the body When given orally, peak plasma levels occur in about 2 hours, and almost complete absorption takes place. When given by the intramuscular route, the drug is fixed to muscle and the peak plasma concentration is delayed, being maximal in 6–10 hours. In the body, the drug is almost completely destroyed and three water-soluble metabolites have been found in human urine. Breakdown is slow and considerable amounts are still present in the body at 72 hours.

INDICATIONS

Phenylbutazone can be used in acute gout and for the treatment of intractable ankylosing spondylitis. It should not be used for long-term treatment.

DOSAGE AND ADMINISTRATION

Phenylbutazone is normally given by mouth in a daily dose of 600–800 mg initially, reducing to a maximum of 400 mg daily. It is given in divided doses after meals. It may also be given by suppository 250 mg once or twice a day. Larger doses are liable to increase the danger of toxic symptoms with little increase in therapeutic effect.

PRECAUTIONS

Phenylbutazone should be avoided in the presence of gastric or duodenal ulceration, and used with caution in cardiac and renal disease. Toxic effects which may occur include skin rashes, renal damage, oedema, depression of the bone marrow, and thrombocytopenia. Weekly white cell counts are advisable during prolonged treatment. The drug should be immediately withdrawn if any of these complications supervene.

Oxyphenbutazone is virtually indistinguishable from phenylbutazone both in therapeutic effect and in side effects.

Azapropazone, although structurally related to phenylbutazone, lacks the toxic effects on the bone marrow. It is about as effective as the propionic acid derivatives such as ibuprofen. It is well tolerated and the dose is 600–1200 mg daily in two, three, or four divided doses.

Feprazone has a terpene group incorporated in the molecule in an attempt to build in the ulcer-healing properties of the terpenes. Peptic ulceration is still, nevertheless, regarded as a contraindication while clinical experience accumulates. It also lacks the haematological toxicity of phenylbutazone. It is given in daily doses of 200–600 mg daily.

Zomepirac sodium

Zomepirac sodium (*BAN*)
Chemical name: sodium [5-(4-chlorobenzoyl)-1,4-dimethylpyrrol-2-yl]acetate dihydrate

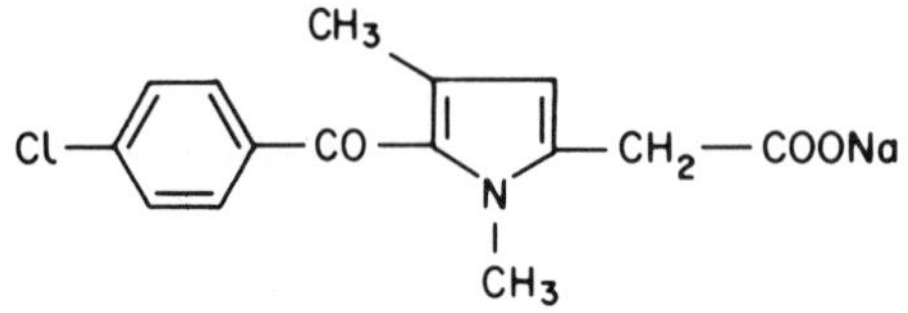

PHARMACOLOGY

Zomepirac sodium is a NSAID which is not only a potent inhibitor of prostaglandin synthetase but is also a moderately potent centrally acting analgesic. It is effective not only in pain of skeletal origin but also in acute pain, such as postoperative pain. Despite evidence of a central action, it has no narcotic or addictive potential. Its effects are not antagonized by naloxone nor does naloxone produce evidence of withdrawal after chronic administration.

INDICATIONS

The drug has been evaluated clinically in a variety of situations: acutely following removal of molar teeth and following meniscectomy, and chronically in the management of osteoarthritis and other rheumatic conditions.

Zomepirac sodium 100 mg is equianalgesic with aspirin 800 mg and pentazocine 100 mg. There are few comparisons with other NSAIDs and no convincing evidence that its considerable extra expense is justified.

DOSAGE AND ADMINISTRATION

Zomepirac sodium can be given in a dose of 50–100 mg orally. Following a single oral dose, onset of analgesia takes about 30 minutes, reaching a peak in 1–2 hours and lasting 4–6 hours. Bigger doses do not seem to be any more effective.

PRECAUTIONS

Cross-sensitivity can occur in patients intolerant to other NSAIDs, in particular so-called aspirin sensitivity. It must be anticipated that it will also inhibit platelet function and raise the bleeding time. There is no prolongation of the prothrombin time.

The most common side effects are related to the gastrointestinal tract, particularly nausea, dyspepsia, diarrhoea, and abdominal pain. There may be an elevation of blood urea and creatinine.

Zomepirac sodium (Zomax) has been temporarily withdrawn, both in the USA and the UK because of sensitivity reactions similar to, but more severe than, those associated with aspirin.

6

Local analgesics

Any agent which, when applied to nervous tissue, can prevent conduction of the nerve impulse in any part of the neurone can be classed as a local anaesthetic. In fact, all true local anaesthetics only produce a reversible depression of conduction. Further, they are commonly used to produce loss of pain with or without loss of touch and other local sensation or nervous control, and therefore the term local analgesic is better than local anaesthetic.

These agents may be injected into the following areas:

1. The spinal theca where all nerve roots in the vicinity are affected – these usually include the motor as well as the sensory roots, and also sympathetic fibres, for example spinal analgesia.
2. The extradural space with a similar effect, for example extradural (epidural) and caudal analgesia.
3. The vicinity of main nerve trunks, for example brachial plexus block, individual nerve block, and field block.
4. The subcutaneous tissues where mainly the sensory fibres from the skin are affected, for example local infiltrations.
5. A suitable limb vein after application of a tourniquet to produce analgesia distal to it – intravenous local analgesia.

Certain analgesics also act on mucous surfaces when applied directly to them.

Pharmacology

The various local analgesics in use today vary in toxicity, potency, and duration of action; their special properties and uses are discussed under their individual headings. They are the water-soluble salts of lipid-soluble substances which vary widely in their chemical constitution. The main groups include the following:

1. Cocaine: a naturally occurring alkaloid, first isolated in 1860, and the first local analgesic to be used.
2. *p*-Aminobenzoic acid derivatives: a large group of compounds including procaine, amethocaine, benzamine, and butacaine.
3. Other synthetic agents, among which must be considered lignocaine, which is an aminoacyl amide; cinchocaine, a quinoline acid derivative; certain aromatic

alcohols, such as benzyl alcohol, which are sometimes used as surface-active local analgesics; and local analgesics of low solubility, such as benzocaine and butylaminobenzoate, used mainly as dusting powders. Many of these drugs have marked chemical resemblance to the *p*-aminobenzoic acid group of drugs.

Many antihistamines, especially certain of the phenothiazines, also have local analgesic properties but are unsuitable for use as they are irritant to tissues.

Prolonged or permanent analgesia can be produced by protoplasmic poisons, such as quinidine, alcohol, phenol, and chlorocresol. These need to be applied close to the nerve and can be used in various sites. Intrathecally, 95 per cent alcohol, 5 per cent phenol in glycerin, and 6–7 per cent phenol in iophendylate have been employed. In other locations aqueous solutions of phenol (5–6 per cent), 5 per cent chlorocresol, and 50 per cent alcohol are generally used. Conduction in nerves can also be blocked by pressure and by low temperatures. These techniques are not suitable for operative procedures.

Chemistry

Most local analgesics are either tertiary amino esters or amides of aromatic acids, with the following basic formulae:

$$R_1CO-OR_2-N\begin{matrix}R_3\\R_4\end{matrix} \quad \text{or} \quad R_1NHCOR_2N\begin{matrix}R_3\\R_4\end{matrix}$$

These molecules consist of three parts, acidic (R_1CO), alcoholic ($-OR_2$) and terminal tertiary amine

$$\left(-N\begin{matrix}R_3\\R_4\end{matrix}\right)$$

Many attempts have been made to produce compounds of greater potency by altering the constituent parts of this molecule. Thus, increasing the chain length of the alcohol or of the groups R_3 and R_4 on the terminal amine produces compounds of increased potency, but usually at the cost of greatly increased toxicity and local irritant properties, and few of the potent local analgesics thus synthesized have been suitable for clinical use.

Local analgesics that are to be injected are prepared as water-soluble salts, usually the hydrochloride, which are stable in solution. After injection it is that fraction of the drug which is present in the cation form which is the active principle. The amount will be determined by the pK_a of the particular drug and the pH of the surrounding tissues.

During recent years interest has developed in an alternative formulation, the carbonated base prepared at a $P\text{CO}_2$ of 700 mmHg (93.3 kPa). These have a relatively high pH of 6.5 compared with the hydrochlorides which have a pH of 6 and those which contain vasoconstrictors whose pH may be as low as 4. They therefore make less demands on the buffering capacity of the tissues and with rapid buffering and diffusion away of the carbon dioxide, free base is deposited rapidly. Clinically, carbonated solutions of lignocaine have been shown to have a shorter latency of onset and greater intensity of blockade than the hydrochloride. In the epidural space the block is more widespread for the same total dose and consequently only about 80 per cent of the usual dose need be employed. This results in lower blood levels in the circulation, and in obstetric cases lower levels also in the fetus.

Carbonated solutions are less prone to tachyphylaxis than the hydrochloride when used for continuous epidural analgesia. The cause of this tachyphylaxis is the increasing acidity of the local tissues due to the deposition of acid salts which are poorly buffered, and this leads to a fall in the proportion of free base. This has been noted particularly with lignocaine but less so with bupivacaine, possibly due to the lower total dose necessary.

Mode of action

On injection into the tissues, the drug will be present in the form of the free base and the positively charged cation. The former is fat soluble and responsible for diffusing through the tissues and the various coverings of the nerves, but it is the cation which is the active principle and responsible for interruption of impulse conduction. This it does by preventing the migration of sodium ions across the nerve membrane, and the mode of action might be related to competition with calcium ions at some receptor site which controls permeability. Thus, although it reduces resting permeability, it produces no change in the resting membrane potential. Local anaesthetics are therefore said to stabilize the nerve membrane.

Fine fibres are blocked before larger ones, and therefore pain, temperature, touch, and motor functions are lost in progressive order. With all analgesics (except cocaine) it is impossible to achieve a completely dissociated sensory block with no motor block. With very low concentrations of cocaine (for example 0.2 per cent) however, sensory block can be achieved without any motor blockade. In a medullated nerve the block only occurs at the nodes of Ranvier.

Other pharmacological actions

Apart from the actions in producing local analgesia, these drugs have important actions on other systems in the body. These are only manifest if absorption is too rapid for destruction and excretion to maintain a safe equilibrium. The side effects most usually encountered are like those of atropine and quinidine.

Central nervous system. Local analgesics can penetrate the blood-brain barrier and exert a similar stabilizing effect on central neurones. They will thus control status epilepticus if given intravenously in suitable doses. Under normal conditions, however, inhibitory neurones are more sensitive to the actions of these drugs than are the excitatory neurones and excitatory phenomena predominate. Overdose leads to tremors and restlessness proceeding to clonic convulsions. Larger doses depress consciousness and ventilation. Cocaine has a special stimulant action on the cortex, increasing mental powers, a fact that renders it a dangerous drug of addiction.

Some local analgesics, especially procaine and lignocaine, have marked general analgesic properties. Even small doses of procaine used in local infiltration produce measurable, although transitory, degrees of general analgesia. Although procaine and lignocaine have been used in continuous intravenous infusions to produce controllable analgesia during surgical operations and the changing of painful dressings, their use in this way is limited by the small margin between the effective dose and that which produces convulsions and severe depression of the cardiovascular system.

Autonomic ganglia and myoneural junction. Local analgesics can produce some degree of blockade of transmission at autonomic ganglia and at myoneural junctions. At both of these sites the block is probably in part an 'anti-release' phenomenon, due to depression of acetylcholine release, and partly a true non-depolarizing competitive block.

Cardiovascular system. Local analgesics are also able to stabilize membrane permeability of excitatory tissue in the heart. They consequently increase the refractory period, prolong conduction time, and depress myocardial excitability. They have thus found a useful role in the control and treatment of ventricular dysrhythmias. Procainamide was originally introduced as a drug with greater stability for this purpose, but lignocaine is now widely employed.

Effects on the fetal heart following paracervical block during labour have also been reported.

All local analgesics except cocaine tend to cause peripheral vasodilatation by a direct action on arterioles; bupivacaine has little effect, whereas cocaine potentiates noradrenaline and causes vasoconstriction in skin and mucosa. Vasodilator effects together with the cardiac action and their tendency to cause blockade of autonomic ganglia tend to result in a fall in blood pressure if large doses or continuous infusions are given.

Local analgesics when given by spinal and epidural routes block preganglionic fibres as they leave the spinal cord in the anterior rami; this too will cause a fall in blood pressure, proportional to the number of nerves affected.

Respiratory system. Central stimulation causes some increase in the rate of respiration, but as the medulla becomes depressed, breathing becomes rapid and shallow. Bronchial musculature is relaxed.

Local analgesics also have an atropine-like spasmolytic effect on smooth muscle and a mild antihistamine action.

Fate in the body. All of the local analgesics are destroyed in the liver. Thus the toxicity of the various agents will vary in inverse proportion to liver function. Procaine and amethocaine are also inactivated by plasma pseudocholinesterase. Those agents which are most slowly broken down will, to a small extent, appear unchanged in the urine.

A large number of local analgesics have been synthesized, but few have stood the test of time. Lignocaine and bupivacaine are the most commonly used agents in Great Britain at present. Prilocaine has a place as a relatively non-toxic agent for intravenous analgesia; cinchocaine and bupivacaine are employed when a long-acting agent is required. Mepivacaine is usefully employed when a vasoconstrictor is contraindicated. Maximum doses and strength of solution are discussed under the appropriate headings of the drugs concerned.

The relative toxicity and potency of these agents to one another are difficult to determine with any accuracy, as they vary with the concentrations employed and with the routes of administration. Much of the experimental work has been done on different animal species and it is not surprising that figures quoted by different workers vary considerably.

PRECAUTIONS

Toxic reactions to local analgesics usually occur only when an excessive amount of the drug has been given; idiosyncrasy can occur, but this diagnosis should be accepted only if minimal doses have been administered and symptoms of overdose can be explained in no other way.

Reactions arise when the blood concentration of the drug reaches toxic levels and this may occur in the following situations:

1. When an absolute overdose is given and the rate of absorption overtakes the rate of breakdown and excretion.
2. When a normal dose is absorbed unduly rapidly, as when the drug is inadvertently injected into a vein, or is introduced into inflamed or highly vascular tissue.
3. When doses safe for other regions are applied topically to mucous surfaces of the respiratory tract where absorption is almost as rapid as when the drug is given intravenously.
4. When destruction is delayed by serious liver disease or by genetic abnormalities, such as plasma pseudocholinesterase in the case of procaine and amethocaine.

As is the case with all drugs, the toxic threshold is considerably reduced in sick, frail, and undernourished patients. Patients suffering from myasthenia gravis are susceptible to the effects of local analgesics, especially when administered intravenously, as the mild neuromuscular block will increase muscular weakness and may depress respiration.

High concentrations of these agents are relatively more toxic dose for dose than weaker ones. A 20 ml injection of a 1 per cent solution, for instance, is considerably less toxic than 10 ml of a 2 per cent solution. In all cases where susceptibility to local analgesics is probable, the maximum dose should be reduced and a weaker solution should be employed.

A vasoconstrictor such as adrenaline is often used with local analgesics to decrease absorption, prolong their action, and decrease bleeding. Adrenaline has little effect on the rate of absorption when amethocaine is used on the mucous membrane of the bronchial tree. Care must be exercised in the amount of adrenaline that is given; serious and sometimes fatal results have followed its use in excessive dose. It is inadvisable (and generally ineffective) to add adrenaline in a subarachnoid block, as ischaemia may damage the spinal cord.

OVERDOSE

In mild cases of overdose, the patient usually exhibits circumoral pallor and becomes anxious and restless, and complains of nausea; the symptoms are transient and will pass off with little or no treatment. In more severe cases, convulsions may occur and respiratory and circulatory failure may follow. In the case of overdose with cocaine, cardiac failure due to ventricular fibrillation may occur suddenly without other symptoms. Syncope has also been reported in amethocaine overdose under similar circumstances.

Treatment. Convulsions should be treated with small divided doses of a short-acting barbiturate such as thiopentone. If they are not controlled by small doses a short-acting muscle relaxant should be given. Respiratory failure will require the administration of oxygen and controlled respiration, if prolonged, by the endotracheal route. Circulatory failure should be treated by the administration of a pressor agent, or if this is ineffective, noradrenaline should be given by intravenous infusion.

Amethocaine hydrochloride

Amethocaine hydrochloride (*BP*) and Tetracaine hydrochloride (*USP*)
Chemical name: 2-dimethylaminoethyl-4-butylaminobenzoate hydrochloride

$$H_9C_4—HN—C_6H_4—CO—O—CH_2—CH_2—N(CH_3)_2 \cdot HCl$$

PHARMACOLOGY

Amethocaine is a local analgesic belonging to the procaine group. By subcutaneous injection it is effective in a 1:4000 solution. Its onset of action is slow (5 minutes or more) but its duration is 2–3 hours.

Its pharmacological effects are similar to those of local analgesics in general; these include a stimulant and later depressant action on the CNS, a quinidine-like action on the heart, and a direct action on blood vessels causing vasodilatation. Like cocaine, it may cause sudden cardiac failure with asystole or ventricular fibrillation, which its quinidine-like action is not strong enough to stop. In contrast with procaine it produces excellent surface analgesia. The 1 per cent solution is approximately equivalent in potency to 10 per cent cocaine.

Detoxication takes place in the body, where it is hydrolysed by plasma cholinesterase, but it is eliminated at a much slower rate than the shorter acting local analgesics such as procaine and lignocaine. *p*-Aminobenzoic acid is a metabolite, and while present in the circulation will inhibit the action of sulphonamides.

INDICATIONS

Amethocaine is used for infiltration analgesia, regional, spinal, and extradural block, and for surface analgesia. It is often mixed with procaine or lignocaine to combine the rapid action of the latter agents with its own prolonged effect.

DOSAGE AND ADMINISTRATION

Unless specifically contraindicated, amethocaine should normally be used with adrenaline. Authorities vary considerably in the strength of solution and total dosage recommended for the different procedures for which this agent is employed. The following are effective and allow a reasonable margin of safety.

Infiltration and regional block. Strengths of solution from 1:1000 to 1:4000 may be employed with adrenaline. Not more than 100 ml (100 mg) of the 1:1000 solution should be used; if a greater volume is required a weaker solution must be given. The 1:4000 solution is reasonably effective and up to 500 ml may be used.

For nerve block a 1:1000 solution is used: up to 30 ml for brachial plexus block and up to 10 ml for individual nerve block, such as intercostal and pudendal.

Surface analgesia. For the cornea, 0.5 or 1 per cent solutions are employed. For the pharynx, trachea, and larynx, up to 8 ml of a 0.5 per cent solution may be used; stronger solutions should be avoided as they are relatively more toxic. The maximum dose is 40 mg. A 1:1000 solution is used for analgesia of the urethra, and a 2 per cent suppository for that of the rectum and anus. Analgesia of the mouth and pharynx can be effected by the sucking of a lozenge (65 mg). It should be started 20 minutes before operation and ejected as soon as analgesia is established. Solutions may be sterilized by boiling or autoclaving but repeated sterilization by these methods causes deterioration. They are rapidly inactivated in the presence of alkalis and many antiseptic solutions.

Spinal block. A 1 per cent solution in 6 per cent dextrose is used, 0.5–2 ml being injected according to the height of analgesia required. Alternatively, the calculated dose of amethocaine crystals (5–20 mg) may be dissolved in CSF and injected similarly.

For extradural block, a 0.15 per cent solution may be employed, 15–50 ml being injected according to the extent of block required.

PRECAUTIONS

Precautions are as for local analgesics in general. Amethocaine is, however, a highly toxic agent and it is important that maximum doses are not exceeded. This applies especially to its use for analgesia of the respiratory passages.

Symptoms and treatment of overdose are discussed on page 213.

Benzocaine

Benzocaine (*BP* and *USP*)
Chemical name: ethyl-4-aminobenzoate

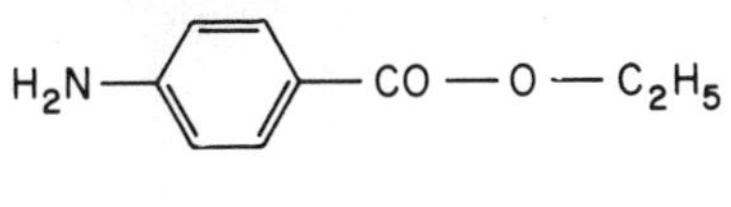

H_2N — CO — O — C_2H_5

PHARMACOLOGY, INDICATIONS AND DOSAGE

Benzocaine is the ethyl ester of *p*-aminobenzoic acid. It has a local analgesic action on mucous surfaces, and is used in various forms for surface analgesia of the mouth and throat, ear, and skin.

Bupivacaine hydrochloride

Bupivacaine hydrochloride (*BP* and *USP*)
Chemical name: (±)-(1-butyl-2-piperidyl) formo-2′,6′-xylidide hydrochloride

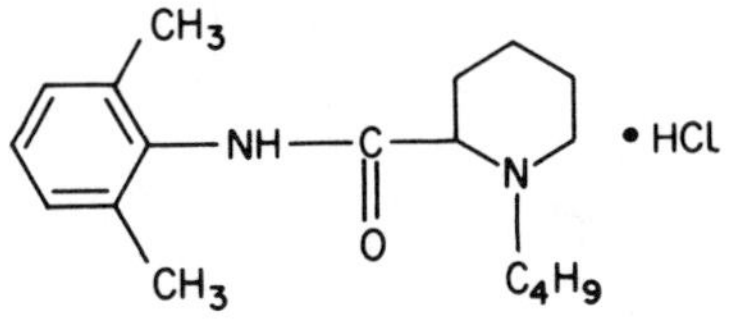

CH_3
NH — C — N • HCL
O
CH_3 C_4H_9

Bupivacaine is chemically related to mepivacaine and differs only in having a butyl side chain in place of a methyl group. Both its potency and toxicity are approximately four times greater than those of lignocaine, so that its therapeutic ratio is similar. It does, however, have a longer duration of action, 3–5 hours for the 0.5 per cent solution with adrenaline given by the epidural route and up to 6 hours after specific nerve blocks.

General systemic effects are similar to those of other local analgesics. No local toxic effects on nerves or surrounding tissues have been reported.

INDICATIONS

It can be used for nerve blocks and is particularly suitable for continuous epidural analgesia in labour. It is also of value for single-dose epidural injections for surgery.

DOSAGE AND ADMINISTRATION

Plain solutions of 0.75, 0.5 and 0.25 per cent are available, and also 0.5 per cent with adrenaline 1:200 000, and 0.25 per cent with adrenaline 1:400 000. Appropriate solutions may be used for all types of nerve blocks. Not more than 150 mg (30 ml of 0.5 per cent solution) should be given at one time or in any 4-hour period.

PRECAUTIONS

These are the same as for lignocaine. Preparations containing adrenaline can only be re-autoclaved once or twice before deterioration of the adrenaline occurs. There is some evidence that it is relatively more toxic on the heart in overdose. It is not, therefore, recommended for use by untrained personnel using Bier's block (*see* page 221).

Cinchocaine hydrochloride

Cinchocaine hydrochloride (*BP*) and Dibucaine hydrochloride (*USP*)
Chemical name: 2-butoxy-*N*-(2-diethylaminoethyl)quinoline-4-carboxamide hydrochloride

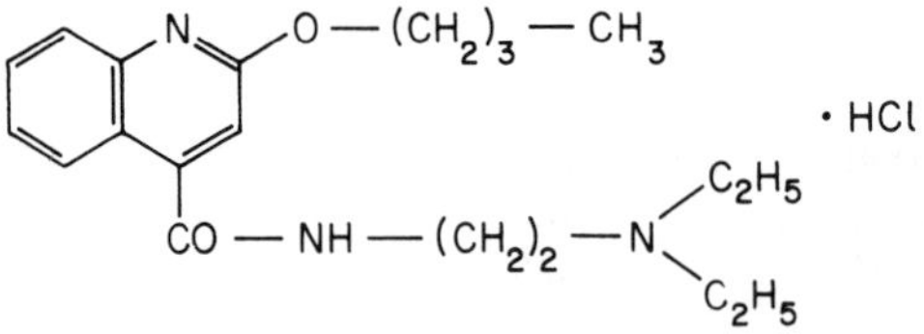

N, $O-(CH_2)_3-CH_3$
$\cdot$ HCl
$CO-NH-(CH_2)_2-N(C_2H_5)_2$

PHARMACOLOGY

Cinchocaine is a quinoline derivative. It is a powerful local analgesic which is effective in concentrations of 1:4000. Its onset of action is slower than that of procaine (3–5 minutes), but its duration is much longer (2–3 hours). It is an effective surface analgesic when applied topically.

Systemic effects produced by cinchocaine are similar to those of other local analgesics. It is detoxicated in the liver, but elimination is much slower than with the short-acting agents such as procaine.

INDICATIONS

Cinchocaine has been used for local infiltration, regional, spinal, and extradural block, and for surface analgesia. It is still extensively used for spinal block.

It is employed in 10^{-5} M concentration as a differential inhibitor which will distinguish between usual and atypical forms of plasma cholinesterase.

DOSAGE AND ADMINISTRATION

Unless otherwise contraindicated, adrenaline should normally be used with cinchocaine to delay absorption.

For local infiltration. Up to 120 ml of a 1:1000 solution or up to 250 ml of a 1:2000 solution may be employed. The suggested maximum dose in healthy adults is 2 mg/kg of body weight. If tissues are highly vascular the dose should be halved.

For nerve blocks. The 1:1000 solution should be used for nerve blocks, 10 ml for individual nerve blocks and up to 30 ml for brachial plexus block.

For spinal analgesia. A 1:200 solution in 6 per cent dextrose is most commonly employed, 0.5–2 ml being injected according to the height of analgesia required. A hypobaric solution, 1:1500 (sp. gr. at 37°C = 1.0036), dose 6–18 ml, is also available. It is rarely employed in Great Britain now as neurological sequelae have been attributed to its use.

For epidural and caudal block. Here 15–50 ml of a 1:600 solution may be given.

For surface analgesia. A 1:1000 solution is used for the cornea and the urethra. For the pharynx, larynx, and trachea, up to 2 ml of a 2 per cent solution or proportionally more of a 1 per cent solution may be applied. Buccal analgesia can be produced by the sucking of a lozenge (1 mg). A 1 per cent ointment is also available for surface application and may be used for the lubrication of endotracheal tubes.

PRECAUTIONS

Precautions are as for other local analgesics, as are also symptoms and treatment of overdosage.

Cocaine

Cocaine (*BP* and *USP*)
Cocaine hydrochloride (*BP* and *USP*)
Chemical name: (1*R*,2*R*,3*s*,5*S*)-2-methoxycarbonyltropan-3-yl benzoate

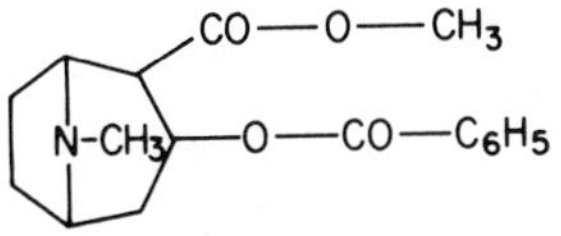

CO—O—CH_3
N-CH_3 —O—CO—C_6H_5

PHARMACOLOGY

Cocaine, methyl benzoylecgonine, an ester of benzoic acid, is an alkaloid obtained from the leaves of *Erythroxylum coca*, a tree found in Peru, Brazil, and other South American countries. The leaves have been chewed by the natives of these countries for centuries to produce euphoria and to increase their capacity for muscular work. Its local analgesic properties were discovered towards the end of the last century; its toxicity, however, was soon found to be too great for general use and an intensive search began for safer substitutes.

Cocaine has many actions in common with other local analgesics; it differs, however, in some respects.

Nervous system. There is marked central stimulation at first, which results in excitement, restlessness, euphoria, and an increase in mental alertness. There is an increased capacity for muscular effort which is due to the loss of feeling of fatigue. Respiratory, vasomotor, and vomiting centres are stimulated, and with increasing dosage convulsions will occur. Later, central stimulation gives place to depression, paralysis of vital centres, and death.

Cocaine blocks the re-uptake of noradrenaline into the presynaptic nerve terminal, the mechanism which is normally responsible for the termination of the action of the transmitter. It is therefore an indirectly acting sympathomimetic agent. Many of the signs of toxicity of cocaine can be explained in terms of excessive sympathetic activity.

Cardiovascular system. Slowing of the heart rate due to central vagal stimulation may occur after small doses. Larger doses induce all the signs of sympathetic stimulation, with tachycardia, peripheral vasoconstriction, and hypertension; these persist until medullary depression or cardiac failure supervene. Ventricular fibrillation may occur quite early.

Respiratory system. Respiratory rate is increased, but depth is unaffected. As the dose is increased, the respiratory centre becomes depressed and respiration becomes rapid and shallow.

Musculature. There is no evidence of direct action on skeletal muscle, but smooth muscle is relaxed. Motor activity is well co-ordinated with small doses of cocaine, but as the dose is increased this activity increases and tremors and convulsive movements appear.

Mucous surfaces. When applied topically, cocaine produces excellent surface analgesia, with intense vasoconstriction. When applied to the eye, mydriasis occurs (sympathomimetic action) and the intraocular pressure is increased, but the effect is less than is seen with atropine. Cocaine has a deleterious action on the cornea, which may become clouded and pitted. This toxic effect is increased by the abolition of the normal protective eyelid reflexes. Because of this damage, and the tendency to produce mydriasis, cocaine has largely been replaced by other local analgesics in ophthalmology.

Fate in the body. Cocaine is absorbed slowly on account of the vasoconstriction which it produces; in spite of this, toxic symptoms readily occur, as it is eliminated relatively slowly. It is mostly detoxicated in the liver, but a small quantity is excreted unchanged by the kidneys.

INDICATIONS

Cocaine can be used with any degree of safety only as a surface analgesic. It is still occasionally used for this purpose in nose and throat surgery and in ophthalmology.

DOSAGE AND ADMINISTRATION

Owing to its vasoconstrictor action, the use of adrenaline with it is not only unnecessary but increases the likelihood of cardiac dysrhythmias and ventricular fibrillation.

For surface analgesia, a 4 per cent solution is used for operations on the eye; 10 and 20 per cent solutions are employed for procedures on the nose and throat. It is stated that the 20 per cent solution is only slightly more toxic than the 10 per cent as absorption is slower. A dose of 100 mg (1.5 mg/kg) of the 10 per cent solution should not be exceeded in fit adults.

PRECAUTIONS

Cocaine is rapidly absorbed from the nose and it is very easy to exceed the recommended dose when administered on gauze or wool plugs. It is advisable to administer a barbiturate before using cocaine, as it not only protects against the toxic effects of the drug but also acts as a sedative.

Cocaine is a drug of addiction; it differs from morphine and similar drugs in that it is taken for the euphoria and pleasing sensations it produces, rather than from the necessity to be free from withdrawal symptoms or pain. Present-day therapeutic uses of cocaine are unlikely to cause addiction.

An overdose of cocaine gives rise to excitement, restlessness, and confusion. Headache, nausea and vomiting, and abdominal pain are common. The pulse rate is increased and respiration is rapid and shallow. The temperature may rise and convulsions, coma, and death may follow. Most, but not all, of these effects can be attributable to sympathetic over-activity, and the logical treatment is to diminish this both by central sedation and by competitive antagonism with adrenergic blocking agents. Both α- and β-receptor blocking agents may be needed. Propranolol 2–5 mg diminishes the tachycardia and protects against the onset of ventricular fibrillation, but has little effect on the hypertension. Phentolamine 5 mg should be given intravenously, and may need to be repeated every 15–20 minutes. Convulsions should be controlled with a small dose of thiopentone; if this is ineffective, muscle relaxants and artificial ventilation will be required. Ventricular fibrillation, probably the most usual cause of sudden death in such cases, should be treated by cardiac massage and electrical defibrillation.

Lignocaine hydrochloride

Lignocaine hydrochloride (*BP*) and Lidocaine hydrochloride (*USP*)
Chemical name: 2-diethylaminoaceto-2′,6′-xylidide hydrochloride

CH_3
—NH—C(=O)—CH_2—N(C_2H_5)(C_2H_5) ·HCl
CH_3

PHARMACOLOGY

Lignocaine is an aminoacyl amide and a derivative of acetanilide. It is an effective local analgesic of slightly greater toxicity in 0.5 per cent solution than procaine, less toxic in weaker solutions, but about one and a half times as toxic in a 2 per cent solution. Its action is more rapid, more intense, and lasts longer.

Its systemic effects are similar to those of procaine; when administered locally it has a tendency to cause vasodilatation and this is normally counteracted by the addition of a vasoconstrictor. Unlike procaine it has a potent analgesic action on mucous surfaces when applied topically. It produces general analgesia when given intravenously, which lasts longer than that of procaine. Less than 10 per cent is excreted in the urine and less than 7 per cent is excreted into the bile. The majority is broken down in the liver to monoethylglycine xylidide, and thence hydrolysed by liver amidases to 2,6-xylidine and 4-hydroxy-2,6-xylidine. Glycine xylidide is also formed. The rate of metabolism is doubled by pretreatment with phenobarbitone.

PHARMACOKINETICS

Following a single rapid intravenous injection, the plasma level declines in two distinct phases. The first phase lasts approximately 30 minutes and exhibits a half-life of approximately 10 minutes. This decline primarily reflects a redistribution of the drug into various body tissues, including the heart. The rapid uptake into the heart is responsible for the immediate onset of antiarrhythmic effect, and the rapid fall in blood levels is probably responsible for the short duration of action following a single intravenous bolus injection. The second phase manifests a half-life of approximately 90–120 minutes and is more representative of the clearance of the drug from the body.

INDICATIONS

Lignocaine is used for the production of local analgesia by infiltration, nerve, epidural, and caudal block and topical application. It has been employed for spinal analgesia, but is not used extensively for this purpose in Great Britain, possibly because this technique is not widely employed. Lignocaine has also been given intravenously to produce general analgesia but this technique is seldom employed at the present time. It is employed for the control of myocardial irritability and ventricular dysrhythmias, particularly in the acute treatment following myocardial infarction. The antiarrhythmic properties of this drug differ distinctly from those of other drugs in that the depressant action on ectopic foci is not accompanied by a significant slowing of the conduction of normal impulses. Furthermore, in normal therapeutic dosage there is no change in myocardial contractility, systemic arterial blood pressure, or peripheral vascular tone.

DOSAGE AND ADMINISTRATION

Adrenaline, unless otherwise contraindicated, is normally used with lignocaine to delay absorption and prolong action.

Infiltration analgesia. A 0.5 per cent solution is commonly employed. The maximum dose is 100 ml (500 mg) with adrenaline and 40 ml (200 mg) without. If the operative field is such that larger amounts are necessary, a 0.25 per cent solution with adrenaline should be used, when 300 ml (750 mg) may safely be given.

Nerve block. A 1 per cent solution is used with adrenaline, up to 10 ml for single nerves and 15–30 ml for brachial plexus block.

Epidural and caudal block. From 15 to 50 ml of a 1.5 per cent solution with adrenaline is used.

Surface analgesia. For the cornea, a 2 per cent solution is used. For the pharynx, larynx, and trachea, a 2 per cent solution, maximum 8 ml, or a 4 per cent solution, maximum 4 ml, may be used. Analgesia of the mouth and pharynx may also be effected by the sucking of a lozenge (250 mg). A 2 per cent jelly is used for the urethra.

A 5 per cent preparation containing hyaluronidase, a 5 per cent ointment, and a 2 per cent jelly are also available for surface application and are useful for the lubrication of endotracheal tubes and instruments used for endoscopy.

Intraveous local analgesia. A self-retaining needle is inserted into a vein in the back of the hand, and the limb is drained of blood by raising it or by applying a rubber bandage. A cuff tourniquet is then applied to the upper arm and blown up to above arterial pressure. Then 25–40 ml of 0.5 per cent lignocaine is injected through the needle. The average dose required is 30 ml. After analgesia has developed a second tourniquet can be applied over analgesic skin if the procedure is likely to be prolonged, and the first cuff deflated. After surgery, all tourniquets are released. The technique can also be used in the lower limb.

Toxic symptoms involving the CNS are not uncommon shortly after deflation of the tourniquet, particularly if the interval since administration is short. They are less likely in the sedated patient and are very rarely serious. In spite of this possible danger, this technique is often employed for the production of analgesia of the upper limb, especially for outpatients. Prilocaine is a preferred drug.

TREATMENT OF DYSRHYTHMIAS

Because of the pharmacokinetic characteristics referred to above, lignocaine takes 6–8 hours to reach a steady plasma level when given by continuous infusion. To obtain and maintain adequate blood levels it is necessary, therefore, to precede the infusion with a loading dose of 50–100 mg given by slow bolus injection. A further two such doses may be given at intervals of 15–20 minutes. The continuous infusion should run at a rate of 2.4 mg/min. A 0.2 per cent solution in 5 per cent dextrose is commonly employed.

SYSTEMIC ANALGESIA

A continuous intravenous infusion of 0.5 per cent lignocaine has been used to provide analgesia for the relief of pain, and to supplement nitrous oxide anaesthesia, the rate of the infusion being adjusted to obtain the desired effect. The management of these techniques is difficult and not without risk as, to be effective, near-toxic doses of lignocaine have to be employed.

PRECAUTIONS

Precautions are as for other local analgesics. Special care is necessary when lignocaine is given by intravenous infusion as near-maximum doses are used in these techniques. The patient must be carefully watched for signs of overdose, treatment for which is the same as for other local analgesics. Preparations should be protected from light. They are stable in the presence of acids and alkalis and can be autoclaved repeatedly. They should not be left in syringes or galley pots containing copper or nickel, as they liberate these ions and the combination is irritating to tissues.

Etidocaine is a long-acting agent with a chemical structure similar to that of lignocaine and bupivacaine. It has been reported on quite widely but not introduced to the UK market. It has four times the potency of lignocaine but only twice the toxicity, thus giving it a better therapeutic ratio. It has a rapid onset of action and a prolonged action which is attributed to high plasma protein binding (94 per cent) and a high oil/water partition coefficient (141). Its most characteristic difference from other agents is its ability to produce intense motor blockade which facilitates surgery. The smallness of the unbound fraction may limit the amount that will cross the placenta. These two factors suggest a possible use in caesarean section. It is used as a 1 or 1.5 per cent solution.

Mepivacaine has properties which place it somewhere between bupivacaine and lignocaine. It is a local analgesic of the amide type, with a rather more rapid onset and longer duration than lignocaine. Its chief advantage is an absence of any vasodilator effect on injection, so that the addition of a vasoconstrictor is unnecessary. Two or 3 per cent solutions are usually employed for nerve blocks; more dilute solutions are used for surface and infiltration analgesia. Solutions may be sterilized by autoclaving. It is available in the UK only in dental cartridges (3 per cent) or in a hyperbaric solution (4 per cent) for spinal anaesthesia.

Prilocaine hydrochloride

Prilocaine hydrochloride (*BP* and *USP*)
Chemical name: 2-propylaminopropiono-2-toluidide hydrochloride

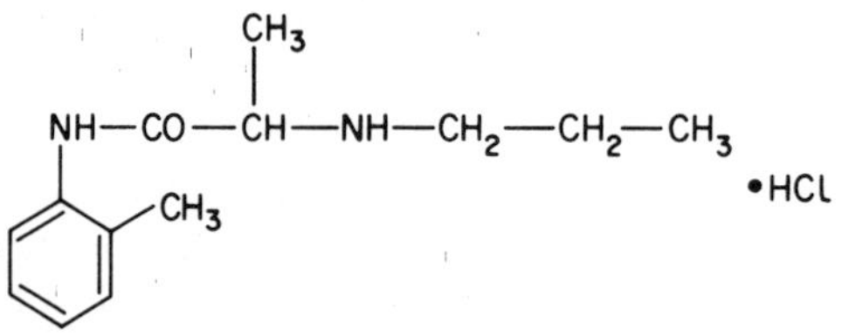

CH_3
NH—CO—CH—NH—CH_2—CH_2—CH_3
CH_3
•HCl

Prilocaine is a local analgesic closely related chemically to lignocaine. It is equally effective as an analgesic, its duration of action is longer, and it is less toxic. It is equally active on mucous surfaces by topical application, and systemic effects also are similar. It is broken down by amidases in the liver.

Prilocaine is an effective local analgesic but is less potent dose for dose than lignocaine. It is less toxic but in large doses cyanosis due to the formation of methaemoglobin may occur. This complication occurs only when doses of the order of 0.9 g are employed. Cyanosis usually disappears within 24 hours. If treatment is urgent, methylene blue 1 mg/kg may be given intravenously.

INDICATIONS
Prilocaine is used for the production of analgesia by infiltration, nerve, epidural, and spinal block, by topical application, and intravenously for limb analgesia, for which purpose it has advantages over lignocaine as it is less toxic.

DOSAGE AND ADMINISTRATION
Prilocaine is available in 0.5–2 per cent solutions, with and without adrenaline, and also with felypressin, an analogue of vasopressin. This powerful vasoconstrictor is without effect on the myocardium and is much to be preferred as a local vasoconstrictor. Doses and volumes employed are similar to those of lignocaine; slightly larger maximum doses may be given – 400 mg in the 0.5 and 1 per cent solutions without adrenaline, 600 mg with adrenaline.

For intravenous analgesia a similar technique may be employed to that described for lignocaine. A 0.5 per cent solution is used.

For spinal use a 5 per cent solution in 6 per cent dextrose is used in a dose of 0.6–2 ml.

Procaine hydrochloride

Procaine hydrochloride (*BP* and *USP*)
Chemical name: 2-diethylaminoethyl-4-aminobenzoate hydrochloride

$$H_2N-C_6H_4-CO-O-CH_2-CH_2-N(C_2H_5)_2 \cdot HCl$$

PHARMACOLOGY

Procaine was first synthesized by Einhorn in 1905. It is a safe and effective local analgesic. It is about one quarter as toxic as cocaine when administered by either the intravenous or subcutaneous routes. The fact that it is not less toxic than cocaine when employed subcutaneously is due to its vasolidator action which allows rapid absorption, cocaine being a vasoconstrictor. Its onset of action is rapid – 2–3 minutes – and its duration is 0.5–1 hour according to the concentration employed.

Procaine has similar systemic actions to other synthetic local analgesics.

Nervous system. Central stimulation occurs at first and is followed later by depression. In contrast to cocaine, there is no euphoria or effect on mental powers. Adequate intravenous infusion will produce a mild degree of general analgesia.

Depression of acetylcholine release causes mild ganglionic blockade.

Cardiovascular system. There is a quinidine-like action on the heart, conduction time being prolonged and irritability decreased. This action requires comparatively large doses and may be accompanied by central stimulation. With increasing dosage the blood pressure falls, an effect due to cardiac depression, peripheral vasodilatation, and mild ganglionic block. The heart rate is increased. When it is desirable to reduce cardiac excitability, procainamide is better because of its longer action.

Respiratory system. The respiratory rate is slightly increased, but as central stimulation gives place to depression, respiration becomes rapid and shallow.

Musculature. Acetylcholine depression results in a mild neuromuscular block and the action of non-depolarizing muscle relaxants is accentuated. Smooth muscle is depressed by direct action and spasm is antagonized because of its atropine-like effect.

Mucous surfaces. Unless employed in concentrations in the region of 20 per cent, procaine has little analgesic action when applied topically.

Fate in the body. On entering the circulation, procaine is hydrolysed by plasma pseudocholinesterase to *p*-aminobenzoic acid and diethylaminoethanol. Of these products of hydrolysis, 80 per cent of the *p*-aminobenzoic acid is excreted in the urine unchanged or in conjugated form, but only 30 per cent of the diethylaminoethanol is excreted by the kidneys, the remainder being metabolized by the liver. The hydrolysis of procaine is very rapid and it is thought that some of its systemic effects, including that of general analgesia, are due to one of its products, probably diethylaminoethanol. Both *p*-aminobenzoic acid and diethylaminoethanol are non-toxic even when given in comparatively large doses, but *p*-aminobenzoic acid antagonizes the sulphonamides and inhibits their action.

As procaine is hydrolysed by plasma pseudocholinesterase, patients with genetic abnormalities of this enzyme may exhibit toxic symptoms following normally safe doses.

INDICATIONS

Procaine is used as a local analgesic for infiltration analgesia and all forms of regional, spinal, and extradural block. Since the introduction of lignocaine it has been employed much less frequently.

DOSAGE AND ADMINISTRATION

Unless specifically contraindicated, procaine should normally be used with adrenaline to delay absorption and prolong its duration of action when used for infiltration analgesia, regional, or extradural block.

Infiltration analgesia. Strengths of solutions commonly used are 0.25–1 per cent. A 0.5 per cent solution is normally adequate for most purposes, but the dose should not exceed 200 ml (1 g); 400 ml or more of the 0.25 per cent solution may be used if larger areas are to be infiltrated.

Single nerve, regional, and extradural block. The 1 per cent solution is usually employed: up to 10 ml for a single nerve block, 30 ml for brachial plexus block, and 15–50 ml for epidural or caudal block.

Spinal analgesia. A 5 per cent solution may be used, 0.5–2 ml according to the height of analgesia required. Alternatively, 50–300 mg of procaine crystals may be dissolved in CSF and injected.

Up to 10 ml of a 1 per cent solution may be given slowly into an artery or vein to relieve spasm.

The long-acting preparation Proctocaine contained benzyl alcohol. This had a destructive action on nerve fibres and it is no longer used.

PRECAUTIONS

Apart from general precautions discussed on page 213, procaine should not be used with sulphonamides as their actions are antagonistic, or with anticholinesterases such as neostigmine which will inhibit its hydrolysis and therefore its excretion.

Symptoms and treatment of overdose are the same as for other local analgesics.

Chloroprocaine hydrochloride was introduced into USA practice in 1952, but has not yet been marketed in the UK. It has become increasingly popular in America for obstetric analgesia because of a very rapid rate of onset. However, it also has a similarly rapid rate of offset and is of relatively short duration. It is metabolized by plasma cholinesterase and claimed therefore to have minimal effects on the fetus.

The chief area of anxiety about the drug is related to reports of persistent or prolonged neurological deficit following its use and some evidence of neurotoxicity.

Local analgesics used in the eye

Oxybuprocaine is probably the most widely used topical agent in the eye. It is twice as potent as amethocaine and has twice the therapeutic ratio. It is less irritant to the conjunctiva in similar concentrations. One drop of 0.4 per cent is sufficient to render the conjunctiva analgesic.

Proxymetacaine causes less initial stinging and may therefore be particularly useful in children. It is used in a concentration of 0.5 per cent. **Lignocaine** (4 per cent) is also effective in this location as is **amethocaine** (0.5 per cent). **Cocaine** (4 per cent) is very effective but is no longer to be recommended for repeated use as it causes clouding and pitting of the cornea, as well as being a powerful mydriatic.

7

Central nervous system stimulants

Drugs with a stimulant action on the CNS can be classified into five groups:

1. *Mood stimulants:* drugs such as caffeine, pemoline, and the amphetamines. The prescribing of some of the drugs of the last group is now restricted by legislation.
2. *Psychotomimetics:* drugs that cause hallucinations such as mescaline and lysergic acid diethylamide (LSD).
3. *Antidepressants:* the principal groups are the monoamine oxidase inhibitors (MAOIs) and the bi-, tri-, and tetracyclic antidepressants.
4. *Analeptics:* a group of drugs ranging from strychnine to nikethamide which have largely fallen into disuse, and one or two such as doxapram which have a limited place.
5. *Specific pathway stimulants:* the most important are drugs used in the treatment of parkinsonism.

Mood stimulants

Several different groups of compounds stimulate mood. They affect all normal people and counteract fatigue, both mental and physical, and suppress appetite. Because of their actions they are potential drugs of abuse, if not of addiction. Amphetamines, dexamphetamine, and methylphenidate are Controlled Drugs (*see* page 46); amphetamine still finds a place in the treatment of narcolepsy.

Pemoline, a milder stimulant, has been recommended as a useful adjunct to antihistamine therapy to counteract the drowsiness caused by these drugs. It is most effective in fatigued individuals and its effects in improving perception and concentration are not accompanied by euphoria. Pemoline 10 mg is equivalent in effect to about 200 mg of caffeine.

Caffeine is a xanthine derivative and shares several properties with other members of this chemical group, such as theophylline. It is a mild stimulant which is used in social beverages world-wide, but is little used in therapeutics. There is a tendency for stimulant effects on the heart to appear at dosage levels that produce a detectable amount of CNS stimulation. Its mode of action may be due to its ability to inhibit the enzyme phosphodiesterase, but it may also affect calcium transport into the cell.

Psychotomimetics

Several classes of drugs with CNS effects can induce illusions, hallucinations, or other alterations in thinking, particularly if given in toxic doses. The terms psychotomimetic, hallucinogenic, or psychedelic are reserved, however, for a group of drugs that regularly induce states of altered perception and thinking which cannot be experienced in any other way except in dreaming.

The term 'mind expanding' has also been used to describe the state produced by these drugs in which there is heightened awareness, unusually vivid sensory experiences, and an inner appreciation of the clarity and portentiousness of the quality of one's thinking. Indeed, there is often more importance attached to the 'meaningfulness' of the thoughts than to their actual meaning.

Drugs producing this state are indolealkylamines such as LSD or phenylethylamines such as mescaline. They produce their mental effects in very low dosage – as little as 20–40 μg. Larger doses produce sympathomimetic effects such as tachycardia, hypertension, tremor, hyperpyrexia, and pupillary dilatation. The duration of action is several hours. These drugs rapidly induce tolerance and psychological dependence but withdrawal phenomena are not seen after abrupt discontinuation. They have no place at present in orthodox therapeutics.

Antidepressants

Depression is a syndrome which is variously classified, but a simple classification is into reactive and endogenous types. Depression may also be a feature of other mental illnesses. Two classes of drugs are predominantly employed in treatment: the MAOIs and the tricyclic group and its close congeners. Apart from potential therapeutic interactions with drugs used by anaesthetists they are of importance because the nature of the illness for which they are prescribed makes them liable to be a frequent cause of self-poisoning. Those using these drugs are also liable to be unconcerned for their proper custody and accidental poisoning of children is therefore not uncommon.

There are two important theories of the mode of action of antidepressant drugs. The catecholamine hypothesis states that depression is associated with a relative or absolute deficiency of catecholamines, especially noradrenaline, at functionally important sites. The indoleamine hypothesis is that depression is due to a functional deficiency in brain indoleamines such as 5-hydroxytryptamine (5-HT). The two theories are not incompatible.

Monoamine oxidase inhibitors

This group of drugs has enjoyed a considerable vogue in the treatment of depression, but their potential toxic effects are such that there is now a tendency to employ them rarely. Tranylcypromine, which has a relatively rapid onset of action, is sometimes prescribed for patients who are severely depressed and a suicide risk, the alternative being in this case electroconvulsive therapy.

An important group of MAOIs are derivatives of hydrazine and include phenelzine, iproniazid, and pargyline. They have little immediate effect on mood, and produce their effect only after a delay of several days' continuous therapy. Tranylcypromine is not related to this group, and produces a much more rapid stimulation which is well maintained.

All these drugs act by forming a stable complex with monoamine oxidase, and this results in an intracellular increase in the biogenic amines – noradrenaline, 5-HT, and dopamine. There is a consequent decrease in the urine of the normal metabolites 3-methoxy-4-hydroxymandelic acid and 5-hydroxyindoleacetic acid, and an increase of metanephrine, normetanephrine, tryptamine, and 5-HT glucuronide, via alternative metabolic pathways. It is not certain how far the intracellular changes in amine concentration are responsible for the antidepressant action.

Apart from the interaction with other drugs, such as the sympathomimetic amines and pethidine, there is always a danger that the patient may eat some food with a high concentration of the amine tyramine. This may lead to a paroxysmal hypertension, severe headache, and even subarachnoid haemorrhage. These drugs have also been the alleged cause of severe liver damage histologically resembling viral hepatitis. Combinations with other antidepressants of the tricyclic type have been condemned, following early reports of serious potentiation of toxic side effects, but other workers continue to use such a combination without ill effect. Careful control of dose is probably important.

Because of the unpredictable toxic effects which can occur, surgical operations should, whenever possible, be postponed until the effects of these drugs have been eliminated. This depends on the generation of fresh enzyme and takes at least 10–14 days. During this time, if necessary, the patient may be transferred to another type of antidepressant. If, however, the operation cannot be postponed, the drugs that must be avoided are pethidine and the sympathomimetic amines, particularly those which release transmitter or which are normally metabolized by monoamine oxidase. Hypotension has been reported following droperidol in a patient receiving an MAOI and this may indicate that any drug with α-adrenergic blocking properties will also exhibit synergism with MAOIs.

Apart from pethidine, other narcotic analgesics may produce undue depression, but morphine and methadone appear to be less likely to cause untoward effects.

Pethidine may cause hypotension, respiratory depression and coma, signs of overdose probably due to interference with its metabolism, or a severe hypertensive crisis with hyperpyrexia, convulsions, sweating, and coma. The mechanism of this reaction has not been elucidated. In this connexion, however, it is of interest that in normal individuals, in the absence of circulatory depressant drugs, intravenous pethidine usually produces an initial rise in blood pressure before a comparable fall, and this toxic response may be, therefore, an idiosyncratic exaggeration of a normal response.

It has been suggested that pethidine 10 mg may be given in cases of doubt to test the patient's response. If no untoward reactions occur this dose may be repeated at 15-minute intervals; a total of 50 mg may be given.

Acute toxic symptoms may be due to overdosage as such, but could also be caused by unsuspected interaction with other drugs. In outpatients this is most likely to be due to tyramine or other active amines in food, or to self-medication with a sympathomimetic amine which may have been taken as a cold cure or a nasal decongestant.

Symptoms of simple overdose or interaction with sympathomimetic amines are referable to the CNS and cardiovascular system. These include restlessness, agitation, hallucinations, severe headaches, convulsions, coma, and hyperpyrexia. Both hypotension and hypertension have been reported. Conservative management, with attention to fluid and electrolyte balance, respiration, and blood pressure usually prove successful. Small doses of thiopentone may be given to control excitement. Hypotension, if severe, may be treated cautiously with minimal doses of noradrenaline.

In hypertensive crises the initial need is for α-adrenergic blockade, and phentolamine is probably the best immediate choice.

Bi-, tri-, and tetracyclic antidepressants

The structural resemblance between these drugs and phenothiazines, when drawn on paper, is somewhat misleading. The replacement of the —S— bridge in promazine by $—CH_2—CH_2—$ in imipramine converts a planar molecule into one that can only be represented in three dimensions.

These drugs are effective in the treatment of endogenous depression. They are generally the first choice, because of the lesser toxic potential. Many of their actions can be explained by their ability to inhibit the uptake of monoamines into the presynaptic terminal. This uptake is an active process by a membrane pump. Pump inhibition varies from one antidepressant to another. For instance, desipramine is a potent inhibitor of noradrenaline uptake, nomifensine of dopamine uptake, and clomipramine of 5-HT uptake.

It has been suggested that inhibition of noradrenaline uptake correlates with psychomotor activation, increase in 5-HT activation with an elevation of mood, and inhibition of dopamine uptake with increased drive. This is too simplistic a view. Uptake of monoamines may not be the only mechanism by which depression is alleviated. They may interfere with the local negative feedback mechanism; for example, amitriptyline and mianserin block presynaptic α-receptors. There is also evidence that chronic therapy with antidepressants alters postsynaptic receptors centrally. In view of the fact that most antidepressants take several weeks to produce their therapeutic effect, this is interesting. They have also been used in the treatment of enuresis in children.

These drugs also have an anticholinergic and and antihistaminc action. These are both central and peripheral, the predominant effect ultimately being one of combined central and peripheral sympathomimetic and anticholinergic actions. However, there may initially be drowsiness. The peripheral anticholinergic actions lead to side effects such as dryness of the mouth, blurring of vision, constipation, and urinary retention. The tricyclics should therefore be avoided in the presence of prostatic hypertrophy and glaucoma. They are also liable to cause hypotension which is probably of central origin. The pharmacological profile differs from drug to drug, for instance amitriptyline initially may cause sedation and has marked anticholinergic activity, while the tetracyclic mianserin has little anticholinergic activity and is less likely to cause cardiac dysrhythmias than drugs like imipramine, since it has little effect on noradrenaline uptake.

The pharmacokinetics of these drugs are of considerable interest and relevance to the management of poisoning. They are unique in having an enormous volume of distribution, something less than 1 per cent of the drug remaining in the circulation, the remainder being bound in the tissues. This makes both dialysis and forced diuresis useless in the treatment of overdose because virtually no drug appears in the dialysate or the urine. The half-life of these drugs is of the order of 2–3 days. Overdose with these drugs produces a very similar CNS picture to that seen with MAOIs, chiefly restlessness, fits, and coma. However, cardiac dysrhythmias and conduction defects are also often seen because of the combination of anticholinergic action with sympathetic stimulation. Severe hypotension is usually a feature and sudden death can occur readily. Conservative and symptomatic management is advocated. Not only is forced diuresis ineffective, but these cardiovascular effects make its employment highly dangerous. Sympathetic stimulating agents are also specifically contraindicated.

Analeptics

Analeptics mainly exert their effects on the brain stem, principally the respiratory and vasomotor centres, but in overdose they will produce cortical convulsions. Although they initially lighten narcosis, this tends to be followed by a central depression which does not yield to further stimulation. Respiratory depression then has to be countered by mechanical means and the blood pressure maintained by agents acting peripherally.

There are two types of analeptics: those which act reflexly through the chemoreceptors in the carotid body, such as doxapram and nikethamide, and those which act directly on the medullary centres, such as picrotoxin and ethamivan. Strychnine is of interest in that it has a marked action on the spinal cord as well as on the higher centres. The mechanism of actions these drugs is believed to be an antagonism to central inhibitory transmitters such as γ-aminobutyric acid (GABA) and glycine. Their actions are thus unlike those of the other types of drugs with central stimulatory actions discussed above.

Analeptics were used routinely in cases of poisoning by depressant drugs, such as the barbiturates, but their effects were uncertain and in severe cases often dangerous as large doses were liable to cause convulsions and, later, increased depression. Amiphenazole was at one time advocated as a compound that would specifically counteract some of the depressant actions of morphine without counteracting the analgesia. Of the analeptics, only doxapram can now be regarded as sufficiently short acting and non-toxic to justify a place in modern therapeutics. It has a place in the management of a few patients in incipient respiratory failure when an intravenous infusion will increase minute volume, reduce arterial carbon dioxide tension, and raise arterial oxygen tension by small but significant increments in doses that do not produce too much in the way of cerebral toxicity. It has also been claimed to reduce markedly the incidence of postoperative pulmonary complications in patients receiving morphine analgesia.

Analeptics should be used with considerable caution. Their action is much shorter than that of the depressant drugs for which they are given and some, like picrotoxin, often have a latent period of action, so that a second dose may be given before the first has had time to act; central depression may return when their effects have worn off. Overdose will cause convulsions and further depression. They increase metabolic rate, which may be dangerous if the patient is already hypoxic following respiratory depression. Other side effects include cardiac dysrhythmias and vomiting.

Analeptics are usually ineffective if the patient is in deep coma. If there is no response to an initial dose, further doses should be withheld.

In the treatment of overdose of analeptics in which convulsions are a feature, thiopentone should be given intravenously in small repeated doses. If serious respiratory embarrassment accompanies convulsions a muscle relaxant may be given and respiration controlled.

Because of their extremely limited place in therapeutics, only two monographs on analeptics are included in this edition, doxapram and one of the traditional analeptics, nikethamide. For their historical interest, short notes are included on others which have little or no place in current therapeutics.

Specific pathway stimulants

Several discrete areas of the brain as well as certain tracts of fibres possess synapses at which a variety of chemicals have been identified as neurotransmitters, including GABA, acetylcholine, noradrenaline, dopamine, and 5-HT. As discussed above it seems likely that the effective treatment of depression is related to stimulation of one or more of at least three of these transmitters. Cyproheptadine, a potent antagonist of both histamine and 5-HT, will stimulate weight gain, either by stimulating appetite or by stimulating the secretion of growth hormone and insulin.

It is difficult to produce adequate CNS effects with such drugs without systemic side effects which may be extremely unpleasant. Furthermore there are few discrete pathological syndromes that can be linked to transmitter defects in the CNS. However, Parkinson's disease and possibly Huntingdon's chorea and schizophrenia are associated with alterations in dopaminergic function.

Dopamine and dopamine receptors

Dopamine is a neurotransmitter, both centrally and peripherally. *Table 7.1* lists some dopaminergic systems found in the mammalian brain. Just as different types of acetylcholine receptors and adrenoceptors have been defined, so there now appear to be different classes of dopamine receptors: D_1 receptors are linked to intracellular adenyl cyclase; D_2 receptors are not. Dopamine receptors are found both presynaptically and postsynaptically.

Table 7.1 Dopaminergic systems found in mammalian brain

System	*Nucleus of origin*	*Sites of termination*
Nigrostriatal	Substantia nigra	Neostriatum
Mesocortical	Ventral tegmental area and substantia nigra	Amygdaloid complex, nucleus accumbens, frontal cortex
Tuberohypophyseal	Periventricular and arcuate hypothalamic nuclei	Pituitary median eminence

Dopamine is metabolized by monoamine oxidase. There are two types of monoamine oxidase: type A which can metabolize adrenaline, noradrenaline, dopamine, and 5-HT, and type B which can only metabolize tyramine and dopamine. The distinction may be of importance since selective inhibition of type B monoamine oxidase would raise brain dopamine levels in preference to other amines.

Of the three dopaminergic systems listed in *Table 7.1*, loss of functional integrity of the nigrostriatal tract leads to parkinsonism; the mesocortical system may be of importance to motivational drive whose loss may be related to schizophrenia and Huntingdon's chorea; the tuberohypophyseal system is of importance in relation to prolactin, the release of which is inhibited by dopamine. The area postrema of the medulla also probably has a dopaminergic innervation: dopamine agonists such as apomorphine cause emesis whereas dopamine antagonists such as the phenothiazones and butyrophenones have antiemetic properties, as well as inhibiting prolactin secretion.

In the periphery, activation of dopamine receptors in blood vessels (for example in the kidney) can cause vasodilatation. Dopamine receptors may be present in the alimentary tract and dopamine antagonists such as metoclopramide can hasten gastric emptying. Dopamine can also increase cardiac contractility although this effect may be mainly mediated through β-adrenoceptors.

Drug treatment of parkinsonism

Parkinsonism is a syndrome characterized by chronic progressive tremor, rigidity, and akinesia which is due to chronic degeneration of dopaminergic pathways between the substantia nigra and the corpus striatum (*Figure 7.1*). Levodopa acts

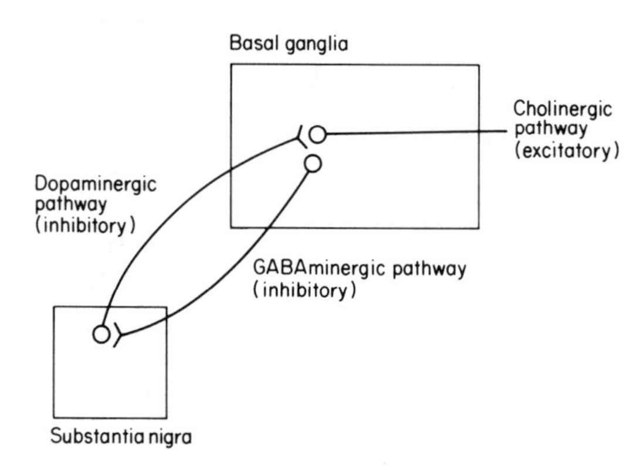

Figure 7.1 Dopaminergic pathways from the substantia nigra have an inhibitory influence on cholinergic cells. Note there is also an inhibitory pathway from the basal ganglia to the substantia nigra

by being converted enzymatically in the CNS into dopamine, thus restoring the integrity of the inhibitory pathway. It also relieves the apathy and depression, giving a feeling of well-being and greater vigour. The action can be complemented by anticholinergic drugs which inhibit the excitatory pathways. Indeed, prior to the use of levodopa, centrally acting antimuscarinic agents were the mainstay of therapy; benzhexol, benztropine, and orphenadrine are three that were commonly used. Such drugs still have a place in the treatment of parkinsonism. They are more effective in the relief of rigidity than tremor. However, they have the disadvantage of producing peripheral toxicity such as blurred vision, a rise in intraocular tension which may precipitate glaucoma, dry mouth, and urinary retention.

Although levodopa is the mainstay of treatment, other drugs with dopamine agonist effects are now available and some are mentioned on page 238, following the monograph on levodopa.

Dothiepin

Dothiepin hydrochloride (*BP*)
Chemical name: 3-(dibenzo[*b,e*]thiepin-11(6*H*)-ylidene)-*NN*-dimethylpropylamine hydrochloride

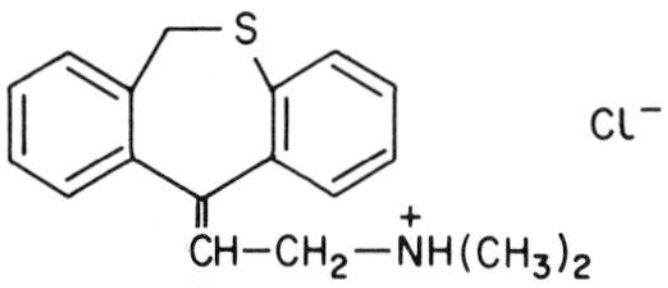

S

Cl^-

$CH{-}CH_2{-}\overset{+}{N}H(CH_3)_2$

PHARMACOLOGY
This tricyclic compound, which is a thio-analogue of amitriptyline, inhibits the re-uptake of noradrenaline, 5-HT, and dopamine. The drug is more potent in inhibiting noradrenaline uptake than 5-HT uptake. *In vitro* studies on rat brain synaptosomes show that it has a potency between imipramine and chlorimipramine in inhibiting dopamine re-uptake. The drug is more potent than imipramine as an anticholinergic agent. It has been shown in animals that the drug can increase the duration of action of thiopentone. It has anxiolytic properties.

Fate in the body. A metabolite of dothiepin, northiaden (the desmethyl derivative), has been studied but appears to be less potent than the parent compound in a number of tests. In man, following a 50-mg dose of the drug, about 50 per cent of the dose is excreted in the urine in 96 hours.

DOSAGE AND ADMINISTRATION
The drug is used in the treatment of depressive illness; 25 mg three times a day is commonly prescribed.

PRECAUTIONS
These are as for imipramine and related drugs; overdosage can produce cardiac dysrhythmias.

Doxapram

Doxapram hydrochloride (*BAN* and *USP*)
Chemical name: 1-ethyl-4-(2-morpholinoethyl)-3,3-diphenylpyrrolidin-2-one hydrochloride

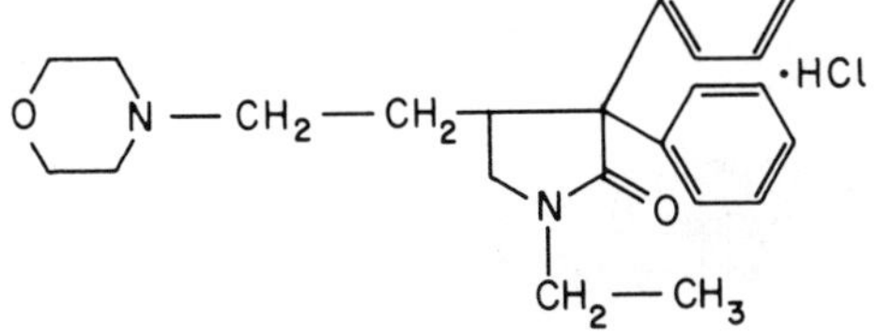

$\cdot HCl$

$O \quad N{-}CH_2{-}CH_2$

$N \quad O$

$CH_2{-}CH_3$

PHARMACOLOGY

Doxapram is a central stimulant which stimulates respiration principally by an action on peripheral chemoreceptors. With low doses there is an increase in tidal volume, but with bigger doses there is also an increase in rate. With larger doses there is a non-specific central stimulation.

These respiratory effects are usually accompanied by a small elevation of the systemic arterial blood pressure and an increase in heart rate. These effects are mediated by the vasomotor centre, resulting in increased sympathetic nervous activity, and can be attenuated by α-adrenoceptor blockade.

The respiratory stimulating effects can be achieved with doses 40–60 times less than those needed to cause convulsions, a therapeutic ratio which is significantly better than that of any other analeptic. With intermediate doses, side effects such as a crawling sensation on the skin, restlessness, warmth, nervousness and nausea may occur. Another centrally mediated effect is a rise in 11-hydroxycorticosteroids which can be prevented (in animals) by hypophysectomy.

In patients with chronic airways disease in respiratory failure there is a significant increase in minute volume and arterial oxygen tension, and a decrease in arterial carbon dioxide tension. The slope of the ventilatory response to carbon dioxide is steeper and displaced to the left.

Rapid administration can cause an increase in cardiac output and a rise in systemic blood pressure, but this is less marked following slow infusion. Side effects such as vomiting, coughing, and apprehension are rare and the liability to convulsions is low.

Doxapram is rapidly inactivated in the body and various metabolites have been identified. Because of rapid inactivation the drug may be safely given by continuous infusion over long periods.

INDICATIONS

Doxapram can be used as a respiratory stimulant in respiratory failure secondary to chronic airways disease; as an analeptic to hasten recovery from anaesthesia; as an antagonist to the depressant effects of analgesics, particularly those with mixed agonist/antagonist properties such as buprenorphine; as an aid to differential diagnosis of postoperative apnoea; and, more controversially, to reduce the incidence of postoperative pulmonary complications.

DOSAGE AND ADMINISTRATION

For the treatment of early respiratory failure, doxapram may be given as a 0.2 per cent solution in 5 per cent dextrose at a rate of 1.5–3 mg/min. It has been given continuously for several days. Postoperatively a dose of 2 mg/kg can be given intravenously to differentiate central depression from other causes of apnoea at the end of anaesthesia. Doses of 0.5–1.0 mg/kg have been recommended to accelerate recovery from anaesthesia. Single doses up to 1.5 mg/kg and infusions of 2 mg/min for 2 hours have been claimed to reduce the incidence of purulent sputum and cough postoperatively after upper abdominal surgery. Less clear-cut results have been achieved after thoracotomy.

PRECAUTIONS

Doxapram is contraindicated in severe hypertension, thyrotoxicosis, status asthmaticus, and significant coronary artery disease. It should be used with caution in patients with epilepsy. Its action is potentiated by MAOIs.

Imipramine

Imipramine hydrochloride (*BP* and *USP*)
Chemical name: 3-(10,11-dihydro-5*H*-dibenz[*b,f*]azepine-5-yl)-*NN*-dimethylpropylamine

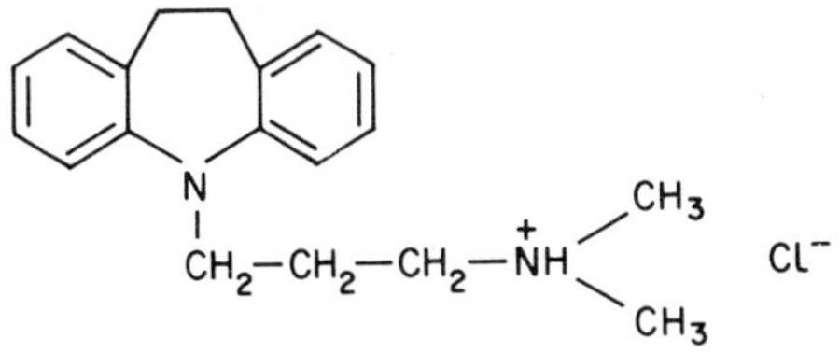

N
$CH_2-CH_2-CH_2-\overset{+}{N}H$ CH_3 CH_3 Cl^-

PHARMACOLOGY

This compound was originally tested as an antipsychotic agent but was found on clinical work to have antidepressant activities. It is a potent inhibitor of both noradrenaline and 5-HT uptake and is an antimuscarinic agent.

Fate in the body. It is readily absorbed from the gastrointestinal tract but it is subject to considerable first-pass hepatic metabolism (approximately 50 per cent). In the plasma it is protein bound (approximately 85 per cent). Demethylation of the side chain leads to the formation of desipramine, a major metabolite which is also active pharmacologically. Ring hydroxylation also occurs leading to pharmacologically inactive compounds. Plasma steady-state levels may vary markedly between patients given the same dose. Thirty-fold differences have been reported.

DOSAGE AND ADMINISTRATION

The drug is normally given orally, dosage being slowly increased (often weekly) from 25 mg to 150–300 mg daily depending on therapeutic response. To test if a patient responds, the drug is initially given for about 6 weeks. About 70 per cent of depressed patients respond to tricyclic drugs.

PRECAUTIONS

The drug can produce a number of adverse effects. These can be grouped as follows:

1. Effects on the autonomic nervous system: dry mouth, constipation, aggravation or initiation of glaucoma, paralysis of accommodation, urinary retention, and tachycardia.
2. Central actions: ataxia, dysrhythmia, convulsions, decreased REM sleep, and fine tremor.
3. Cardiovascular effects: imipramine has an atropine-like action and inhibits noradrenaline uptake; both these effects can initiate changes in cardiac function and thus it is not surprising that in large doses cardiac dysrhythmias can occur, for example ventricular flutter and atrial fibrillation; in therapeutic doses the ECG may show prolongation of the QT interval, ST depression, and a flattened T wave.

A number of drug interactions can occur. Imipramine can be potentiated by MAOIs. Treatment with these drugs is normally stopped 14 days before initiating imipramine therapy. The effects of anticholinergic drugs are increased and antiparkinsonian drugs may interact with imipramine and related compounds to produce an agitated hyperpyrexic patient who may convulse. Imipramine antagonizes the antihypertensive action of clonidine and also that of adrenergic neurone blockers like guanethidine. It achieves the latter effect by blocking the uptake of the adrenergic neurone blocker into the presynaptic nerve ending of the sympathetic neurone.

Other tricyclic-type antidepressants

Amitriptyline and clomipramine are potent inhibitors of 5-HT uptake but less effective than imipramine in inhibiting noradrenaline uptake. Like imipramine they have atropine-like effects. Clomipramine can raise plasma prolactin levels, an effect probably mediated by inhibition of 5-HT uptake in the hypothalamus.

Iprindole, which differs chemically from the tricyclics in having an indole nucleus, inhibits noradrenaline uptake centrally. It has only a tenth of the activity of imipramine as an anticholinergic agent. Some patients have developed a cholestatic jaundice while on the drug.

Maprotiline is a tetracyclic antidepressant. It is well absorbed from the gut but undergoes hepatic first-pass metabolism; peak plasma levels are reached at about 10–15 hours after oral administration. It is a more potent inhibitor of noradrenaline uptake but a less potent inhibitor of 5-HT uptake than imipramine. Its adverse effects are similar to imipramine. It can, in overdose, induce cardiac dysrhythmias and is contraindicated in patients with ischaemic heart disease.

Mianserin is another tetracyclic antidepressant. It can antagonize the peripheral effects of 5-HT in isolated preparations, but does not inhibit noradrenaline, dopamine, or 5-HT uptake by neurones. It is not a sympathomimetic and has no appreciable antimuscarinic actions. It increases noradrenaline turnover, possibly by an action on presynaptic α-adrenoceptors. It has antihistamine H_1 activity and hence it is not surprising that it can cause sedation. It is less likely than many other antidepressants to have cardiotoxic effects in overdose because it does not interfere with catecholamine uptake; for the same reason effects of adrenergic neurone blocking drugs are not diminished.

Nomifensine is an interesting antidepressant, being a derivative of tetrahydroisoquinoline. It is a potent inhibitor of the re-uptake of both noradrenaline and dopamine. In addition, it causes dopamine release. Since it can raise, by two mechanisms, the concentrations of dopamine at the receptor site, it has been used in parkinsonian patients and shown to produce symptomatic improvement. It has a short half-life, plasma $t_{1/2}$ being approximately 1–2 hours. The drug may be useful in depressed patients where the predominant features are apathy and retardation. It has an activating effect thought to be due to its effect in increasing central dopaminergic activity; however, agitated depressives can be made worse.

Viloxazine is a bicyclic antidepressant. It is a potent inhibitor of noradrenaline uptake with little effect on 5-HT uptake. It has less anticholinergic activity than imipramine. It may produce postural hypotension after an initial increase in blood pressure. Epileptic seizures have also occurred during therapy, as has jaundice.

Levodopa

Levodopa (*BP* and *USP*)
Chemical name: (−)-3-(3,4-dihydroxyphenyl)-L-alanine

NH_2
HO— —CH_2—C— COOH
H
HO

PHARMACOLOGY

Levodopa is practically inert: its main effects are produced by the product of its decarboxylation, dopamine. About 95 per cent of an oral dose is decarboxylated in the periphery but the dopamine that is produced, although responsible for side effects, does not cross the blood-brain barrier. Consequently, large doses need to be given to ensure that sufficient levodopa penetrates the brain. Levodopa may be given in combination with carbidopa which inhibits the peripheral decarboxylation of levodopa by an action on the enzyme L-amino acid decarboxylase. Carbidopa, however, does not penetrate the brain. By limiting only the extracerebral decarboxylation, more levodopa is available to penetrate the brain and the adverse side effects caused by systemic dopamine are reduced.

Central nervous system. It is believed that levodopa produces its effects by enhancing the transmitter stores in the degenerating dopaminergic pathways between the corpus striatum and substantia nigra. This relieves the tremor, rigidity, and akinesia. Levodopa also relieves the mental apathy associated with parkinsonism and gives a sense of well-being. In a significant proportion of patients, psychiatric disturbances occur, ranging from agitation and insomnia to hypomania and frank psychosis. These symptoms tend to be dose dependent.

Cardiovascular system. The dopamine produced systemically exerts both α- and β-stimulating effects on adrenoceptors. This is largely abolished by the administration of carbidopa. Orthostatic hypotension is also a feature and is not so modified; it is believed to be a centrally mediated effect of CNS dopamine. Tolerance to these side effects tends to develop after several months.

Gastrointestinal system. Nausea, vomiting, and anorexia are common and are due to stimulation of the chemoreceptor trigger zone, another dopaminergic area of the brain.

Endocrine systems. Levodopa inhibits the secretion of prolactin, but stimulates the production of growth hormone. Some effects on insulin and glucose metabolism are probably secondary to the increased levels of growth hormone.

ABSORPTION, FATE, AND EXCRETION

Levodopa is rapidly absorbed from the gut: the majority is decarboxylated in the gut and liver by L-amino acid decarboxylase, so that little unchanged drug reaches the circulation. This metabolism can be markedly influenced by the concurrent administration of the inhibitors carbidopa and benserazide hydrochloride.

Metabolism of dopamine is principally to 3,4-dihydroxyphenylacetic acid (DOPAC) and 3-methoxy-4-hydroxyphenylacetic acid (homovanillic acid or HVA). The metabolites are excreted in the urine.

INDICATIONS

Levodopa is used in the treatment of parkinsonism; the majority of such cases are caused by 'idiopathic' degeneration, but a diminishing number are the late consequence of the pandemic of encephalitis lethargica following the First World War. It is not effective in the treatment of parkinson-like extrapyramidal reactions to drugs such as the butyrophenones and some phenothiazines which have strong dopamine antagonist effects.

DOSAGE AND ADMINISTRATION

Initial dosage is 0.5–1 g daily in divided doses, gradually increasing to about 2.5–3 g daily in 2–3 weeks. Full benefit may not be reached for 3–4 months, when dose levels may range from 3–6 g daily. It may be given in combination with carbidopa in a ratio of 10:1, when the total dose must be reduced by 75 per cent.

PRECAUTIONS

The majority of patients experience side effects but fortunately tolerance usually develops to most of them. The commonest early effects are nausea, vomiting, and orthostatic hypotension. Cardiac dysrhythmias occur, particularly in patients with pre-existing conduction defects. Psychiatric disturbance is a significant late consequence. Levodopa may interfere with diabetic management. It is contraindicated in narrow-angle glaucoma. It should not be given to nursing mothers; even if lactation is not inhibited it appears in the milk. There is animal evidence of teratogenicity. Stimulation of melanocyte-stimulating hormone may lead to growth of melanomas.

Pyridoxine (even in the amounts found in over-the-counter vitamin pills) increases peripheral decarboxylase activity and diminishes the amount of free levodopa available for penetration of the brain. Discontinuation of therapy for 6–24 hours prior to anaesthesia is recommended although no untoward reactions have been reported.

Other dopamine agonists

Amantidine was introduced as an antiviral agent. It was tried in a patient with parkinsonism who also had influenza and an improvement in her parkinsonism was noted. It probably acts indirectly, causing the release of endogenous dopamine from the presynaptic nerve terminals in the basal ganglia.

Selegiline is an inhibitor of monoamine oxidase type B. It has been shown to cause some clinical improvement in patients with parkinsonism. The usual dose is 5–10 mg daily and it can be combined with levodopa plus a peripheral dopa decarboxylase inhibitor.

Bromocriptine is a semisynthetic ergot derivative which has dopamine agonist properties. As might be expected, it can inhibit prolactin release and is used in the treatment of prolactin-secreting pituitary tumours. It is useful in the treatment of parkinsonism also. In parkinsonism, bromocriptine has been shown to improve tremor, rigidity, and akinesia but can induce severe vomiting. Bromocriptine appears to be of value in patients who have a variable response to levodopa due to fluctuating plasma levels. However, it causes a higher incidence of neurological and psychiatric disturbances such as dyskinesia and hallucination. The drug is given in an initial dose of 2.5 mg twice daily, increasing gradually.

Lithium

Lithium carbonate (*BP* and *USP*)
Chemical formula: Li_2CO_3

PHARMACOLOGY

This toxic compound is an extremely useful drug in maniacal states and can be used in the prophylaxis of recurrent affective disorders. Its mechanism of action is not known. As an ion, it can compete with sodium and potassium ions in some cellular processes. Acute lithium treatment has been shown in animals to accelerate noradrenaline turnover and increase 5-HT synthesis, but chronic treatment produces a fall in 5-HT and dopamine turnover. Following oral administration peak plasma levels occur about 4 hours after dosing. In young adults the $t_{1/2}$ is about 19 hours but this is increased in the elderly. Up to 36 hours has been reported, hence cumulation can occur. The drug is almost completely excreted by the kidney.

INDICATIONS

Lithium produces an improvement in about 70 per cent of patients with acute mania. It is an antidepressant, being more effective in patients with a history of bipolar depression, that is those with a history of mania in the past.

DOSAGE AND ADMINISTRATION

Lithium carbonate is usually initially prescribed in a dosage of 600–900 mg daily in divided doses. The plasma level is monitored and the dose may be slowly increased. Doses of 1500–2400 mg daily arc quitc common. Clinical improvement usually occurs in about 3 weeks.

PRECAUTIONS

It is important to monitor plasma lithium concentrations, which should be maintained between 0.8–1.2 mmol/ℓ. If plasma concentrations rise to between 1.5 and 3.0 mmol/ℓ, diarrhoea, weakness, drowsiness, thirst, and ataxia can occur. A further rise in plasma levels to 3–5 mmol/ℓ can cause confusional states, convulsions, and coma, and lead to death.

Dose-independent toxicity can also occur; about 10 per cent of patients on chronic therapy have evidence of thyroid deficiency. The drug is thought to inhibit adenyl cyclase and this decreases thyroid efficiency. It can also induce nephrogenic diabetes insipidus by preventing the antidiuretic hormone mediating its effect on the collecting duct through adenyl cyclase.

Cardiac effects can occur even in the therapeutic range. A common finding is T-wave changes in the ECG (intracellular potassium replaced by lithium). Myocardial infarction and cardiac failure are contraindications to lithium therapy.

Lithium should be stopped 48–72 hours before surgery involving a muscle relaxant. In patients with renal failure or renal tubular disease the drug is contraindicated. Thiazide diuretics can precipitate lithium toxicity by reducing lithium clearance. Lithium may enhance extrapyramidal effects and tardive dyskinesias produced by butyrophenones and phenothiazines.

Nikethamide

Nikethamide (*BP*)
Chemical name: *NN*-diethylpyridine-3-carboxyamide

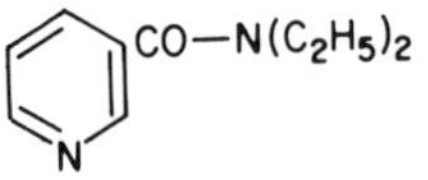

$$\text{(pyridine ring)-CO-N}(C_2H_5)_2$$

PHARMACOLOGY

Nikethamide is a cerebral stimulant and analeptic. Its action on the medulla is mainly due to its stimulatory effect on the chemoreceptors in the carotid and aortic bodies. Respiration is stimulated, the effect being more marked in the presence of central depression due to drugs. The margin between the therapeutic effect and toxic symptoms is wide, but convulsions follow excessive dosage and death from respiratory failure may occur later. The myocardium may be depressed, but large doses are said to increase cardiac output and coronary flow; stimulation of the vasomotor centre will cause vasoconstriction and a rise in blood pressure. Its action is not as powerful as picrotoxin, but its duration of action is a little longer. After intravenous injection it is rapidly destroyed in the body.

Nikethamide is now mainly used as a stimulant when the cause of apnoea is uncertain, but may be due to overdose with centrally acting drugs. It has also been employed as a respiratory stimulant to improve ventilation in chronic bronchitis. Although it may improve the mental state of the patient, it does not produce any important increase in ventilation. Although recommended in the past as a cardiovascular stimulant, it should not be used for this purpose. It is not effective except in large doses, and any myocardial weakness may be intensified.

Nikethamide is well absorbed when given by mouth but its stimulant action is not appreciable by this route. It is usually given intravenously in a dose of 0.25–1 g (1–4 ml of a 25 per cent solution).

Amiphenazole hydrochloride was originally claimed to be a specific antagonist to certain depressant actions of morphine but this has not been substantiated. Its actions are similar to those of doxapram but the therapeutic margin is less. The intravenous dose is 150 mg.

Bemegride was introduced as a specific antagonist to the barbiturates to which it is structurally closely related (*see* page 98) but there is no reliable evidence to support this in man. The intravenous dose is 25–50 mg.

Strychnine is no longer employed except possibly as an ingredient in a few brands of 'tonic'. It is an alkaloid obtained from *Nux vomica* and the seeds of other species of *Strychnos*. In small doses strychnine stimulates the flow of saliva and, reflexly, that of gastric juice. It has thus been used to promote appetite. It selectively depresses inhibitory synapses, and this produces marked over-activity of the CNS, particularly of the spinal cord. The sensations of touch, smell, and hearing are all increased in acuity, as is vision; and the field of vision, particularly for blue, is enlarged. Increasing doses stimulate all parts of the brain, having a marked facilitative action on central synapses. Exaggerated reflex responses are produced by small doses, the motor component being augmented and the inhibitor diminished; with larger doses there is symmetrical contraction of flexor and extensor muscles. The body is rigid, head bent back and back arched, in the typical opisthotonos position. Fewer than five convulsions may be fatal, the cause of death being asphyxia from spasm of the intercostal muscles. The convulsions last about 1 minute and then all the muscles relax.

Overdose causes convulsions and asphyxia, and treatment must be immediate if the patient is to survive; thiopentone should be given intravenously until convulsions are controlled, or a muscle relaxant may be given immediately following the thiopentone and repeated as required, supplemented, of course, by controlled ventilation.

Vanillic acid diethylamide is closely related structurally to nikethamide. Its actions are similar and it is used for similar purposes. The adult dose is 5–10 ml of 5 per cent solution intravenously. It can also be given intramuscularly or by mouth.

8

Histamine, antihistamines; drugs affecting bronchial calibre

Histamine

Histamine is the oldest and most familiar of a group of substances that share the common property of being naturally occurring agents with intense pharmacological actions, predominantly at the local site of release. This group also includes serotonin (5-hydroxytryptamine, 5-HT), 'slow-reacting substance in anaphylaxis' (SRS-A), the prostaglandins, angiotensin, and the various kinins. They have been referred to as local hormones, but the generic term, *autacoid* (Greek, *autos*—self, and *akos*—medicine) is now being applied to such substances. The more important of these (other than histamine) are discussed in Chapter 16.

Histamine is found in almost all mammalian tissues (Greek, *histos* – tissue) particularly in the mast cells where, like heparin, it is present in high concentration. In allergic and anaphylactic reactions, both substances are liberated together.

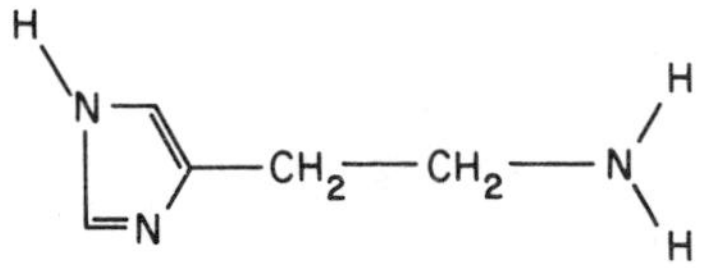

Figure 8.1 Structural formula of histamine

It is an intensely active substance biologically, producing responses on suitable isolated tissues in concentrations much less than 1 part in 10^6. Histamine is present in an inactive form in intracellular particles (like adrenaline), and is liberated in trauma, by certain drugs and other substances, from the tissues. It is found widely in nature, not only in animal tissues but also in plant and vegetable cells, in nettle stings, and the stings of certain insects such as wasps.

The chief actions of histamine are contraction of plain muscle and dilatation and increased permability of capillaries. It also stimulates secretions, especially of the oxyntic cells of the stomach, and causes secretion of adrenaline from the medulla of the adrenal glands.

These actions are mediated by two types of receptors, which have been named H_1 and H_2. H_2-receptors are involved in the release of acid in the stomach and in some of the cardiovascular effects of histamine. H_1-receptors mediate all the other actions of histamine discussed below. Both types of receptors can be blocked by appropriate competitive antagonists.

The actions of this drug have been intensively studied, but even now its true physiological role is uncertain. In man, the highest concentrations are found in the skin, intestine, and lung – parts in contact with the outside world. It has been suggested that the vasodilatation it produces may reduce the pathogenicity of invading organisms.

Action on plain muscle

Histamine was first isolated from ergot, and its action studied on the uterus, which it stimulates in most species whether this organ is isolated or *in situ*. It has a direct stimulant action on bronchiolar muscle which is unrelated to nervous innervation and usually not blocked by atropine. The guinea-pig is particularly sensitive to it, and as little as 0.1 mg will cause death from bronchoconstriction and oedema of the mucosa. This action of the drug is commonly used for testing the protective power of antihistamine drugs. In the normal human subject the bronchoconstrictor action of histamine is negligible, but patients with bronchial asthma, bronchitis, emphysema, and even cardiac asthma are much more sensitive to it as, in them, it exerts a bronchoconstrictor action. Its action on other plain muscle, except in the cardiovascular system, is of little importance.

Cardiovascular system

The action of histamine on the heart is negligible, but it is powerful on the capillaries and arterioles. An intravenous injection causes a sharp fall in blood pressure and a rise in CSF pressure. This is followed by an intense headache of short duration, after which the pressure changes subside.

The action of histamine on the capillaries can be demonstrated in human skin if a scratch is made through a drop of histamine solution. The triple response which follows causes capillaries to dilate in the traumatized area, a weal due to increased permeability of the vessels permitting plasma to escape, and a flare consisting of dilated arterioles surrounding the weal. The flare is produced by an axon reflex through sensory nerves which can be blocked by local analgesics. If histamine is injected into the skin it causes itching, and pain if acetylcholine is injected with it. Both of these substances are found in the stinging nettle.

In some animals, histamine may cause a rise in the blood pressure through its vasoconstrictor action on the arterioles and almost complete absence of capillary effect as seen in man. Histamine shock can be produced readily in animals after large doses have been injected. The fall in blood pressure is pronounced and persistent due to excessive capillary dilatation, and much plasma escapes into the tissues, causing a diminished circulating blood volume and reduced cardiac output. Owing to haemoconcentration, haemoglobin estimations will give a falsely high reading.

The hypotensive effects of histamine are potentiated by anaesthetic agents that increase sympathetic activity. This is presumably due to histamine blocking the vasoconstrictor effects on the capillaries of the skin and mucous membranes, while the vasolidator effect on muscle blood vessels is unaffected.

Alimentary system

When given by mouth, histamine produces no pharmacological effects, probably because it is acetylated in the intestine. Marked stimulation of gastric secretion occurs in response to an injection of histamine subcutaneously, and 1 mg given this way is used as a test clinically for gastric function.

Peptic ulceration can be produced by continuous administration of large doses of histamine. Although gastrin and histamine are now known to be different substances, the former may act by liberating the latter. Histamine can cause an increase in salivary secretions and in those of the pancreas and intestine. These effects are not marked in man and seem to be cholinergic mechanisms as they are potentiated by physostigmine and abolished by atropine.

The plain muscle of the gut is not particularly affected by histamine *in vivo*, but it is a very powerful stimulant of mammalian intestine, especially guinea-pig ileum, in an isolated tissue bath.

Liberation of histamine

Histamine is released by a wide variety of drugs and physicochemical insults.

Physical and chemical damage. Any mechanical, thermal, or radiant injury, if severe enough to cause tissue damage, will liberate histamine. Some chemicals, such as bile salts and detergents, will also release histamine by direct injury.

Anaphylaxis and allergy. These reactions have a basic mechanism in common. This involves an interaction between a specific antigen and a cell-bound antibody. The latter is an immunoglobulin of the IgE type in man. Antigens are usually proteins that are foreign to the individual but may be other large molecules or complexes formed by the combination of a small reactive molecule with a protein. Many drugs can form such complexes and are then called haptens. The intensity of the anaphylactic reaction depends on the portal of entry of the antigen. If it enters parenterally, as with the case of a drug, a foreign serum, or the saliva of a biting insect, systemic anaphylaxis supervenes and this is due to the explosive release of histamine from storage granules in a large number of tissues as well as other agents such as 5-HT, SRS-A, and plasma kinins. If the reaction takes place at an exposed mucosal surface the reaction is much milder and restricted to that tissue. Such restrictions give rise to hay fever, conjunctivitis, asthma, urticaria, and gastrointestinal upsets.

Drugs and macromolecules. Apart from their potentiality for initiating an antigen–antibody response, many chemicals, including numerous therapeutic agents, have the capacity for eliciting histamine release directly. Among them are antibiotic bases, quaternary ammonium compounds such as tubocurarine, piperidine derivatives, and morphine derivatives. In the clinical situation it can be difficult to decide whether a drug releases histamine directly, or indirectly by a hypersensitivity mechanism.

Venoms and toxins. Many sorts of venoms and toxins release histamine; this property so far transcends the other pharmacological actions that they have been called histamine liberators. The histamine released is that bound in the granules, and non-mast cell histamine is not depleted.

Synthesis, storage, and metabolism

Ingested histamine is largely bound and subsequently destroyed by the liver and lungs or excreted in the urine. Tissue histamine is largely synthesized *in situ* by decarboxylation of histidine. In tissue mast cells and circulating basophils histamine is synthesized and stored in a complex with heparin in membrane-bound storage granules. The turnover rate in this site is slow. Histamine is also found in substantial amounts in many tissues outside the mast cells where it undergoes a brisk turnover.

There are two main routes of enzymatic breakdown: (1) methylation, followed by oxidation to methylindoleacetic acid; (2) oxidation by diamine oxidase. The relative roles of these enzymes in the metabolism of endogenous histamine have not been established.

Histamine activity is increased by oxygen and oestrogens and is inhibited by cyanides, hydroxylamine, phenylhydrazine, and isoniazid. Diamine oxidase activity increases during the first trimester of pregnancy and stays elevated until term. Its origin is the placenta but its function is not clear.

Antihistamines

The term antihistamine is commonly used alone when synthetic competitive antihistamines active at H_1-receptors is meant. There are, of course, other ways in which the actions of histamine can be opposed: physiological antagonism of the effects of histamine on capillaries can be achieved by adrenaline and on bronchial tone by β-stimulating adrenergic agents such as salbutamol.

Antihistamines specifically prevent released histamine from affecting cells by blocking the receptors upon which it normally exerts its effect. There are now drugs that are specific for both H_1- and H_2-receptors. The former are the traditional antihistamines such as mepyramine and promethazine; the latter is typified by cimetidine.

H_1-receptor antihistamines

These drugs, introduced by Bovet in 1944, are given to control the principal effects of released histamine in allergic conditions such as hay fever, urticaria, dermatoses, serum sickness, and reactions to drugs and blood transfusions. They are frequently used, however, solely for their pharmacological actions *other* than as antihistamines. It is a matter of perspective as to whether or not to regard these actions as side effects. Clearly drowsiness is an unwanted side effect when trying to control hay fever; equally, depression of the vomiting centre is the desired therapeutic effect if vomiting associated with radiotherapy is being treated. Additional effects are possessed by all antihistamines in varying degrees and consist of the following.

Central depression, which may either be predominantly a hypnotic or tranquillizing effect or may be more specific. The most important of these effects is on the vomiting centre, making them suitable agents in treating motion sickness or other causes of nausea and vomiting not due to reflex stimulation via the chemoreceptor trigger zone. Another useful action is as a vestibular sedative; cinnarizine possesses this property and is effective in vertigo due to Ménière's disease and in the treatment of tinnitus.

Anticholinergic action, which is antimuscarinic or atropine-like, includes the drying-up of secretions, relaxation of smooth muscle, and an increase in heart rate. The prolongation of the refractory period of the atria of the heart – the so-called quinidine-like action – is also believed to be due partly to an anticholinergic action.

Antiadrenergic action, which often passes unnoticed, is, however, marked with some drugs, for example chlorpromazine, and hypotension is a feature.

Local analgesic action, which is of course not apparent when an antihistamine drug is given by mouth or parenterally; it is, however, a definite action of this group of agents. Their effectiveness locally in pruritus may be due as much to this effect, which is long lasting, as to the antihistamine action.

Certain H_1-receptor antihistamines, cyclizine and meclozine in particular, have been suspected of having teratogenic properties. Evidence is still inconclusive, but it would be wise to avoid their use during the early months of pregnancy.

Cases of overdose so far reported in the literature reveal symptoms of general depression and should be treated symptomatically.

The drugs in this category which have been included in the monograph section are ones with strong antihistamine activity at H_1-receptor sites. They are used primarily in the treatment of allergic conditions but some are also useful antiemetics. The phenothiazines, many of which also have some degree of antihistamine effect, are now almost entirely used for their tranquillizing and sedative action and are considered in Chapter 3.

H_2-receptor antihistamines

The earlier compounds in this category have been abandoned because of toxic effects, particularly on the bone marrow. Cimetidine and ranitidine are believed to be free of this liability. The principal therapeutic effect is to inhibit both basal and stimulated gastric secretion of acid. There is also some reduction in pepsin output. Any effect on H_2-receptors in the circulation is not apparent after clinical doses although they may become apparent in overdose. Agents of this type are used in conditions where suppression of gastric acidity is required, such as peptic ulceration, reflux oesophagitis, and the Zollinger–Ellison syndrome.

Inhibitors of histamine release

Ideally, one would like to be able to inhibit the release not only of histamine, but also the other autacoids active in anaphylactic and allergic reactions. This is generally an unattainable objective at present. However, substances are now being developed which prevent the release of histamine and this is an important therapeutic approach in asthma and some other allergic conditions. The only drug of this type available at present is sodium cromoglycate, which is used prophylactically for both asthma and allergic rhinitis.

Bronchoconstrictors

A bronchoconstrictor is an agent that causes any degree of constriction of the smooth muscle of the bronchial tree. Some can bring this about via the nervous system, either by increasing vagal action or by decreasing that of the sympathetic, and others affect the bronchial muscle directly.

Bronchoconstriction by drugs acting through the nervous system may be initiated at any link in the reflex arc. The important sites are at receptors (irritants), at the postganglionic vagal nerve endings (inhibitors of cholinesterase), and at the vagal centre in the medulla (morphine). The infiltration of local analgesic solutions to the relevant portion of the sympathetic chain would increase bronchial tone by removing the dilator action of the sympathetic. A similar effect can be produced by β-adrenoceptor blocking agents which block bronchodilator receptors. None of these mechanisms produce severe bronchospasm in normal individuals, although they may cause measurable changes in airway resistance. They can be more serious in patients with existing abnormal bronchial tone.

Drugs that can cause bronchoconstriction by a direct muscular effect are theoretically all those that are general stimulants of plain muscle, but fortunately comparatively few have a marked effect upon bronchial muscle. The most important is histamine, which can be liberated in the body by a number of substances, as discussed above.

Bronchodilators

Bronchodilators are drugs that decrease the tone of the muscle of the bronchial tree and so lessen respiratory resistance. Their importance lies in their ability to overcome bronchoconstriction and their efforts are usefully reinforced by drugs that diminish secretion or reduce mucosal engorgement by causing vasoconstriction.

The most important members act directly on the muscle to promote relaxation, or achieve this by potentiating the effects of noradrenaline being liberated normally at the sympathetic nerve endings. Powerful examples of the latter are sympathomimetic amines such as adrenaline, isoprenaline, and ephedrine, and of the former theophylline is the most active of the xanthine derivatives. The nitrites also exert a direct action but lower the blood pressure in effective doses; papaverine is ineffective. Ether in anaesthetic concentrations, although irritant, relaxes bronchial tone, although it is possible that it is the liberation of adrenaline which is responsible for the bronchodilatation.

Since bronchial tone is the result of a balance between parasympathetic and sympathetic activity, specific antagonists of the muscarinic actions of the acetylcholine liberated at vagal nerve endings will act as bronchodilators. This is the mechanism of the bronchodilator activity of atropine and hyoscine; these drugs will also oppose the muscarinic actions of other choline esters upon the bronchial tree, but they are not very effective in bronchial asthma. However, more recent derivatives, deptropine (page 306) and ipratropium (page 308), are claimed to be effective in the treatment of this condition.

Competitive antihistamines will relieve bronchoconstriction caused by histamine. In the case of asthma, antihistamines fail to prevent bronchoconstriction. The reason usually advanced is that competitive inhibition by specific antihistamines is impossible because the histamine is intrinsic, which means that it is liberated directly in or on the effector cells of the tissue concerned and obtains immediate and intimate contact with receptors from a vantage point which a competitive antagonist cannot attain.

In this situation, however, universal β-receptor stimulating drugs, such as adrenaline, and selective β_2-stimulators, such as salbutamol and terbutaline, are effective, as are drugs acting directly on the bronchial smooth muscle.

In the treatment of asthma, drugs are best given by inhalation. Several types of inhaler system are available. To reach the bronchioles the drug should be delivered in particle sizes of 2–4 μm. Larger particles are deposited in the upper airway; smaller ones enter the alveoli or are exhaled. Pressurized inhalers deliver a metered dose of 25–100 μl suspended in a fluorocarbon propellant. Dry powder inhalers are less convenient but are sometimes preferred. In the intensive care situation, various nebulizers, such as ultrasonic nebulizers, may be employed.

Mucolytic agents

In many clinical situations ventilation difficulties are caused not so much by bronchospasm as by tenacious secretions, and in such circumstances mucolytic therapy may be beneficial. Enzymes such as chymotrypsin can digest sputum *in vitro*, but their clinical use has not been satisfactory. Some preparations related to amino acids are available as aerosols or as oral preparations, such as acetylcysteine and carboxymethylcysteine. These principally affect sputum volume and viscosity. The volume of mucus may initially increase so greatly that endotracheal suction becomes necessary to maintain an adequate airway. The compounds, being related to proteins, may be attended by undesirable reactions such as fever when given by inhalation.

Another agent which has a specific action on sputum is bromhexine, an alkaloid derived from the plant *Adhatoda vasica*. This appears to break down mucopolysaccharide fibres and reduce sputum viscosity.

While the effects of bromhexine are relatively easy to demonstrate *in vitro,* there are problems *in vivo*, and clinical studies have been conflicting. Whereas there may be an increase in sputum volume and a reduction in viscosity, improvements in ventilatory capacity are hard to demonstrate. No serious side effects have been encountered and most authors have felt that the drug was beneficial, and it has been occasionally tried in patients with postoperative chest infection and 'flail' chests.

While drug therapy may prove to have a place in the therapy of viscid secretions, it must not be overlooked that adequate hydration of the patients and humidification of the inspired air have been shown to have a dramatic influence on sputum viscosity, and such simple non-specific lines of therapy should not be overlooked.

Theophylline and Aminophylline

Theophylline (*BP*) and Aminophylline (*BP* and *USP*)
Chemical constitution: aminophylline is a mixture of theophylline and ethylenediamine, its composition approximating to the formula
$(C_7H_8O_2N_4)_2 \cdot C_2H_4(NH_2)_2 \cdot 2H_2O$

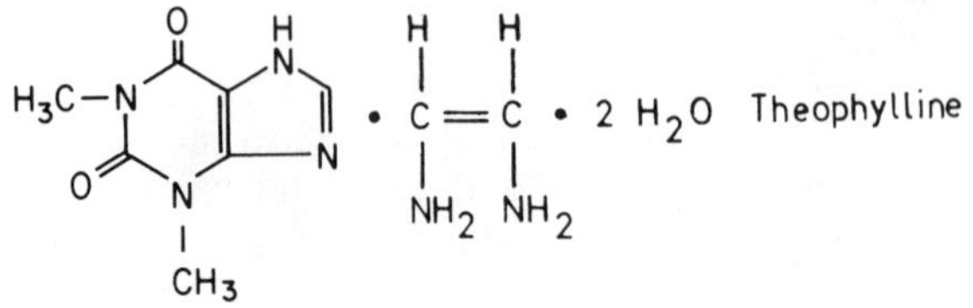

Theophylline

PHARMACOLOGY

Theophylline is a dimethylxanthine, sharing properties with caffeine and theobromine. In this group – the xanthine derivatives – differences in action are of degree only, all being stimulants of the CNS and the heart, relaxants of smooth muscle, and diuretics by direct action on the kidney.

Central nervous system. The activity of theophylline is not great enough for it to be of use against central depressants. It does, however, have a stimulant action on the respiratory centre, which may be valuable in connexion with its bronchodilator action. In overdose it can cause agitation and even convulsions.

Cardiovascular system. The force of the heartbeat is increased and output rises. The rate of beat is slightly raised, being the resultant of a direct effect offset by vagal stimulation centrally. Coronary vessels are dilated, but it is conjectural whether the increased blood flow is in excess of that demanded by the extra cardiac work. Central vasomotor stimulation acts against direct peripheral vasodilatation, which predominates in general, but cerebrovascular resistance increases and cerebral blood flow falls. The resultant of the various opposing cardiovascular actions upon blood pressure is usually a slight rise.

In common with other methylxanthines, theophylline is an inhibitor of the enzyme phosphodiesterase, and therefore allows tissue levels of cyclic AMP to increase. It therefore closely reproduces the effects of β-adrenergic stimulation which increase cyclic AMP levels by stimulating its elaboration. A rise in cyclic AMP in lung tissue leads to bronchial smooth muscle relaxation. Its toxic effects in other tissues are probably related to a similar mechanism.

Extravascular smooth muscle. The most important site of action is bronchial smooth muscle, which is dilated, often in asthmatics refractory even to adrenaline. Biliary spasm is also relieved and there is a transient suppression of activity of the muscle of the small and large bowel.

The kidney. Renal blood flow is increased and this will increase urine output in conditions of poor renal blood flow. Probably of more importance is the direct depression of tubular reabsorption of electrolyte by an unknown mechanism. Tubular secretion of potassium is not affected.

Fate in the body. Xanthines are well absorbed following administration by oral, rectal, or parenteral routes. They are irritant and some preparations attempt to overcome this disadvantage by combination with choline, glycine, or other organic bases. When given by rectum or intramuscularly, effective blood levels are reached in 30–60 minutes. Appreciable blood levels remain for over 6 hours, but its activity is over more quickly. Little unchanged theophylline reaches the urine, most of it being demethylated and oxidized to methyluric acid.

INDICATIONS

Aminophylline is used mainly in the treatment of asthma and bronchospasm. It possesses a combination of pharmacological actions particularly suited to geriatric patients.

DOSAGE AND ADMINISTRATION

Aminophylline may be given orally in a dose of 100–200 mg by tablet, in an elixir (containing about 80 mg/5 ml), or by rectum in the form of a suppository; these are available in at least five strengths and confusion about dose may lead to overdose. Suppositories should rarely be needed now that well-tested, oral, slow-release preparations are available. It may also be given slowly intravenously when a rapid response is required. It has been specifically recommended for the relief of bronchospasm associated with the carcinoid syndrome, by virtue of its ability to antagonize both 5-HT and histamine.

The dosage and rate of administration are crucial in obtaining a maximal therapeutic effect with the minimum of toxic side effects. Bronchodilatation can be first detected at a plasma level of about 5 µg/ml and increases as the plasma level increases to about 15–20 µg/ml. Toxic effects start to appear in this range. The optimum level appears to be 10–12 µg/ml and this can be achieved by giving a loading dose of 5.6 mg/kg over 15–30 minutes, followed by 0.9 mg/kg per hour. Users of tobacco and alcohol need bigger doses to achieve the same serum concentration. Patients in heart failure need less.

PRECAUTIONS

Rapid administration can lead to agitation, convulsions, tachycardia, hypotension, and cardiac arrest. It has been suggested that if used in combination with a β_2-agonist there is an enhanced danger of fatal cardiac dysrhythmias (Wilson, Sutherland and Thomas, 1981).

Wilson, J. D., Sutherland, D. C. and Thomas, A. C. (1981) Has the change to beta-agonists combined with oral theophylline increased cases of fatal asthma? *Lancet,* **1,** 1235

Other theophylline derivatives include diprophylline, acepifylline, and etamiphylline. They can all be given orally and by suppository and the first two by injection. Reported experience with these is not extensive but they seem to offer little in the way of practical advantages.

Chlorpheniramine maleate

Chlorpheniramine maleate (*BP* and *USP*)
Chemical name: (3-*p*-chlorophenyl-3-pyrid-2′-ylpropyl) dimethylamine hydrogen maleate

Chlorpheniramine is a highly effective antihistamine, acting competitively at H_1-receptors with a rapid action and duration of effect lasting 4–6 hours. Side effects are minimal, dizziness and drowsiness being rarely encountered. It is used in the prophylaxis and treatment of a wide range of allergic disorders and of drug and blood transfusion reactions.

Chlorpheniramine is given by mouth in tablet form in a dose of 4 mg three to four times a day. In severe cases of allergic and drug reactions 10–20 mg may be given intramuscularly, or intravenously in an emergency. For prophylactic use in patients subject to allergic reactions 10 mg may be injected intravenously immediately before a blood transfusion, or mixed with penicillin in the syringe prior to injection.

Cimetidine

Cimetidine (*BAN*)
Chemical name: 2-cyano-1-methyl-3-[2-(5-methylimidazol-4-ylmethylthio)ethyl] guanidine

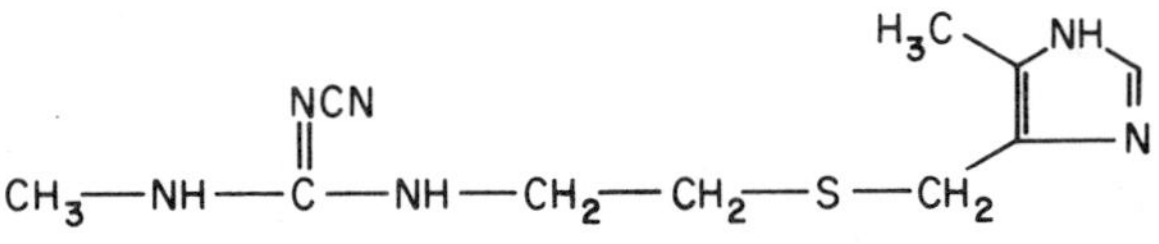

H_3C NH N

NCN
||
CH_3—NH—C—NH—CH_2—CH_2—S—CH_2

PHARMACOLOGY

Cimetidine is a competitive antagonist of H_2-receptors. It thus inhibits both basal and stimulated secretion of gastric acid and reduces pepsin output. It does not affect the H_1-receptors in bronchial, vascular, or intestinal smooth muscle. It is rapidly absorbed from the duodenum and effective blood levels are maintained for several hours after a single oral dose. It is largely excreted unchanged in the urine. It causes a small rise in serum creatinine. It may be given by intravenous infusion if necessary.

INDICATIONS

It is indicated in peptic ulceration of all kinds, reflux oesophagitis, and any condition where reduction of gastric acid secretion is likely to be beneficial. It is also of value in the management of the Zollinger–Ellison syndrome. It is used to raise the intragastric pH in obstetric patients, but is being replaced by ranitidine.

DOSAGE AND ADMINISTRATION

The normal dose is 1 g per day, 200 mg with each meal and 400 mg at bed-time, but may be increased to 1.6 g per day. By continuous intravenous infusion, 2 g may be given over 24 hours in electrolyte or dextrose solutions.

PRECAUTIONS

Dosage must be reduced in the presence of impaired renal function. It may reduce the rate of metabolism of drugs, notably phenytoin, by an effect on cytochrome P450-mediated pathways. Cimetidine crosses the placenta and is excreted in the milk. Its safety in human pregnancy has not been tested but it is not teratogenic in animals. Mild and transient diarrhoea and muscle pains have been reported. It blocks androgen receptors, and gynaecomastia and impotence have occasionally been reported. Overdose is unlikely; up to 1000 times the therapeutic dose is not lethal in animals. The reduction of gastric acidity allows the proliferation of bacteria, and respiratory infection with such organisms has been noted in patients in intensive care units receiving cimetidine while on artificial ventilators.

Ranitidine closely resembles cimetidine: it is much longer acting but its pharmacological effects are equally effective in clinical studies. It is more potent on a weight for weight basis and the effective dose is 160 mg twice a day. No important adverse reactions have been identified and there are some differences which may or may not prove to be of importance. It does not block androgen receptors nor cause any rise in serum creatinine. It does not interact with cytochrome P450 and thus should have no effect on the metabolism of phenytoin or other drugs broken down in this pathway. Since it is as effective as cimetidine in reducing gastric acidity it is likely to allow bacterial proliferation to a similar extent.

Sodium cromoglycate

Sodium cromoglycate (*BP*)
Chemical name: sodium 5,5′-(2-hydroxytrimethylenedioxy)bis(4-oxo-4*H*-chromene-2-carboxylate)

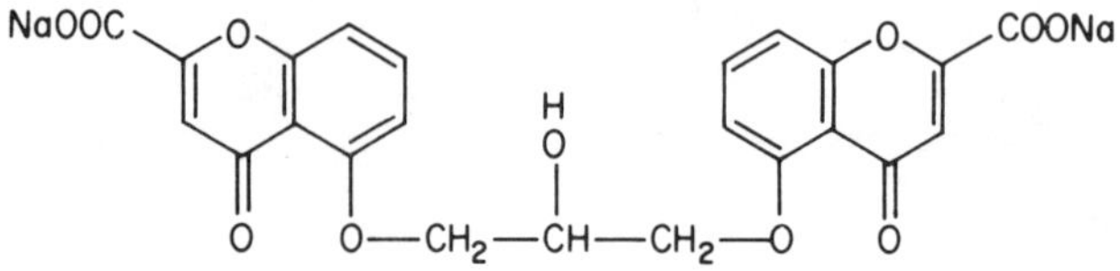

NaOOC COONa
H
O
O O—CH_2—CH—CH_2—O O

PHARMACOLOGY

Sodium cromoglycate has no direct action on bronchial smooth muscle, nor does it inhibit the direct action of bronchoconstrictor drugs. Its mode of action is to prevent the release of histamine and SRS-A from mast cells in human lung as a consequence of IgE-mediated allergic responses. Both histamine and SRS-A are potent bronchial spasmogens. It therefore prevents the immediate and late asthmatic response to allergens.

Cromoglycate does not inhibit the antigen–antibody reaction itself, but appears to suppress the release of histamine which is a consequence of this reaction. Moreover, this suppression of release is not universal. The actions of histamine liberators (*see* page 244) are unaffected, and mast-cell mediated histamine release in other tissues, such as skin, is not blocked. The drug is, however, effective on the nasal mucosa.

INDICATIONS

Sodium cromoglycate is indicated in the prophylaxis of bronchial asthma, particularly where there is good reason to think that an allergic response to an inhaled allergen is implicated. It is also indicated for the prophylaxis of allergic rhinitis.

The use of the drug is entirely prophylactic and not therapeutic.

DOSAGE AND ADMINISTRATION

For the prevention of asthma the drug is normally given as a powder by inhalation from a single-dose 20-mg cartridge ('Spincap') in a specially designed turbovibratory inhaler. This dose should be inhaled four to eight times a day. It may be combined with a small dose of isoprenaline (0.1 mg) to counteract the immediate transient bronchospasm which may follow the inhalation of a dry powder. In the prophylaxis of allergic rhinitis it may be given as 2 per cent nasal drops. It is important for the patient to understand that the preparations must be taken regularly, and not in response to symptoms.

PRECAUTIONS

There are no specific contraindications. Cromoglycate powder may irritate the throat and trachea. Therapy may permit a reduction in concomitant steroid dosage; this should be reinstituted before sodium cromoglycate is withdrawn.

Cyclizine salts

Cyclizine hydrochloride (*BP* and *USP*) and Cyclizine lactate (*USP*)
Chemical name: 1-diphenylmethl-4-methylpiperazine

Cyclizine is a competitive antihistamine acting at H_1-receptors whose main action is on the vomiting centre, which it depresses. Its action is potent and prolonged; it begins within a few minutes of administration, and is stated to cause side effects in only 5 per cent of cases.

It has been suspected of producing teratogenic effects. Evidence is conflicting, but it would be safer not to use it during the early stages of pregnancy.

It is used in the prevention of travel sickness, in the treatment of vertigo (Ménière's syndrome), and combined with analgesics and ergotamine to prevent the emetic side effects of these drugs.

Cyclizine is given by mouth in tablet form in doses of 50 mg up to three times a day. Children aged 6–10 years may be given half this dose.

Dimenhydrinate

Dimenhydrinate (*BP* and *USP*)
Chemical name: the diphanhydramine salt of 8-chloratheophylline (theoclic acid)

Dimenhydrinate is a competitive antihistamine of moderate potency acting at H_1-receptors. It has powerful antiemetic properties, and is used almost entirely in the treatment and prevention of vomiting and vertigo.

In the prevention of vomiting associated with anaesthesia 50 mg may be given by mouth 1 hour before operation and repeated at the end of operation if necessary. A similar dose is given to prevent travel sickness, taken 30 minutes before departure, and it may be repeated 4-hourly if required. Larger doses are sometimes necessary.

Vomiting associated with irradiation, toxaemias of pregnancy, carcinomatosis, and drugs such as nitrogen mustard, morphine and its derivatives may be treated orally with 50–100 mg, repeated 4-hourly as required, the dose then being adjusted to control symptoms. A dose of 50 mg may be given intramuscularly if the tablets cannot be retained in the stomach. If a more rapid response is necessary, dimenhydrinate 50 mg in 10 ml of isotonic saline may be given slowly intravenously; if given rapidly it may cause venous irritation. Drowsiness is commonly associated with the administration of this drug, and the patient must be duly cautioned.

Diphenhydramine hydrochloride

Diphenhydramine hydrochloride (*BP* and *USP*)
Chemical name: 2-benzhydryloxy-NN-dimethylethylamine hydrochloride

Diphenhydramine is a competitive antihistamine acting at H_1-receptors and has been used in all the common allergic conditions such as hay fever, urticaria, and the dermatoses. It was one of the earliest available, clinically, and is one of the most sedative and least active antihistamines, lasting less than 5 hours when given orally. The incidence of side effects is about 60 per cent, especially drowsiness, and it tends to be used now more as a sedative than an antihistamine.

The usual dose is 50 mg by mouth, repeated as necessary up to three or four times a day. A cream may be applied by local application in the treatment of skin conditions and pruritus.

As drowsiness is usual during treatment, patients must be duly warned.

The drug is one component of several proprietary formulations with the hypnotic methaqualone. The synergistic hypnotic effect is very striking and is discussed under methaqualone.

Diphenhydramine is one of the many sedative drugs that have been shown to increase the synthesis of hepatic microsomal enzymes.

Meclozine hydrochloride

Meclozine hydrochloride (*BP*) and Meclizine hydrochloride (*USP*)
Chemical name: 1-*p*-chlorodiphenylmethyl-4-*m*-methylbenzylpiperazine dihydrochloride

Meclozine is a competitive antihistamine acting on H_1-receptors with marked antiemetic action which lasts for 12–24 hours. Side effects are said to be rare.

It has been widely investigated for teratogenic effects and the data sheet allows its use during early pregnancy. It can also be used for radiation and travel sickness, and in the treatment of urticaria, dermatoses, and allergic reactions.

Meclozine is given by mouth in tablet form, 25 mg combined with pyridoxine 50 mg. Up to 100 mg a day may be given in divided doses if necessary.

Mepyramine maleate

Mepyramine maleate (*BP*) and Pyrilamine maleate (*USP*)
Chemical name: *N*-*p*-methoxybenzyl-*N′N′*-dimethyl-*N*-pyrid-2-ylethylenediamine hydrogen
maleate

Mepyramine maleate is a competitive antihistamine acting at H_1-receptors and, although slightly less potent than promethazine and shorter in action, its effects last for 8–16 hours and it is still one of the most active of this group in use. Side effects may occur in about 20 per cent of cases. They include drowsiness, mild headache, and visual disturbances, which may be marked, and sometimes gastric irritation occurs.

It is used for the treatment of hay fever, urticaria, and anaphylactic reactions and is given by mouth in tablet form or as an elixir. The commencing adult dose is 300 mg daily in divided doses, and the maximum dose should not exceed 1 g daily. It can also be given slowly intravenously, 50 mg of a 2.5 per cent solution, but should only be used in emergency by this route.

Salbutamol

Salbutamol (*BP*) and Albuterol (*USAN*)
Chemical name: 1-(4-hydroxy-3-hydroxymethylphenyl)-2-(tert-butylamino)ethanol

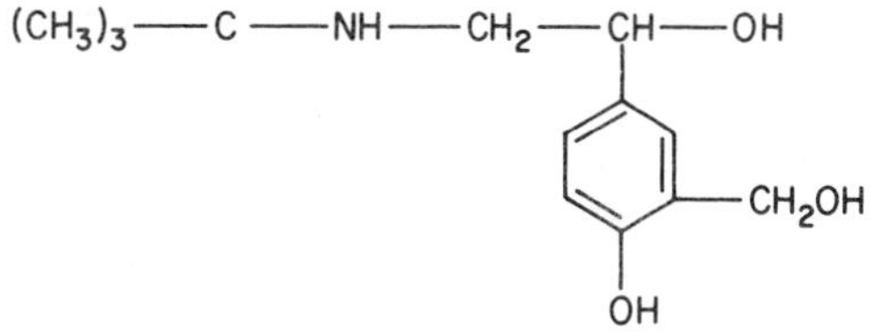

$(CH_3)_3$—C—NH—CH_2—CH—OH

CH_2OH

OH

PHARMACOLOGY
Salbutamol is a selective β-adrenergic stimulant which has little or no action on β_1-receptors. It belongs to a new series of agents in which the —OH group in position 3 of isoprenaline is replaced by a —CH_2OH group. It resulted from research to find a β-adrenergic stimulant free from action on the heart. From a therapeutic point of view, it certainly appears to have a highly selective action on bronchial musculature, lack of effect on the myocardium, and a long duration of action, when administered in the usual way by an aerosol inhaler. However, when given intravenously it produces much less apparent selectivity. Its long action after inhalation may therefore simply indicate that absorption is very poor from the inhalation site, and thus the effect on the heart is slight. By the intravenous route the drug reaches both sites indiscriminately and thus its true nature becomes apparent. In all species so far tested, salbutamol is a more potent bronchodilator than isoprenaline when administered by aerosol or by mouth and about equally active intravenously.

Studies on asthmatic volunteers using a whole-body plethysmograph show that doses of 100 μg of salbutamol by inhalation produced a substantial and almost immediate reduction in airway resistance for several hours. In normal volunteers doses of up to 400 μg by inhalation have no effect on heart rate, ECG, or blood pressure. In the same subjects 200 μg of isoprenaline has marked cardiovascular effects. Its duration of action is 4–6 hours because it is not metabolized by catechol-*O*-methyl transferase, the enzyme which rapidly inactivates isoprenaline in the body.

Onset of action is rapid by inhalation and near-maximal bronchodilatation occurs within 5 minutes. Side effects are not seen with normal therapeutic dosage. Doses greatly in excess of those needed for full bronchodilatation may cause short-lived secondary effects, such as peripheral vasodilatation, minor increase in pulse rate, and skeletal muscle tremor.

INDICATIONS
Salbutamol may be used in the treatment of asthma and all other types of bronchospasm. It is also used to inhibit uterine activity in premature labour.

DOSAGE AND ADMINISTRATION
Salbutamol is administered from a metered aerosol inhaler, delivering 100 μg at each inhalation. As the duration of action is at least 4 hours, the number of

inhalations should not exceed eight in any 24-hour period. It can be given as a slow intravenous injection in a dose of 2–4 μg/kg and by mouth in amounts of 2–4 mg three to four times a day.

PRECAUTIONS

If a previously effective treatment lasts for less than 3 hours, diagnosis and therapy should be reconsidered. Like that of ephedrine when administered regularly by mouth, the bronchodilator effect of salbutamol gradually wanes after a period of 1–3 weeks of continuous therapy. As with other β-stimulants, therefore, it is advisable to reserve its use for the relief of acute asthmatic symptoms, and not to attempt to maintain continuous bronchodilatation.

Terbutaline is similar to salbutamol in that it selectively stimulates the β-receptors in the bronchial musculature while affecting the β_1-receptors in the heart to a lesser extent. Its action reaches a peak in 30 minutes after subcutaneous injection and in 2–3 hours after oral administration. Its duration of action after a single oral dose of 5 mg is similar to salbutamol 5 mg orally, and of the order of 5–6 hours. The normal dose is 2–4 mg three times a day.

Triprolidine hydrochloride

Triprolidine hydrochloride (*BP* and *USP*)
Chemical name: (*E*)-2-[3-(pyrrolidin-1-yl)-1-*p*-tolylprop-1-enyl]pyridine hydrochloride

Triprolidine is a competitive antihistamine acting at H_1-receptors. It is the most potent of the antihistamines and is stated to be 10 times more so than promethazine, although its side effects are less marked. It reaches its maximal activity in 3 hours and is of shorter duration than promethazine, lasting about 12 hours. It is used in the treatment of the common allergic conditions, including hay fever, the dermatoses, and urticaria. The recommended dose is 2.5 mg three times a day by mouth, but doses up to 16 mg may be given if necessary.

9

Neuromuscular blocking agents

Muscle tone, a form of partial tetanus, is thought to be maintained by continuous nervous impulses originating in the anterior horn cells of the spinal cord.

Complete muscular paralysis can be produced by blocking these impulses centrally by deep general anaesthesia, peripherally through nerve block by local analgesics, or by blocking myoneural transmission by certain specific drugs; these latter are known as muscle relaxants, myoneural, or neuromuscular blocking drugs. Of these terms, neuromuscular blocking drug is to be preferred, being the term that most accurately describes the mode of action.

Some degree of muscular relaxation can also be obtained by drugs acting on the spinal cord, such as mephenesin, diazepam, and chlorpromazine. The rigidity of parkinsonism is also relieved by drugs acting centrally.

Agents that act on the muscle itself are also now available and are of some value in relieving spasticity. Because of its special importance to anaesthetists, a monograph on dantrolene is included; this drug is *not* a neuromuscular blocking agent but is included in this chapter for the sake of convenience.

Physiology of neuromuscular transmission

At the junctional region between nerve and muscle there is a specialized portion of muscle membrane known as the motor end-plate. Under resting conditions selective permeability enables an unequal distribution of ions to be maintained between the inside and outside of the cell. The primary ionic disequilibrium is due to the active extrusion of Na^+ from the cell, a process that requires energy. The electrical gradient that results induces an unequal distribution of K^+, so that the intracellular concentration of this ion is higher than the extracellular. This, of course, tends partly to neutralize the intracellular electronegativity that would result from the unequal Na^+ distribution, but the concentration gradient that develops limits the extent of the K^+ influx. The net result of this ionic distribution is a difference of electrical potential across the membrane of the cell so that the inside is about −90 mV.

The arrival of a motor nerve impulse results in the release of acetylcholine from storage vesicles in the nerve terminal, but there is a delay of about 1 ms between the crest of the nerve action potential and the release of transmitter. The mechanism that couples depolarization to release is sensitive to the concentration of Ca^{2+} and Mg^{2+}. The released acetylcholine reacts with receptors in the end-plate to cause a breakdown of the impermeability of the membrane to Na^+, followed by an outward migration of K^+. This loss of polarization constitutes the end-plate potential, and the end-plate is said to be 'depolarized'.

The end-plate potential is a non-propagated potential, but if it exceeds about 45 mV the membrane potential is reduced from about −90 mV to about −45 mV, and the adjoining muscle fibre membrane is 'short-circuited'. This potential, which is propagated along the fibre and causes it to contract, is known as the propagated action potential.

Within a few milliseconds of its release, acetylcholine is hydrolysed to almost totally inactive choline and acetic acid. The cell membrane regains its original impermeability to Na^+, this being extruded from the cell and partially replaced by K^+, and the end-plate and muscle fibre become repolarized.

Neuromuscular block

Interference with the mechanism described above will stop nerve impulses which arrive at the motor end-plate from causing contraction of the muscle fibre. The following main types of block are recognized.

Deficiency block

Two types of deficiency block are theoretically possible: interference with synthesis of transmitter and interference with its release. Hemicholinium and triethylcholine act competitively on the synthesis of acetylcholine and are antagonized by choline. Their effects are slow in onset, being manifest only as the presynaptic store of transmitter is depleted. Many drugs, including botulinus toxin, local anaesthetics, neomycin, kanamycin, and streptomycin, as well as calcium deficiency and magnesium excess, diminish the quantal release of acetylcholine per nerve impulse, and may enhance clinical block produced by competitive receptor blocking drugs.

Competitive block

In competitive block the agents compete with acetylcholine for the end-plate receptors, but once attached to them they do not cause depolarization. They are often, therefore, referred to as non-depolarizing blocking drugs. This terminology is not to be recommended, since it merely describes what the drug does *not* do. Once such a drug occupies a significant number of receptors, there are fewer receptors to which acetylcholine can become attached and consequently a lower end-plate potential follows a nerve impulse. If sufficient blocking drug is present, the end-plate potential will fail to reach the triggering threshold, and neuromuscular block occurs.

Drugs that cause neuromuscular block by this mechanism include tubocurarine, gallamine, alcuronium, pancuronium, and fazadinium. Their action can be opposed by increasing the local concentration of acetylcholine, and this can be brought about by giving anticholinesterases, such as neostigmine. Their action is enhanced when there is a diminution of the presynaptic quantal release of acetylcholine, as in myasthenia, or in the presence of certain antibiotics. Competitive blockade is enhanced by volatile anaesthetics in a concentration-dependent manner. Even anaesthetics that do not by themselves appear to have an effect on neuromuscular transmission always potentiate competitive blocking agents.

Depolarization block

Drugs producing this form of block, such as decamethonium and suxamethonium, are agonists of acetylcholine at end-plate receptors but, unlike acetylcholine, the depolarization caused by these drugs persists for more than a few milliseconds. The initial depolarization produced causes a muscular contraction, seen as a short period of muscular fasciculation. Action potential records show that this is the result of repetitive firing of the muscle fibres. This may be a reflex initiated by the sudden depolarization of the muscle spindle.

If depolarizing drugs are applied for prolonged periods, partial repolarization of the end-plate takes place. Nevertheless, the persistence of neuromuscular blockade in the clinical situation is normally associated with continuing depolarization. Another consequence of a long-continuing depolarization is the development of an area of reduced excitability of the surrounding muscle membrane which is associated with loss of potassium.

Dual block

This term was introduced by Zaimis (1953) to describe the actions of tridecamethonium in chicks, in which an initial muscle contracture is followed by a flaccid paralysis. The initial contracture is predominantly due to an action on the muscle membrane. A 'dual' action has since been described in some muscles in some species (but not in man) where the phenomenon is undoubtedly due to the action of the drug at the end-plate. In some muscles this response is the normal response to a normal dose, unlike the allegedly analogous situation in man which requires large doses, prolonged administration, or an abnormality of muscle. For example, some myasthenic muscles undoubtedly exhibit a dual response to decamethonium.

Desensitization block

This term was introduced by Thesleff (1955) and renamed receptor inactivation by Nastuk, Manthey and Gissen (1966), and was used to describe a condition in which application of a depolarizing drug causes the end-plate to become refractory to chemical stimulation. This phenomenon is relatively easy to produce in isolated muscle if unphysiologically high concentrations of drugs are given. It is probable that potassium loss is an important factor in its development. If large doses of suxamethonium are given for a prolonged period some evidence of desensitization can be elicited.

Phase I and II block

These terms have been borrowed from a 'two-phase' action of decamethonium in certain selected *in vitro* muscle preparations. The first phase is a neuromuscular block which lasts a few minutes and then recovers spontaneously even in the continued presence of the drug. After 15–30 minutes a progressive block develops which reaches a steady state in about 30 minutes and persists for hours if undisturbed. Suxamethonium or acetylcholine (in the presence of a cholinesterase inhibitor) can produce a similar effect in these special circumstances. These unphysiological conditions are unlikely to be of much relevance to any clinical situation.

The relevance to clinical practice of these three abnormal types of response to depolarizing drugs is still debated, as is the best descriptive term for the clinical syndrome. Increasingly, Phase I and Phase II is the terminology being employed.

The existence of a Phase II type of block in man has been denied by some pharmacologists but there is a general acceptance by anaesthetists that in clinical practice the characteristics of neuromuscular blockade produced by depolarizing blocking drugs can change with time, particularly if the drugs have been used in high dosage or over a long period and develop some of the characteristics of competitive blockade. The signs that have been thought to indicate the late development of a competitive blockade have been the demonstration of post-tetanic potentiation and 'fade' (*see* page 262), a change in the response to a train-of-four (TOF) stimuli (*see* page 261), and reversal of the block by anticholinesterases. These signs have been demonstrable in cases of prolonged paralysis after suxamethonium, particularly when there is some evidence of recovery. A simple explanation of these phenomena should not be overlooked. At this stage a proportion of end-plates may have recovered from the block and will then demonstrate these phenomena even though the majority of the muscle still remains paralysed.

Another possible explanation is provided by some evidence in cats, the neuromuscular junction of which resembles man in its responses to drugs. In this species, large doses of depolarizing drugs impair prejunctional release of acetylcholine; if this is also true in man this would explain the fade, the post-tetanic facilitation, and the response to cholinesterase inhibitors.

Measurement of neuromuscular blockade

Direct measurement is now almost universally employed, the commonest practice being to stimulate the ulnar nerve and record the response of the abductor pollicis or the muscles of the hypothenar eminence. The response to nerve stimulation can be measured in two ways, either by recording integrated action potentials from surface or needle electrodes, or by measuring the muscle tension developed during the contraction. It is important to realize that these two measurements are not comparable because they do not measure the same thing. The action potential provides a measure of the electrical activity generated in a limited number of muscle fibres whereas the tension measures the response of the whole muscle.

While the introduction of direct measurements has enabled both qualitative and quantitative aspects of neuromuscular blockade to be recorded readily, the employment of a wide range of techniques of stimulation has led to a good deal of confusion. If the compound action potential is measured, it is essential to ensure that the electrodes cannot move and therefore the muscle must be tested in isometric contraction.

When muscle contraction is recorded, a force transducer is used. It is essential to ensure that the direction of movement of the transducer is aligned with the pull exerted by the muscle and that the resting tension is kept constant. The motor nerve may be stimulated with either needle or surface electrodes. The stimulus duration should be less than 0.2 ms; longer stimuli can result in double stimulation or repetitive firing of the muscle. The intensity of the stimulus must produce a maximal response. The pattern of stimulation also can influence the results; tetanus should be at a frequency of 30–50 Hz; single stimuli may be applied at intervals of 2–5 seconds. Tetanic stimuli should not be applied more frequently than at 5-minute intervals.

The chief clinical application of such measurements is in the assessment of residual neuromuscular blockade. In this situation it is likely that baseline measurements will not be available. To circumvent this difficulty, Ali, Utting and

Gray (1971) described a technique of using a TOF supramaximal stimuli in 2 seconds, followed by an interval of 10–12 seconds. This technique of assessment has several advantages. Unlike tetanus, the stimuli are acceptable in the conscious patient and do not alter the character or intensity of the block. Different types of neuromuscular block produce characteristic responses and baseline values are not essential to the assessment.

During a competitive blockade (*Figure 9.1*) there is a progressive reduction in the height of the response to the four stimuli. The ratio of the fourth twitch to the first has been called the TOF ratio. The greater the intensity of the blockade, the smaller this ratio. During recovery this ratio increases again: when it reaches 0.70–0.75 a single twitch (or the first of the four) will have returned to the control value (C in *Figure 9.2*) and tetanic fade (*see* below) will not be demonstrable. In contrast, a partial depolarizing block shows well-sustained twitches at all levels of block. Both this test and the phenomena originally observed by Churchill-Davidson and Christie (1959) are interpretable in terms of underlying mechanisms, some of

Non-depolarizing neuromuscular block

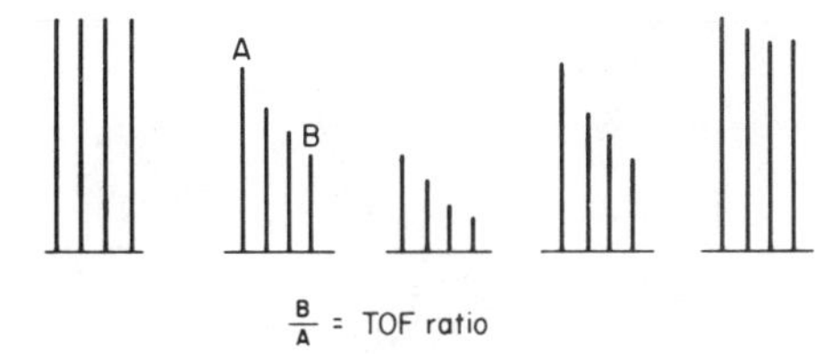

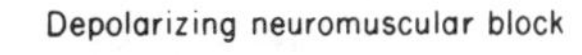

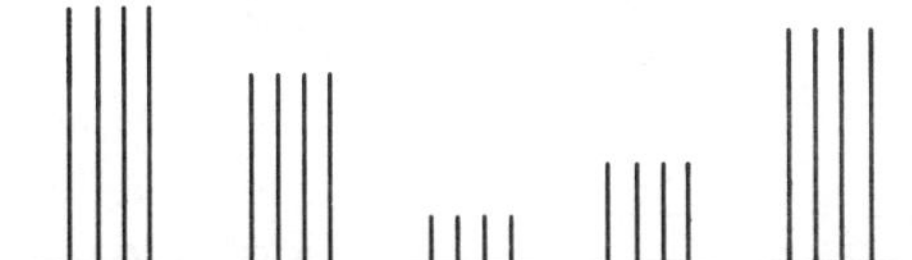

Figure 9.1 A diagrammatic representation of the response to train-of-four (TOF) nerve stimulation. The upper trace shows the response to a moderate dose of a competitive agent demonstrating a TOF ratio (*see* text) of about 0.4 at the height of the block. The lower trace shows the effect of partial depolarizing block with an unchanged TOF ratio of 1.0

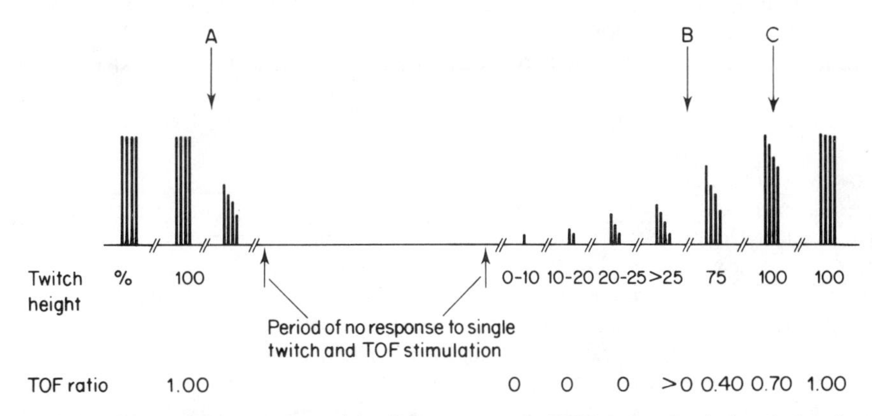

Figure 9.2 A diagrammatic representation of the response to TOF nerve stimulation during the onset and recovery from an intense competitive neuromuscular block. A = injection of relaxant; B = injection of neostigmine

which are related to the normal behaviour of muscle and some of which are presynaptic in origin. Some descriptive terms are used by different authors to mean different things and some precision is desirable.

Post-tetanic potentiation is an increase in twitch tension which occurs physiologically in normal muscle following tetanic stimulation. It is unassociated with any change in the muscle action potential, thus indicating that the effect is due to a change in the contractile properties of the muscle.

Post-tetanic 'decurarization' is associated with an increase in the compound muscle action potential as well as in the muscle tension, in response to a single stimulus following tetanic stimulation during partial competitive neuromuscular block. The increase in the muscle action potential indicates that more muscle fibres are firing; this is due to the effects of the tetanus on presynaptic mechanisms and is discussed below.

Tetanic fade occurs physiologically in fatigued muscle or when unphysiologically fast rates of motor nerve stimulation are used. It is, however, readily demonstrated in the presence of competitive blocking drugs at normal rates of stimulation.

Post-tetanic fade is the waning of the post-tetanic decurarization induced by a tetanic burst of stimuli.

Post-tetanic facilitation is a term used by some authors to describe both post-tetanic decurarization and post-tetanic potentiation. There is some logic in this in that the phenomenon presumably is a summation of both processes. It should not be forgotten, however, that two different mechanisms underlie it. Post-tetanic potentiation is a physiologically normal event, whereas post-tetanic decurarization depends on a presynaptic action which is made obvious by the presence of a partial competitive neuromuscular blockade.

Under normal conditions the store of transmitter in the nerve terminal is sufficient for many thousands of impulses, but a considerable amount is not available for immediate release. The immediately accessible fraction is readily depleted by a sequence of impulses, and an early decline in end-plate potential size during a tetanic burst is the manifestation of this. However, since the end-plate potential is much in excess of threshold, this reduction is not clinically obvious. When the end-plate potential is reduced by the presence of a competitive blocking drug, a reduction in end-plate potential will result in it falling below threshold in some fibres, and increasing weakness or 'fade' will result.

However, the nerve potentials have a further important presynaptic action, in that each impulse facilitates the release of acetylcholine by a subsequent impulse. During a tetanic burst this facilitation is proceeding to a marked extent, even though the exhaustion of the readily available fraction disguises it. Following the tetanus, the facilitation persists for a short period, and single impulses during this time will release larger quanta of transmitter, with a consequent increase in end-plate potential which may now reach threshold and trigger an action potential in a previously unresponsive fibre. There is thus recruitment of muscle fibres with an increase in the compound action potential and in the developed tension leading to post-tetanic decurarization. This facilitation of transmitter release is transitory and the response soon fades off again. The rapidity of the fade is enhanced by the fact that the facilitated release exhausts the readily available fraction even more quickly. These features are illustrated in the top panel of *Figure 9.3* which shows the characteristic electromyographic picture of a competitive block which exhibits fade and post-tetanic decurarization.

In the presence of depolarizing drugs a variety of responses may be seen. If the block is intense the end-plate will be insensitive and no transmission will occur.

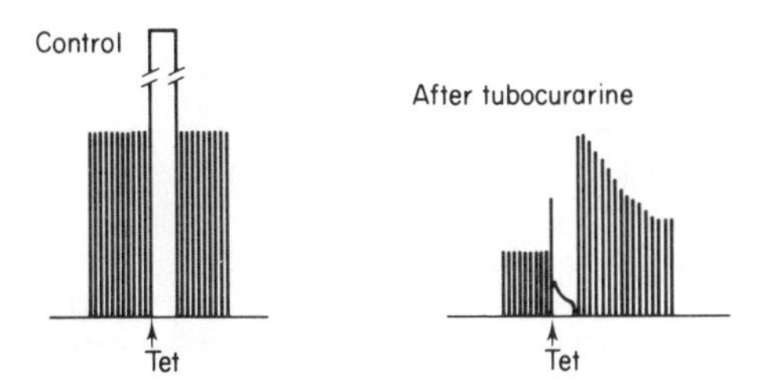

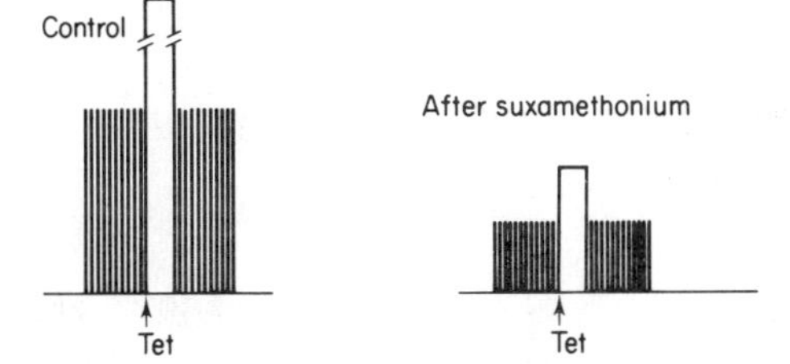

Figure 9.3 A diagrammatic representation of the response to tetanic and post-tetanic single twitch stimulation. Upper panel, control and following a subparalysing dose of tubocurarine; lower panel, control and after a subparalysing dose of suxamethonium. Tet = a tetanic burst 50 Hz for 5 seconds

With incomplete blocking concentrations, however, the presence of the drug lowers the threshold for triggering an action potential and smaller quanta of acetylcholine are adequate for transmission. As a consequence, even the reduced quanta available during repetitive stimulation maintain good tone in those muscle fibres whose end-plates have not been depolarized. The clinical manifestation, then, is either of complete block or of a weak response that is well sustained and unaffected by tetanic stimulation. This situation is illustrated in the lower panel of *Figure 9.3*.

Pharmacokinetics of relaxants

All the clinically used neuromuscular blocking drugs are quaternary ammonium compounds which are fully ionized at normal body pH. They are largely lipid insoluble, and therefore do not cross cell membranes, and are largely confined to the extracellular fluid. The distribution and metabolic fate differ from drug to drug. Suxamethonium is rapidly hydrolysed by plasma cholinesterase; the rate of decay of the pharmacological effect (twitch depression) is unaffected by the initial dose. Decamethonium is excreted unchanged in the urine.

The competitive relaxants undergo both renal excretion and hepatic metabolism, but the relative importance of these two routes differs from drug to drug. Gallamine is heavily dependent on renal excretion but the other drugs currently available have sufficient hepatic metabolism to be usable in renal failure, at least with moderate doses. The new relaxants, vecuronium and atracurium, are both preferable, however, being even less dependent on the renal route.

After intravenous administration the plasma drug concentrations decline in two phases: an initial rapid fall due to redistribution (described by the distribution half-life $t_{1/2}^{\alpha}$) and a slower fall due to elimination (the elimination half-life $t_{1/2}^{\beta}$). Both are exponential in character. The volume of distribution at steady state ($V_{d(ss)}$) is small and varies from 200–450 ml/kg. These terms, plus a value for *clearance* (*Cl*, the volume of plasma from which all the relaxant is removed in unit time), are sufficient to describe the pharmacokinetics of any competitive relaxant.

Clinical use of relaxants

During the last 25 years muscle relaxants have come to be employed routinely in major surgery and to a considerable extent for even minor surgical procedures, the main advantage being that with their aid lighter levels of anaesthesia may be employed. The use of nitrous oxide and oxygen alone for the maintenance of anaesthesia was once widely practised but most anaesthetists now prefer to use some other supplement in order to guarantee amnesia and to minimize autonomic and hormonal responses.

The competitive blocking drugs are more commonly used for major surgical operations as their duration of action is longer (20–45 minutes); the shorter acting depolarizing agents are more often employed for short procedures, such as endoscopies, bronchoscopies, and manipulations, when only a brief period of relaxation is required. These latter drugs have also been used in repeated doses or by intravenous infusion for major operations, but have the disadvantage that a dual block inevitably develops.

The sensitivity of different muscle groups to relaxant drugs varies considerably; thus, the muscles of the eyelids are paralysed most easily, and then relaxation of the limbs and jaws, intercostals, and abdominal muscles follows with increasing dosage, and finally the diaphragm will be paralysed. There is considerable overlapping of these effects, and even small doses insufficient to produce abdominal relaxation may depress respiration.

Residual weakness due to competitive agents should be treated with neostigmine preceded by atropine. In the case of that due to depolarizing drugs, artificial respiration should be continued until ventilation is adequate.

It has been common practice in recent years to use suxamethonium for intubation, and later to give a long-acting competitive relaxant for maintenance of relaxation during operation. This practice rarely gives rise to complications. Suxamethonium has also been given following the administration of a competitive blocking drug to provide relaxation for the closure of the peritoneum. However, this practice may lead to difficulties if neostigmine is given to reverse the competitive block before the suxamethonium has been metabolized or the end-plate regained its normal sensitivity, and is not recommended as a routine practice.

A fall in temperature enhances the effect of depolarizing relaxants but diminishes the effect of competitive relaxants. As a consequence, higher doses of tubocurarine may be necessary during hypothermia, and these will be excessive when the patient's temperature rises.

Apart from their use in anaesthesia for general surgery and obstetrics, muscle relaxants are used to minimize the convulsions in electroconvulsive therapy, and in the treatment of tetanus.

Katz and colleagues (1969) described apparent differences in the response of patients in London and New York to muscle relaxants. The duration of action of suxamethonium was less in British patients, as were the magnitude and duration of action of tubocurarine. United States Air Force personnel stationed in London retained their American pattern of response. No explanation for these differences has yet been forthcoming.

Prolonged apnoea and respiratory depression

A wide variety of circumstances can be responsible for prolonged apnoea or respiratory depression after the use of neuromuscular blocking drugs. Some are not directly due to the action of the drugs themselves, but to the facility they give to disguise other errors of technique. Thus, in the absence of the usual indications, an overdose of centrally acting narcotic or anaesthetic agent may be given, leading to central depression. Likewise, hyperventilation may be imposed on the patient leading to respiratory alkalosis. Thus, before a neuromuscular blocking drug is held responsible, myoneural block should be demonstrated with a peripheral nerve stimulator.

Possible causes of a continuing block should be considered in relation to the type of muscle relaxant employed; that is competitive, depolarizing, or a mixture of both.

After competitive muscle relaxants

Metabolic acidosis

Better management of fluid and electrolytes and the preoperative correction of metabolic acidosis has resulted in the virtual disappearance of a syndrome originally described as 'neostigmine-resistant' curarization. Three features dominated the clinical picture:

1. Inadequacy of respiration accompanied by a tracheal 'tug';
2. Tachycardia, hypotension, and raised central venous pressure;
3. Coma or semi-coma.

The onset of this syndrome in the immediate postoperative period led to the belief that penetration of the CNS by the relaxant might be involved. It seems more likely that the probable sequence was as follows: preoperative dehydration and metabolic acidosis in an elderly patient with limited ventilatory reserve was just compensated by respiratory alkalosis. At the end of operation, however, a painful incision and a continuing distension caused the compensatory respiratory alkalosis to be replaced by a complicating respiratory acidosis which led to a rapid fall in pH.

Inadequate respiration unresponsive to neostigmine, particularly if accompanied by coma and cardiovascular depression, calls for continued ventilation, assessment of acid–base state, and appropriate alkali therapy. Both intravascular and extracellular fluid and electrolyte therapy should be critically reappraised, with central venous pressure and ECG monitoring. Undoubtedly many such patients have died with a diagnosis of 'postoperative collapse' or other euphemisms, and the outcome has been excused on the grounds that the patients were too ill to withstand the effects of the operation.

Myasthenia gravis–myasthenic syndrome
Latent myasthenia gravis may first be manifest by unexpected sensitivity to competitive relaxants, as may be the myasthenic syndrome, associated with carcinoma of the bronchus.

Antibiotics
The antibiotics neomycin, streptomycin, and kanamycin can cause neuromuscular blockade which is similar to that produced by high concentrations of magnesium, or by calcium deficiency. It is thus presynaptic and is due to a reduction in the amount of transmitter released by each nerve impulse. The block is usually only clinically significant when the end-plate potential is simultaneously reduced by competitive blocking agents. Neostigmine may restore transmission. Calcium gluconate will produce further improvement.

After depolarizing agents

Overdose
The continuance of high circulating levels of depolarizing relaxants can lead to the onset of a dual block in some patients. This is rarely accompanied by apnoea but may cause neuromuscular inadequancy lasting for up to an hour or more.

Low plasma cholinesterase
This can lead to a prolonged action of suxamethonium, but is unlikely to be clinically significant until the level falls to around 10–15 per cent of the normal level. This only occurs in severe liver disease, or in the presence of cholinesterase inhibitors.

Atypical enzyme
Complete apnoea for periods in excess of 5–10 minutes in fit individuals after a normal dose of suxamethonium may indicate the presence of an atypical plasma cholinesterase. These are genetically determined variants which do not metabolize suxamethonium. This was first demonstrated using as an enzyme inhibitor the local anaesthetic dibucaine (cinchocaine). In the presence of a 10^{-5} M concentration of this substance, the enzyme is about 80 per cent inhibited in 97 per cent of the population, who are believed to be homozygous for the 'usual' gene, which is responsible for the elaboration of the 'usual' enzyme. About 0.03 per cent of the population are homozygous for an atypical gene, and their enzyme is resistant to inhibition by dibucaine, being only about 20–25 per cent inhibited: 3 per cent of the population are heterozygous and are believed to have both types of enzyme in their serum. Their cholinesterase activity is about 60 per cent inhibited. The percentage inhibition of cholinesterase activity in the presence of a 10^{-5} M concentration of dibucaine is called the dibucaine number.

Sodium fluoride is also a differential inhibitor of cholinesterase variants, and the fluoride number can be similarly determined. By using this test, a subgroup of cases has been delineated within the atypical group which is unusually resistant to fluoride, but not particularly to dibucaine. A 'silent' gene which fails to elaborate any enzyme has also been discovered.

Concurrent administration of cholinesterase inhibitors
Ecothiopate in eye drops can be absorbed in sufficient amounts to affect plasma cholinesterase levels, and prolonged apnoea after suxamethonium has been reported. Some cancer chemotherapeutic agents have also been implicated. Patients suffering from poisoning by organophosphorus cholinesterase inhibitors would exhibit sensitivity to suxamethonium in addition to other derangements of neuromuscular function.

After mixtures of relaxants

There is no convincing evidence that there are any syndromes associated with mixtures of both types of relaxants beyond those which could have occurred with either type given alone. Indeed, elements of both kinds of block may be present in different muscle fibres. In such a situation, any associated physiological disturbance should be corrected and time should be allowed for the dual block to 'cure' itself. Further pharmacological interference is capable of worsening the situation.

Muscle rigidity and spasm

Muscle tone can be influenced by other mechanisms than blocking the neuromuscular junction. The rigidity and tremor of parkinsonism can best be relieved by levodopa, which is believed to act by restoring the level of dopamine in certain motor pathways in the brain. This is discussed in more detail in Chapter 7. Symptoms can also be relieved by the use of anticholinergic agents that penetrate the brain.

There are now many centrally acting drugs available for the relief of muscle spasm. Mephenesin is the oldest and best studied drug of this type but has been superseded by newer congeners such as orphenadrine, methocarbamol, and metaxalone. In animals these drugs diminish experimental hypertonia and protect against convulsive agents. In man, they can be employed to relieve spasticity, particularly associated with trauma and inflammation. They are all sedatives in large doses.

A third site of action for influencing muscle tone is the muscle itself. Dantrolene represents a class of muscle relaxant acting at this site. Its importance for anaesthetists is that it is effective in the treatment of malignant hyperpyrexia, an inherited condition associated with abnormal muscle metabolism. It is also given orally in spastic conditions such as those resulting from multiple sclerosis, spinal cord injury, stroke, and cerebral palsy.

Ali, H. H., Utting, J. E. and Gray, T. C. (1971) Quantitative assessment of residual antidepolarizing block (part II), *British Journal of Anaesthesia,* **43**, 478

Churchill-Davidson, H. C. and Christie, T. H. (1959) The diagnosis of neuromuscular block in man. *British Journal of Anaesthesia,* **31,** 290

Katz, R. L., Norman, J., Seed, R. F. and Conrad, L. (1969) A comparison of the effects of suxamethonium and tubocurarine in patients in London and New York. *British Journal of Anaesthesia,* **41,** 1041

Nastuk, W. L., Manthey, A. A. and Gissen, A. J. (1966) Activation and inactivation of post-junctional membrane receptors. *Annals of the New York Academy of Sciences,* **137,** 999

Thesleff, S. (1955) The mode of neuromuscular block caused by acetylcholine, nicotine, decamethonium and succinylcholine. *Acta Physiologica Scandinavica,* **34,** 218

Zaimis, E. (1953) Motor end-plate differences as a determining factor in the mode of action in neuromuscular blocking substances. *Journal of Physiology,* **122,** 238

Alcuronium chloride

Alcuronium chloride (*BAN* and *USAN*)
Chemical name: NN′-diallylbisnortoxiferinium dichloride

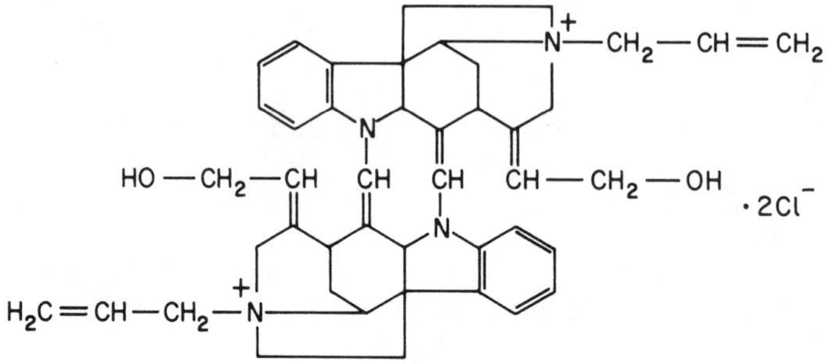

Alcuronium is a derivative of calabash curare alkaloid C-toxiferine-I and is prepared from toxiferine by the substitution of an allyl radical in each of the two quaternary ammonium groups.

It is a competitive muscle relaxant, about twice as potent as tubocurarine, but its duration of action is slightly longer. As with tubocurarine, hypotension may follow its use. Indeed, it is very difficult to distinguish between the cardiovascular effects of alcuronium and tubocurarine. There is usually a small fall in mean blood pressure and a slight rise in pulse rate. Alcuronium is bound to serum albumin.

Alcuronium can be used in any situation in which any other competitive relaxant could be employed and 10–20 mg may be given intravenously, depending on the site of operation and degree of relaxation required; further doses of 3–5 mg can be given as necessary. If halothane is being used for the maintenance of anaesthesia smaller doses will be required. Alcuronium is effectively antagonized by neostigmine. Precautions are the same as for other muscle relaxants.

Atracurium dibesylate

Atracurium dibesylate (*BAN*)
Chemical name: 2,2′-(3,11-dioxo-4,10-dioxatridecylene)-bis-[6,7-dimethoyl-1(3,4-dimethoxy-benzyl)-2-methyl-1,2,3,4-tetrahydroisoquinolinium] dibenzenesulphonate

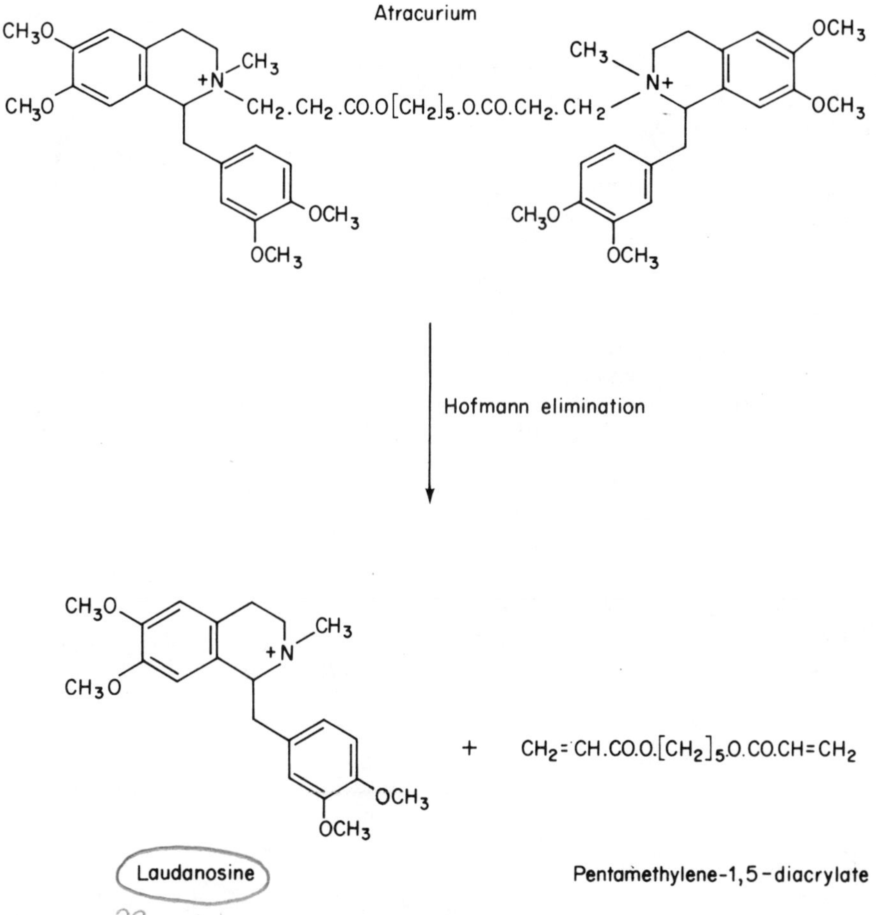

Atracurium
CH3O
CH3O
CH3
+N
CH2.CH2.CO.O[CH2]5.O.CO.CH2.CH2
CH3
N+
OCH3
OCH3
OCH3
OCH3
CH3O
OCH3
Hofmann elimination
CH3O
CH3O
CH3
+N
OCH3
OCH3
+
CH2=CH.CO.O.[CH2]5.O.CO.CH=CH2
Laudanosine
Pentamethylene-1,5-diacrylate

?? could -> convulsions

PHARMACOLOGY

Atracurium is a highly specific, competitive, neuromuscular blocking agent which undergoes spontaneous breakdown into inactive fragments at body temperature and at physiological pH. This 'Hofmann elimination' is illustrated above. It has a relatively short onset of action and it is claimed that intubation can be achieved in 1.5–2 minutes with doses of 0.6 mg/kg. The duration of action depends on the dose and lies between about 20 and 40 minutes for doses of 0.3–0.6 mg/kg. Supplementary doses of one third as much extend the duration of action for an equal time. Such doses are not cumulative and have a similar effect.

Cardiovascular system. There is normally little histamine release with recommended doses although it has been reported. There is also little effect on autonomic ganglia (Payne and Hughes, 1981). However, cases of severe bradycardia during surgery have been reported (Carter, 1983).

Respiratory system. Effects are similar to those with other muscle relaxants. There should be little risk of bronchospasm.

Muscular system. Striated muscles are paralysed by a competitive action at the myoneural junction. Onset is claimed to be more rapid than with tubocurarine, but this may be related to the use of non-equipotent doses. Duration of effective action is dose dependent and lies between 20 and 40 minutes. The duration of action can be extended by further supplements in a predictable way. The blockade terminates spontaneously within about 30–40 minutes of the last dose. Recovery can be hastened by the administration of neostigmine, preceded by atropine or another antimuscarinic drug. Recovery from full blockade takes 10 minutes.

Placental barrier. Placental transfer of significant quantities of drug is unlikely.

Fate in the body. Hofmann elimination (*see* above) is the principal mode of breakdown; the breakdown products are inactive. There is also a breakdown pathway by non-specific esterases. Termination of action is thus unaffected by renal or hepatic failure and it has been used successfully in anephric patients (Hunter, Jones and Utting, 1982).

INDICATIONS

Atracurium may be used in any situation in which other competitive muscle relaxants could be used but would seem to be particularly indicated in the presence of renal or hepatic failure. Its relative lack of cardiovascular effects would also appear to be an advantage in many clinical situations.

DOSAGE AND ADMINISTRATION

The initial intravenous dose lies between 0.3 and 0.6 mg/kg. The latter dose is necessary when the patient is to be intubated; a smaller dose can be used when the drug is given after intubation under suxamethonium. The doses for children over the age of 1 year can be calculated on the same dose/body weight basis. Supplementary doses lie between 0.1 and 0.2 mg/kg, depending on the duration of action required. Dosage should be reduced by about one third in the presence of hypothermia to 25°C. Changes in body pH within the physiological range seem to have little effect. The action is potentiated by halothane and by aminoglycoside antibiotics.

Carter, M. L. (1983) Bradycardia after the use of atracurium. *British Medical Journal*, **3**, 247

Hunter, J. M., Jones, R. S. and Utting, J. E. (1982) Use of the muscle relaxant atracurium in anephric patients: preliminary communication. *Journal of the Royal Society of Medicine*, **75**, 336

Payne, J. P. and Hughes, R. (1981) Evaluation of atracurium in anaesthetized man. *British Journal of Anaesthesia*, **53**, 45

Dantrolene sodium

Dantrolene (*BAN*)
Chemical name: 1-(5-*p*-nitrophenylfurfurylideneamino)hydantoin

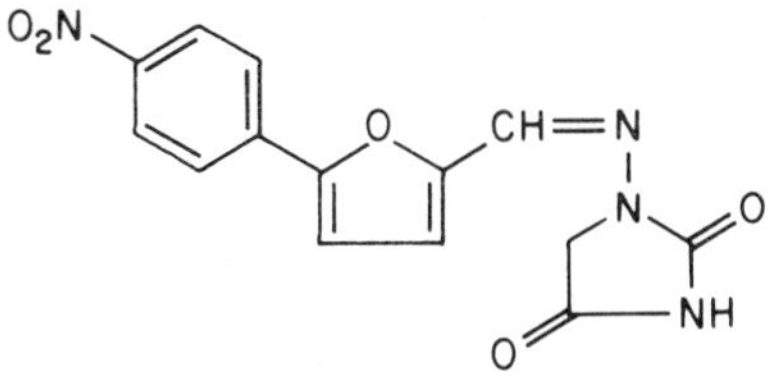

The drug is presented as a dry orange-coloured powder, consisting of dantrolene 20 mg, mannitol 3 g, and sufficient sodium hydroxide to make a solution of approximate pH 9.5. It is also available in tablet form.

PHARMACOLOGY

Dantrolene uncouples excitation–contraction coupling in isolated muscle preparations, probably by interfering with the release of ionic calcium from the sarcoplasmic reticulum. In the malignant hyperpyrexia syndrome, triggering agents, notably suxamethonium, halothane, and other volatile inhalational agents, cause a rise in myoplasmic calcium, although it is not absolutely certain whether this is due to accelerated release from the sarcoplasmic reticulum or failure of this structure to re-accumulate it. The effectiveness of dantrolene in preventing and treating the condition in susceptible pigs (a syndrome that is believed to be the same as the human one) suggests the former possibility.

Dantrolene has no action on neuromuscular transmission, the membrane action potential, or muscle excitability. However, it diminishes the force of contraction of muscles stimulated via the motor nerve. Reflex contractions are affected more than voluntary ones.

INDICATIONS

The drug can be given by mouth in spastic conditions such as those resulting from multiple sclerosis, spinal cord injury, cardiovascular accident, and cerebral palsy. It is given intravenously in the treatment of the malignant hyperpyrexia syndrome.

DOSAGE AND ADMINISTRATION

For the treatment of spasticity, 25 mg daily should be administered initially, increasing cautiously up to a maximum of 400 mg/day. Doses above 225 mg a day are rarely required to achieve the maximum therapeutic effect.

For the treatment of malignant hyperpyrexia it is given by intravenous injection in a dose of 1 mg/kg, repeated if necessary up to 10 mg/kg. The average dose which has been required to reverse the syndrome has been in the region of 2–3 mg/kg. This drug has not been recommended for use as a prophylactic agent in known susceptible individuals, avoidance of all triggering agents being preferred.

PRECAUTIONS

The prognosis of untreated malignant hyperpyrexia is so poor that consideration of potential toxic effects is of no relevance when the drug is used acutely.

Dantrolene is potentially hepatotoxic and liver function tests should be performed before starting chronic therapy and thereafter at intervals. Other common side effects are drowsiness, weakness, fatigue, and diarrhoea.

Fazadinium bromide (This drug has been withdrawn since this edition was prepared)

Fazadinium bromide (*BAN*)
Chemical name: 1,1′-azobis(3-methyl-2-phenyl-1*H*-imidazo[1,2-*a*]pyridinium) dibromide

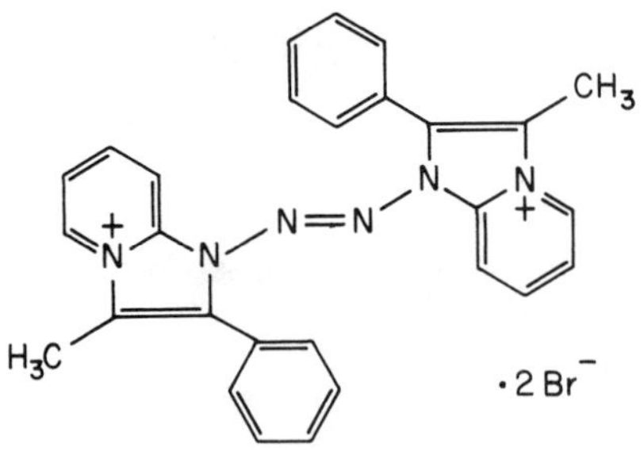

PHARMACOLOGY

Fazadinium is a rapidly acting, long-lasting competitive neuromuscular blocking agent. After an average initial intravous dose it acts within 60 seconds and its duration of action is about 40 minutes.

Cardiovascular system. Heart rate and cardiac output rise and there is an accompanying significant fall in stroke volume, central venous pressure, and systemic vascular resistance.Tachycardia may be quite marked and blood pressure may then rise. It is likely that these changes are due to ganglion blockade. Atropine increases these effects. There is no evidence of histamine release.

Respiratory system. Effects on respiration are similar to those with other muscle relaxants. The degree of paralysis of respiratory muscles is dose dependent.

Muscular system. Striated muscles are paralysed by a competitive action at the myoneural junction. Onset of action is more rapid than with tubocurarine. After a dose of 0.75 mg/kg intubation is possible within 60 seconds and the duration of action is about 40 minutes. Larger doses will shorten the time of onset of action and lengthen the duration of action. Paralysis is readily reversed by neostigmine in about 3 minutes.

Placental barrier. Placental transfer, should it occur, is minimal. No clinical effects on the infant following caesarean section have been reported.

Fate in the body. Fazadinium is eliminated mainly by excretion in the urine, but some hepatic metabolism also occurs.

INDICATIONS

Fazadinium can be used in clinical situations in which other competitive muscle relaxants are indicated. Its relatively quick onset of action led to it being promoted as an alternative to suxamethonium for rapid intubation but this does not seem to have become popular in practice.

DOSAGE AND ADMINISTRATION

The initial intravenous dose is 0.75–1 mg/kg or up to 75 mg for an average adult. Increments may be given as required.

PRECAUTIONS

These are similar to those for gallamine. Fazadinium is not a suitable drug for use in the presence of renal failure or for cardiac surgery. If it is so used, the greatest care should be exercised. Fazadinium solution (15 mg/ml) is bright yellow and stains the skin. It has a pH of 3.2–4.3 and should not be mixed with alkaline solutions, including thiopentone.

Gallamine triethiodide

Gallamine triethiodide (*BP* and *USP*)
Chemical name: 2,2′,2′′-(benzene-1,2,3-triyltrioxy)tris(tetraethylammonium) tri-iodide

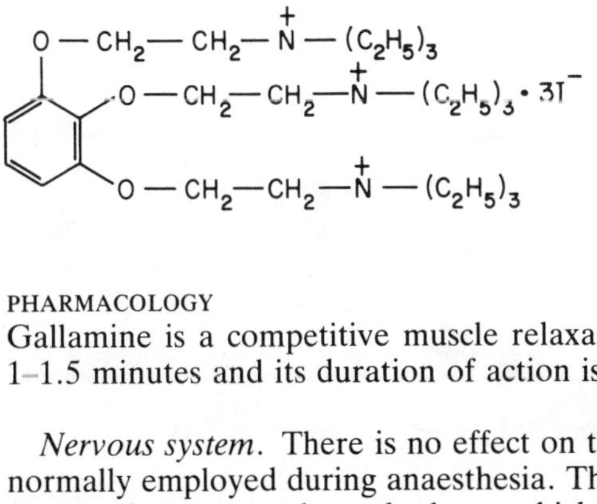

$O-CH_2-CH_2-\overset{+}{N}-(C_2H_5)_3$
$O-CH_2-CH_2-\overset{+}{N}-(C_2H_5)_3 \cdot 3I^-$
$O-CH_2-CH_2-\overset{+}{N}-(C_2H_5)_3$

PHARMACOLOGY

Gallamine is a competitive muscle relaxant. When given intravenously it acts in 1–1.5 minutes and its duration of action is 20–30 minutes.

Nervous system. There is no effect on the CNS or sympathetic ganglia in doses normally employed during anaesthesia. There is, however, an inhibitory action on the vagal nerve supply to the heart which results in tachycardia.

Cardiovascular system. The increased heart rate is occasionally accompanied by cardiac irregularities. Blood pressure usually remains unchanged but it may be increased if hypotension associated with bradycardia is already present.

Respiratory system. There is no action apart from depression of the muscles of respiration. Bronchospasm due to histamine release is extremely rare.

Muscular system. Relaxation of striated muscle follows a competitive blockade of the neuromuscular junction where this drug competes with acetylcholine.

Placental barrier. Appreciable amounts of gallamine cross the placenta, but the infant's ventilation is not affected clinically.

Fate in the body. Negligible amounts of gallamine are excreted in the absence of renal function. Gallamine is bound to serum albumin and the increase in potency in man with increasing pH which has been described is probably related to changes in this binding. Sensitivity occurs in myasthenia gravis, and in the presence of anaesthetics with a curare-like action such as ether.

INDICATIONS

The indications for the use of gallamine are similar to those for tubocurarine, but its briefer action has made it popular for short operations. However, if a full paralysing dose is still present at the end of the procedure, gallamine is in fact more difficult to reverse with neostigmine than an equipotent dose of tubocurarine or pancuronium.

DOSAGE AND ADMINISTRATION

Gallamine is normally given intravenously. It is approximately one sixth as potent as tubocurarine and may be substituted in proportionate dose in all the relaxant techniques described for tubocurarine.

An initial dose of 80–120 mg intravenously will produce full relaxation in 1.5–2 minutes. Duration of apnoea is variable but may last up to 10 minutes. Respiratory inadequacy lasts much longer.

Supplementary doses of 20–40 mg are given as required. These will be necessary at more frequent intervals than when tubocurarine is being used.

PRECAUTIONS

Gallamine should not be used in patients suffering from myasthenia gravis, in the presence of renal failure, or in cardiac surgery and serious heart disease where tachycardia is undesirable.

Pancuronium bromide

Pancuronium bromide (*BP* and *USAN*)
Chemical name: 1,1′-(3α,17β-diacetoxy-5α-androstan-2β,16β-ylene)bis (1-methylpiperidinium) dibromide

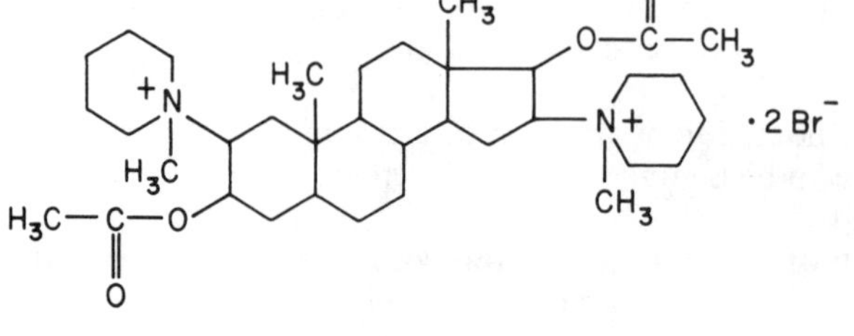

PHARMACOLOGY

Pancuronium is a synthetic muscle relaxant, and is a bisquaternary aminosteroid without hormonal activity. Since its introduction it has achieved wide popularity as a competitive muscle relaxant for routine use with a duration of action comparable to tubocurarine.

Nervous system. As with other relaxants of this type, the drug does not cross the blood-brain barrier. There is a mild vagolytic action on the heart but no evidence of ganglion blockade in normal doses.

Cardiovascular system. Pancuronium causes a moderate rise in pulse rate of about 20 per cent, a rise in arterial blood pressure of 10–20 per cent, and an increase in cardiac output. There is no change in peripheral vascular resistance. None of these changes is seen in atropinized patients, thus indicating that the mechanism is due to a vagolytic effect of the drug.

Respiratory system. Pancuronium appears to be free of histamine-releasing properties and has been used satisfactorily in patients with high bronchial reactivity, although bronchospasm has been reported very occasionally. Respiratory muscles are depressed or paralysed depending on the size of the dose.

Muscular system. Relaxation of striated muscle follows a competitive blockade of the neuromuscular junction. The onset of paralysis is quicker than with tubocurarine; after a dose of 0.15 mg/kg it is usually possible to intubate within 1.5 minutes. Paralysis is readily reversed by neostigmine, except within 10–20 minutes of a paralysing dose. It increases the tone of the lower oesophageal sphincter.

Kidney. Pancuronium can be used satisfactorily in cases of renal failure, although most of the dose is normally excreted via the kidney. It has been recommended for intubation and maintenance in renal transplantation but is being replaced by atracurium for this indication.

Placental barrier. Some pancuronium can be detected in the fetal blood, but no clinical effects on the fetus have been reported, and it may be used for operative obstetrics.

Fate in the body. Eighty-seven per cent of a clinical dose is protein bound. The majority of the drug is broken down in the liver and excreted in the bile. It has been reported that some patients with liver disease show resistance to the drug but the reason for this is not clear. Moderate degrees of hyperventilation do not affect recovery time but a severe respiratory acidosis slows recovery.

INDICATIONS

These are the same as for tubocurarine or alcuronium. Because of its effects on the cardiovascular system, its lack of effect on sympathetic ganglia, and the absence of any histamine-releasing effect, it has been recommended as the relaxant of choice in poor-risk and emergency cases. In fact, it is widely used in the UK for any surgical procedure requiring muscle relaxation.

DOSAGE AND ADMINISTRATION

Pancuronium is only given intravenously. Dose-response curves show that the potency relative to tubocurarine depends on the absolute dose level, and pancuronium becomes relatively more potent as the doses are increased. Early work suggested that pancuronium is about five times as potent as tubocurarine but at the dose levels necessary to just produce total paralysis it may be as much as seven times as potent as tubocurarine, and difficulty in reversing its action could have been due to relative overdose. Initial doses should not exceed 0.1 mg/kg.

PRECAUTIONS

Pancuronium will trigger malignant hyperpyrexia in pigs but there have been no cases reported in man. As with other relaxants of this type, it should be avoided in cases of myasthenia gravis; its actions can be antagonized by neostigmine preceded by an antimuscarinic parasympatholytic agent.

Vecuronium is the monoquaternary homologue of pancuronium, with which it shares many features. Despite featuring in the anaesthetic literature for several years, it has only recently been marketed in the UK.

It has a lower affinity for the receptor than pancuronium; it has a more rapid onset, shorter duration of action, and more rapid offset and can possibly be more easily antagonized by neostigmine. Indeed, it may also be successfully reversed by edrophonium. Like pancuronium, vecuronium has low histamine-releasing properties. However, it has little or no ganglion-blocking action and the dose required to produce vagal blockade is very much greater than that required for neuromuscular blockade. This gives it somewhat different actions on the cardiovascular system. There tends to be a fall in pulse rate, no change in blood pressure, and less rise in blood pressure during intubation.

It is slightly more potent than pancuronium and five times as potent as atracurium. Lower doses are needed in the elderly.

The pharmacokinetics and clinical effects of vecuronium have been found to be unchanged in the presence of renal failure as excretion is mainly biliary, suggesting that it, too, would be an appropriate drug in this condition. It is potentiated by a previous dose of suxamethonium.

It is supplied as a powder: once mixed it must be used within 24 hours.

Suxamethonium salts

Suxamethonium bromide (*BP*)
Suxamethonium chloride (*BP*) and Succinylcholine chloride (*USP*)
Chemical name: 2,2′-succinyldioxybis(ethyltriethylammonium) dibromide and dichloride

$$\begin{array}{l} CH_2-CO-O-(CH_2)_2-\overset{+}{N}(CH_3)_3 \\ | \qquad\qquad\qquad\qquad\qquad\qquad\qquad \cdot 2Cl^- \text{ (and } 2Br^-\text{)} \\ CH_2-CO-O-(CH_2)_2-\overset{+}{N}(CH_3)_3 \end{array}$$

Aqueous solutions of suxamethonium salts hydrolyse slowly with loss of potency; this hydrolysis takes place more rapidly at tropical temperatures and it is preferable that prepared injections should be stored in a refrigerator. The dry powders retain their potency for much longer periods. The rate of hydrolysis is markedly increased in alkaline media. It should not be mixed with intravenous induction agents.

PHARMACOLOGY

Suxamethonium is a short-acting depolarizing muscle relaxant, most commonly used as the chloride. When given intravenously it acts within 30 seconds, with duration of effect up to 5 minutes.

Nervous system. Suxamethonium has no action on the CNS. In spite of its chemical similarity to acetylcholine its action on autonomic effector organs is not great, but muscarinic actions are sometimes observed.

Cardiovascular system. There is no direct action on the heart, but vagal stimulation may cause bradycardia and a fall in blood pressure. This is more likely to occur after large doses or when the dose is repeated. Dysrhythmias and temporary cardiac arrest may also occur. Atropine given previously will prevent these effects and stop them when present.

Circulatory arrest has been reported when suxamethonium is used in burned patients. This is due to an acute rise in serum K^+. This rise is common in burns and injured patients and is maximal between the 21st and 56th day after injury.

Hypotension associated with a skin rash and other evidence of an anaphylactic reaction has also been reported. This seems to be very rare indeed.

Muscular system. There is a rapid, profound and almost synchronous neuromuscular block of all skeletal muscle, usually preceded by fasciculation, due to depolarization of the motor end-plate. Sometimes, especially when large doses are given, the initial depolarizing block is followed by one with features resembling a competitive block, the so-called 'dual' or 'desensitization' block. This may result in prolonged action and the block, when fully established, can usually be antagonized by an anticholinesterase, such as edrophonium or neostigmine. The onset is dose (cumulative) dependent, not time dependent.

Suxamethonium has an abnormal effect in many muscular diseases, including myotonia (in which it may cause contracture) and polymyositis. It is also one of the drugs which trigger the malignant hyperpyrexia syndrome.

Respiratory system. Apart from paralysis of the muscles of respiration, there may be some increase in bronchial secretions. Bronchospasm has been reported in a few isolated cases, in some of which evidence of histamine release was also obtained. An anaphylactic response has occasionally been reported in which bronchospasm was a feature.

Alimentary tract. There may be some increase in bowel movement, and in gastric and salivary secretions due to muscarinic action. This may be inhibited by atropine.

Uterus and placental barrier. There is no change in intrauterine pressure with either intermittent or continuous administration. Suxamethonium does not reach the fetal circulation.

The eye. The administration of suxamethonium causes an abrupt and short-lived rise in intraocular pressure which returns to normal within 6 minutes. This is principally due to contracture (that is, spasm) of the extraocular muscles and is a consequence of their multiple innervation. However, the rise does not occur in the majority of patients with glaucoma, which suggests that changes in arterial and venous pressure are also of importance.

Elimination. Suxamethonium is hydrolysed by plasma cholinesterase into succinylmonocholine and choline; the former is further broken down to succinic acid and choline and about 2 per cent is excreted unchanged in the urine. Suxamethonium is hydrolysed to the monocholine six times faster than the monocholine to succinic acid and choline. The monocholine therefore accumulates temporarily; it has some neuromuscular blocking action but it is about one twentieth of that of suxamethonium.

Low cholinesterase activity, which may be due to liver disease, malnutrition, poisoning with organophosphorus compounds, or genetic factors, will cause delay in elimination of the drug and thus a prolongation of its action. Resistance to its effects occurs in mild myasthenia gravis and in the neonate. Longer periods of paralysis can be produced by combining it with reversible cholinesterase inhibitors such as tacrine and hexafluorenium.

INDICATIONS

Suxamethonium is used whenever profound relaxation of skeletal muscles is required for short periods. It is, therefore, particularly useful in endoscopies, manipulations, and electroconvulsive therapy, and as an aid to tracheal intubation. It can be used for longer operations by repeated doses or by intravenous infusion.

DOSAGE AND ADMINISTRATION

Suxamethonium salts are ineffective by mouth, and although normally given intravenously they can be used intramuscularly – the latter method can be employed in infants and small children when suitable veins cannot be found.

The average dose for the production of full relaxation for 2–4 minutes in the normal healthy adult is about 50 mg (0.75–1 mg/kg). Supplementary doses of 20–30 mg may be given as required.

Doses recommended for neonates and infants vary considerably. Neonates may be given an initial dose of 1–2 mg as required. The total dose should not exceed 50 mg. A single dose of 2 mg/kg may be given intramuscularly for intubation, but should not be repeated owing to the danger of prolonged action. Children may be given 1 mg/kg intravenously, with supplementary doses about one third of the original dose. Infants and small children may require an initial dose of 2 mg/kg.

When suxamethonium is given by intravenous infusion for long operations, a 0.15 per cent or a 0.1 per cent solution may be used.

PRECAUTIONS

Suxamethonium is contraindicated in severe liver disease, in burned patients, in those with large degenerating muscle masses, for example paraplegia of recent onset and major limb trauma, and in patients known to be liable to the malignant hyperpyrexia syndrome. Its use is best avoided in advanced myasthenia gravis. Premedication with atropine is advisable to prevent excessive bronchial secretions, bradycardia, and other muscarinic effects. It is inadvisable in uraemic patients, particularly those with high serum K^+ in whom a further rise in K^+ may occur.

Suxamethonium should not be given to patients with a penetrating injury of the eye or while the globe is open. Suxamethonium is also absolutely contraindicated in patients with myotonia, who develop a rigidity which renders inflation of the lungs impossible.

Complications following the use of suxamethonium include muscle pains in the postoperative period and prolonged partial blockade or apnoea. Muscle pains similar in nature to the aches and discomfort following strenuous exercise occur in the immediate postoperative period and may last for several days. There is usually little inconvenience to patients who are confined to bed after operation, but ambulant patients may suffer considerable discomfort, although they are said to be comparatively uncommon in pregnant women. These pains do not appear to be related to the size of the dose of suxamethonium given or the amount of fasciculation following the initial injection. They can be prevented by giving small doses of a competitive relaxant (not fazadinium) just prior to the injection of suxamethonium. Thiopentone given just previously also exerts a considerable protective effect. It is better to avoid the use of suxamethonium in outpatients and make sure that inpatients remain in bed for at least 24 hours following operation. Muscle fasciculation is also associated with rises in serum creatine phosphokinase, a muscle enzyme, and with rises in serum K^+. This rise also can be diminished by pretreatment with a small dose of a competitive muscle relaxant. The response is greater in traumatized and burned patients; the magnitude of the rise depends on the interval since injury.

Large doses or prolonged administration of suxamethonium lead to a change in the character of the block. The characteristics of a Phase II block appear gradually and not all of them develop simultaneously. The onset seems to be both time and dose dependent and the underlying mechanisms are still unclear. The development of Phase II block can be detected by TOF stimuli (*Figure 9.4*). A relatively

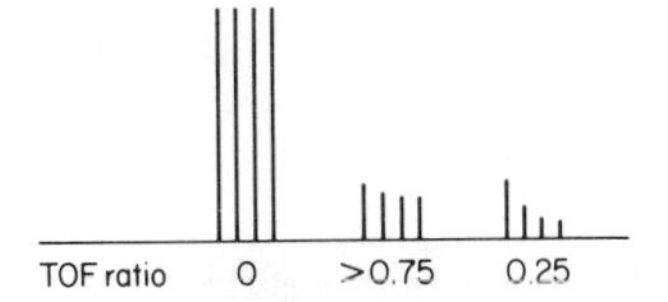

Figure 9.4 A diagrammatic representation of the development of a Phase II block with a TOF ratio changing from over 0.75 to 0.25

well-sustained partial block with a TOF ratio of over 0.75 changes to a TOF ratio of much less. It seems clear from the examination of case reports that the administration of neostigmine in the early stages of a prolonged block was responsible for the very long apnoeas reported, but that when the block exhibited well-developed characteristics of a Phase II block, neostigmine restored normal function.

Decamethonium is no longer commercially available in Great Britain. It is a depolarizing muscle relaxant. Its action lasts for 15–20 minutes and is preceded by fasciculation. It is approximately five times as potent as tubocurarine. There is no action on the CNS, but depression of autonomic ganglia may cause a fall in blood pressure, bradycardia, and dilatation of the pupil. Dual block and muscle pains may occur. It is excreted in the urine and it does not cross the placenta.

Tubocurarine chloride

Tubocurarine chloride (*BP* and *USP*)
Synonym: (D)-tubocurarine chloride
Chemical name: (+)-7′,12′′,-dihydroxy-6,6-dimethoxy-2,2′,2′-trimethyltubocuraranium dichloride

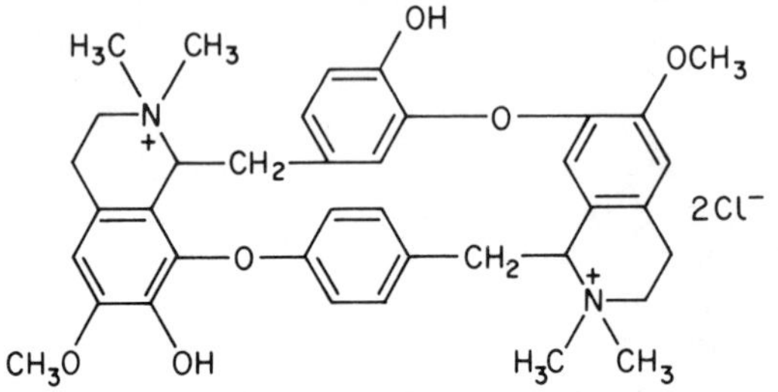

HISTORY

Curare has been known since the beginning of the sixteenth century under the names of uiraery, urari, ourari, wourari, and wourali. It was first obtained from the bark of various species of *Strychnos*, but more recently it has been extracted from *Chondrodendron tomentosum*, a member of the family *Menispermaceae*. It has been stored in a variety of receptacles – calabash, pot and tube (hollow bamboo canes) – hence the names under which it is described. Most of the experimental investigations have been carried out with tube curare, and it was from this source that the first purified extract and the active principle D-tubocurarine were first obtained.

Curare was first described as an arrow poison in 1516 by Ascorio Sforza in his history of the new world (*De Orbe Novo*) based on letters from explorers who had travelled in what is now Brazil. Similar observations were made by Sir Walter Raleigh in 1595 and Humboldt in 1807. In 1812, Charles Waterton described in detail the effects of curare on animals and his experiment in resuscitating a paralysed donkey with assisted respiration by means of a pair of bellows. Two years later he and Brodie suggested that this drug had a toxic effect on the myoneural mechanism, but it was not until some 40 years later that Claude Bernard proved by his classic experiments that this was in fact true.

The next landmark in the history of curare was in 1935 when King isolated the active principle D-tubocurarine; during the previous 50 years curare had been of interest only to physiologists, and apart from its use in the treatment of tetanic spasms in 1878 found no clinical use. Even the isolation of D-tubocurarine bore no fruit immediately, but Palmer of the Middlesex Hospital used it in 1939 to control the spasms of electroconvulsive therapy. At about the same time, Gill returned to the USA from South America with a large quantity of tube curare, from which was extracted the commercial product Intocostrin. Bennet used this preparation in electroconvulsive therapy, and Griffiths and Johnson in Canada were the first to use it for the production of relaxation in anaesthesia in 1942. In Great Britain much of the pioneer work concerning the use of this drug in anaesthesia was done by Gray and Halton of Liverpool.

The substance D-tubocurarine chloride is now known officially as tubocurarine; its preparations are extracted as the chloride from *Chondrodendron tomentosum* and are standardized by chemical assay.

Tubocurarine is a competitive muscle relaxant which when given intravenously takes up to 3 minutes to act, and its effect lasts for 30–40 minutes.

Nervous system. Tubocurarine, being a quaternary ammonium compound and fully ionized, does not pass the blood-brain barrier and has little effect on the CNS. Autonomic ganglia are little affected in doses normally given to produce neuromuscular block. The effect on sympathetic ganglia is somewhat greater than on the parasympathetic. Even so, a fall in blood pressure is not uncommon immediately following a bolus dose.

The effect of tubocurarine is therefore selective on the autonomic system according to the dose. It should be noted that while it is antagonistic to certain nicotinic actions of acetylcholine, antagonism to muscarinic actions has not been recorded.

Cardiovascular system. There is no direct action on the heart. A 15–20 per cent fall in blood pressure is usual and is due to blocking of sympathetic ganglia. This is occasionally severe, and can be markedly potentiated by halothane or chloroform anaesthesia. Heart rate may increase by 10 per cent and there is no significant change in cardiac output. Total peripheral resistance falls.

Muscular system. Relaxation of striated muscle follows a competitive blockade of the neuromuscular junction where this drug competes with acetylcholine. Very small doses are said to decrease muscle tone without loss of voluntary control – the so-called 'lissive effect'.

There is no direct effect on plain muscle; this is only affected by any action that there may be on the autonomic system or by histamine release. Uterine muscle is not affected.

Respiratory system. Apart from depression or paralysis of the muscles of respiration, bronchospasm may occur due to histamine release. It is a rare occurrence.

Alimentary tract. There is normally little effect on bowel movement, the gut is usually quiet, but the effect is variable. This probably depends on whether sympathetic or parasympathetic tone predominates following the partial blocking of these systems. The sphincters at the cardiac end of the stomach and upper end of the oesophagus are said to be unaffected, but stomach contents undoubtedly may gravitate into the pharynx during operations in the Trendelenburg position.

Placental barrier. There is no evidence that tubocurarine passes through the placenta from mother to child.

Fate in the body. Under normal circumstances about two thirds of a dose is excreted within a few hours in the urine, the remainder being metabolized in the liver. In the presence of renal failure metabolic removal by the liver is able to deal with normal doses. Although normal doses have been shown to be clinically safe in the presence of renal failure, pharmacodynamic studies suggest that large or repeated doses will lead to prolonged curarization and this has been reported.

Larger doses of tubocurarine than those normally required are sometimes necessary when liver function is impaired, and this can be ascribed to the low albumin/globulin ratios which may occur and the ability of serum globulins to bind tubocurarine.

Sensitivity occurs in neonates, in the presence of electrolyte disturbance, myasthenia gravis, and of anaesthetics such as ether which have a curare-like action themselves.

INDICATIONS

Despite the introduction of other agents that are more specific to the neuromuscular junction, tubocurarine is still a commonly used muscle relaxant and has played its part in balanced anaesthesia for many years. It is particularly useful in long abdominal and thoracic operations where full muscle relaxation or control of respiration are necessary. The tendency for the pulse rate and blood pressure to fall (as opposed to the cardiovascular responses to pancuronium) are not necessarily a disadvantage. It may be safely used in obstetrics. Although a proportion of tubocurarine is excreted unchanged by the kidneys it may be safely used in renal disease if dosage is carefully controlled.

Tubocurarine is also used in the treatment of tetanus and in the past has been employed in the diagnosis of myasthenia gravis, and in the treatment of various spastic disorders.

DOSAGE AND ADMINISTRATION

Tubocurarine is, for all practical purposes, inactive by mouth, absorption from mucous surfaces being extremely slow. Intramuscularly its effect is variable and delayed. It is normally given intravenously.

The methods and doses employed by individual anaesthetists in the administration of tubocurarine vary considerably. Initial doses of 15–30 mg are most commonly used, with supplementary doses of 5–10 mg when required to maintain apnoea and full muscular relaxation. Some authorities advocate the use of an initial test dose of 5 mg in the conscious patient to determine the susceptibility of the patient towards the drug, a procedure which may be of value when the use of very large doses is contemplated.

It has often been stated that supplementary doses of tubocurarine should not be given less than 30 minutes before the end of operation, in order to avoid terminal respiratory depression. However, in most patients who have had large doses of tubocurarine over a long period of time, residual curarization is inevitable, and will require reversal with neostigmine. The use of 5–10 mg of tubocurarine to facilitate abdominal closure will not materially affect the ease of reversal of curarization, and is preferable to deepening anaesthesia or giving a short-acting depolarizing agent such as suxamethonium.

Tubocurarine can be used with safety in neonates provided that the dose is carefully controlled. The average initial dose is 0.317 mg/kg on the first day of life, rising to approximately 0.528 mg/kg at 1 month. From then onwards the dose appropriate for infants and children is 0.62 mg/kg.

The intramuscular use of tubocurarine in anaesthesia is not recommended.

Tubocurarine is used in the treatment of tetanus for the control of spasms. It is given in repeated doses intravenously or intramuscularly, combined with intermittent positive pressure respiration and sedation.

PRECAUTIONS

Tubocurarine is non-toxic in the doses likely to be employed during anaesthesia; it is, however, contraindicated in myasthenia gravis. The importance of maintaining efficient respiratory exchange cannot be overemphasized.

Postoperative respiratory depression due to tubocurarine is effectively antagonized by anticholinesterases such as neostigmine. Atropine 0.6–1.2 mg should be given intravenously with 2–3 mg of neostigmine. Additional neostigmine may be given until muscle power is normal; 2–3 mg is usually sufficient and 5 mg should not be exceeded. Edrophonium also antagonizes tubocurarine, but its effect is transient and respiratory depression is liable to recur when its effects have worn off.

10

Parasympathomimetic and cholinergic agents; anticholinesterases

These are drugs which have a similar effect to that of stimulation of the parasympathetic system (fibres in the third, seventh, ninth, and tenth cranial nerves, and sacral fibres from the spinal cord). Stimulation of this system may be expected to produce the following effects: constriction of plain muscle of the alimentary tract and detrusor muscle of the bladder; relaxation of sphincters; constriction of bronchial musculature; slowing of the heart and lowering of the blood pressure with dilatation of certain vessels; miosis; promotion of salivary, bronchial, gastric, and mucous secretions; stimulation of the pregnant uterus; and contraction of the ciliary muscle of the eye (the lens is now set for near vision and by the opening of the canal of Schlemm intraocular drainage is improved, thus causing a fall in intraocular pressure, *Figure 10.1*).

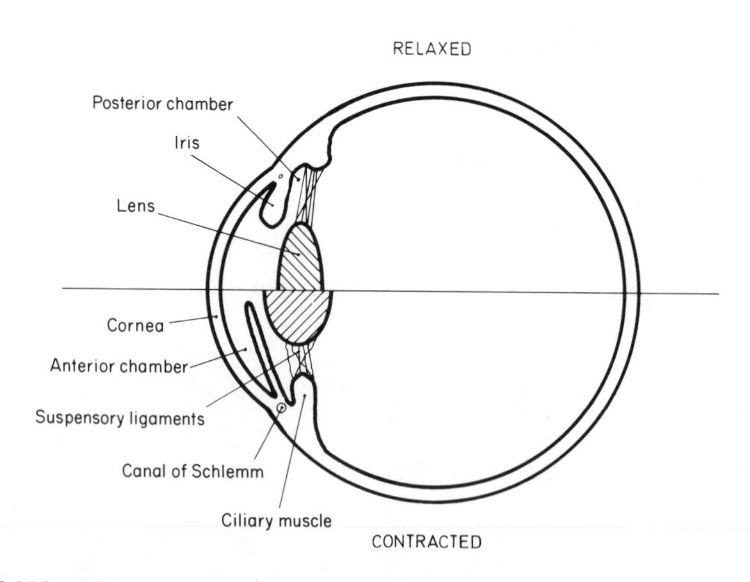

Figure 10.1 Muscarinic agonists contract the ciliary muscle thereby relaxing the suspensory ligament, setting the lens for near vision. They also contract the circular muscle of the iris, thereby constricting the pupil and opening the canal of Schlemm

Drug action

Cholinergic drugs have the same effects as acetylcholine (*see* below). Some act directly upon effector cells and others indirectly by blocking cholinesterases, so that at sites where acetylcholine is being liberated by nervous activity it persists longer and in a higher concentration than usual. The latter group are the anticholinesterases which exhibit, by virtue of the way they act, both muscarinic and nicotinic actions of acetylcholine. A not uncommon error is to use the adjective cholinergic and parasympathomimetic synonymously. Parasympathomimetic refers only to those effects of acetylcholine or cholinergic agents at parasympathetic effectors, whereas cholinergic can refer to any acetylcholine-like actions, be they muscarinic or nicotinic, and therefore includes actions upon all autonomic ganglia, sympathetic and parasympathetic, upon the neuromuscular junctions of striated muscle, and upon cholinergic sympathetic effectors such as sweat glands and the adrenal medulla.

Parasympathetic stimulation is an unwanted action during anaesthesia, as it increases salivary and bronchial secretions, slows the heart rate, and increases myocardial irritability. Certain anaesthetics have this effect, for example chloroform, cyclopropane, and halothane, and it is usual practice to use atropine to block these muscarinic effects. Excess parasympathetic activity is only helpful in an emergency such as fainting or neurogenic shock, when it is of a protective nature.

Acetylcholine

$$CH_3-\underset{\underset{O}{\|}}{C}-O-CH_2-CH_2-\overset{+}{N}\begin{matrix}CH_3\\CH_3\\CH_3\end{matrix}$$

Acetylcholine is a normal body constituent of the greatest importance. It may also be artificially synthesized from choline. It is the chemical transmitter of nerve impulses at:

1. The synapses in all autonomic ganglia, both sympathetic and parasympathetic, and the endings of the preganglionic sympathetic fibres in the adrenal medulla;
2. All postganglionic parasympathetic nerve endings;
3. Postganglionic sympathetic nerve endings in the uterus and sweat glands;
4. The end-plates of motor nerves to striated muscle.

Its role at CNS synapses is not fully elucidated, although it is undoubtedly the transmitter at some. The administration of physostigmine, a cholinesterase inhibitor, causes general arousal. Morphine-like drugs may act by inhibiting acetylcholine release. Acetylcholine also probably has actions as a 'local hormone' controlling the rhythmic activity of atrial muscle and of cilia.

In tissues, at the relevant nerve endings, it is present combined as an inactive precursor from which it is liberated when a nerve impulse arrives. By its own direct action the acetylcholine then transmits the nerve impulse to postganglionic fibres, by stimulating the cell bodies of the post ganglionic neurones; to the autonomic effector organ, by stimulating or depressing its cells directly; and to the motor end-plate of striated muscle, by depolarizing it. Immediately after a nerve impulse has taken effect acetylcholine is hydrolysed by acetylcholinesterase into choline, with only 1/500 to 1/1000 of the original activity, and acetate. The mechanism of this reaction is discussed in detail on page 290. Choline-acetylase catalyses their resynthesis to acetylcholine, and further combination, probably with a protein, yields the precursor again. The effect of acetylcholine may be increased with anticholinesterases, such as neostigmine, which inhibit the hydrolysis of acetylcholine and thus allow it to persist and to reach a higher concentration when liberated. In the body, there is no store of acetylcholine, comparable to that of adrenaline and noradrenaline in the adrenal medulla. Acetylcholine is believed to be stored in small agranular vesicles in the terminal varicosities of cholinergic nerves. Each agranular vesicle is thought to contain about 10^5 molecules of acetylcholine (*Figure 10.2*).

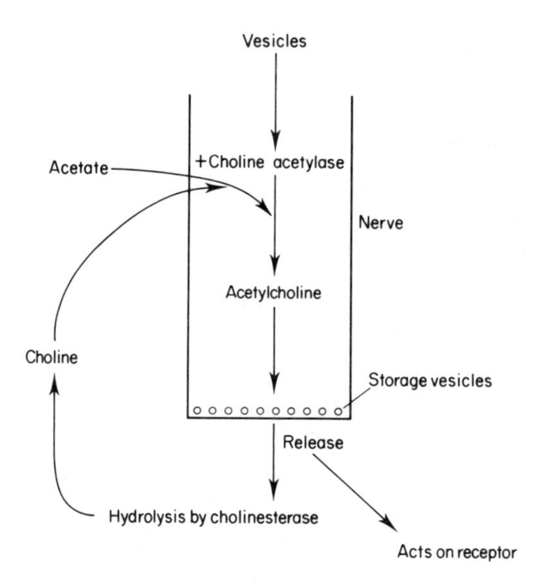

Figure 10.2 Acetylcholine is formed from choline and acetate. It is stored in vesicles and hydrolysed by cholinesterase

Two main classes of acetylcholine action are recognized, muscarinic and nicotinic, so called since they mimic those of muscarine and nicotine, the effects of which were known before those of acetylcholine.

The muscarinic actions of acetylcholine are those upon autonomic effector organs and imitate the effect of parasympathetic stimulation and the sympathetic function of sweating. They are antagonized by the belladonna alkaloids, their semisynthetic derivatives, and synthetic substitutes. Muscarinic effects are elicited with much smaller doses of injected acetylcholine than are necessary to evoke nicotinic actions and, in fact, unless muscarinic effects are inhibited (for example by atropine) the nicotinic effects may be completely masked.

Many other drugs possessing atropine-like actions, such as pethidine, methadone, and procaine, and some other local analgesics, chlorpromazine, and the antihistamines, can antagonize, or partially so, these muscarine-like effects.

Injected acetylcholine shows muscarine-like effects and these are easier to block by atropine than is stimulation of a parasympathetic nerve such as the vagus. Vasodilator responses are elicited by smaller doses of acetylcholine than are cardiac slowing effects, so that a small fall in blood pressure is brought about by peripheral vasodilatation while a greater fall with a bigger dose is caused by cardiac slowing as well.

The nicotinic actions are caused by stimulation of the cell bodies of autonomic postganglionic neurones, the adrenal medullary cells, and the motor end-plates of striated muscle. Persistence of acetylcholine (or nicotine) at these sites finally produces depression there. Antagonists of nicotinic actions usually act much more strongly at one of these types of site than at another. Thus, tubocurarine inhibits neuromuscular transmission in striated muscle in doses that have no demonstrable effect upon autonomic ganglia or the adrenal medulla. On the other hand, hexamethonium and pentamethonium salts have no effect upon neuromuscular transmission when used in doses that inhibit transmission to a high degree in autonomic ganglia.

When nicotinic effects are obtained from injected acetylcholine, it is those upon autonomic ganglia and the adrenal medulla which are mainly in evidence; the neuromuscular effects, when evident, consist of fibrillary twitchings of striated muscle followed by a transient loss of power. Fortunately, when anticholinesterases are used their nicotinic effects are well in evidence at the neuromuscular junction of striated muscle, where useful antagonism may thus be achieved to curare-like drugs. At muscarinic sites excessive effects may then be countered by atropine or hyoscine; the latter drug, however, has little effect on blocking the cardiac vagus in normal doses.

The actions of acetylcholine alone are too brief and too widespread to be of clinical use. After an anticholinesterase any administered acetylcholine would have a more lasting but still very widespread action. Synthetic derivatives which are more stable and possess some slight specificity (*see* carbachol and methacholine) are often used clinically. The commonly used derivative, suxamethonium, is highly specific in action as a depolarizing neuromuscular blocking agent. It consists of a combination of two molecules of acetylcholine.

Carbachol

Carbachol (*BPC* and *USP*)
Chemical name: (2-carbamoyloxyethyl)trimethylammonium chloride

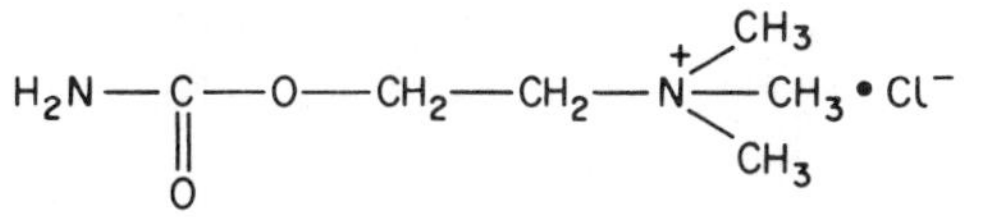

$$H_2N-\underset{\underset{O}{\|}}{C}-O-CH_2-CH_2-\overset{+}{N}(CH_3)_3 \cdot Cl^-$$

PHARMACOLOGY

Carbachol is an ester of choline, having an action like acetylcholine, but longer lasting and thus suitable for clinical use. This is because it is completely resistant to destruction by cholinesterase. Thus its action is more persistent and it is active orally, although less certain than by injection. As with acetylcholine, carbachol has both muscarinic and nicotinic actions and, because of the latter, it is more dangerous to use than methacholine; atropine will antagonize the muscarinic but not the nicotinic effects, which are then unmasked.

Carbachol stimulates the parasympathetic system, dilates the peripheral blood vessels, causes bradycardia, and so lowers blood pressure. If, however, muscarinic effects are inhibited by atropine, the blood pressure will rise as sympathetic ganglia are stimulated and adrenaline and noradrenaline are released.

There is a marked increase in intestinal activity, and bladder tone and exocrine secretions are increased.

INDICATIONS

Carbachol has largely been superseded as a therapeutic agent. It has been used to relieve the symptoms of intermittent claudication, Raynaud's disease, and arterial spasm in hypertension. It has been used in paroxysmal tachycardia, but methacholine is safer; it has been superseded by bethanechol for the treatment of postoperative retention of urine and intestinal atony because of its relatively higher component of nictonic activity at autonomic ganglia. It can be used to reduce intraocular pressure when used as eye drops. A proprietary preparation contains 3 per cent carbachol.

DOSAGE AND ADMINISTRATION

Oral administration, 1–4 mg; subcutaneous injection, 0.25–0.5 mg up to three times daily.

PRECAUTIONS

It is not advisable to use the drug in patients suffering from shock or bronchial asthma as it may worsen these conditions. Its use is also contraindicated in acute cardiac failure and in peptic ulcer. It should not be given by the intravenous route.

Minor side effects are often seen, such as salivation, sweating, nausea, shivering, and faintness. Overdosage can cause bronchoconstriction, cardiovascular collapse, and cardiac arrest. Untoward effects respond readily to the hypodermic injection of atropine sulphate 0.6 mg. If large accidental doses have been taken, care must be exercised in the dose of atropine given, as there may be a sudden and dangerous rise in arterial blood pressure.

Methacholine salts

Methacholine chloride (*USP*) and Methacholine bromide (*USP*)
Chemical name: 2-(acetoxypropyl)trimethylammonium chloride

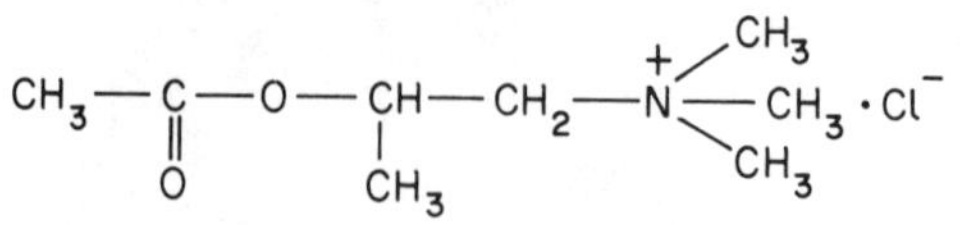

$$CH_3{-}C({=}O){-}O{-}CH(CH_3){-}CH_2{-}\overset{+}{N}(CH_3)_3 \cdot Cl^-$$

PHARMACOLOGY

Methacholine chloride has actions similar to the muscarinic effects of acetylcholine. It is more stable than the latter drug because it is a poor substrate for cholinesterase and thus more slowly broken down. It is 10–20 times more potent by subcutaneous injection; it simulates the stimulation of parasympathetic postganglionic fibres and opposes many effects of adrenaline. It is a safer drug than carbachol as its nicotinic action is much less marked. Its effect is mainly on the cardiovascular system. It slows the heart and dilates peripheral blood vessels, the combined effects lowering blood pressure. Intestinal tone is increased and the activity of the salivary and sweat glands is stimulated.

INDICATIONS
It is used to terminate attacks of paroxysmal tachycardia when these do not respond to usual measures, and in the treatment of Raynaud's disease and other vasospastic conditions.

DOSAGE AND ADMINISTRATION
By mouth, 100–200 mg; subcutaneously, 10–25 mg.

PRECAUTIONS
Methacholine should be used with care in elderly and hypertensive patients; it should not be given to those with bronchial asthma, or those who are seriously ill, and should be avoided in cases of thyrotoxicosis, coronary occlusion, or Addison's disease. Prolonged use of the drug is inadvisable. Untoward effects are due to excessive parasympathetic stimulation; nausea and vomiting are common with overdosage and precede flushing, sweating, and increased salivation. Transient heart block is a rare occurrence, but care should be taken in hypertensive patients who may react to the drug by a sudden and marked fall in blood pressure. Overdose should be treated with atropine 0.6 mg.

Bethanechol chloride is another choline ester which is resistant to cholinesterase and which has predominantly muscarinic actions. In normal doses, however, it does not slow the heart or lower the blood pressure. It can be used for the treatment of urinary retention, ileus, gastric atony, and megacolon. Optimal dosage lies between 30 and 60 mg daily in divided doses. Precautions are as for methacholine.

Furtrethonium iodide is a muscarinic agonist which has been used to contract the bladder in non-obstructive urinary retention. The usual dose is 5 mg subcutaneously.

Pilocarpine is an alkaloid obtained from the leaves of a South American shrub, *Pilocarpus*. It acts primarily at the muscarinic receptors of autonomic effector cells, but also has some ganglionic action. Given systemically, it mimics general cholinergic stimulation, stimulating the smooth muscle of the intestinal tract, bronchi, bladder, and gall bladder, and the secretion of sweat, gastric juice, saliva, tears, and pancreatic juice. It has somewhat anomalous actions on the cardiovascular system because of its nicotinic actions at the sympathetic ganglia.

It is now used solely in the treatment of glaucoma. Pupillary constriction and spasm of accommodation lead to a fall in intraocular pressure after an initial transient rise. The miosis persists for several hours although the ability to accommodate for near vision returns in about 2 hours. It is given as 1–4 per cent eye drops. It is often combined synergistically with physostigmine.

Anticholinesterases

Cholinesterases are of two types: acetylcholinesterase, also known as true, specific, e-type, red cell cholinesterase; and plasma cholinesterase, also known as pseudo, non-specific, butyro, s-type cholinesterase. They differ in their location and behaviour towards substrates and inhibitors. Acetylcholinesterase occurs in red cells and at the endings of all cholinergic neurones. 'Plasma' cholinesterase also occurs in the liver. Acetylcholine is a more specific substrate for acetylcholinesterase than plasma cholinesterase and the reverse applies to butyrylcholine.

Anticholinesterases are cholinergic in their action as they inhibit or inactivate cholinesterases which normally hydrolyse acetylcholine, and consequently they raise the concentration and duration of acetylcholine at all sites at which it is being released. The most noticeable effects are muscarinic ones, since these are evoked by lower concentrations of acetylcholine than are necessary for nicotinic actions. Nicotinic actions can usually be produced safely only when the patient is protected by atropine or hyoscine from excessive muscarinic effects. A familiar example is the use of neostigmine to restore transmission at the neuromuscular junction after blockade with a competitive blocking agent, while atropine prevents untoward muscarinic effects upon the heart, bronchial tree, and intestine. It should be noted that excessive amounts of acetylcholine persisting at the motor end-plates of skeletal muscle produce a persistent localized depolarization of the muscle membrane, analogous to that produced by blocking agents such as decamethonium or suxamethonium salts. To understand the cholinesterase inhibitors it is first necessary to understand the enzyme itself.

Acetylcholinesterase

Acetylcholinesterase is widely distributed in the body, and is found wherever acetylcholine is the chemical transmitter.

This enzyme can be prepared in a purified form but has not been crystallized. It is a polymeric protein, each unit of which has a molecular weight of about 240 000.

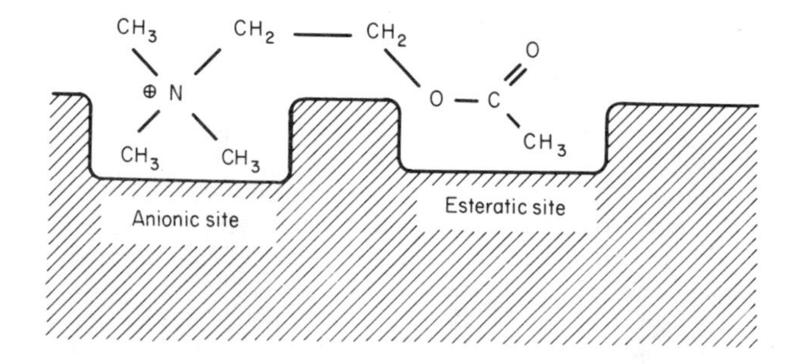

Figure 10.3 Anionic and esteratic binding sites of acetylcholinesterase. Acetylcholine bound to active sites. Initial binding to anionic site by ionic bond between charged nitrogen and ionized carboxylic group; also van der Waals' bonds. The esteratic site contains a glutamic-acid-serine-alanine sequence. The serine hydroxyl is involved in the breaking of the ester linkage

The active site on the enzyme is composed of two sub-sites, the anionic site and the esteratic site, which are so arranged that they are complementary to the natural substrate acetylcholine. The anionic site binds the N^+ of acetylcholine and this locates the ester linkage in the region of the esteratic site (*Figure 10.3*). Thus, the enzyme has an optimum substrate concentration, and is less effective against longer chain choline esters.

The steps in the hydrolysis of acetylcholine can be outlined diagrammatically as follows:

E +	S $\leftrightharpoons$	ES $\rightarrow$	E(Acid) +	P_1 $\rightarrow$	E +	P_2
Enzyme:	Substrate:	Enzyme substrate complex:	Inter-mediate compound:	First product:	Enzyme:	econd product:
cholin-esterase	acetyl-choline	Michaelis–Menten complex	acetylated enzyme	choline	cholin-esterase	acetic acid

Attraction between enzyme and substrate depends on electrical, intermolecular, and hydrophobic binding forces. Hydrolysis begins with electron transfer at the esteratic site with the formation of an acetylated enzyme (the intermediate compound) and choline (first product). The half-life of the acetylated enzyme is only 42 μs, but until it is hydrolysed the active site is inhibited.

Although it has such an evanescent existence, the acetylated enzyme is of importance in understanding the action of acid-transferring cholinesterase inhibitors such as neostigmine, physostigmine, and organophosphate compounds.

Classification of cholinesterase inhibitors

Inhibitors of acetylcholinesterase can be classified as either prosthetic or oxydiaphoretic. The latter are also known as acid-transferring inhibitors. Prosthetic inhibitors have an affinity for the anionic site on the enzyme, and by their presence impede the union of enzyme and substrate. They may be regarded therefore as reversible competitive inhibitors of the enzyme. They contain a cationic group, usually a quaternary nitrogen. Examples include tetraethylammonium, edrophonium, and tetrahydroaminacrine.

Prosthetic inhibitors such as edrophonium and tacrine form a relatively stable enzyme–substrate complex, the inhibitor molecule merely preventing enzyme and acetylcholine approximating correctly. The reaction between enzyme and inhibitor is in dynamic equilibrium, and the degree of inhibition depends on the concentrations of the three components and the binding affinity between enzyme and inhibitor.

In contrast, the acid-transferring inhibitors act as substrate substitutes for the enzyme. The initial formation of an enzyme–substrate complex (Michaelis–Menten complex) proceeds in the same way as the initial reaction between enzyme and acetylcholine. Likewise, the next stage of formation of an intermediate acid–enzyme compound and first split product also proceeds normally. However, at this stage the intermediate acid–enzyme compound cannot be hydrolysed to release the acid radical and reconstituted enzyme with the rapidity that the acetyl radical can be split off during hydrolysis of acetylcholine. The enzyme is thus inactivated, and the time course of the inhibition depends on the rate at which the hydrolysis takes place. With carbamates such as neostigmine and physostigmine this reaction takes place in a matter of minutes or hours, and such inhibitors used to be called 'reversible'. With the so-called 'irreversible' organophosphate inhibitors the hydrolysis takes days or weeks, but can be markedly speeded up by certain compounds such as pralidoxime iodide.

Acid-transferring inhibitors will also react with plasma cholinesterase. Prosthetic inhibitors, however, are relatively less effective, because this enzyme lacks an anionic site.

Both classes of anticholinesterases exhibit excitatory and inhibitory actions on the CNS if given in suitable doses.

Organophosphate compounds

Organophosphate compounds, which have been developed in recent years for use in chemical warfare and as insecticides, are acid-transferring inhibitors of cholinesterase, the acid radical–enzyme complex formed having a negligible rate of hydrolysis. The insecticides, parathion, EPN, and OMPA differ from the nerve gases in that the active cholinesterase inhibitor is only produced as a consequence of metabolism. Malathion is a selective insecticide because it undergoes considerable metabolism in mammals and birds to an inactive compound by enzymes which insects lack. The nerve gases have extremely high lipid solubility so that absorption can occur from any site in or on the body, including intact skin. This high lipid solubility ensures that they cross the blood-brain barrier very easily and thus produce powerful effects on the CNS.

Treatment of poisoning requires atropine 2 mg intravenously, repeated every 30–60 minutes as required. This will relieve muscarinic effects such as bradycardia, hypotension, salivation, and bronchospasm. Smaller doses at less frequent intervals may be necessary for several days in severe cases. Central actions, convulsions, and nicotinic effects such as muscle weakness will be relieved only by specific therapy of the cholinesterase lesion. Hydrolysis of the acid radical–enzyme can be achieved, particularly with parathion, by pralidoxime iodide or the more soluble methanesulphonate. A dose of 1 g is given intravenously, repeated after 30 minutes if the condition has not improved. A maintenance dose may be given intramuscularly or subcutaneously if signs of poisoning persist. Such reactivators need to be given *early*, because the phosphorylated cholinesterase undergoes 'ageing' and becomes refractory to reversal. Some organophosphate agents are inherently more difficult to reverse by this means. Barbiturates and benzodiazepines have also been employed to produce sedation and control convulsions. Artificial respiration may be necessary in the early stages of treatment.

The skin and clothing of patients poisoned by these agents may be highly contaminated and those handling them should wear gloves. The patient's clothing should be removed and destroyed and the skin washed with soap and water. If the agent has been ingested the stomach should be washed out with a solution of sodium bicarbonate.

Ecothiopate (echothiophate in the USA) is the only organophosphate compound used medicinally. It is used in the treatment of glaucoma, but systemic absorption has been reported to prolong the action of suxamethonium.

Myasthenia gravis

Myasthenia gravis is an autoimmune disease. In many cases antibodies to acetylcholine receptor protein are present in the patient's serum. It presents as a syndrome of increased fatiguability of striated muscles.

For many years the principal effective drug therapy has been the regular use of an anticholinesterase which prevents the breakdown of the reduced quanta of acetylcholine, so that sufficient transmitter reaches the postsynaptic region of the neuromuscular junction. In recent years treatment has tended more towards immunosuppression with the use of prednisone and immunosuppressive drugs such as azathioprine. Many patients are now manageable on such a regimen without the use of anticholinesterases. The beneficial effects of such agents are associated with a fall in acetylcholine receptor protein antibodies. Thymectomy can also produce a fall.

When anticholinesterase therapy is employed, neostigmine 15 mg orally or 1 mg intramuscularly three times a day, increasing to four or more times a day, is the standard initial treatment. It may be convenient to change to pyridostigmine which has a longer duration of action; 60 mg orally is equivalent to 15 mg of neostigmine orally. Other drugs that may be of benefit are ambenonium, 5–25 mg three or four times a day, and distigmine, 5 mg two to four times a day. On occasions it is necessary to determine whether muscle weakness is due to inadequate therapy or to the development of cholinergic crisis, and edrophonium 2–10 mg intravenously may be employed for this purpose.

The suppression of cholinesterase by these drugs is non-specific, and unwanted muscarinic effects in glands and smooth muscle also occur. Such parasympathetic excitation may give rise to colic, diarrhoea, nausea, salivation, and miosis. If the dose is excessive, the drugs may cross the blood-brain barrier, giving rise to confusion and coma. The muscarinic effects can be prevented by atropine-like drugs, although in the presence of atropine it is even easier to give an overdose of anticholinesterase with its potentially dangerous cerebral effects. They also affect the miosis, and thus interfere with a useful index of anticholinesterase activity. With the exception of edrophonium, parenteral atropine should be given when anticholinesterases are given parenterally. For those on routine oral maintenance, 0.6 mg orally twice daily is usually sufficient to control muscarinic side effects.

Myasthenic syndrome

The myasthenic syndrome is most commonly found in a small proportion of patients with bronchogenic carcinoma. It may be due to defective release of stored acetylcholine and, as might be expected, anticholinesterases can give rise to some improvement. Guanidine, which acts by prolonging the action potential (due to its effect in delaying the time at which increase in sodium ion permeability is switched off), has been found of use also. It should be given in divided doses of about 20–30 mg/kg per day, a reasonable schedule being 250 mg three or four times a day. Full benefit may not occur until treatment has been continued for several days. No commercial preparation is currently available. Side effects, such as diarrhoea, restlessness or agitation, salivation, and tremor, can be corrected with atropine.

Edrophonium chloride

Edrophonium chloride (*BP* and *USP*)
Chemical name: ethyl(3-hydroxyphenyl)dimethylammonium chloride

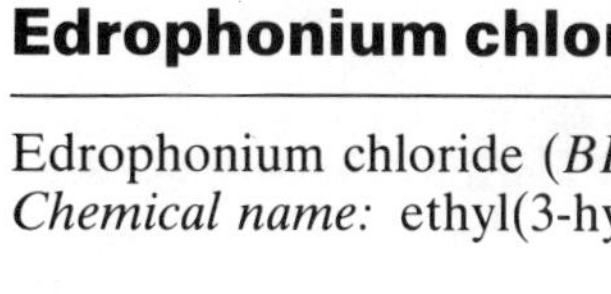

PHARMACOLOGY

Edrophonium is a cholinergic agent which functions mainly by direct action but also as a prosthetic cholinesterase inhibitor. Its action on skeletal muscle is more marked than on ganglia and visceral effector organs. A small intravenous dose will cause fasciculation of muscle fibres, but excessive doses produce neuromuscular block and death from peripheral respiratory paralysis will result. There is little effect on the cardiovascular system, and muscarinic actions in general are mild. Its duration of action is short, and is only effective for upwards of 10 minutes. It is rapidly destroyed in the body.

INDICATIONS

Edrophonium is used to antagonize the effects of tubocurarine and other competitive neuromuscular blocking agents, for the diagnosis and assessment of therapy in myasthenia gravis, in the differential diagnosis between myasthenic weakness and cholinergic crisis, and to assess the progress of a dual block after depolarizing muscle relaxants such as suxamethonium.

DOSAGE AND ADMINISTRATION

Edrophonium, although normally given intravenously, can also be given intramuscularly or subcutaneously.

As an antagonist to a competitive neuromuscular blocking agent, 10–20 mg may be given intravenously, preceded a few minutes previously by atropine 0.6–1.2 mg. As its effects are transient, further doses of edrophonium may be required at about 10-minute intervals if respiratory depression occurs.

In suspected dual block 10 mg is given intravenously (preceded by atropine). If the threshold has returned to near normal, muscle power and respiration will improve. If the block is still predominantly depolarizing there will be either no improvement or actual intensification of the block, although any deterioration may be preceded by a transitory improvement.

In the diagnosis of myasthenia gravis, up to 10 mg is given slowly intravenously over a period of 30 seconds. In the presence of this condition there is a marked increase in muscle strength within 1 minute, which returns to its original state in 5–15 minutes. In the assessment of anticholinesterase therapy, and in differentiating inadequate therapy from cholinergic crisis, edrophonium 1 mg is given initially, and is repeated after 1 minute if no action is observed. Inadequate cholinergic therapy is apparent if there is improvement in myasthenic symptoms; patients in incipient cholinergic crisis, provided that they have not received atropine, exhibit marked muscarinic side effects and an increase in weakness.

In contrast to neostigmine, an overdose of edrophonium in normal individuals causes a preponderance of nicotinic effects, muscle fasciculation gives place to depression and peripheral respiratory failure will ensue. This will require controlled respiration while the effects of the drug, usually only transient, wear off.

Ambenonium chloride is a reversible anticholinesterase used in the treatment of myasthenia gravis. It can be given orally in doses from 5–25 mg three or four times daily, treatment commencing usually with a dose of 5 mg, increasing if necessary. A very careful watch on patients is necessary in view of the possibility of producing cholinergic crisis. Patients vary considerably in their requirements. Atropine is normally contraindicated as it can mask the onset of a cholinergic crisis, usually manifest by abdominal pain, diarrhoea, vomiting, and excessive salivation. If such signs of overdosage occur, atropine 0.5–1 mg intravenously can be given, plus supportive measures such as artificial respiration.

Neostigmine salts

Neostigmine bromide (*BP* and *USP*)
Neostigmine methylsulphate (*BP*) and Neostigmine methylsulfate (*USP*)
Chemical name: 3-(dimethylcarbamoyloxy)-*NNN*-trimethylanilinium bromide or methylsulphate

PHARMACOLOGY

Neostigmine is an acid-transferring cholinesterase inhibitor. It is a quaternary ammonium compound and is therefore poorly absorbed by mouth and largely confined to the extracellular fluid phase.

Nervous system. By inhibiting normal hydrolysis of acetylcholine at the sites at which it is released, neostigmine raises its concentration and duration of action. This action thus excites or inhibits those parts of the nervous system where transmission is cholinergic. It also has presynaptic actions and increases the rate of repetitive firing following a single nerve impulse. This also contributes to the build-up of acetylcholine at the end-plates.

In normal doses there is no consistent action on the CNS, although the potentiation of narcotic analgesics may be such an effect. On the autonomic system its actions are clear-cut and both muscarinic and nicotinic effects are evident. The former result from stimulation of the effector organs of postganglionic parasympathctic nerve endings and of postganglionic sympathetic nerve endings in the uterus and sweat glands; the latter from stimulation after small doses and depression after large doses of all autonomic ganglia, cells of the adrenal medulla, and the motor end-plates of skeletal muscle fibres. Muscarinic effects predominate but can be blocked by atropine.

Cardiovascular system. Peripheral vagal stimulation will cause bradycardia, some degree of vasodilatation, and a fall in blood pressure. Cardiac dysrhythmias and arrest may follow large doses, especially in the presence of hypercapnia. If atropine is given, blood pressure and pulse rate may rise as a result of stimulation of sympathetic ganglia and adrenaline release (nicotinic effect).

Respiratory system. There is little effect on respiration, but bronchi are constricted and secretions are increased.

Skeletal muscle. Neostigmine prolongs and intensifies local depolarization produced at the end-plate by acetylcholine. This is due mainly to the increased concentration of acetylcholine present but also to the direct action of neostigmine itself. A small dose will increase the muscle contraction produced by a single maximal nerve stimulation; larger doses or repeated stimulation may cause depression. Fasciculation of groups of muscle fibres may also result. This is due to repetitive firing of the motor neurone. The various actions on skeletal muscle are increased by adrenaline, slightly reduced by atropine, and antagonized by competitive neuromuscular blocking drugs. In myasthenia gravis the strength of muscle contractions is increased.

Smooth muscle. Neostigmine stimulates smooth muscle; peristalsis of the stomach, intestine, ureter, and bile duct are increased and may give rise to colic. The bladder and the bowel may be emptied.

Other actions of neostigmine include sweating, salivation, and increase in mucous and other exocrine secretions. The pupil is constricted. There is evidence that neostigmine increases the intensity and duration of action of analgesics; how this effect is brought about has not yet been determined but is possibly by an increase in the pain threshold. Its cholinergic action is also beneficial when employed with analgesics as it prevents constipation and atony of the bladder.

INDICATIONS

Neostigmine is used to antagonize the effects of competitive neuromuscular blocking drugs and in the treatment of atony of the intestinal tract (paralytic ileus), atony of the bladder, myasthenia gravis, glaucoma, and sinus tachycardia. It has also been employed to potentiate the effect of analgesics and the relaxation of muscle spasm.

DOSAGE AND ADMINISTRATION

Neostigmine is given by mouth as the bromide, and parenterally or intravenously as the methylsulphate. The poor lipid solubility accounts for the very high ratio (15:1) of oral to parenteral dose for comparable effects.

There have been several investigations directed at devising the safest way in which to reverse the residual paralysis of muscle relaxants. The different effects of relaxant drugs in the USA and Great Britain (*see* page 265) may account for some of the conflicting conclusions drawn. The prevailing view at present is that there is no advantage in giving the atropine much before the neostigmine, and indeed this practice may in some circumstances precipitate both tachycardia and more serious dysrhythmias. The recommended ratio of doses of atropine and neostigmine ranges from 1:2 to 1:3.3. In Great Britain doses below 2.5 mg are rarely used, and should not exceed 5 mg. Serious dysrhythmias can occur in the presence of respiratory acidosis, and hypoventialtion should be avoided during its administration. There is general agreement that the appropriate mixtures of atropine and neostigmine should be injected slowly over about 60 seconds. The actions of neostigmine develop more slowly than those of atropine, and an initial moderate tachycardia may give way to a bradycardia, particularly when the ratio of neostigmine to atropine exceeds 3:1.

In the treatment of intestinal and bladder atony, 15–30 mg may be given by mouth, or 0.5–1 mg parenterally if a more rapid effect is desirable. In an emergency, 0.5 mg can be given intravenously. Oral and parenteral doses may be repeated every 4–6 hours. A similar parenteral dose may be given to control sinus tachycardia.

The initial regimen for a recently diagnosed case of myasthenia gravis is neostigmine 15 mg orally three times a day, increasing to four or more, up to say 2-hourly according to tolerance; 15 mg orally is approximately equivalent to 1 mg parenterally. Atropine in appropriate dosage may be necessary to control muscarinic side effects. In the treatment of glaucoma one drop of a 3 per cent solution may be instilled into the eye and repeated every 10 minutes for up to 12 doses.

A dose of 0.5 mg may be given intramuscularly with morphine and similar analgesics to potentiate their analgesic action.

PRECAUTIONS

Atropine should always be given prior to or with neostigmine when it is given intravenously, and when nicotinic effects only are required, as muscarinic actions are uncomfortable and can be dangerous when excessive. It should be repeated if bradycardia becomes marked (pulse rate below 60).

Neostigmine should be used with particular care in the presence of asthma and heart disease. It augments the action of depolarizing muscle relaxants and must not be used in an attempt to reverse their effects unless an unequivocal improvement has been demonstrated to a test dose of edrophonium (*see* suxamethonium).

Overdose of neostigmine may cause sudden death due to cardiac arrest, but otherwise is characterized by restlessness, weakness, muscular twitchings, dysarthria, pin-point pupils, nystagmus, sweating, salivation, nausea and vomiting, colic, defaecation, and a desire to urinate. The pulse is weak and rapid and accompanied by hypotension. Respiration is embarrassed by bronchospasm and excessive secretions, and death due to respiratory paralysis and pulmonary oedema may follow. Treatment with atropine will antagonize the muscarinic effects and bronchospasm and excessive secretions are thus inhibited. Muscular twitchings are not affected but may be relieved by small doses of tubocurarine; if respiration is consequently depressed it must be assisted or controlled.

Care must be taken in the treatment of myasthenia gravis not to give an overdose, as this will increase muscular weakness rather than decrease it.

Physostigmine salts

Physostigmine salicylate (*BP* and *USP*)
Physostigmine sulphate (*BP*) and Physostigmine sulfate (*USP*)
Chemical name: (3a*S*,8a*R*)-1,2,3,3a,8,8a-hexahydro-1,3a,8-trimethylpyrrolo-[2,3-*b*]indol-5-yl methylcarbamate

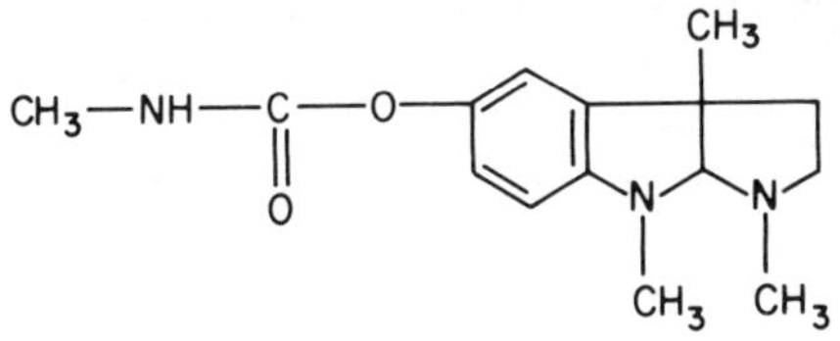

PHARMACOLOGY

Physostigmine is an alkaloid obtained from the calabar bean, the seed of *Physostigma venenosum*, which is indigenous in West Africa, where it has long been used as an ordeal poison. It has been known to physiologists since the middle of the last century, when it was first introduced into England. It is an anticholinesterase whose properties resemble those of neostigmine. However, it is not a quaternary compound and, being lipid soluble, it crosses the blood-brain barrier, the placenta, and penetrates the eyes. It is more potent than neostigmine and has a greater effect on the CNS and cardiovascular system.

It is destroyed in the body by hydrolysis and is eliminated in about 2 hours.

INDICATIONS

Physostigmine was first used in the treatment of myasthenia gravis in 1931 because of the striking resemblance between this condition and the effects of curare, but has since been displaced by neostigmine and pyridostigmine. It is unsuitable for reversing neuromuscular blockade because of its widespread actions on other systems.

Physostigmine has been used (in increments of 0.5 mg) to reverse some of the sedative effects of CNS depressants, including atropine, hyoscine, the phenothiazines, benzodiazepines and tricyclic antidepressants. It is also likely to be the subject of renewed interest as a result of recent reports on its ability to antagonize central effects of other agents. Balmer and Whyte (1977) have shown that physostigmine is able to reverse the psychotomimetic side effects of ketamine without reversing the analgesia, and Toro-Matos *et al.* (1980) have shown that it shortens the recovery time following ketamine. Henderson and Holmes (1976) reported that, after a latent interval of 2–10 minutes, 2 mg physostigmine produced a rapid and sustained awakening in patients in coma under the influence of sodium γ-hydroxybutyrate. Weinstock and her colleagues (1980, 1982) have shown that physostigmine antagonizes morphine-induced respiratory depression but not analgesia. In postoperative patients 1 mg physostigmine intravenously abolished the somnolent effect of morphine and restored respiratory rate, without diminishing the analgesia. Such patients had been pretreated with *N*-butyl-hyoscine to prevent the peripheral effects of physostigmine and droperidol to prevent vomiting induced by physostigmine or morphine.

A 1 per cent solution of physostigmine salicylate is used as a local application to relieve intraocular tension in the treatment of glaucoma.

Balmer, H. G. R. and Whyte, S. R. (1977) Antagonism of ketamine by physostigmine. *British Journal of Anaesthesia,* **49,** 510

Henderson, R. S. and Holmes, C. McK. (1976) Reversal of the anaesthetic action of sodium gamma-hydroxybutyrate. *Anaesthesia and Intensive Care,* **4,** 351

Toros-Matos, A., Rendon-Platas, A. M., Avila-Valdez, E. and Villarreal-Guzman, A. (1980) Physostigmine antagonises ketamine. *Anesthesia and Analgesia,* **59,** 764

Weinstock, M., Roll, D., Enez, E. and Bahar, M. (1980) Physostigmine antagonises morphine-induced respiratory depression but not analgesia in dogs and rabbits. *British Journal of Anaesthesia,* **52,** 1171

Weinstock, M., Davidson, J. T., Rosin, A. J. and Schnieden, H. (1982) Effect of physostigmine on morphine-induced postoperative pain and somnolence. *British Journal of Anaesthesia,* **54,** 429

Pyridostigmine bromide

Pyridostigmine bromide (*BP* and *USP*)
Chemical name: 3-dimethylcarbamoyloxy-1-methylpyridinium bromide

CH_3 — N^+ (pyridinium ring) —O—C(=O)—N(CH_3)$_2$ · Br^-

PHARMACOLOGY

Pyridostigmine is a pyridine analogue of neostigmine. Compared with the latter it is 25–50 per cent less potent. It has less nicotinic action on voluntary muscle, although its onset and duration of action are longer. Its muscarinic action on viscera is weaker.

INDICATIONS

It may be used for similar purposes to neostigmine. It is less satisfactory as an antagonist to curare-like drugs, but it is more useful when a prolonged action is required, as in myasthenia gravis.

DOSAGE AND ADMINISTRATION

Pyridostigmine may be given by mouth, intramuscularly, and intravenously. By mouth, 60 mg is approximately equivalent to 15 mg of neostigmine; by injection 1 mg has a similar effect to 0.5 mg of neostigmine. As an antagonist to competitive muscle relaxants, an initial dose of 2–5 mg may be given intravenously, preceded by atropine 1.2 mg. At least 10 minutes should be allowed to elapse for the drug to take effect before a supplementary dose is given, and the total dose should not exceed 10 mg.

Distigmine bromide is an acid-transferring inhibitor of cholinesterase with a slow onset and prolonged duration of action. After a single intramuscular injection, inhibition of cholinesterase reaches a maximum in 9 hours and persists for approximately 24 hours. It may be used in conjunction with shorter acting but similar agents in myasthenia gravis, particularly to control morning weakness, in doses of 5–10 mg orally twice a day. It can also be used for urinary retention or ileus. Intramuscularly, the dose is 0.5 mg every 24 hours. Muscarinic side effects are similar to those with other anticholinesterases, and can be controlled with atropine; overdose should be similarly treated. Precautions and contraindications are likewise the same as for neostigmine or pyridostigmine, and include all conditions in which acetylcholine potentiation would be undesirable.

Tacrine hydrochloride (This drug has been withdrawn since this edition was prepared)

Tacrine hydrochloride (*BAN*)
Chemical name: 1,2,3,4-tetrahydroacridin-9-ylamine hydrochloride

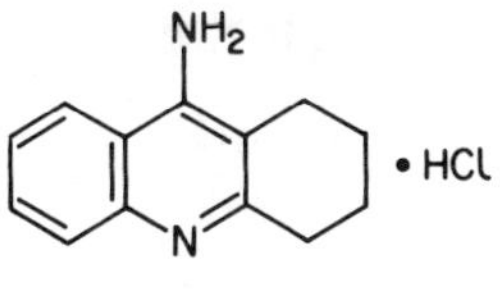

NH_2 • HCl

PHARMACOLOGY

Tacrine is a central stimulant with marked effect on the respiratory centre and convulsions have been reported in animals following large doses. Vomiting, although rare, may also follow its use. It is a non-specific antagonist to the depressant action of morphine, barbiturates, and similar drugs.

Tacrine also has strong anticholinesterase and mild anti-choline-acetylase activity; it potentiates the action of suxamethonium and antagonizes that of competitive muscle relaxants. Parasympathetic (muscarinic) effects will occur, notably bradycardia, unless the patient is adequately atropinized. If the drug is used to prolong the action of suxamethonium, dual block is as likely to develop as when a comparable degree of depolarization block is achieved by other means.

INDICATIONS

Tacrine can be used to prevent respiratory depression and promote wakefulness when large doses of morphine are required in the treatment of chronic pain and for extending the action of suxamethonium.

DOSAGE AND ADMINISTRATION

When used in conjunction with morphine and similar drugs in the treatment of intractable pain, 10–30 mg of tacrine is given intramuscularly with the selected analgesic drug. The dose of each is adjusted until analgesia without depression is obtained. The mixture is repeated 6-hourly. Tacrine is inadequate to reverse neuromuscular blockade by competitive relaxants.

To prolong the neuromuscular block produced by suxamethonium, 15 mg of tacrine is usually given before or with an initial dose of 20–30 mg of suxamethonium. Supplementary doses of 10 mg suxamethonium are given as required. When these have to be repeated at intervals of less than 5–6 minutes a further 10 mg of tacrine may be given.

PRECAUTIONS

Full atropinization is essential before tacrine is given with suxamethonium.

11

Parasympathetic antagonists and anticholinergic agents

The terms, parasympathetic antagonists and anticholinergic agents, overlap to a great extent, but not entirely. The anatomical and functional basis for the difference can be seen by reference to *Figure 11.1*. With the exception of some sympathetic postganglionic nerve endings (which are adrenergic), the transmitter at all preganglionic and postganglionic nerve endings is acetylcholine. Its action at ganglia is nicotinic and that on effector cells is muscarinic. Antagonists at the former are the ganglion-blocking drugs such as hexamethonium, and at the latter atropine and its derivatives. The transmitter at the neuromuscular junction is also acetylcholine and is antagonized at this site by competitive neuromuscular blocking agents such as tubocurarine. Acetylcholine is also a transmitter in certain pathways in the CNS.

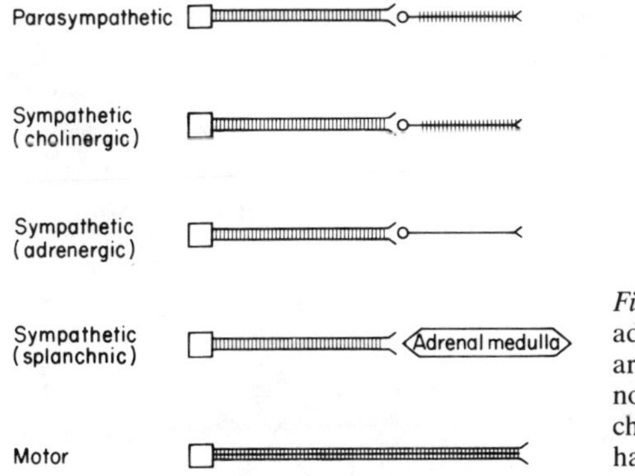

Figure 11.1 Chemical transmitters in cholinergic and adrenergic nerves. Medullated preganglionic fibres are indicated by double lines; postganglionic non-medullated fibres are indicated by single lines; cholinergic transmission is indicated by cross-hatching

Thus, any drug that interferes with the action of acetylcholine as a chemical transmitter can be classed as an anticholinergic agent. It may act by interfering with the release of acetylcholine, by competing with released acetylcholine for the cell receptors or, in the case of the motor end-plates of striated muscle and the nerve cell bodies of autonomic ganglia, by prolonged depolarization which renders them inactive.

Anticholinergic agents do not always inhibit transmission equally at the different sites of cholinergic activity and these differences are due to different degrees of penetration to different sites and different affinities for the various receptors. The most extreme examples are quaternary ammonium compounds such as tubocurarine and hyoscine butylbromide, which do not cross lipid membranes and therefore have no effect on the CNS or eye.

No class of drug is a pure parasympathetic antagonist. While the belladonna alkaloids (atropine and hyoscine) inhibit transmission at all parasympathetically innervated effector cells, they also block transmission to the sweat glands which, although cholinergic, are innervated by the sympathetic nervous system; they are antimuscarinic in action. They are used in premedication as antisialogogues, and to antagonize the unwanted muscarinic action of anticholinesterases when these are required for their nicotinic effect at the motor end-plates of striated muscles.

The parasympathetic pathway can also be blocked at the ganglia, but ganglion-blocking agents affect sympathetic ganglia as well, and antinicotinic action is marked.

Atropine-like action is found in many classes of therapeutic substances which are considered in chapters 3, 5, 6 and 7.

Synthetic atropine-like compounds

Synthetic atropine-like drugs usually have the basic structure shown in *Figure 11.2*. They may be divided into two types, tertiary amines and quarternary ammonium compounds. The former include many that are used therapeutically for their mydriatic and cycloplegic actions on the eye, for example homatropine. Others,

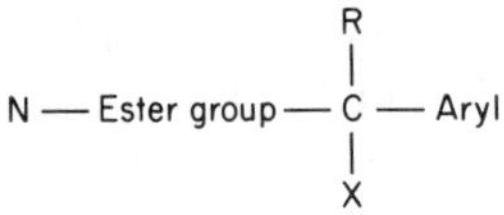

```
                      R
                      |
N — Ester group — C — Aryl
                      |
                      X
```

Figure 11.2 Structure of atropine-like compounds. N may be tertiary or quaternary; X may be alkyl, —H, —OH, —CN, —$CONH_2$, or —COOR; R may be hydroxymethyl, cyclohexyl, or phenyl; aryl group may be phenyl or phenyl-containing polycyclic group

such as dicyclomine and piperidolate, are used for their antispasmodic action on the gut. Such compounds, in addition to being muscarinic antagonists, have other non-specific relaxant effects with papaverine-like or local anaesthetic properties. Tertiary amines can cross the blood–brain barrier and thus have central actions. Quarternary amines, however, are ionized substances and cannot easily cross the blood–brain barrier. Examples are ambutonium, dibutoline, glycopyrronium bromide, ipratropium, lachesine, and tricyclamol.

Belladonna alkaloids

Belladonna alkaloids are widely distributed in nature, particularly in the deadly nightshade (*Atropa belladonna*) which yields mainly the alkaloids atropine and hyoscyamine, while hyoscine is found chiefly in the shrub henbane (*Hyoscyamus niger*). The naturally occurring belladonna alkaloids consist of organic esters of tropic acid with organic bases such as tropine and scopine. The synthetic alkaloids contain mandelic rather than tropic acid combined with a simpler organic base. Homatropine is a synthetic alkaloid consisting of a combination of tropine with mandelic acid.

Atropine is a racemic substance, DL-hyoscyamine, and owes its peripheral effects against the muscarinic actions of choline esters mainly to the L-hyoscyamine. The *laevo*-isomer of hyoscine is also much more active than the *dextro*-isomer. Atropine is closely related chemically to cocaine, and in fact has weak local analgesic actions.

Belladonna alkaloids are so called because of their mydriatic effect, which is seen especially when a solution is instilled into the conjunctival sac. This mydriasis is part of their action as antagonists of the muscarinic actions of acetylcholine and of other choline esters. Their other shared effects include various excitant and depressant actions upon the CNS and an indirect vasodilator action upon the skin vessels, especially those of the blush area.

Hyoscine differs from atropine mainly in having central depressant actions of a sedative nature without causing any preliminary excitatory effects, except in rare instances. Peripherally, it is the more potent in antimuscarinic activity upon the ciliary muscle, the constrictor pupillae, and the gastrointestinal, bronchial, and sweat glands, whereas atropine is the more potent upon the bronchial and gastrointestinal musculature and on the heart.

The usefulness of such drugs depends on their variability of action on different end-organs. Small doses which depress salivary secretion and palmar sweating do not necessarily accelerate the heart or slow micturition. The time course of these drugs varies with the different end-organs studied. The changes in heart rate, salivary secretion and sweating begin and end sooner than those affecting the pupil and accommodation. The peak effect on the heart rate and salivary secretion tends to occur sooner with increasing dosage, but that on the iris and ciliary muscle always occurs later, perhaps because the aqueous humour may be acting as a reservoir for these drugs.

Acceleration of the heart is frequently preceded by slowing, indicating that these drugs have a dual action and that the central effect seems to take place before the peripheral action. In healthy young adults, when vagal tone is greatest, the influence on rate is most marked.

Atropine and hyoscine usually increase the heart rate when given intravenously in sufficient doses although both drugs decrease the heart rate in small doses.

Antiparkinsonian drugs

Anticholinergic agents were the mainstay of treatment for many years but have been relegated to a secondary role by levodopa (*see* Chapter 7). They are, however, still much more effective than levodopa for the control of drug-induced parkinsonism and dystonias. Synthetic anticholinergic agents with selective central actions still have a place as supporting therapy when the side effects of levodopa prevent optimum dosage being used.

For many years benztropine, which combines the chemical and pharmacological features of atropine and diphenhydramine, was the drug of choice. It reduces tremor and rigidity and depression, as well as secondary problems such as excessive salivation and hyperhidrosis. Peripheral cholinergic effects such as dry mouth, loss of accommodation, constipation, and urinary retention usually limit dosage, even though these are less prominent than with the natural alkaloids. Overdose produces typical central symptoms of atropine intoxication. Newer drugs such as benzhexol and benapryzine produce milder side effects and are particularly suitable for combination with levodopa therapy.

Mydriatics

Antimuscarinic agents are used topically in ophthalmology to produce dilatation of the pupil (mydriasis) and to paralyse accommodation (cycloplegia). The latter requires higher concentrations or more prolonged application and so is invariably accompanied by pupil dilatation.

Atropine is prone to produce local irritation and tends to have too long an action for most purposes. Homatropine is shorter acting and its effects can be more readily reversed by physostigmine although usually not completely. Cyclopentolate has mydriatic and cycloplegic actions, the effects of which can last for 24 hours. If dilatation of the pupil only is required, eucatropine or tropicamide may be used. These drugs also have a much shorter duration of action. They can be supplemented by sympathomimetic agents such as phenylephrine. Mydriasis produced by the shorter acting agents can be effectively reversed by pilocarpine (4 per cent) drops; the effects of atropine and hyoscine are more difficult to reverse completely.

Mydriatics are contraindicated in narrow-angle glaucoma. Systemic absorption of drugs after conjunctival application is minimal, although drugs reaching the nasal mucosa via the nasolacrimal duct are readily absorbed.

Atropine

Atropine (*BPC 1973, USP*)
Atropine sulphate (*BP*) and Atropine sulfate (*USP*)
Synonym: (DL)-hyoscyamine

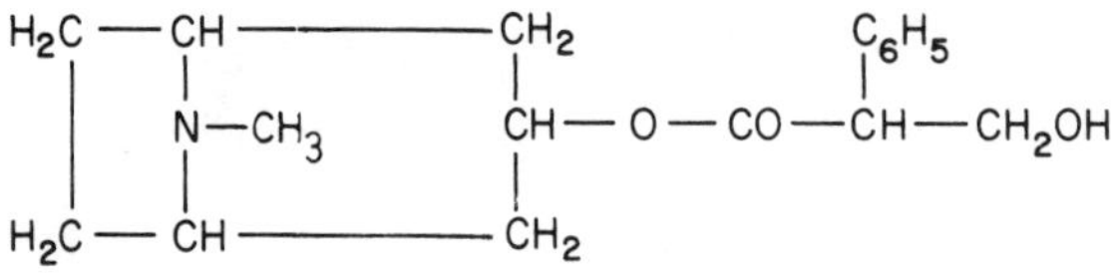

```
H2C — CH ———————— CH2          C6H5
 |     |           |            |
 |    N—CH3        CH — O — CO — CH — CH2OH
 |     |           |
H2C — CH ———————— CH2
```

PHARMACOLOGY

A full discussion of the properties and chemical aspects of atropine will be found under Belladonna alkaloids (*see* page 302), where comparison with hyoscine and hyoscyamine is made. Its main actions are on the central and autonomic nervous systems.

Central nervous system. Certain cerebral and medullary centres are stimulated and subsequently depressed by high dosage. An exception is apparent in parkinsonism where the ability to diminish tremor may be a purely depressant action as no initial stimulation occurs. In general, the central stimulant actions are elicited to a marked degree only by doses that have a pronounced antimuscarinic effect peripherally, but some authorities maintain that even small doses may produce an initial powerful vagal stimulation with obvious cardiac slowing. This does not occur after intravenous injection of doses exceeding 0.5 mg.

Autonomic system. The muscarinic actions of acetylcholine and other choline esters are inhibited. This is also true of nearly all cholinergic nerves and is the basis of the use of atropine in depressing important secretory activity, much smooth muscle, and the effect of the vagus on the heart. Sweating is prevented and body temperature rises, skin blood vessels are dilated, particularly in the blush area.

Cardiovascular system. The main action of atropine is on the heart rate, which it usually increases by inhibiting the cardiac vagus peripherally; occasionally central slowing occurs initially after subcutaneous injection but not when adequate doses are given intravenously. Blood pressure is unchanged, but if already depressed by vagal activity due to reflex or drug action it will be raised.

Respiratory system. Minute volume is slightly increased due to central stimulation. Bronchial musculature is relaxed and secretions are reduced. There is an increase in both the anatomical and physiological dead space but blood gas tensions are not affected.

Absorption and fate in the body. Atropine is rapidly absorbed from the gastrointestinal tract, from the eye, and even slightly from the intact skin; it quickly disappears from the circulation and is distributed throughout the tissues. It is mainly broken down by enzyme hydrolysis in the tissues or liver to tropine and tropic acid; about 13 per cent (after oral administration) is excreted by the kidneys within 12 hours. Traces appear in sweat and milk, which may affect a breast-fed baby. It crosses the placenta and reaches the fetus.

INDICATIONS

Atropine is used to diminish salivary and bronchial secretions during anaesthesia, to protect the heart from vagal inhibition, and to antagonize the muscarinic action of anticholinesterases, such as neostigmine, given to reverse the effects of the competitive muscle relaxants. It may be used to raise the blood pressure in hypotension associated with bradycardia due to vagal stimulation during operations on the neck, chest, and upper abdomen. It is also given to allay the pain caused by spasm in renal and other forms of colic and in the treatment of asthma, to control spasm of the pyloric and cardiac sphincters, and is given with vegetable purgatives to prevent griping. Its control of gastric secretion in cases of peptic ulcer is variable.

Atropine is also used locally in the eye where a prolonged action is required as a mydriatic and cycloplegic, in iritis to immobilize the iris and ciliary muscle and to prevent or break down adhesions. Dilatation of the pupil will occur in 30 minutes and lasts for about a week; paralysis of accommodation takes 1–2 hours but wears off in half this time. Perhaps of more interest to anaesthetists is the use of atropine to reverse hypercapnia during enflurane anaesthesia (Wamba and Sadkova, 1979).

DOSAGE AND ADMINISTRATION

For premedication, 0.3–0.6 mg may be given subcutaneously or intramuscularly 0.5–1 hour before operation, or intravenously immediately before induction of anaesthesia.

In the treatment of hypotension associated with bradycardia, atropine 0.3–0.6 mg may be given intravenously.

In the reversal of residual paralysis of competitive neuromuscular blocking agents, it is given prior to or with neostigmine to antagonize its muscarinic effects; 0.6–1.2 mg is given, in conjunction with neostigmine 2.5 mg. Oral doses of 0.6 mg are sometimes necessary to control the side effects of therapy with anticholinesterases in myasthenia gravis.

For the relief of pain due to renal and other forms of colic, atropine 0.6 mg may be given subcutaneously.

PRECAUTIONS

Atropine as a premedicant is best avoided where there is marked tachycardia such as may occur in thyrotoxicosis, cardiovascular disease, and in cardiac surgery.

Hyoscine or promethazine, which have little or no accelerating effect on the heart rate when given subcutaneously, may be substituted. Atropine premedication should also be avoided in hyperpyrexial patients when the operating theatre temperature exceeds 27.5°C; inhibition of sweating and increase in metabolic rate may give rise to hyperthermia and possibly to convulsions, especially in children.

When intraocular pressure is raised, as in glaucoma, atropine must not be used as it can precipitate an attack, but if mydriasis is necessary, one of the sympathomimetic amines such as ephedrine should be employed.

Atropine in overdose gives rise to dilatation of the pupils and blurred vision, dryness of the mouth, difficulty in swallowing, restlessness, and delirium; convulsions followed by central depression may also occur. Treatment should include gastric lavage if the atropine was taken by mouth. Repeated small doses of thiopentone (100 mg) or diazepam (0.1 mg/kg) may be given slowly intravenously to control convulsions; neostigmine, 1–2 mg intravenously, will antagonize the peripheral antimuscarinic effects of this agent. Central depression may require supportive therapy, including assisted respiration and the administration of pressor agents.

Wamba, W. M. and Sadkova, J. (1979) Atropine reversal of hypercarbia during enflurane anaesthesia. *British Journal of Anaesthesia,* **51,** 221

Atropine methonitrate has the same antispasmodic properties as atropine, but being a quaternary compound it fails to penetrate the CNS and the eye. It is accordingly less toxic. It is used mainly in the treatment of pylorospasm of infants and congenital hypertrophic pyloric stenosis.

Deptropine citrate has antihistamine and antiserotonin activity and thus has bronchodilator and antiallergic properties. An increase in forced expiratory volume in one second has been demonstrated on injection, particularly when combined with isoprenaline.

It diminishes secretions in the bronchial tract, and protects against histamine or acetylcholine-induced bronchospasm in sensitive individuals. Doses that reduce secretions do not have an effect on heart rate. It has little sedative effect on the CNS. It has been used as a drying agent for premedication.

Deptropine citrate 1–2 mg may be given intramuscularly as an anticholinergic agent when an antisialogogue is required. Oral therapy with doses of 1–3 mg daily may be given for allergic rhinitis or bronchitis. Side effects are those which would be expected from its peripheral antimuscarinic actions.

Glycopyrronium bromide

Glycopyrronium bromide (*BAN*) and Glycopyrrolate (*USP*)
Chemical name: 3-(α-cyclopentylmandeloyloxy)-1,1-dimethylpyrrolidinium bromide

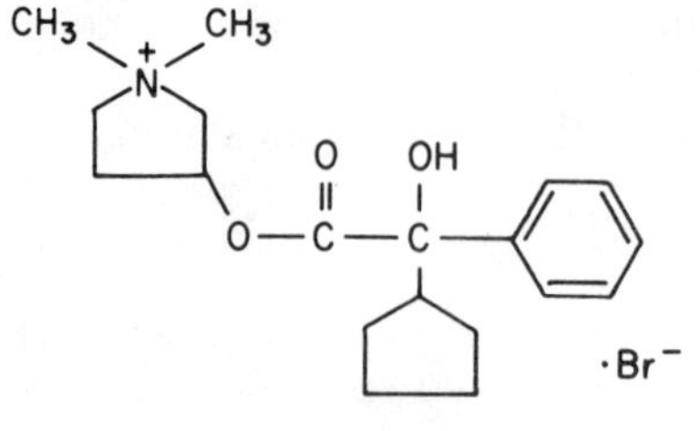

PHARMACOLOGY

Glycopyrronium bromide is a potent long-acting muscarinic antagonist, five to six times as potent as atropine. Being a quaternary compound, it only weakly penetrates the blood–brain barrier, the placenta, and the eye. In anaesthetized patients, intravenous glycopyrronium bromide is approximately twice as potent as atropine in producing a dose-related increase in heart rate. Thus it is possible to control secretions with doses that do not cause marked changes in heart rate (Mirakhur, Jones and Dundee, 1981). Because of its longer duration of action, it has been recommended for preventing the muscarinic actions of neostigmine.

INDICATIONS AND DOSAGE

Glycopyrronium bromide may be used for the reduction of secretions and other antimuscarinic effects. For premedication, 0.2–0.4 mg may be given intravenously prior to anaesthesia. The dose in children is 0.004–0.008 mg/kg. For reversal of competitive neuromuscular block, 0.2 mg with each milligram of neostigmine may be used, and repeated if necessary.

PRECAUTIONS AND SIDE EFFECTS

If dosage is excessive, antisialagogue action can be unpleasant. Overdosage produces peripheral rather than central atropine-like effects. As quaternary ammonium anticholinergics may block end-plate nicotinic receptors, it is contraindicated in myasthenia gravis. Overdose may be relieved by small doses of neostigmine 1 mg per milligram of glycopyrronium bromide previously given.

Mirakhur, R. H., Jones, C. J. and Dundee, J. W. (1981) Effects of intravenous administration of glycopyrrolate and atropine in anaesthetised patients. *Anaesthesia*, **36**, 277

Hyoscine hydrobromide

Hyoscine hydrobromide (*BP*) and Scopolamine hydrobromide (*USP*)
Synonym: (L)-hyoscine hydrobromide

```
                                          C6H5
  HC——CH————————— CH2                      |
 / |   |+           |                      |
O  |  HN—CH3        CH—O—CO—CH—CH2OH  ·Br⁻
 \ |   |            |
  HC——CH————————— CH2
```

PHARMACOLOGY

Hyoscine is an alkaloid resembling atropine, found in the same group of plants, and with central and peripheral actions. These alkaloids are compared above (*see* page 302). The peripheral actions of hyoscine resemble those of atropine. It blocks the action of acetylcholine liberated at parasympathetic postganglionic nerve endings and, in fact, at any site where this exhibits muscarine-like effects. Its effect on the heart rate is variable: when given subcutaneously it tends to cause a decrease by central stimulation of the vagus; when given intravenously heart rate is decreased by small doses and increased by large doses. It is a powerful antisialogogue, requiring only one third the dose of atropine to produce the same effect.

The central actions of hyoscine differ from those of atropine in that they do not produce initial stimulation and excitement, but depress the cortex from the start, especially the motor areas. Hyoscine also affects other parts of the brain causing amnesia, which fact was used in the combination of hyoscine with morphine to produce 'twilight sleep'. When used as a premedicant for caesarean section under ultralight anaesthesia, there is a lower incidence of awareness than when atropine is used. It effectively controls motion sickness and diminishes the emetic effects of morphine-like drugs.

Hyoscine occasionally produces excitement and restlessness, chiefly in elderly patients. In therapeutic doses it usually causes drowsiness and dreamless sleep, amnesia, and sometimes euphoria. In normal subjects it increases respiratory rate and volume, as does atropine, but when respiration is depressed with morphine, hyoscine is better in counteracting this than atropine.

When used in place of atropine in equivalent antisialogogic doses, there is less rise in pulse rate and blood pressure during surgical stimulation.

In general, hyoscine tends to be used for its central actions, and atropine for peripheral ones.

Like atropine, hyoscine is rapidly absorbed and distributed throughout body tissues. It is almost entirely broken down in the body, only about 1 per cent appearing in the urine.

INDICATIONS

Hyoscine is used as a sedative and antisialogogue in premedication and in the treatment of motion sickness. It has also been used as a sedative in general medicine to calm the excited patient and induce sleep, especially in the acute mania of delirium tremens, and in the symptomatic treatment of paralysis agitans and postencephalitic parkinsonism.

DOSAGE AND ADMINISTRATION

For premedication, 0.2–0.4 mg may be given subcutaneously 0.5–1 hour before operation, usually combined with pethidine or morphine or one of its derivatives. Hyoscine may cause depression or excitement in the elderly. Smaller doses may be given, but it is better to substitute atropine in those over the age of 60 years.

Oral preparations are available for premedication in children but they are less effective as drying agents than atropine by this route.

As a general sedative, doses up to 0.6 mg are given and repeated as required. In the acute mania of delirium tremens 1.2 mg may be given alone or combined with morphine 20 mg.

PRECAUTIONS

Precautions to be noted are the same as for atropine. Central stimulation prior to depression is, however, usually absent; drowsiness leading to coma ensues.

Ipratropium bromide is an interesting anticholinergic agent since it is used in the treatment of bronchoconstriction when this is thought to be due to vagal over-activity. The drug is given by a metered inhaler, each metered dose containing 0.02 mg of ipratropium bromide. A contraindication is known sensitivity to atropine. If absorbed from the lungs it might be expected to produce other antimuscarinic effects and urinary retention has been reported. It has been used to produce bronchodilation in patients on β-blocking drugs and in the treatment of chronic reversible airways obstruction. It has been reported to be somewhat less effective than β_2-adrenoceptor agonist drugs such as salbutamol or fenoterol in patients with asthma, but at least as effective as these agents in bronchitis (Pakes *et al.*, 1980)

Pakes, G. E., Brogden, R. N., Heel, R. C., Speight, T. M. and Avery, G. S. (1980) Ipratropium bromide: a review of its pharmacological properties and therapeutic efficiency in asthma and chronic bronchitis. *Drugs,* **20,** 237

Propantheline bromide

Propantheline bromide (*BP* and *USP*)
Chemical name: di-isopropylmethyl[2-(xanthen-9-ylcarbonyloxy)ethyl]ammonium bromide

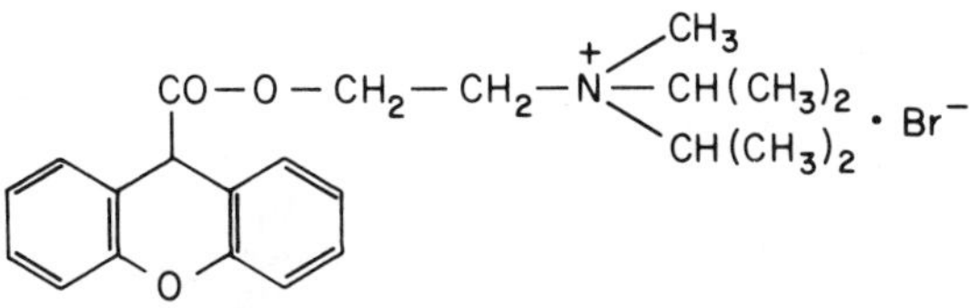

$$\text{(xanthen-9-yl)}-CO-O-CH_2-CH_2-\overset{+}{N}(CH_3)(CH(CH_3)_2)(CH(CH_3)_2) \cdot Br^-$$

PHARMACOLOGY

A number of synthetic quaternary ammonium compounds, methantheline, oxyphenonium, and propantheline, have been shown to antagonize the muscarinic actions of acetylcholine. Propantheline is about three times as active as methantheline as an anticholinergic agent, and its ganglion-blocking activity is also greater. Undesirable side effects are usually less marked than with atropine when given in doses sufficient to depress gastric secretion and motility, but they can be troublesome.

INDICATIONS

Propantheline has been used either alone or with phenobarbitone in the symptomatic treatment of peptic ulcer. It can be used in pancreatitis, intestinal and biliary colic, pylorospasm, bladder spasm, hyperhidrosis, excessive salivation, and in vomiting of pregnancy.

DOSAGE AND ADMINISTRATION

A dose of 15–30 mg is given three times a day by mouth, the evening dose being greater or twice that of the others. For rapid relief of symptoms, 30 mg may be dissolved in 10 ml of isotonic saline and given intravenously. Propantheline can also be given intramuscularly.

PRECAUTIONS

As with atropine, propantheline should not be given to patients with glaucoma. It is also contraindicated in pyloric obstruction and in prostatic enlargement as retention of urine is likely to follow its use. It should always be used cautiously in elderly patients and is best avoided in conditions in which a rise in heart rate could be harmful.

Symptoms of overdose are similar to those of atropine and should be treated on similar lines. Neostigmine 2 mg may be given intravenously to antagonize its effects.

12

Cardiovascular drugs

Before discussing in this and the next chapter the action of drugs on the cardiovascular system, the following brief physiological summary of the factors that control cardiac function and blood pressure is presented to indicate their possible modes of action. The major determining factors in the maintenance of blood pressure are the cardiac output and the peripheral resistance. Other important factors are the elasticity of the arteries and the volume of blood in the circulation. Both the cardiac output and peripheral resistance can vary in response to nervous stimuli.

Nervous control of cardiac function and blood pressure

In the CNS, autonomic cardiovascular representation occurs in the cerebral cortex, the hypothalamus, the medulla oblongata, and the spinal cord, the most active motor control being from the medullary centres (vasomotor, cardioaccelerator, and vagal). These are connected by catecholaminergic and serotonergic tracts. The nucleus tractus solitarius (NTS) in the medulla has an important role (*Figure 12.1*). Stimulation of neurones arising from this nucleus causes inhibition of the

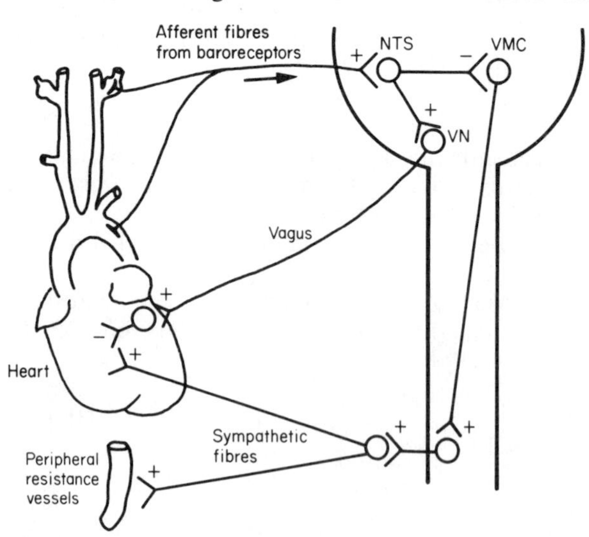

Figure 12.1 The baroreflex pathway. NTS = nucleus of the tractus solitarius; VMC = vasomotor centre; VN = vagal nuclei

vasomotor centre; the transmitter here may be adrenaline. From the vasomotor centre there is a facilitatory noradrenergic pathway to efferent sympathetic neurones in the spinal cord and, in addition, there may be a facilitatory serotonergic pathway.

All efferent autonomic fibres, including the cardiovascular, are relayed at synapses in the autonomic ganglia, except those fibres to the adrenal medulla. All these preganglionic fibres, including those to the adrenal medulla, are cholinergic. The acetylcholine that they release excites the cell bodies of the postganglionic fibres and so transmits nerve impulses; it also directly stimulates the adrenal medulla to liberate a mixture of adrenaline and noradrenaline.

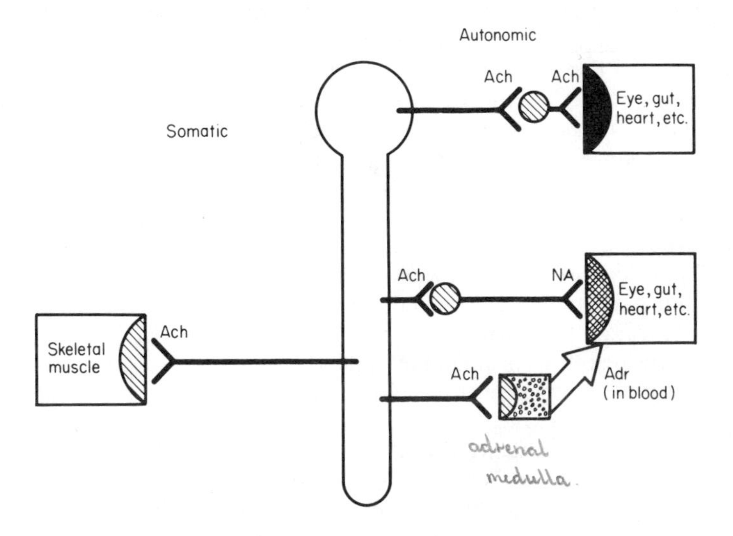

Figure 12.2 Diagram of the peripheral nervous system. Ach = acetylcholine; Adr = adrenaline; NA = noradrenaline; ▧ = nicotinic cholinoceptor; ■ = muscarinic cholinoceptor; ▩ = adrenoceptors

Postganglionic fibres may be cholinergic or adrenergic (*Figure 12.2*). In the cardiovascular system postganglionic cholinergic fibres are parasympathetic (vagal); they slow the heart and dilate certain blood vessels. Postganglionic adrenergic fibres are sympathetic; they accelerate the heart, increase the force of contraction of cardiac muscle, and constrict or dilate blood vessels according to their site (vasoconstrictor to skin and mucous membranes, vasodilator in voluntary muscle). Sympathetic cholinergic vasodilator fibres have been reported; they could be involved in emotional responses like blushing.

Normally, heart rate is under the influence of the vagus and therefore block of vagal transmission will have an obvious effect, the rate being increased. Sympathetic tone opposes that of the vagus but is less powerful. If vagal and sympathetic influences are both blocked concurrently, the rate is increased. The 'intrinsic' heart rate so produced decreases progressively with age.

Blood pressure

In the reflex autonomic control of the arterial blood pressure, the most important afferent fibres run from baroreceptors in the carotid sinuses and aortic arch.

Chemoreceptors in the carotid bodies are of much less importance in cardiovascular control but of major importance in respiratory regulation. Other receptors are present in the pulmonary circulation and the heart but their significance in circulatory control is not yet clear. The aortic and carotid baroreceptors discharge afferent impulses to the CNS with increasing frequency as pressure rises. This results in efferent impulses via the vagi to slow the heart, and probably inhibition of cardiac sympathetic tone as well. While constrictor tone from the vasomotor centre is inhibited, vasodilator tone may be applied instead. Carotid body chemoreceptors are stimulated by excess of carbon dioxide or lack of oxygen to produce a reflex increase in the cardiac rate and vascular tone.

Through this system of reflexly controlled humoral transmitters the autonomic nervous system regulates cardiac output and peripheral resistance. The blood pressure varies as the product of these and so is kept within normal limits by their appropriate adjustment. Peripheral resistance depends mainly on the tone of the arterioles and can be varied independently in different organs, so the total peripheral resistance is the resultant of these values.

Cardiac output

Cardiac output depends upon the venous return and the force and frequency of the heartbeat, but particularly upon venous return, for without an increase in this no increase in cardiac force or rate can avail. However, decreased ventricular contractility, by resulting in a smaller ejected volume in systole, would diminish output. Extreme changes in rate alone can cause output to fall, for severe bradycardia allows diastole to continue after maximum ventricular filling is completed, and marked tachycardia may allow too short a time for adequate ventricular filling. On the other hand, diminished venous return by itself, resulting from venous pooling by dilatation of capillaries and veins, is bound to diminish cardiac output, yet an increased venous return, achieved by raised capillary and venous tone, will increase cardiac output in proportion only, provided that the myocardium can respond. It should be remembered that up to a certain level the force of contraction, and therefore the stroke volume, although variable by sympathetic control, adjusts itself to the input load automatically and without nervous regulation (Starling's law).

Renin–angiotensin system

There are also non-nervous control mechanisms that influence blood pressure, particularly over the long term. The most important of these is the renin–angiotensin system.

Renin is a protein (molecular weight about 40 000) which is secreted from juxtaglomerular cells that are found in the walls of the afferent arterioles in response to a fall in arteriolar pressure. Its plasma half-life is about 20 minutes. While in the bloodstream it acts on plasma angiotensinogen, changing it to the decapeptide angiotensin I. This has little pressor activity. Angiotensin I is converted to angiotensin II by converting enzyme (*Figure 12.3*), the main site of conversion being the lung. Angiotensin II is not only an extremely potent

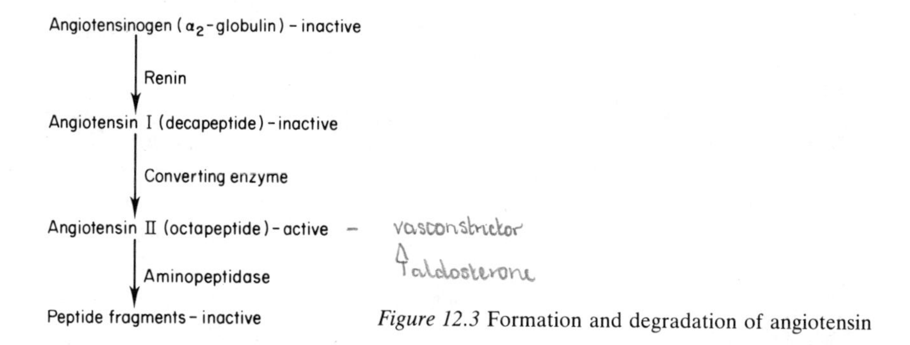

Figure 12.3 Formation and degradation of angiotensin

vasoconstrictor but also induces the release of aldosterone. Angiotensin II has a plasma half-life of about 1 minute. Aldosterone, by causing salt retention, will tend to increase the plasma volume.

The myocardium

The myocardium consists of the heart muscle of the atria and ventricles and their blood supply through the coronary arteries. The latter are most important and resemble certain vessels in the kidney and brain in that they have no vasoconstrictor nerves. When, therefore, there is a rise in systemic blood pressure, the organs they supply benefit and are not affected as they might be by a compensatory vasoconstriction. The coronary blood flow is increased by some of the sympathomimetic amines, such as adrenaline, isoprenaline, and to a lesser extent by noradrenaline and ephedrine. Other drugs with a direct relaxant action on the plain muscle in the arterioles, such as the nitrites and xanthines, particularly theophylline with ethylene diamine (aminophylline), are used for this effect therapeutically in angina pectoris and in any other condition where coronary dilatation is advisable. Coronary constriction will occur only by the action of drugs on the plain muscle of the arterioles direct, such as when vasopressin is released by the posterior pituitary gland in neurogenic shock.

The heart muscle consists of an anastomosis of quadrilateral cells, joined longitudinally to form fibres, connected to neighbouring cells by short bridges. The muscle fibres in the right and left atria are continuous, so that an impulse will spread over both atria simultaneously, but these are separated from the ventricles, whose muscle fibres are also continuous, by a fibrotendinous ring (A-V ring). The pacemaker of the heart is the sinoatrial node (S-A node), situated at the junction of the right atrium and the superior vena cava, and this can be influenced by an increase in vagal tone, which will cause slowing.

Heart muscle has the intrinsic property of rhythmical contraction, which originates in the S-A node, spreads over the atria, and stimulates the A-V node so that an impulse passes down the A-V bundle to the ventricles, causing their contraction. The A-V bundle, or bundle of His, passes across the A-V ring, enters the interventricular septum and divides into right and left branches supplying the ventricles. The bundle continues as Purkinje fibres, forming a plexus beneath the endocardium of each ventricle. By this system the number of atrial impulses reaching the ventricle is regulated, the maximum number possible in the mammalian heart being about 270/min. When the number is in excess of this, some degree of heart block will be present which can be greatly increased by the action of digoxin.

There are certain marked differences between heart muscle and other types of muscle. There is an 'all or none' response, so that above the threshold level, an increase in the intensity of the stimulus does not cause an increase in the force of contraction. Conduction is delayed from atria to ventricles so that they always contract in the right order; the refractory period differs from that of skeletal muscle, it lasts much longer, as long as the phase of contraction, so that there is no summation of contractions or tetanus. Whether the heart rate is slowed by the vagus or increased by the sympathetic, the refractory period of the heart muscle gets shorter as the rate alters in either direction, which means it gets more excitable and conduction of impulse is more rapid through the myocardium. These three features, length of refractory period, excitability, and rate of conduction, must always be influenced in the same direction owing to their inherent relationship.

Under normal physiological conditions the heart beats regularly under the balanced influences of the parasympathetic and sympathetic systems. The mammalian heart has an inherent ability to retain its rhythmicity. This rhythmicity is determined by the spontaneous rate of depolarization of the cardiac cell membrane. Tachycardia will occur if the rate of depolarization is increased by inotropic agents, for example. If their effect is excessive, some dysrhythmia may ensue. On the other hand, local anaesthetics, by stabilizing the cardiac cell membrane, reduce the rate of depolarization and tend both to slow the rate and reduce the number of ectopic beats (*see* page 378).

The cardiac cycle commences with atrial systole (simultaneous contraction of both atria), then after a short pause, due to delayed conduction down the A-V bundle, ventricular systole (simultaneous contraction of both ventricles) follows; each chamber relaxes after contraction which constitutes diastole. At a rate of 72 beats per minute the cardiac cycle occupies 0.8 s, of which ventricular systole occupies 0.3 s and ventricular diastole 0.5 s. When the atria are not contracting, as in atrial fibrillation, the ventricles fill slowly. Ventricular filling depends on the difference between the atrial and ventricular pressures and on the length of diastole. Gravity may make a small contribution.

Hypothermia has a marked effect on cardiac function. The rate is slowed and irritability of the myocardium is increased. Ventricular extrasystoles commonly occur below 28°C, and below 25°C ventricular fibrillation and cardiac arrest may be expected. The cause of this increase in irritability has not been determined, but it has been suggested that hypoxia, hypercapnia, changes in electrolyte balance (calcium:potassium ratio), or increased sensitivity to adrenaline and noradrenaline may be responsible.

Pressor agents and vasoconstrictors

Pressor agents are those which raise the blood pressure. They usually act by causing vasoconstriction, as with noradrenaline, thus increasing peripheral resistance, but some also increase cardiac output or act predominantly in this way, for example adrenaline.

Vasoconstrictors can act on the arterioles and small veins by several mechanisms: by stimulation of the vasomotor centre, by a central stimulant action releasing adrenaline and noradrenaline from the adrenal medulla, by direct action on the plain muscle in the arterioles, or by acting at vasoconstrictor nerve endings or receptors.

Central stimulants are not specifically employed as pressor agents, although several sympathomimetic amines that are used for their adrenergic action also have a central stimulatory effect. Drugs that stimulate sympathetic ganglia are not suitable for producing vasoconstriction as they have undesirable side effects. Stimulation is followed by depression and hypotension.

Vasopressin which acts directly on the muscle of the arterioles is a powerful pressor drug but is no longer used as it causes constriction of the coronary arteries and cardiac ischaemia. Angiotensin amide, a synthetic agent, was thought not to have this effect. It is an extremely potent short-acting pressor agent, and is rapidly broken down by peptides in the blood.

In practice, the drugs most commonly employed are the sympathomimetic agents (*see* below). They act by stimulating the heart, by causing vasoconstriction, or by a combination of both effects. The precise mode of action of some members of this group is still uncertain, experimental evidence is conflicting, and the effects of individual drugs often vary with the dose, the route by which they are given, and the state of the circulation at the time.

Pressor agents are used to raise the blood pressure in simple hypotension or when it is associated with circulatory failure, in spinal and caudal analgesia, in the removal of chromaffin tissue tumours, in overdose of ganglion-blocking agents, and in coronary thrombosis.

It must be remembered that the action of these drugs is of little avail in circulatory failure due to blood loss. This loss must first be replaced with whole blood, plasma, or a plasma substitute. Pressor agents are most effective when hypotension is caused by vasodilatation due to central depression, spinal or ganglion block. In the former case, their use may be unnecessary if anoxia is prevented or removed. Patients under the effects of choloroform, cyclopropane, halothane, or trichloroethylene anaesthesia should not be given pressor drugs that increase the irritability of the heart. Methoxamine and mephentermine are probably the safest.

Certain vasoconstrictors such as adrenaline and felypressin are also used locally with local analgesics to diminish their rate of absorption and increase their duration of action. They may be used alone locally to diminish bleeding and to decongest the nasal mucosa.

Sympathomimetic agents

Sympathomimetic agents, often referred to loosely as adrenergic agents, induce the same responses from various tissues as do adrenaline and noradrenaline. These tissues are those innervated by sympathetic postganglionic fibres whose impulses are transmitted at their nerve endings by the liberation of noradrenaline.

Two major classifications are in vogue at present. Drugs can be classified in relation to the receptors with which they interact. For instance, noradrenaline is a potent α-adrenoceptor agonist, whereas adrenaline is an agonist at both α- and β-adrenoceptors (*see* below). An alternative classification is to divide sympathomimetic drugs into two categories labelled direct or indirect. Drugs that depend on the release of noradrenaline from the presynaptic nerve terminal of the postganglionic fibres of the sympathetic system are then described as indirectly acting.

Reserpine, a drug obtained from the plant *Rauwolfia serpentina*, can cause an almost complete loss of noradrenaline from adrenergic nerves. It releases noradrenaline from its bound stores in the presynaptic nerve ending into the cytoplasm, where most of it is broken down by monoamine oxidase (MAO). It can be shown that in reserpinized animals in which almost complete loss of noradrenaline occurs, tyramine, amphetamine, methylamphetamine, and mephentermine have very little action. Such results suggest that they are mainly indirectly acting sympathomimetic agents. Moreover, indirectly acting sympathomimetic agents have to penetrate the adrenergic nerve terminal to produce their effects. To do so they utilize the re-uptake process normally used by noradrenaline. Indirectly acting sympathomimetic drugs will, therefore, have their action inhibited by re-uptake inhibitors such as imipramine, while the action of directly acting ones will be potentiated. Destruction of the adrenergic neurone by postganglionic denervation or by immunosympathectomy will also inhibit the effects of indirectly acting sympathomimetic drugs.

Using such techniques, sympathomimetic drugs fall on a spectrum from fully directly acting to fully indirectly acting. Noradrenaline, adrenaline, and phenylephrine fall at the directly acting end, amphetamine and tyramine towards the indirectly acting end of the spectrum, while in between fall drugs like methoxamine, metaraminol, and ephedrine.

Adrenoceptors

Dale first suggested in 1906 that sympathetic nervous activity was mediated by two different receptors, when he showed that the normal pressor response of the cat to adrenaline could be reversed by ergot and that vasoconstrictor fibres were blocked while vasodilator fibres were unaffected.

Ahlquist (1948) studied the relative potency of a number of catecholamines on different tissues. He noted that on some tissues, for example heart muscle, isoprenaline was more potent than noradrenaline, while in others, for example peripheral blood vessels, noradrenaline was more potent than isoprenaline. Using

Table 12.1 Types of adrenoceptors in various tissues

Tissue	*Receptor present*
Vascular smooth muscle (skin)	α_1
Vascular smooth muscle (splanchnic area)	α_1
Radial muscle, iris	α_1
Vas deferens	α_1
Intestinal smooth muscle	α_1 and β_1
Heart	β_1
Bronchial smooth muscle	β_2
Blood vessels to skeletal muscle	β_2
Uterus (relaxation)	β_2
Liver (glycogenolysis)	β_2
Presynaptic terminal sympathetic nerve	α_2

as a criterion the differential response to agonists, Ahlquist suggested that there were two types of adrenoceptor. These he called α-receptors and β-receptors. The development of selective antagonists has lent support to this subdivision. Since then β-adrenoceptors have been reclassified into β_1- and β_2-adrenoceptors, and α-adrenoceptors subdivided into α_1- and α_2-types. *Table 12.1* lists some sites where α- and β-adrenoceptors are found.

Following nerve stimulation, noradrenaline released into the synaptic cleft can inhibit further release from the nerve by acting on presynaptic receptors to cause presynaptic inhibition (*Figure 12.4*). Langer (1974) has suggested that these

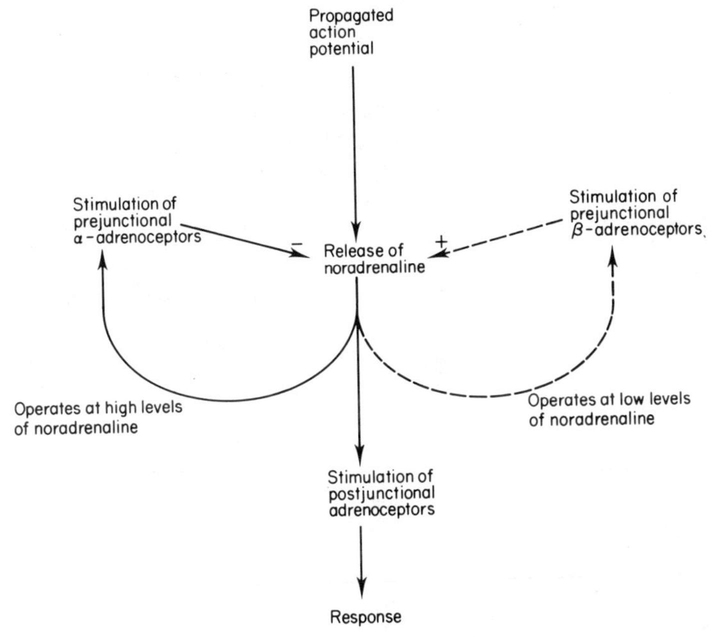

Figure 12.4 Modulation of noradrenaline release by feedback mechanisms operating upon prejunctional adrenoceptors

presynaptic α-adrenoceptors be referred to as α_2-adrenoceptors and postsynaptic α-adrenoceptors as α_1. Since then, although there is an increasing amount of evidence for the existence of more than one type of α-adrenoceptor, the anatomical distinction is not so clear-cut since α_2-adrenoceptors can also be found postsynaptically.

Although drugs that stimulate adrenoceptors are often referred to as sympathomimetic amines, the effects are not completely identical with sympathetic stimulation because some postganglionic sympathetic fibres are cholinergic – notably those to the sweat glands.

Catecholamines, a term also frequently used as synonymous with sympathomimetic, is in fact a classification on purely chemical grounds. It refers to those sympathomimetic amines that have hydroxyl groups in the 3- and 4-positions in the benzene ring (*Table 12.2*) since *o*-dihydroxybenzene is called catechol. Noradrenaline, adrenaline, dopamine, and isoprenaline are truly catecholamines whereas phenylephrine and metaraminol are not. As a group they are basic substances forming salts. The structure–activity relationships of these compounds have been closely studied, and their actions can largely be determined from their formulae depending on the presence or absence of certain groupings (*see Table 12.2*).

The various sympathomimetic agents in common use include ephedrine, methylamphetamine, methoxamine, phenylephrine, isoprenaline, mephentermine, and salbutamol, and their actions vary according to whether they produce a mainly α- or β-response or a mixture of the two. A mixed response such as that produced by adrenaline causes some degree of central stimulation, vasoconstriction in some blood vessels, dilatation in others, cardiac stimulation, bronchial dilatation, and intestinal inhibition with an increase in the tone of the sphincters. A sympathomimetic agent that appears to have no stimulant effect on the CNS in the dosage generally used is fenfluramine, which is used in the treatment of obesity. In addition to its anorectic effect, fenfluramine is claimed to increase the uptake of glucose by muscle and thus to reduce the glucose available for conversion to lipid.

Sympathomimetic drugs are used for the action or actions that mainly predominate; thus, those with strong pressor action are used to raise the blood pressure in the treatment of hypotension, and those with good bronchodilator action are used in the treatment of asthma and bronchospasm.

Table 12.2 Basic structure and effect of replacing certain hydrogen atoms on the activity of sympathomimetic amines

Drug	*Ring position* 2	3	4	5	β-Carbon	α-Carbon	Amine
Dopamine		OH	OH				
Noradrenaline		OH	OH		OH		
Adrenaline		OH	OH		OH		CH_3
Isoprenaline		OH	OH		OH		$CH(CH_3)_2$
Orciprenaline		OH		OH	OH		$CH(CH_3)_2$
Terbutaline		OH		OH	OH		$C(CH_3)_3$
Salbutamol		CH_2OH	OH		OH		$C(CH_3)_3$
Phenylephrine		OH			OH		CH_3
Metaraminol		OH			OH	CH_3	
Methoxamine	OCH_3			OCH_3	OH	CH_3	
Ephedrine					OH	CH_3	CH_3
(Dex)amphetamine						CH_3	
Methylamphetamine						CH_3	CH_3
Mephentermine						$(CH_3)_2$	CH_3
*Notes**		*b, c*	*c*		*a*	*d*	*e*

* *a* An —OH group on the β-carbon atom favours direct action on receptors.

b An increasing number of —OH groups in the ring increases direct action on receptors. A decreasing number of —OH groups favours indirect (transmitter releasing) action.

c Drugs with —OH groups at both 3- and 4-positions can be metabolized by COMT (*see* page 322).

d Drugs *without* substitution on the α-carbon atoms can be metabolized by monoamine oxidases. Therefore, drugs *without* —OH groups on positions 3 and 4 in the ring, and *with* substitutions on the α-carbon atom, are either metabolized to an inactive compound before excretion (for example, mephentermine) or excreted unchanged in the urine (for example, ephedrine).

e Increasing size of substitution on the amine group increases action at β-adrenoceptors.

Table 12.3 Principal actions of some sympathomimetic amines

Drug	*Receptors stimulated*	*Mode of action*	*Cardiac*			*Venous constriction*	*Total peripheral resistance*	*Blood pressure*	*Renal blood flow*	*Broncho-dilatation*	*CNS stimula-tion*
			Out-put	*Rate*	*Irrit-ability*						
Noradrenaline	Mainly α	Direct	0/−*	−	+	+	+	+	−	0	0
Adrenaline	α and β	Direct	+	+	+	+	−	+	−	+	+
Isoprenaline and orciprenaline	Mainly β	Direct	+	+	+	+	−	−	?	+	+
Salbutamol	Mainly β_2	Direct	0	0	0	?	0	0	0	+	0
Phenylephrine	Mainly α	Direct	0/−	−	0/+	+	+	+	−	+	0
Metaraminol	α and β	Direct and indirect	+	−	?+	+	+	+	−	0	0
Methoxamine	α (β-block)	Direct	−	−	0	+	+	+	−	0	0
Ephedrine	α and β	Indirect mainly	+	+	+	+	+/−	+	+/−	+	+
Methylamphetamine	α and β	Indirect	+	+	+	+	+/−	+	+	0	+
Mephentermine	α and β	Indirect	+	+/0	0	+	+	+	+	0	0/+

* In an *in vivo* situation rate and force of cardiac contraction can be reduced by reflex inhibition consequent on rise in mean arterial pressure

The excitatory actions (α-effects), with the exception of that upon the heart, are reduced or eliminated by the α-adrenoceptor blocking agents. The inhibitory actions, bronchodilator actions, and excitatory effects on the heart (β-effects) are reduced or antagonized by the various types of β-adrenoceptor blocking agents.

Symptoms of overdose with these drugs will vary with the predominant action of the individual drug concerned. They may be mainly those connected with central stimulation – anxiety, apprehension, restlessness, and possibly convulsions; or hypertension and cardiovascular collapse – tachycardia, palpitation, cardiac pain, and syncope. Treatment must be symptomatic, using α-adrenoceptor blocking agents to control hypertension, and β-adrenoceptor blocking agents to control cardiac irritability and dysrhythmias.

Drugs which, although they are closely related chemically to the catecholamines, are used predominantly for other purposes (for example, salbutamol as a bronchodilator), are considered in their appropriate chapters.

The principal actions of sympathomimetic amines are summarized in *Table 12.3*.

Ahlquist, R. P. (1948) Study of adrenotropic receptors. *American Journal of Physiology,* **153,** 586
Dale, H. H. (1906) On some physiological actions of ergot. *Journal of Physiology,* **34,** 163
Langer, S. Z. (1974) Presynaptic regulation of catecholamine release. *Biochemistry and Pharmacology,* **23,** 1793

Adrenaline

Adrenaline (*BP*) and Epinephrine (*USP*)
Adrenaline acid tartrate (*BP*) and Epinephrine bitartrate (*USP*)
Chemical name: (*R*)-1-(3,4-dihydroxyphenyl)-2-methylaminoethanol
For structural formula *see Table 12.2*, p. 318

PHYSICAL CHARACTERISTICS

Commercial preparations of adrenaline contain a stabilizer (potassium metabisulphate, 0.1 per cent); this enables them to be sterilized by autoclaving. Repeated autoclaving, however, causes deterioration.

PHARMACOLOGY

Adrenaline is a most important naturally occurring hormone. It can also be synthesized. In the body it is produced from tyrosine by the following enzymatic processes:

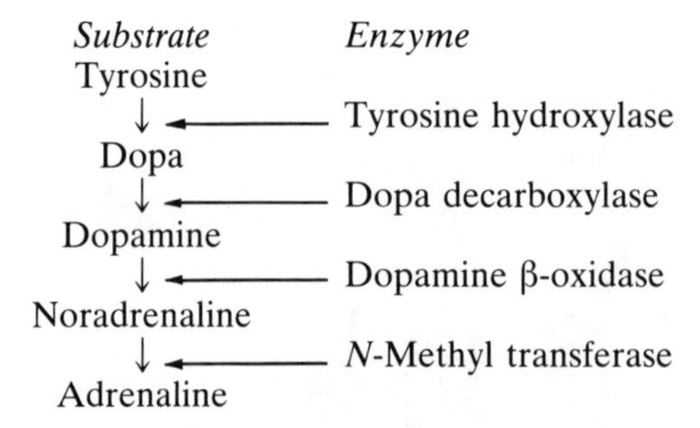

There are other biosynthetic pathways but the above is the main route. In the adult, adrenaline forms about 80 per cent of the catecholamines in the adrenal medulla, the remainder being noradrenaline, but in infancy it is noradrenaline that predominates. There is evidence that adrenaline and noradrenaline are contained in different cells. They are liberated by acetylcholine, in its role of chemical transmitter, by impulses from the autonomic preganglionic fibres supplying the medullary cells. Thus, the adrenal medulla is essentially a sympathetic ganglion with postganglionic neurones replaced by a histologically different type of cell. This comparison is justifiable both on embryological and pharmacological grounds. In contrast, the mixture of catecholamines liberated at adrenergic nerve endings has a minute proportion of adrenaline and a large proportion of noradrenaline. Adrenaline accounts for less than 10 per cent of the catecholamines extractable from tissues other than the adrenal medulla, and probably occurs in them in scattered chromaffin cells. Adrenaline has both α- and β-effects.

In general, it is true to say that the effects of adrenaline, with the exception of sweating, are the same as those of sympathetic activity, but adrenaline may be thought of more as an extra hormone mainly called forth from the adrenal medulla for use in physiological emergency. The ordinary requirements of sympathetic tone are controlled by noradrenaline liberated at adrenergic nerve endings. In the CNS there is some evidence that there are adrenergic neurones as well as the more widely accepted noradrenergic neurones.

Mode of action. Adrenaline has an action both on the cell membrane and on intracellular metabolism by increasing the production of cyclic AMP. It does so by stimulating the enzyme adenyl cyclase which converts ATP into cyclic AMP. Adrenaline causes sodium to leave the cell and reduces the sodium uptake of the cell. It also enters the cell itself and increases energy production. In the case of smooth muscle, most of this energy is taken up to stabilize the inherently unstable cell membrane, whereas with voluntary muscle, whose membrane is inherently stable, the energy is available for contraction. This explains how adrenaline inhibits intestinal muscle and enhances contraction of voluntary muscle.

Central nervous system. There is little effect in small doses. Larger doses have a stimulating effect on the cerebral cortex and medulla and may cause excitement, apprehension, headache, and tremors. Compared with its congeners, ephedrine and amphetamine, its analeptic effect is minimal and of no use clinically.

The EEG spectrum is similar to that produced by attention, but the effect is more marked than that caused by caffeine or amphetamine.

Cardiovascular system. The action of adrenaline upon the circulation varies according to the size of the dose, the route by which it is given, and the prevailing state of the circulation. The smallest effective doses raise the systolic blood pressure, but cause a slight fall in diastolic pressure. This latter effect is caused by a decrease in overall peripheral resistance, vasodilatation of the vessels of the skeletal muscles and liver more than counterbalancing vasoconstriction of the vessels of the skin and mucosae.

In spite of this drop in peripheral resistance, the systolic pressure increases. This is due to the rise in cardiac output which results from increased heart rate and force of beat, caused both by the direct effect of adrenaline on the heart and by the increased venous return initiated by the constrictor action of adrenaline upon the veins.

Large doses of adrenaline cause vasoconstriction even in skeletal muscle, and the overall peripheral resistance is then increased, so that both systolic and diastolic pressures rise.

It should be noted that the degree of change in heart rate is a resultant of the opposing forces of the direct cardiac action of adrenaline and the depressor reflex evoked by the rise in mean arterial blood pressure. Rarely, reflex cardiac slowing may predominate and, conversely, the rise in heart rate and mean blood pressure will be much greater if the reflex arc is weakened at any point, as by block of the vagi or the autonomic ganglia. In complete atrioventricular block adrenaline increases the ventricular as well as the atrial rate even if the block is not overcome by the improvement in conduction which adrenaline also achieves.

Wherever capillaries are constricted their permeability is decreased and the leakage of plasma protein into tissue fluids as a result of allergic reactions is opposed. Capillary constriction also retards the absorption of solutions containing adrenaline. Large doses of adrenaline, or the accidental intravenous injection of doses intended to be subcutaneous, can cause cardiac dysrhythmias which may lead to ventricular fibrillation; acute pulmonary oedema may also occur due to left ventricular failure and to a direct action on the pulmonary epithelium. These complications may also occur from small doses if the heart is more sensitive than usual to adrenaline as the result of the action of certain other drugs, for example chloroform and cyclopropane. Coronary vessels are said to be dilated by adrenaline, but the evidence is not conclusive. It appears that β_2-adrenoceptors mediating vasodilatation are present in the smaller arteries and arterioles, while α-adrenoceptors mediating constriction are present in the larger coronary arteries. Cocaine potentiates the action of adrenaline, and even on a mucous membrane the action of these two drugs together is not advisable.

Respiratory system. Smooth muscle of the bronchi and bronchioles is inhibited by adrenaline and relaxes. The vascular action of adrenaline on the mucosa and the reduction of bronchial secretion will also improve the airway. The central action of adrenaline in causing respiratory stimulation is not great enough, in proportion to all its other actions, to be of use.

Other effects. Adrenaline causes dilatation of the pupil and secretion of tears if it reaches the eye via the bloodstream, but not when instilled into the conjunctival sac, except in hyperexcitability of the sympathetic system in acute pancreatitis, in which it has been used as a diagnostic test (Loewi's), and in thyrotoxicosis.

The movements of the stomach and intestine are inhibited and the fundus of the bladder relaxed, but the ileocolic sphincter and that of the bladder are contracted. It increases the rate of recovery of skeletal muscle in fatigue, and will sensitize ganglion cells to the action of acetylcholine. The parturient uterus in women is relaxed, while in most other species the pregnant uterus is contracted.

Metabolism. Stimulation by adrenaline is expensive in terms of tissue requirements of oxygen as the usual doses of adrenaline can increase the body's total consumption by 20–30 per cent; cardiac efficiency is probably lowered, in spite of the fact that cardiac output is increased, since the extra oxygen uptake is out of proportion to the increased work done. Blood sugar is raised mainly by increased breakdown of muscle and liver glycogen, and glycosuria may occur. High levels of adrenaline in the blood can cause the release of corticotrophin (ACTH) and sometimes of histamine.

Fate in the body. Adrenaline is rapidly inactivated by the enzyme catechol-*O*-methyl transferase (COMT; *see Figure 12.5*) which replaces the hydrogen atom of

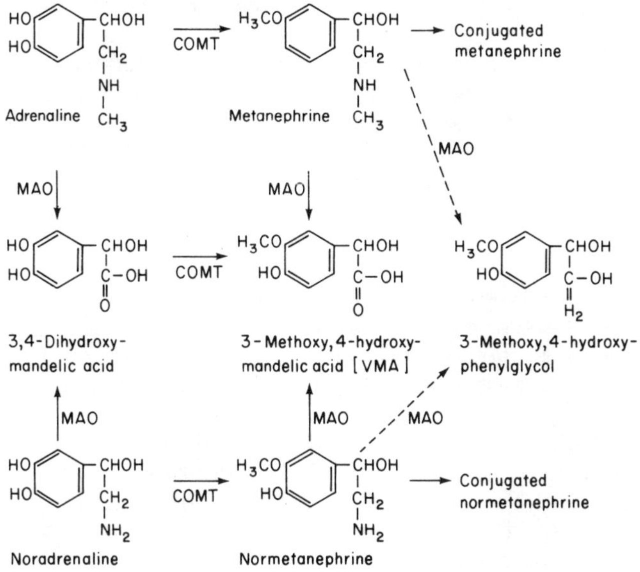

Figure 12.5 Pathways for metabolism of adrenaline and noradrenaline. MAO = monoamine oxidase; COMT = catechol-*O*-methyl transferase

the hydroxyl group in the *meta*-position with a methyl group. Oxidative deamination by MAO (*see also* page 420) also plays a part, although a subsidiary one, in its inactivation. These two processes result in the appearance of 3-methoxy-4-hydroxymandelic acid in the urine (*Figure 12.5*). The level of this substance in the urine is a useful test in the diagnosis of phaeochromocytoma. Large amounts of adrenaline and noradrenaline also appear in the urine when this condition is present.

Antagonists. The α-effects of adrenaline are antagonized by α-adrenoceptor blocking agents, such as phentolamine, tolazoline, and phenoxybenzamine; the β-effects are antagonized by β-adrenoceptor blocking agents, such as acebutolol, oxprenolol, and propranolol.

INDICATIONS

Adrenaline is employed to produce vasoconstriction in local analgesia, broncho-dilatation in asthma, in the treatment of hay fever, and in the various forms of allergy including that following incompatible blood transfusion.

DOSAGE AND ADMINISTRATION

In local infiltration analgesia and nerve block a final strength of solution in the region of 1:200 000 is commonly used, although concentrations down to 1:500 000 are fairly effective. A 1:200 000 solution may be obtained by adding 0.5 ml of 1:1000 adrenaline to 100 ml of the selected analgesic solution. For surface analgesia 0.05–0.1 ml of 1:1000 adrenaline may be added to 1 ml of the analgesic agent: this concentration produces efficient vasoconstriction, but the rate of absorption of the analgesic is not retarded. It has been suggested that this effect can be achieved on mucous surfaces only by using adrenaline a few minutes before the analgesic is applied.

In asthma the patient may inhale the spray of a 1:100 solution of adrenaline or be given a subcutaneous injection of up to 0.5 ml of the 1:1000 solution. The latter dose and method of administration are also suitable in the treatment of serum reactions and the various forms of allergy. In anaphylactic shock accompanied by severe hypotension, 0.2–0.4 ml may be given slowly intravenously, and preferably diluted.

PRECAUTIONS

Great care must be exercised in its use in the presence of hypertension, hyperthyroidism, and severe heart disease.

It must not be given intravenously in strengths exceeding 1:250 000, and when used in the treatment of asthma and serum reactions and in conjunction with local analgesics the total dose given at one administration should not exceed 500 μg.

Adrenaline should not be used in solutions of local analgesics in ring block of the finger as the consequent vasoconstriction is likely to cause gangrene of the tissues distal to the injection. The danger of impairing the blood supply to the cord also contraindicates its use in spinal analgesia. It is best avoided in solutions used for local infiltration for the extraction of teeth as it may give rise to a 'dry socket'.

Overdose of adrenaline produces a feeling of anxiety and apprehension, pallor, and tachycardia; circulatory collapse and syncope may follow. In mild cases recovery is rapid, but should arrest of the circulation occur, cardiac massage must be carried out immediately; the use of a defibrillator will also be necessary.

Adrenaline in the presence of anaesthetic agents. The interaction between adrenaline and volatile anaesthetics, which has been recognized since 1895, presents a common problem with many agents including halothane, chloroform, trichloroethylene, and cyclopropane.

The actual mechanism is believed to be an increased automaticity in the ventricular conducting system. Stimulation of β-adrenoceptors by the catecholamine can be inferred from the specific protective effect of β-adrenoceptor blockade. Hypercapnia and hypoxia have a potent aggravating effect, but the chief determinant is the effective dose of adrenaline reaching the heart. This depends on the total dose, the concentration, and the vascularity of the site, or route of injection. Adrenaline can be safely administered with halothane if the following points are observed:

1. There should be no hypoxia or hypercapnia;
2. Solutions should be no stronger than 1:200 000;
3. The total dose should not be more than the equivalent of 20 ml of 1:200 000 in 10 minutes, or 30 ml in an hour.

In the case of cyclopropane and chloroform, however, the threshold seems to be lower and the combination of adrenaline with these agents should be avoided. However, if these restrictions cannot be strictly followed, a prophylactic injection of practolol, 1–2 mg, may be given intravenously. Whether or not such prophylactic action can be justified, any ventricular dysrhythmias that occur may be treated with practolol if they cannot be abolished by reducing vapour strength and correcting hypoventilation.

Amphetamine and dexamphetamine

Amphetamine sulphate (*BP*) and Amphetamine sulfate (*USP*)
Dexamphetamine sulphate (*BP*) and Dextroamphetamine sulfate (*USP*)
Chemical names: (±)-α-methylphenethylamine sulphate
(+)-α-methylphenethylamine sulphate
For structural formulae *see Table 12.2,* p. 318.

PHARMACOLOGY
Amphetamine is a congener of adrenaline, being racemic 2-aminopropylbenzene. The *dextro*-isomer (dexamphetamine) is twice as potent as amphetamine, and four times as potent as the *laevo*-isomer. In general, its actions resemble those of ephedrine and like it, it is an indirectly acting sympathomimetic agent, but it is more powerful on the CNS and less so at all other sites. It has both α- and β-effects and is an inhibitor of MAO.

It causes less restlessness and apprehension than ephedrine, fatigue is abolished, wakefulness is promoted and more work can be done, there is increased initiative rather than ability and mistakes may occur more frequently. In the usual oral doses there is little cardiovascular effect, but the blood pressure is usually slightly raised. Tolerance is not accompanied by greater rates of excretion or destruction. Because of its CNS-stimulating properties, it is a drug of dependence and has been in the past one of the 'dopes' commonly taken by athletes to improve their performance. Chronic abuse can produce antisocial behaviour in dependent persons and even schizophrenia-like states. About half of an oral dose is deaminated in the liver and the other half is excreted unchanged in the urine in slightly more than 2 days.

Dexamphetamine sulphate has identical but more powerful actions, with a similar dose range. Amphetamine and dexamphetamine are among those drugs which may be lawfully in the possession of only a few authorized categories of user.

INDICATIONS
Owing to its tendency to cause addiction, therapeutic uses tend to be limited now to narcolepsy and postencephalitic parkinsonism.

DOSAGE AND ADMINISTRATION
The official dose of the sulphate is 2.5–10 mg orally. It will prevent sleep if administered too late in the day.

Ephedrine

Ephedrine (*BP*), Ephedrine hydrochloride (*BP* and *USP*) and Ephedrine sulfate (*USP*)
Chemical name: (1*R*,2*S*)-2-methylamino-1-phenylpropan-1-ol
For structural formula *see Table 12.2,* p. 318

PHARMACOLOGY
Ephedrine is a sympathomimetic amine and is the active principle of the Chinese plant *Ma Huang*, known and used for centuries in the East. It was introduced to Europe in 1923 and is now produced synthetically. It has α- and β-effects and acts

both directly and indirectly; as with amphetamine, tachyphylaxis is marked. It is an inhibitor of MAO.

Central nervous system. There is considerable stimulation of the cerebral cortex and medulla, but this is not as marked as with amphetamine, although wakefulness may occur and there is some analeptic effect on the unconscious. Ephedrine stimulates the spinal cord and enhances spinal reflexes.

Cardiovascular system. Cardiac output and rate are increased and repeated frequent doses or a single very large dose may result in depression of the heart. Vasoconstriction is almost balanced by vasodilatation and overall peripheral resistance is little changed; diastolic blood pressure is increased but less so than systolic blood pressure. There is also an increase in cardiac irritability. Vessels of mucous membranes are constricted following local application, but this action is not so marked after systemic administration. Cerebral blood flow is reduced as is blood flow through the kidneys. Coronary vessels are stated to be dilated, but the increased blood flow through them may be due to the increase in cardiac output.

Respiratory system. There is dilatation of the bronchial tree due to inhibition of the muscles of the bronchi and bronchioles. Respiration is stimulated, especially if drug-induced depression is present.

Alimentary system and urinary tract. There is inhibition of smooth muscle and increase in tone of the sphincters of the alimentary tract and the bladder. The drug may cause retention of urine, especially when there is an enlarged prostate.

Fate in the body. It inhibits MAO and is not destroyed by it. It is excreted unchanged in the urine within 24 hours.

INDICATIONS

Ephedrine is less commonly used for its pressor action but it is still occasionally used in the prophylactic treatment of asthma. Many proprietary preparations contain ephedrine mixed with other bronchodilator drugs and are sold in considerable quantities. It may also be used as a local application to reduce congestion of the nasal mucosa during colds and hay fever, and prior to the passage of a nasal endotracheal tube to prevent bleeding from abrasions. If a vasopressor is needed in obstetric practice, it is the drug of choice as it does not reduce uterine blood flow. It has a limited place in a few cases of myasthenia gravis.

DOSAGE AND ADMINISTRATION

Ephedrine hydrochloride is active by mouth, and may also be given intramuscularly; duration of action may be up to an hour or more.

The treatment of asthma is usually by the oral route in doses of 30–60 mg, repeated as required. Tolerance may be shown to repeated doses.

For the relief of nasal congestion and the production of vasoconstriction to aid the passage of a nasal endotracheal tube, a 1 per cent solution in water or liquid paraffin may be used.

PRECAUTIONS

Ephedrine produces a number of cardiovascular side effects which contraindicate its use in myocardial or coronary disease. It should also be used with care in cases of even moderate hypertension. As it is apt to cause wakefulness it should not be given late in the day.

Overdose causes anxiety, apprehension, restlessness, tachycardia, palpitations, and hypertension. Treatment should be sedation with barbiturates in sufficient dose to control the symptoms.

Isoprenaline salts

Isoprenaline sulphate (*BP*) and Isoproterenol sulfate (*USP*)
Isoprenaline hydrochloride (*BP*) and Isoproterenol hydrochloride (*USP*)
Chemical name: 1-(3,4-dihydroxyphenyl)-2-isopropylaminoethanol
For structural formula *see Table 12.2,* p. 318

PHARMACOLOGY

Isoprenaline is a catecholamine closely allied to adrenaline. It has powerful stimulant effects on all β-adrenoceptors but only very weak actions on α-adrenoceptors.

Central nervous system. There is a mild stimulatory effect on the cerebral cortex.

Cardiovascular system. Isoprenaline has a powerful cardiac stimulating action and accelerates the heart rate. It produces marked peripheral vasodilatation. Effects on blood pressure are variable; usually there is a moderate fall in systolic and a greater fall in diastolic pressure. This results from the peripheral vasodilatation more than overcoming the effects of the increase in cardiac output. These observations also apply to therapeutic doses of isoprenaline given by aerosol. However, heavy users of isoprenaline aerosols are relatively resistant to the cardiac stimulant effects of isoprenaline. In dogs, cardiac depression may follow the cardiac stimulant action of isoprenaline in the presence of anoxia, and it has also been suggested that in the presence of raised pulmonary artery pressure, β-stimulants can also cause cardiac depression. There is normally no vasoconstriction except when the drug is applied locally to mucous surfaces.

Respiratory system. There is a marked dilatation of bronchial muscle, even more effective than that of adrenaline. The rate and depth of respiration are slightly increased. Isoprenaline inhibits the release of histamine from passively sensitized human lung to a much greater extent than salbutamol, orciprenaline, or sodium cromoglycate. This suggests that it is of particular use in bronchospasm associated with anaphylactic reactions. Isoprenaline, like orciprenaline, while improving airway resistance may cause a fall in arterial oxygen tension and raise the tension of carbon dioxide. This effect is thought to be due to an aggravation of the existing ventilation/perfusion inequality present in asthmatic subjects. Worsening of airway obstruction with prolonged use of isoprenaline in heavy doses and an improvement on withdrawal of the drug has been reported. It has been postulated that this could be due to the accumulation of 3-methoxyisoprenaline, a β-blocking metabolite, although it has not been possible to produce demonstrable changes in respiratory function in man with this substance. However, it has been suggested that tolerance may also develop to other β-stimulants which do not form 3-methoxy derivatives, and may be a problem with all β-stimulant drugs. Prolonged heavy dosage may lead to decreasing response of the receptors, and this may also reduce the effect of the patient's own sympathetic nervous system and produce increasing bronchoconstriction.

Alimentary system. Ulceration in the buccal mucosa has been reported after sublingual absorption. There is some inhibition of peristaltic action and of the tone of the intestine.

Metabolism. Isoprenaline stimulates metabolism and increases oxygen consumption and carbon dioxide production.

Fate in the body. The metabolic fate of isoprenaline is similar to that of adrenaline.

INDICATIONS

Isoprenaline is chiefly used in the treatment of bronchospasm, and for this purpose is administered as a metered dose from an aerosol spray. It may also be used in the treatment of bradycardia and hypotension due to heart block, as a cardiac stimulant following cardiac arrest, and in the management of cardiogenic and endotoxic shock in patients who do not respond to fluid replacement and acid–base correction.

DOSAGE AND ADMINISTRATION

For the treatment of asthma, isoprenaline may be given in the form of sublingual tablets containing 10 or 20 mg or by the inhalation of a 1 per cent spray from a nebulizer or proprietary pressurized spray delivering a metered dose. For heart block 5-mg suppositories may be given every 3–4 hours or in emergency 25 μg (0.5 ml of 1:20 000 solution) intravenously. In the management of shock an infusion of isoprenaline 1 mg in 500 ml of 5 per cent dextrose may be given, at a rate of 2–4 μg/min.

PRECAUTIONS

Side effects, which occasionally are severe, include tachycardia, palpitations and precordial pain, dizziness, faintness, headache, tremor, weakness, and sometimes nausea and vomiting.

The death rate from asthma increased in England and Wales in the years following the widespread introduction of pressurized isoprenaline aerosols for the treatment of this condition. In the age-group 5–64 years the death rate in males doubled and in the age-group 5–34 years it trebled; in the age-group 10–14 years it increased eight-fold. A review of deaths certified as due to asthma showed that a high percentage of these patients had been using pressurized aerosols containing isoprenaline.

There are at least four possible mechanisms by which isoprenaline might affect asthma mortality:

1. Cardiac stimulation giving rise to dysrhythmias;
2. A fall in arterial Po_2 despite an improvement in airway resistance due to changes in ventilation/perfusion inequalities;
3. Excessive doses causing increased airways obstruction;
4. Cardiac depression under conditions of anoxia and right heart strain.

Isoprenaline should be given intravenously only in cases of emergency. It should be used with the greatest caution in thyrotoxicosis and in the presence of serious cardiovascular disease, such as acute coronary disease and cardiac asthma. It may be used alternately with adrenaline, but not at the same time.

Orciprenaline differs from isoprenaline only in having both the hydroxyl groups of its benzene ring in the *meta*-position instead of having one in the *para*-position. Its actions are similar but it has a longer duration of action and it is active by mouth. It may be given as 20-mg tablets three times a day or by the inhalation of a 5 per cent spray. Proprietary pressurized sprays delivering a metered dose are also available. Toxic effects are less marked than those of isoprenaline but deaths have been recorded following the excessive use of sprays. The total dose should not exceed 100 mg a day.

Isoetharine combines the *N*-isopropyl group associated with the excellent bronchodilator action of isoprenaline with an ethyl group on the α-carbon atom, where substitution at this point is associated with less cardiovascular activity. Isoetharine hydrochloride has been formulated in a special porous plastic matrix. By this means, the release of the isoetharine is controlled, giving a duration of action of 4–6 hours. Isoetharine is used for the relief of bronchospasm in asthma, in chronic bronchitis, and in pulmonary emphysema. In normal dosage, one 10-mg tablet three or four times a day has negligible effects on heart rate and blood pressure.

Mephentermine sulphate (This drug has been withdrawn since this edition was prepared)

Mephentermine sulphate (*BP*) and Mephentermine sulfate (*USP*)
Chemical name: *N*αα-trimethylphenethylamine sulphate
For structural formula *see Table 12.2,* p. 318

PHARMACOLOGY

Mephentermine is closely related chemically to methylamphetamine. It has α- and β-effects and its action at nerve endings is indirect. Tachyphylaxis occurs with repeated injections.

Central nervous system. It is a mild cerebral stimulant with about half the activity of amphetamine.

Cardiovascular system. Mephentermine increases arterial pressure and systemic vascular resistance, but produces little change in cardiac output. It has considerable β-effects, which become more obvious in the presence of atropine. The combination results in marked increases in cardiac output and heart rate, and greater increases in arterial pressure and ventricular work. Thus, the existing state of autonomic balance will markedly influence the effects of the drug and this could account for discrepancies between various studies of its actions. The drug has a relatively slow onset (4 minutes after intravenous injection) and prolonged peak action lasting 1–2 hours. Compared with methoxamine it produces a relatively greater increase in arterial pressure with less disturbance to other circulatory parameters.

Respiratory system. There is no effect on bronchial musculature or on respiration.

Fate in the body. Mephentermine is metabolized in the body by *N*-demethylation to normephentermine; *p*-hydroxynormephentermine may be formed by subsequent *p*-hydroxylation.

INDICATIONS

Mephentermine is used in the control of circulatory failure and hypotension when a pressor agent with both α- and β-actions is desirable. It has also been used to maintain blood pressure following cardiac infarction, and as an inhalant to reduce nasal congestion. It can safely be used in the presence of cyclopropane and halothane, and may be useful in maintaining blood pressure after the withdrawal of a noradrenaline infusion.

DOSAGE AND ADMINISTRATION

Mephentermine may be given intramuscularly or intravenously. When given intramuscularly it acts in 5–15 minutes and lasts for 1–2 hours; when given intravenously it acts more quickly and lasts for 30–45 minutes.

In the treatment of hypotension, 15 mg may be given intramuscularly, or slowly intravenously; if ineffective, this dose may be repeated, and supplementary doses are given as necessary. Mephentermine can be given by intravenous infusion, 30 mg in 100 ml of 5 per cent dextrose. A 0.5 per cent solution is inhaled or instilled into the nose to relieve congestion.

PRECAUTIONS

Mephentermine should be used cautiously in severe cardiovascular disease and hypotension. Overdose will produce symptoms of extreme hypertension – headache, vomiting, and palpitations; drugs that interfere with the uptake of mephentermine into the noradrenergic nerve terminal, such as the tricyclic antidepressants, will inhibit its activity.

Metaraminol tartrate

Metaraminol tartrate (*BP*) and Metaraminol bitartrate (*USP*)
Chemical name: (−)-2-amino-1-(3-hydroxyphenyl)propan-1-ol hydrogen tartrate
For structural formula *see Table 12.2*, p. 318

PHARMACOLOGY

Metaraminol has both α- and β-effects, and its action at adrenoceptors is mixed: both direct and indirect actions are demonstrable.

Cardiovascular system. Cardiac output and force are increased and there is an increase in peripheral resistance. The combination of these factors causes a well-sustained rise in blood pressure. Coronary blood flow is increased. The heart rate is slowed, especially after intramuscular injection.

Respiratory system. There may be moderate slowing of respiration with some increase in depth.

INDICATIONS

Metaraminol is used in the treatment of hypotension due to circulatory failure, myocardial infarction, spinal analgesia, and overdose of ganglion-blocking agents.

DOSAGE AND ADMINISTRATION

It may be given subcutaneously, intramuscularly, or intravenously. When given intravenously, it acts in 1–3 minutes, and lasts for about 25 minutes. Intramuscularly it acts in 5–10 minutes and lasts for an hour or more. Dosage is 2–10 mg given intramuscularly, and 1.5–5 mg intravenously. Administration should not be repeated until it is certain that the full effect of the previous dose has been produced.

PRECAUTIONS

Metaraminol should be used with caution in patients with hypertension, severe heart disease, or hyperthyroidism.

Methoxamine hydrochloride

Methoxamine hydrochloride (*BPC* and *USP*)
Chemical name: 2-amino-1-(2,5-dimethoxyphenyl)propan-1-ol hydrochloride
For structural formula *see Table 12.2,* p. 318

PHARMACOLOGY

Methoxamine is a sympathomimetic agent whose agonist actions are mediated solely at α-adrenoceptors. It produces some blockade of β-adrenoceptors. Its action at α-adrenoceptors is mainly direct but some degree of indirect action has also been demonstrated.

Central nervous system. There is no stimulatory action.

Cardiovascular system. Cardiac output is probably decreased, and there is no effect on force or irritability. Heart rate is slowed: this was originally thought to be due to vagal action initiated by baroreceptors, but is probably due to β-adrenoceptor blockade. Peripheral vessels are markedly constricted by direct action, and there is an overall increase in peripheral resistance, consequently both systolic and diastolic blood pressures are increased; renal blood flow is reduced.

Other systems. There is no effect on bronchial musculature and respiration is not stimulated.

Inhibitory action on the intestinal musculature is not marked.

INDICATIONS

Methoxamine is used in the treatment of hypotension associated with circulatory failure, the prevention of hypotension during spinal analgesia, and in the control of blood pressure during anaesthesia in which hypotensive techniques are involved. As it does not increase the irritability of heart muscle, it may be used during anaesthesia with chloroform, cyclopropane, and trichloroethylene. Methoxamine has also been used in the treatment of paroxysmal tachycardia, and overdose with ganglion-blocking drugs.

DOSAGE AND ADMINISTRATION

Methoxamine may be given by the intramuscular or intravenous route. It acts within 2 minutes when given intravenously and lasts for about an hour; when given intramuscularly it takes up to 20 minutes to act but lasts somewhat longer.

In the treatment of hypotension of moderate degree due to circulatory failure 10–15 mg may be given intramuscularly; in more severe cases 5–10 mg may be given slowly intravenously. Blood loss must, of course, be replaced.

In the treatment of paroxysmal tachycardia, 10–20 mg may be given intramuscularly.

PRECAUTIONS

Methoxamine should not be given in severe myocardial or coronary disease or to patients on MAO inhibitors and extreme care must be exercised when it is administered to patients with hypertension or hyperthyroidism. The effect of small doses should first be noted. If supplementary doses are considered necessary, they must not be given until the previous dose has had time to take full effect.

Overdose with methoxamine will produce an undesirably high blood pressure, excessive slowing of the heart, headache and projectile vomiting, a desire to empty the bladder and a marked pilomotor response. An α-adrenoceptor blocking agent such as phentolamine (5 mg) will relieve hypertension, otherwise treatment should be symptomatic.

Methylamphetamine hydrochloride

Methylamphetamine hydrochloride
Chemical name: (+)-*N*α-dimethylphenylethylamine hydrochloride
For structural formula *see Table 12.2,* p. 318

PHARMACOLOGY

Methylamphetamine is a derivative of amphetamine and has similar properties, but is more rapid in effect and acts for a longer period of time. It is an indirectly acting sympathomimetic drug which has both α- and β-effects. Its action on the cardiovascular system is more prolonged and therefore more useful, but weaker, than that of amphetamine, whereas in equal dosage it has double the stimulant effect on the CNS.

Central nervous system. There is marked central stimulation and it produces an elevation of mood and general euphoria. It causes wakefulness and has some analeptic effect on the unconscious. Prolonged cerebral stimulation is followed by depression.

Cardiovascular system. As with adrenaline there is an increase in cardiac output, force, rate, and irritability. This is accompanied by peripheral vasoconstriction, although overall peripheral resistance may be increased or unchanged. Renal blood flow is increased. Systolic blood pressure is increased, but the rise in the diastolic pressure is less marked.

Respiratory system. There is no effect on bronchial musculature, but respiration is stimulated.

Gastrointestinal tract. There is no inhibitory action on the plain muscle of the alimentary tract. Like amphetamine, it reduces appetite.

Fate in the body. Recovery from overdose may take several days as it is excreted in the urine very slowly. Elimination can be increased by making the urine more acidic.

INDICATIONS

Methylamphetamine is used as a pressor agent in the control of hypotension when both α- and β-actions are required. It will maintain blood pressure after withdrawal of a noradrenaline infusion.

DOSAGE AND ADMINISTRATION

Methylamphetamine is active by mouth, but when a more rapid effect is required it is given intramuscularly or intravenously.

In moderate hypotension 15–20 mg is given intramuscularly. In more severe cases 10–15 mg should be given intravenously, followed by 15–20 mg intramuscularly. Any blood loss must of course be replaced. Ten minutes should be allowed for the drug to take effect if given intravenously, or 20 minutes if given intramuscularly, before giving a supplement. Injection of methylamphetamine can only be dispensed from a hospital pharmacy. It can cause dependence of the amphetamine type.

PRECAUTIONS

Methylamphetamine should not be given to patients suffering from myocardial or coronary disease, and it should be used with caution in hypertension and hyperthyroidism. It should be remembered that the analeptic action of this agent will temporarily lighten the level of anaesthesia when used during operation.

Overdose will produce hypertension, tachycardia, excitement, restlessness, and convulsions. Treatment, as in the case of amphetamine, should be by sedation, and an α-adrenoceptor blocking agent such as phentolamine (5 mg) should be given if hypertension reaches dangerous levels.

Naphazoline salts

Naphazoline nitrate (*BP*) and Naphazoline hydrochloride (*USP*)
Chemical name: 2-(1-naphthylmethyl)-2-imidazoline

Naphazoline, an imidazoline derivative, is a powerful vasoconstrictor. When applied to mucous surfaces its action is rapid (2–3 minutes) and its effect lasts from 4–6 hours. It differs from other sympathomimetic drugs in producing CNS depression in place of stimulation.

The naphazoline salts are used to relieve nasal congestion in acute rhinitis, sinusitis, and hay fever, and may be employed prior to the passage of a nasal endotracheal tube to prevent bleeding. They are normally administered as 1:2000 aqueous solutions by means of a nebulizer, or 2–3 drops may be instilled into the nose. When used with local analgesics on mucous surfaces 2–4 drops may be added to 1 ml of the selected agent. Naphazoline should not be used parenterally. Excessive dosage could cause a rise in blood pressure, so it should be used cautiously in cardiovascular disease, but this has not been reported after local application.

Noradrenaline acid tartrate

Noradrenaline acid tartrate (*BP*) and Levarterenol bitartrate (*USP*)
Chemical name: (*R*)-2-amino-1-(3,4-dihydroxyphenyl)ethanol hydrogen tartrate
For structural formula *see Table 12.2*, p. 318

PHARMACOLOGY

Like adrenaline, noradrenaline is an important naturally occurring hormone, and it can be synthesized artificially. In the body it is derived from the amino acid tyrosine via dopa and dopamine. In the adult it forms about 10–20 per cent of the catecholamines in the adrenal medulla, the remainder being adrenaline; in infancy the proportion of noradrenaline exceeds that of adrenaline. These hormones are contained in different cells, but both are liberated by acetylcholine, in its role of chemical transmitter, by impulses from the autonomic preganglionic fibres supplying the medullary cells. In the catecholamines liberated at adrenergic nerve endings more than 90 per cent is noradrenaline, and a similar proportion is extractable from tissues other than the adrenal medulla, probably in scattered chromaffin cells. Noradrenaline has powerful α-effects and weak β-effects. It is the chemical transmitter released by postganglionic nerve fibres of the sympathetic system and is responsible for normal sympathetic tone, and the stimulation of effector cells. It is stored in granules in nerve axons and is also released by indirectly acting adrenergic agents such as mephentermine and methylamphetamine, whose pressor and other effects are due to this action.

Central nervous system. In contrast to adrenaline there is no central stimulation of the cerebral cortex.

Cardiovascular system. Cardiac output is unchanged, but the contractile force and the irritability of the heart are slightly increased, but not to the same extent as that produced by adrenaline. Heart rate is usually decreased, due to the effect of the increased blood pressure on the baroreceptors. There is constriction of all peripheral vessels and an increase in venous pressure producing an increase in overall resistance and consequent rise in systolic and diastolic blood pressures. Renal, hepatic, and cerebral blood flow are reduced, but there is evidence, although not conclusive, that the coronary vessels are dilated. Muscle blood flow is reduced.

Respiratory system. There is little effect on bronchial muscle. Rate and depth of respiration are increased slightly.

Plain muscle. Noradrenaline has a weaker inhibitory action on plain muscle than adrenaline, but it stimulates contractions of the uterus in late pregnancy and labour.

Elimination. As with adrenaline, it is rapidly inactivated by the enzyme catechol-*O*-methyl transferase. Oxidation and deamination also play a part in its degradation.

INDICATIONS

Noradrenaline is used in the treatment of hypotension in circulatory failure, and following operations for the removal of chromaffin cell tumours. It has also been used successfully in the treatment of severe hypotension associated with coronary thrombosis. It will overcome the hypotensive action of reversible adrenoceptor blocking agents although not that of irreversible agents such as phenoxybenzamine. However, a direct α-stimulating drug without cardiac effects such as methoxamine, is now regarded as more appropriate.

DOSAGE AND ADMINISTRATION

Noradrenaline is given by intravenous infusion, 2 mg being added to 500 ml of 5 per cent dextrose solution; this gives a concentration of 4 μg/ml. The infusion is started at 2 ml/min (about 40 drops), the blood pressure is taken at the end of 30 seconds and the infusion rate is adjusted accordingly. A continual check of blood pressure readings and rate of flow is necessary, at 1-minute intervals at first, but less frequently as the blood pressure becomes stabilized. In case of extreme hypotension the strength of the solution may be doubled; if there is no response following the rapid infusion of this solution it is unlikely that increasing the dose further will be of any avail. Stronger solutions (up to 16 mg/ℓ) given at a proportionately slower rate may be used in conditions in which fluid intake must be restricted.

If a noradrenaline infusion is abruptly stopped, hypotension, often severe, will result. This is due to a rapid increase in the vascular bed (relaxation after previous intense constriction) which causes the circulatory blood volume to become inadequate. Hypotension may be prevented by giving a blood, plasma, or dextran transfusion as the noradrenaline infusion is being withdrawn. Indirectly acting pressor drugs that release noradrenaline, such as methylamphetamine or mephentermine, have been recommended to maintain blood pressure following the withdrawal of a noradrenaline infusion. These drugs appear to be effective under these circumstances but the administration of blood or other plasma expander is a more logical procedure.

PRECAUTIONS

Noradrenaline must not be injected subcutaneously even in dilute solutions. Care is necessary to avoid leakage from the infusion around the intravenous needle, as gangrene of the skin may result, and as this agent is liable to diffuse through the vein wall it is safer to infuse into a central vein. Local treatment of extravasation is as for dopamine.

Dextrose 5 per cent is the only solution commonly available that is sufficiently acidic to protect noradrenaline from oxidation. It is advisable, therefore, that noradrenaline should not be mixed with isotonic saline, blood, or plasma.

Noradrenaline, although less likely to cause ventricular fibrillation than adrenaline, should not be used during chloroform, trichloroethylene, or cyclopropane anaesthesia, and it should be used with the utmost caution in patients suffering from hypertension or serious heart disease. Because of its local effect on tissues and the difficulties associated with its withdrawal, noradrenaline cannot be used with impunity, but it may prove life saving when other pressor drugs, such as mephentermine and methoxamine, are ineffective.

Overdose of noradrenaline produces intense vasoconstriction and hypertension. These effects pass with the withdrawal of the infusion: α-adrenoceptor blocking agents antagonize its effects.

Phenylephrine hydrochloride

Phenylephrine hydrochloride (*BP* and *USP*)
Chemical name: (*S*)-1-(3-hydroxyphenyl)-2-methylaminoethanol hydrochloride
For structural formula *see Table 12.2,* p. 318

PHARMACOLOGY
Phenylephrine, like noradrenaline, has strong α- and weak β-effects. Its action at α-adrenoceptors is direct.

Central nervous system. There is no effect on the cerebral cortex.

Cardiovascular system. There is little or no effect on cardiac output, force or rate, but irritability is slightly increased. The heart rate is slowed due to stimulation of the baroreceptors, an effect that can be antagonized by atropine. Blood pressure is increased due to vasoconstriction causing an increase in overall peripheral resistance.

Local application causes constriction of the vessels of mucous membranes. It is irritant and may cause local discomfort or even local necrosis if it leaks from the vein being injected.

Respiratory system. There is some degree of bronchial dilatation due to relaxation of the smooth muscle of the bronchial tree. It is considerably less effective than adrenaline or isoprenaline.

INDICATIONS
Phenylephrine is used in the treatment of circulatory failure and of hypotension due to excessive doses of vasodilators. It has also been used in the treatment of paroxysmal tachycardia, as a local application for the relief of nasal congestion, and to produce mydriasis. It is effective in combating hypotension due to chlorpromazine. Because it has a lower β-agonist activity than noradrenaline it is probably a safer agent to use to raise the blood pressure in patients given a halogenated anaesthetic.

DOSAGE AND ADMINISTRATION
Phenylephrine may be given intramuscularly or intravenously in the form of an infusion. By the intramuscular route it takes 10–15 minutes to act and its effect lasts up to 1 hour.

In the treatment of hypotension due to circulatory failure, 5 mg may be given intramuscularly, 0.5 mg intravenously, or an infusion containing 10 mg in 500 ml of 5 per cent dextrose may be set up and started at 40–60 drops/min and controlled in the same way as a noradrenaline infusion.

Solutions containing 0.5–1 per cent of phenylephrine are used to relieve nasal congestion, 2–3 drops being instilled into the nose.

In the treatment of paroxysmal tachycardia, 5 mg is given intramuscularly. For the production of mydriasis, 2.5–10 per cent solutions may be employed; a suitable local analgesic should first be instilled into the eye to avoid irritation.

PRECAUTIONS
Phenylephrine should not be given in severe myocardial or coronary disease, and special care is necessary when it is administered to patients with hypertension.

Overdose causes hypertension, palpitations, headache, and vomiting. Treatment should be symptomatic; α-adrenoceptor blocking agents will relieve excessive hypertension.

Hypotensive agents and vasodilators

Drugs that lower arterial blood pressure can do so theoretically in a number of ways (*Figure 12.6*) but only a few of these are exploited therapeutically. They either produce peripheral dilatation by central or peripheral actions which lower

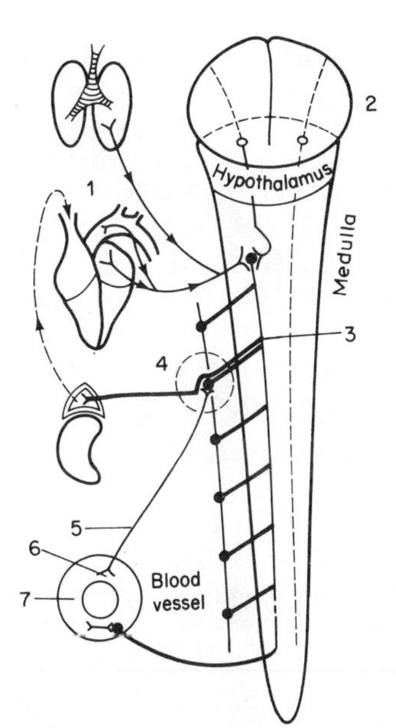

Figure 12.6 Diagram to show sites of action of vasodilators. Preganglionic medullated fibres are shown in thick lines; postganglionic non-medullated are in thin lines; afferent fibres are drawn thinly with arrow marks indicating direction of impulse. The figures indicate the sites of action of drugs producing vasodilatation; (1) afferent receptors; (2) hypothalamus and medulla; (3) preganglionic fibres; (4) autonomic ganglia; (5) sympathetic neurones; (6) adrenoceptors; (7) vascular smooth muscle

peripheral resistance and affect tone of capacitance vessels, or act by diminishing the force of cardiac contraction and output. The sites of action of these drugs are as follows:

1. Afferent receptors in the heart, lungs, and great vessels (veratrum alkaloids).
2. Hypothalamus and medulla:
   (*a*) general depression (anaesthetics and barbiturates)
   (*b*) α-adrenoceptors (clonidine, methyldopa).
3. Preganglionic sympathetic fibres as they leave the spinal cord (local analgesics used for spinal and epidural analgesia).
4. Cholinergic receptors:
   (*a*) nicotinic, in autonomic ganglia (ganglion blockers)
   (*b*) muscarinic (anticholinesterases and methacholine).
5. Sympathetic neurones (guanethidine, bethanidine).
6. Adrenoceptors:
   (*a*) α-adrenoceptor blocking drugs (phenoxybenzamine)
   (*b*) β-adrenoceptor blocking drugs (propranolol).
7. Vascular smooth muscle (thiazide diuretics, nitrites, diazoxide, hydralazine).

When drugs are widely employed in therapy, relevant monographs are described in each section of this chapter. Those relevant to spinal and epidural analgesia and the cholinomimetics are discussed in Chapters 6 and 10, respectively.

Historical development

When barbiturates became generally available they were used in combination with bed-rest to treat hypertension. The principle of sedation is still important in this condition but is now usually obtained by tranquillizers such as the benzodiazepines. The first peripherally acting vasodilators were the nitrites, but they were too toxic over a long period and control of blood pressure was difficult.

The ganglion-blocking agents were the first effective drugs to be employed for the control of hypertension and began the emphasis on drugs with a peripheral effect for this purpose. Early drugs such as hexamethonium had to be given by injection and were unselective, affecting all autonomic ganglia. The actions on the parasympathetic ganglia produced effects that were neither useful nor wanted. Since then many classes of compounds acting peripherally have been developed, either acting by blockade of sympathetic neurones or blocking adrenoceptors. The most recent research has revealed mechanisms for antihypertensive action hitherto unsuspected, acting principally through the α-adrenoceptors in the hypothalamus or medulla. The need to avoid parenteral administration has never been an inhibitory factor in anaesthesia and so both ganglion-blocking drugs and nitrites are still widely employed for the induction of peroperative hypotension.

Stimulants of the depressor reflexes

The veratrum alkaloids act at afferent sites via receptors in the heart, lungs, and great vessels and also have a central action. Because of the undependable and mild nature of their action they are rarely employed.

Hypothalamic and medullary depressants

Clonidine, levodopa and methyldopa owe their hypotensive action primarily to the fact that directly or indirectly they stimulate α-adrenoceptors in the brain. Hypothalamic α-adrenoceptors are inhibitory and cause a decrease in outflow from the vasomotor centres. Medullary α-adrenoceptors are concerned with blood pressure control. The nucleus solitarius in the medulla is probably implicated. Micro-injections of noradrenaline, α-methylnoradrenaline, and clonidine into this region result in a fall in blood pressure and heart rate; α-adrenoceptor blocking agents given into the same region can inhibit these effects.

Methyldopa also has peripheral actions in that it acts as a false substrate for noradrenaline elaboration, leading to the formation of a false transmitter (α-methylnoradrenaline). However, this mechanism, although generally adduced to be the mechanism of action, was always an unsatisfactory explanation because α-methylnoradrenaline was equipotent with noradrenaline as a vasoconstrictor. Also, it was not more tightly bound and thus released in smaller quantities by nerve impulses.

Levodopa is not used to produce hypotension but may do so as a side effect because of its tendency to increase the availability of stimulators of α-adrenoceptors in the brain such as noradrenaline.

Clonidine hydrochloride

Clonidine hydrochloride (*BP* and *USAN*)
Chemical name: 2,6-dichloro-*N*-(imidazolin-2-ylidene)aniline hydrochloride

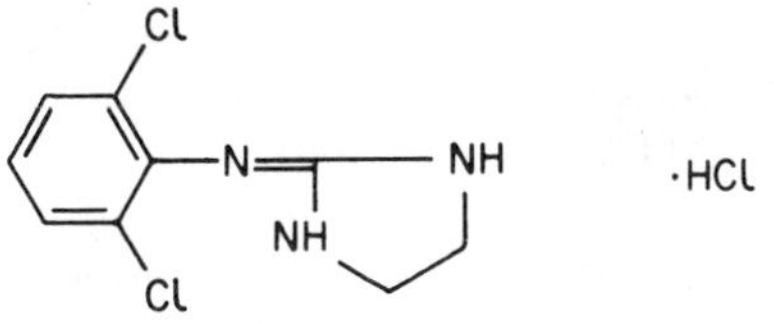

PHARMACOLOGY

Clonidine hydrochloride is an imidazoline derivative, chemically related to tolazoline and phentolamine, and causes a fall in blood pressure accompanied by bradycardia and a fall in cardiac output. The fall in systolic pressure is more marked than the fall in diastolic pressure. In patients on oral therapy, peripheral resistance is little affected.

Clonidine has a complex action as yet ill understood. Contributing to its hypotensive effect is postsynaptic stimulation of α-adrenoceptors in the medulla, and stimulation of presynaptic α-adrenoceptors, both centrally and peripherally. It may also interact with dopaminergic and tryptaminergic neurones centrally.

Clonidine owes its hypotensive action to its ability to stimulate α-adrenoceptors in the brain. These receptors are inhibitory and cause a decrease in outflow from the vasomotor centre. Any interruption of the pathways from the vasomotor centre interferes with its action. With prolonged treatment vascular smooth muscle develops a reduced ability to respond to catecholamines and angiotensin and this may contribute to the hypotensive action.

Following rapid intravenous injection, however, there is an initial rise in blood pressure due to direct α-adrenoceptor stimulant action, and this can be blocked by an α-adrenoceptor blocking agent, such as phentolamine. After oral administration, plasma levels reach a peak in 3 hours and decline with a half-life of 20 hours.

Clonidine is of interest because normal homeostatic cardiovascular reflexes are preserved, thus avoiding the problems of postural hypotension and hypotension on exercise. Diuretics given simultaneously act synergistically and enable the dose of clonidine to be reduced.

Renal blood flow and glomerular filtration rate are maintained; there is a reduction in Na^+ and Cl^- excretion, but K^+ excretion is unaffected.

INDICATIONS

The principal indication for clonidine hydrochloride is in cases of essential hypertension when it is usually combined with a diuretic such as chlorthalidone. It has also been found effective as a prophylactic in small doses in cases of migraine, particularly in those who give a history of migraine associated with particular foods, such as chocolate, cheese, alcohol, and citrus fruits.

DOSAGE

In the treatment of essential hypertension the dose is 200–300 μg daily in divided doses. This dose is gradually increased on alternate days until a satisfactory reduction in blood pressure is achieved. Doses in excess of 1 mg/day may be required on occasions.

For the prophylaxis of migraine the dose is 25 μg twice daily, increasing up to 75 μg twice daily. Larger doses may cause hypotension.

PRECAUTIONS

On withdrawal of the drug, metabolites of catecholamines increase markedly and this may be associated with rebound hypertension. The drug should, therefore, not be withdrawn abruptly prior to surgery. Patients on treatment are more sensitive to parenterally administered catecholamines. It should be used with caution in patients with Raynaud's phenomenon or thromboangiitis obliterans, who are unusually sensitive to any effects of endogenous or exogenous catecholamines. Clonidine would be expected to potentiate agents that lower blood pressure by ganglion blockade or direct action on the vessels and in which central vasomotor mechanisms normally act to try and limit the fall in blood pressure. Nevertheless, because of the danger of rebound hypertension it is normally inadvisable to stop therapy suddenly prior to giving an anaesthetic. Rebound hypertension due to sudden withdrawal of clonidine may be treated by administration of phentolamine or by re-introduction of clonidine.

Initially sedation and dry mouth are encountered in a proportion of patients. The effects are seldom severe, usually subside in 2–3 weeks and the sedative effect may be beneficial in the early stages. It may aggravate depressive illness. In the early stage of treatment there may be a little fluid retention and weight gain on occasions, which are usually transient and may be controlled with diuretics. It commonly causes skin rashes and constipation. Other occasional side effects include dizziness, headache, nocturnal unrest, nausea, euphoria, constipation and, rarely, impotence.

Guanfacine is an analogue of clonidine. There is evidence that like clonidine it stimulates α-adrenoceptors centrally. Bioavailability (measured by comparing the areas under the plasma level curves following oral and intravenous dosing) was close to 100 per cent, suggesting lack of first-pass effect and very good absorption of the drug. The elimination half-life after oral administration is about 21 hours. Clinically the drug appears to be less sedative than clonidine and less likely to produce rebound hypertension. Tolerance to it can occur. For the treatment of essential hypertension doses of 3–6 mg daily have been used.

Methyldopa

Methyldopa (*BP* and *USP*)
Chemical name: (−)-2-amino-2-(3,4-dihydroxybenzyl) propionic acid

$$(HO)_2C_6H_3{-}CH_2{-}C(CH_3)(NH_2){-}COOH$$

PHARMACOLOGY

Methyldopa has a powerful hypotensive action which is more marked in the hypertensive subject. The fall in blood pressure is most marked in the erect posture and during exercise. There is still uncertainty as to its mechanism of action. It provides an alternative substrate to dopa and is converted in the body to α-methylnoradrenaline, which replaces the normal transmitter, noradrenaline, at storage sites in the nerve terminal. It was originally believed that this had a weaker action than noradrenaline and therefore functioned as a 'false transmitter', but in fact its pressor properties are hardly less than those of noradrenaline. It is now clear that its principal site of action is centrally, where its metabolite, α-methylnoradrenaline, stimulates α-adrenoceptors, for instance, in the region of the nucleus solitarius in the medulla. These α-adrenoceptors appear to be inhibitory and cause a decrease in outflow from the vasomotor centre. No major redistribution of cardiac output occurs and renal blood flow and glomerular filtration are well maintained.

The *laevo*-isomer of methyldopa inhibits dopa decarboxylase activity and thereby diminishes synthesis and storage of noradrenaline. It is unlikely that this effect is of relevance to its clinical actions since other inhibitors of this enzyme fail to produce hypotension.

Normal sensitivity is retained to both directly and indirectly acting pressor amines.

Methyldopa regularly produces sedation, and occasionally mental depression. Postural hypotension, although less frequent and less severe than with guanethidine or ganglion blockade, may occur.

On rare occasions, abnormalities in liver chemistry and granulocytopenia have been noted, but these conditions disappear on withdrawal of the drug. Autoimmune haemolytic anaemia has also been reported. The direct Coombs' test is positive. Rapid remission usually occurs when the drug is stopped or if steroids are given.

INDICATIONS

Methyldopa is used in the treatment of hypertension, either alone or in combination with diuretics.

DOSAGE AND ADMINISTRATION

Methyldopa is given orally in daily doses of 0.5–2 g. Commencing with 250 mg three times a day, the dose is gradually increased after 48 hours until an adequate response has been achieved. If the blood pressure cannot be controlled by a daily dose of 2 g or tolerance occurs, a thiazide compound may be given in combination.

PRECAUTIONS

Methyldopa is contraindicated in phaeochromocytoma and active liver disease, and regular blood examinations should be undertaken in order to detect the onset of anaemia.

Ganglion-blocking agents

Transmission through autonomic ganglia, both sympathetic and parasympathetic, is effected by means of acetylcholine. This is released when preganglionic nerve impulses reach the synapses, and it activates receptors on the cell bodies of the postganglionic neurones. Drugs that interfere with transmission at this site are known as ganglion-blocking agents.

Classification

A large number of compounds are capable of interfering with transmission through ganglia. They can be divided into the following two main groups:

1. Substances that resemble acetylcholine and act by mimicking it, competing with it, or allowing it to accumulate. This group includes the following classes of substances:
   (*a*) Substances whose properties must be very similar to acetylcholine, and which imitate its action at synapses. The depolarization produced is initially associated with increased excitability but depolarization persists and so re-excitation of the neurone cannot take place and this constitutes a block. Such substances are tetramethylammonium, nicotine, and decamethonium salts.
   (*b*) Substances that compete with acetylcholine for ganglion cell receptors but do not stimulate them, such as tetraethylammonium, pentamethonium, hexamethonium, and pentolinium.
   (*c*) Anticholinesterases: the block produced by these substances is usually due to competition for the receptors between the anticholinesterase and acetylcholine, rather than to persistent depolarization by accumulation of acetylcholine.
2. Substances that do not resemble acetylcholine and probably act on preganglionic nerve endings or on effector cells, changing some of the properties essential for normal transmission. This group contains a large number of miscellaneous compounds whose ganglion-blocking activity is small in comparison with their main pharmacological action; examples of such compounds include the general anaesthetics, local analgesics, barbiturates, many antihistamines, and atropine. This group also contains some highly specific ganglion-blocking agents, such as mecamylamine (a diamine), trimetaphan (a thiophanium derivative), and phenactropinium chloride.

Effects

The ganglion-blocking agents are non-specific and block both sympathetic and parasympathetic ganglia equally. The only practical method of blocking specific ganglia is by local infiltration with a local analgesic (as in stellate-ganglion block). Blocking of the sympathetic ganglia diminishes the number of impulses reaching the vasomotor fibres to the blood vessels, the accelerator fibres to the heart, inhibitory fibres to the smooth muscle of the alimentary tract, constrictor fibres to its sphincters, secretory fibres to the adrenals and to sweat glands, dilator fibres to the iris, inhibitory fibres to the wall of the bladder, constrictor fibres to its internal sphincter, and dilator fibres to the bronchial musculature.

Parasympathetic block similarly affects secretory fibres to the salivary glands, mucous glands of the bronchial tree and alimentary tract, decelerator fibres to the heart, constrictor fibres to the smooth muscle of the alimentary tract, constrictor fibres to the iris, and fibres responsible for the erection of the penis.

The overall effects on particular organs or systems depend on whether the autonomic activity of the system is predominantly sympathetic or parasympathetic. Thus, the overall effect on peripheral vessels is vasodilatation, due to release from predominant constrictor sympathetic control, while the effect on the alimentary tract can be so severe as to cause a paralytic ileus due to absence of parasympathetic motor impulses.

Uses of ganglion-blocking agents

With the introduction of drugs that produce vasodilatation by specific action on sympathetic nervous transmission, or selective depression of the vasomotor centre, the use of ganglion-blocking drugs in the treatment of hypertension has declined and they are now rarely employed for this purpose. They do, however, continue to be used for the production of controlled hypotension during surgery.

Chlorothiazide and related compounds increase the hypotensive effect of ganglion-blocking drugs and other vasodilators. This is due partially to a decrease in circulating blood volume and partially to a direct effect on peripheral circulatory tone. This action of these diuretic drugs is often used in the treatment of hypertension, by giving one of them together with the selected antihypertensive drug.

Patients who are under treatment with ganglion-blocking drugs, especially long-acting ones, occasionally become more hypotensive during anaesthesia. This situation rarely gives cause for alarm and can be readily controlled, if necessary, by the administration of an appropriate pressor agent.

Controlled hypotension

Ganglion-blocking drugs are used with the aid of the gravitational effects of posture to produce a relatively ischaemic operative field during surgery. After the patient is anaesthetized the chosen drug is given and the patient is postured so that the operative field is well above heart level. Drug action produces vasodilatation, venous pooling, and a fall in cardiac output. The posture of the patient causes blood to be drained from the operative site to dependent parts. Local pressure at the site of operation will fall about 20 mmHg (2.7 kPa) for every 25 cm above heart level.

Overdosage

In the conscious subject the effects of mild overdosage with ganglion-blocking agents are dryness of the mouth, mydriasis, paralysis of accommodation, difficulty in micturition, mild gastrointestinal disturbances, postural hypotension, muscular weakness, and diminished sexual potency. Larger doses may cause marked hypotension with syncope due to cerebral anaemia, paralytic ileus, and urinary retention.

The treatment of overdosage should be symptomatic. An excessive degree of hypotension is best treated by pressor agents, such as mephentermine. Intestinal inhibition will usually respond to an anticholinesterase such as neostigmine.

Hexamethonium salts

Hexamethonium bromide, iodide, and tartrate (*BAN*)
Chemical name: *NN'*-hexamethylenebis(trimethylammonium) dihydrogen tartrate, dibromide, and diiodide

Hexamethonium inhibits transmission in autonomic ganglia by the competitive inhibition of acetylcholine. Its poor and irregular absorption from the gastrointestinal tract makes parenteral administration a necessity. Within the body it is distributed in the extracellular fluid and it is excreted unchanged by the kidneys, solely by the glomeruli. Sixty per cent of a dose reaches the urine in 3 hours and 90 per cent in 24 hours. A tolerance to its action develops within the first few weeks of continuous use. For controlled hypotension 10–40 mg is given slowly intravenously. Half doses should be given to the frail and the elderly.

Pentolinium is a ganglion-blocking agent with very similar properties to those of hexamethonium, but with the advantage of being better absorbed when taken by mouth.

In the treatment of hypertension 10–20 mg may be given orally three times a day. Daily increments of 10–20 mg are added until the desired fall in blood pressure is obtained.

In the control of hypotension during anaesthesia, 2.5–10 mg should be given intravenously when anaesthesia has been established. Reduced doses should be given to the frail and the elderly.

Trimetaphan camsylate

Trimetaphan camsylate (*BAN*) and Trimethaphan camsylate (*USP*)
Chemical name: 4,6-dibenzyl-1-thionia-4,6-diazatricyclo[6,3,0,$0^{3,7}$]undecan-5-one (+)-camphor-10-sulphonate

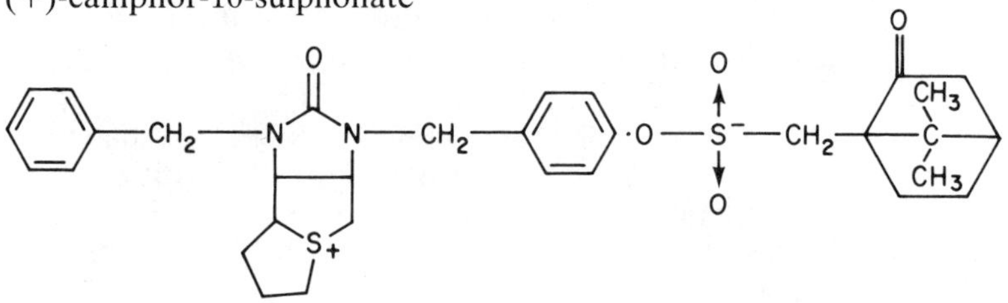

PHARMACOLOGY

Trimetaphan is a ganglion-blocking agent with a very rapid onset (1–3 minutes) and short duration of action (5–15 minutes) after single intravenously injected doses. Following continuous administration tachyphylaxis has been reported and the fall in blood pressure may persist for up to 30 minutes after discontinuing the administration. In this respect it is distinctly inferior to sodium nitroprusside. In supine spontaneously ventilating patients under light halothane anaesthesia the principal mode of action is a lowering of arterial peripheral resistance, although when big falls in arterial pressure are induced, there are significant falls in cardiac output. When a slight head-up tilt is used, more marked falls in cardiac output occur without further change in peripheral resistance, suggesting pooling in capacitance vessels and a fall in venous return. A compensatory tachycardia is sometimes seen.

The drug is partly broken down by enzymatic hydrolysis and partly excreted unchanged in the urine. If the blood pressure is lowered so much that glomerular filtration ceases, excretion cannot occur, and this may account for the prolonged action which may follow.

It is mainly used for the production of controlled hypotension, but has also been used to improve perfusion during and after cardiac surgery.

DOSAGE AND ADMINISTRATION

Trimetaphan can be given by repeated intravenous injection, but it is more usually given by continuous intravenous infusion. In either case the patient is first anaesthetized and positioned on the operating table. When the intermittent intravenous technique is used, an initial dose of 50 mg in 5 per cent solution may be given, followed by doses of 10–30 mg at intervals of 10–15 minutes to maintain the desired level of hypotension.

For continuous intravenous infusion, a 0.1 per cent solution in 5 per cent dextrose or isotonic saline is used, started at a rate of about 60 drops/min (3–4 ml). Frequent blood pressure readings are taken, and the rate of infusion is adjusted to maintain the blood pressure at the required level. Weaker solutions are recommended for the frail and the elderly, but children or infants, who are more resistant to this drug, may be given a 0.2 per cent solution.

Excessive hypotension can usually be controlled by reducing the rate of the infusion. If this fails, the head of the operating table should be lowered; in emergency a pressor drug such as mephentermine or methoxamine should be given.

PRECAUTIONS

Trimetaphan is incompatible with thiopentone, gallamine, strongly alkaline solutions, iodides, and bromides.

Adrenoceptor blocking agents

When Dale in 1906 showed that sympathetic nervous activity was mediated by two different receptors and Ahlquist named them α and β (*see* page 316) the only blocking agents available were those that blocked α-adrenoceptors. Since then drugs that block β-adrenoceptors have been discovered, and also those that produce blockade by interfering with the release of noradrenaline from stores in adrenergic nerve axons. The latest developments include drugs that block some β-adrenoceptors selectively and some that block both α- and β-adrenoceptors.

This has followed the recognition that the β-adrenoceptors could be divided into β_1- and β_2-groups. Heart muscle contains β_1-adrenoceptors; bronchi, arteries, uterus, and skeletal muscle contain β_2-adrenoceptors. It has been postulated that the enzyme adenyl cyclase is the actual β-adrenoceptor, although it seems more likely that the enzyme just has β-adrenoceptors on it. The evidence, however, is conflicting. In liver and fatty tissue, adenyl cyclase mediates the responses of glycolysis and lipolysis to catecholamines. Metabolic effects in liver due to this enzyme are also fairly well established. Using affinity labels for α- and β-adrenoceptors, a protein fraction with a high affinity for isoprenaline has been isolated from heart and liver, and a lipoprotein, with a high affinity for noradrenaline, from the smooth muscle of the splenic capsule.

α-Adrenoceptor blocking agents

These drugs block the α-responses of adrenaline and other sympathomimetic amines. General systemic effects produced include dilatation of peripheral vessels causing orthostatic hypotension with compensatory tachycardia, congestion of mucous membranes, constriction of the pupil, and sometimes intestinal over-activity or colic due possibly to preponderance of vagal action. In addition, each of these blocking agents can produce side effects by direct actions either on effector organs or through the CNS, and these may sometimes modify their main action.

In general, circulating adrenaline and noradrenaline are more easily antagonized than are the effects of adrenergic nerve stimulation, a difference that has been attributed to the more intimate nature of the contact between nerve and effector cell.

These drugs act as competitive antagonists for catecholamines and sympathomimetic amines at α-adrenoceptors of the sympathetic nervous system. In most cases both the agonists and antagonists have a comparable affinity for the receptor, and increasing the dose of either will overcome the action of the other. However, this is not the case with phenoxybenzamine. Once an adequate block has been established a massive dose of a sympathomimetic agent is ineffective until the effect of the blocking compound is terminated by metabolism.

There are four main groups of drugs that block α-adrenoceptors:

1. Imidazolines, such as tolazoline and phentolamine;
2. Benzodioxans, which are chemically related to adrenaline, such as piperoxan;
3. Chloroethylamines, which are chemically related to the nitrogen mustards – these include dibenamine and phenoxybenzamine;
4. Ergot alkaloids and their dihydro-derivatives, except ergometrine.

The ergot alkaloids are included solely for historical interest, as their direct actions on the CNS and smooth muscle are so great that doses demonstrating adrenoceptor blockade in man cannot safely be used. Other drugs that block α-adrenoceptors include chlorpromazine and droperidol.

α-Adrenoceptor blocking agents may be employed in the diagnosis and treatment of peripheral vascular disease in which there is increased sympathetic tone. They differ in specificity, freedom from side effects, speed of onset and duration of action, so the choice for any given purpose must be in the light of these factors. Except when used in conjunction with other hypotensive drugs, they are of little use in the treatment of essential or malignant hypertension or for the production of controlled hypotension. In the treatment of hypertension a useful reduction in blood pressure cannot be obtained without causing unpleasant side effects; also, the action of many of these agents is too transient. The development of labetalol shows, however, that α-adrenoceptor blockade, when combined with β-blockade, can be an effective treatment for hypertension. α-Adrenoceptor blocking agents are, however, effective in the control of the hypertensive episodes that often occur during the removal of chromaffin tissue tumours. Now that the metabolites of catecholamines can be readily estimated in the urine, α-adrenoceptor blocking agents are rarely used in the diagnosis of chromaffin tumours.

Monographs on the commonly used α-adrenoceptor blocking drugs follow. β-Adrenoceptor blockers are more commonly employed to modify the force of contraction of the heart or influence rate or rhythm; accordingly they are dealt with in Chapter 13.

Dale, H. H. (1906) On some physiological actions of ergot. *Journal of Physiology,* **153,** 163

Phenoxybenzamine hydrochloride

Phenoxybenzamine hydrochloride (*BP* and *USP*)
Chemical name: *N*-(2-chloroethyl)-*N*-(1-methyl-2-phenoxyethyl)-benzylamine hydrochloride

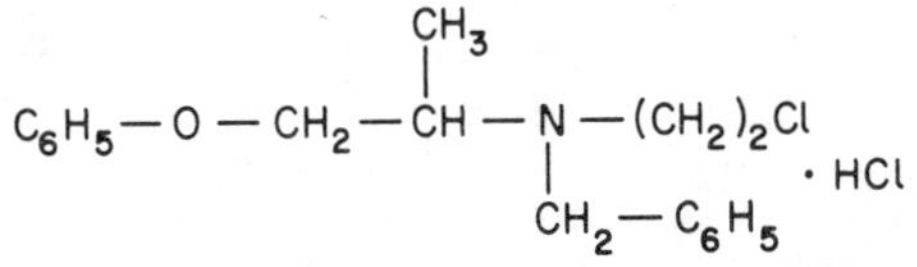

$$C_6H_5-O-CH_2-CH(CH_3)-N(CH_2-C_6H_5)-(CH_2)_2Cl \cdot HCl$$

PHARMACOLOGY

Phenoxybenzamine is a chloroethylene derivative and is related to the nitrogen mustards. It is a powerful α-adrenoceptor blocking agent.

During administration, α-stimulating amines compete for the receptors, indicating that the initial attracting forces are of the same kind. However, once a block is established it cannot be reversed by other adrenoceptor stimulators (agonists) indicating the formation of a non-dissociating stable bond at or near the receptor. This is an example of a non-equilibrium blockade. This is clinically detected, however, only when the number of unblocked receptors has been reduced very considerably, and with moderate doses sufficient receptors remain unblocked for some response of the tissue to normal agonists to be demonstrable. Onset of action is slow and it may take up to an hour for the drug to reach its full effect following intravenous injection. This delay is due to conversion of the drug into an active metabolite in the body. The block is very persistent, and decreases only slowly over 3–4 days. The major effects are on the cardiovascular system. In normal recumbent subjects there is a slight fall in diastolic pressure, but a marked postural hypotension occurs. The effect on blood pressure is greater in hypertensive subjects, and precipitous falls occur in the presence of even moderate hypovolaemia. Drugs such as morphine may have a similar effect.

Changes in blood flow depend on the existing pattern of α-adrenergic activity. Cerebral and coronary blood flows will be unchanged unless blood pressure falls below a critical level; muscle and skin flows tend to be increased. If splanchnic flow is much reduced, as in vasoconstricted states, phenoxybenzamine will cause an increase, which will be limited only by unmasked hypovolaemia.

The chronotropic and inotropic effects of catecholamines on the heart are not blocked, but the drug exhibits a considerable antidysrhythmic action, and will block cyclopropane/adrenaline-induced dysrhythmias.

Side effects may be troublesome. An initial central stimulation on rapid administration may cause nausea and vomiting. With slow intravenous administration sedation is usually seen. Postural hypotension and reflex tachycardia occur, but are limited if the circulatory volume is increased. Giddiness, nasal congestion, and fatigue are common.

INDICATIONS

Phenoxybenzamine is used in the treatment of peripheral vascular disease where vessel tone is abnormally increased, and in the control of hypertension in phaeochromocytoma.

It may also be used in peripheral cardiovascular failure to improve perfusion which is impaired by intense vasoconstriction.

DOSAGE AND ADMINISTRATION

Phenoxybenzamine may be given by mouth or intravenously by infusion.

In the treatment of the above conditions, 20 mg by mouth three to four times a day is usually effective, but doses up to 120 mg may be required; 0.5–2 mg/kg may be given in 300 ml of 5 per cent dextrose solution if the intravenous route is employed.

In the preoperative preparation of cases of phaeochromocytoma, α-adrenoceptor blockade should be progressively induced over 3 days prior to operation, and the blood volume increased *pari passu* by blood or plasma volume expanders. Central venous pressure monitoring should be used as a guide. A similar approach is necessary in the treatment of 'shock' associated with intense vasoconstriction, although the time course is much shorter.

PRECAUTIONS

Ambulant patients being treated with this agent should be warned about its side effects and advised accordingly.

Patients treated intravenously need central venous pressure monitoring and facilities for active therapy. Since the block cannot be reversed pharmacologically, potentially lethal hypotension must be controlled by transfusion and posture.

Phenoxybenzamine therapy may lead to uncontrolled β-stimulation in a hypertensive crisis associated with an adrenaline-secreting phaeochromocytoma.

Phentolamine mesylate

Phentolamine mesylate (*BP* and *USP*)
Chemical name: 3-[*N*-(2-imidazolin-2-ylmethyl)-*p*-toluidino]phenol methane-sulphonate

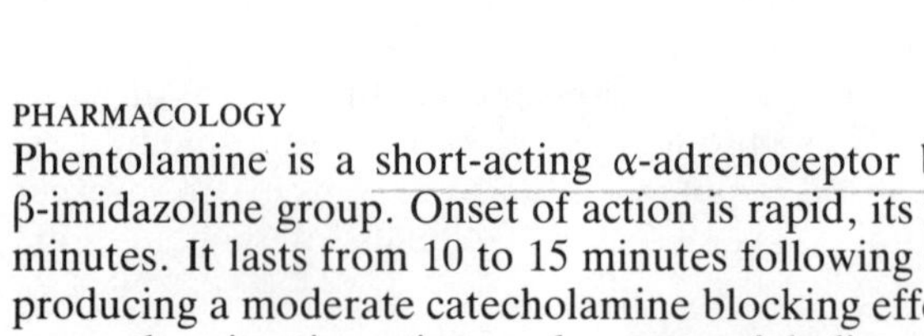

PHARMACOLOGY

Phentolamine is a short-acting α-adrenoceptor blocking agent belonging to the β-imidazoline group. Onset of action is rapid, its full effect being reached within 2 minutes. It lasts from 10 to 15 minutes following intravenous injection. As well as producing a moderate catecholamine blocking effect, phentolamine also has a mild sympathomimetic action and a powerful direct vasodilator action on vascular smooth muscle. Following intravenous infusion it produces a reduction in peripheral resistance and blood pressure, an increase in cardiac output and heart rate, and a decrease in stroke volume and cardiopulmonary blood volume.

Side effects which may occur include sweating, apprehension, palpitation, nausea, diarrhoea, and nasal congestion.

INDICATIONS

Phentolamine is used in the control of blood pressure during surgery for phaeochromocytoma. It can also be used for the diagnosis of this condition if facilities for estimating catecholamines in the urine are not available. It has also been used for the treatment of peripheral vascular disease, for the relief of arterial spasm, and as an antidote in the treatment of overdose of adrenaline and other sympathomimetic amines. It may be of value in the treatment of toxic reactions between MAO inhibitors and tyramine-containing foods.

DOSAGE AND ADMINISTRATION

Phentolamine may be given by mouth, intramuscularly, intravenously, or intra-arterially.

For the diagnosis of phaeochromocytoma, 5 mg of the methanesulphonate is given intravenously. The patient should be lying at rest and have had no sedation for 24 hours. A fall of 35 mmHg (5 kPa) in systolic blood pressure and 25 mmHg (3.4 kPa) in diastolic blood pressure indicates a positive result. Blood pressure readings must be taken at 30-second intervals at first as the fall may last only a few minutes. For several reasons false results may be obtained and the estimation of urinary catecholamines should always be undertaken when possible.

For the control of blood pressure during surgery, 5 mg may be given intravenously a few minutes, or intramuscularly 30 minutes, before induction of anaesthesia. This should ensure a smooth induction. Further doses of 5 mg are given during operation as necessary to control excessive hypertension, especially that likely to occur when the tumour is being handled by the surgeon.

When used for the treatment of vascular disease, 20–40 mg of the hydrochloride is given three to four times a day by mouth; alternatively, 5–10 mg can be given intra-arterially, intravenously, or intramuscularly, repeated as required. Larger doses are sometimes necessary. For adrenaline overdose, 5–10 mg should be injected intravenously immediately. Speed is important.

PRECAUTIONS

Ambulant patients should be warned about the side effects of this drug, and it should be avoided in serious heart disease and affections of the gastrointestinal tract.

Prazosin hydrochloride

Prazosin hydrochloride

Chemical name: 2-[4-(2-furoyl)piperazin-1-yl]-6,7-dimethoxyquinazolin-4-ylamine hydrochloride

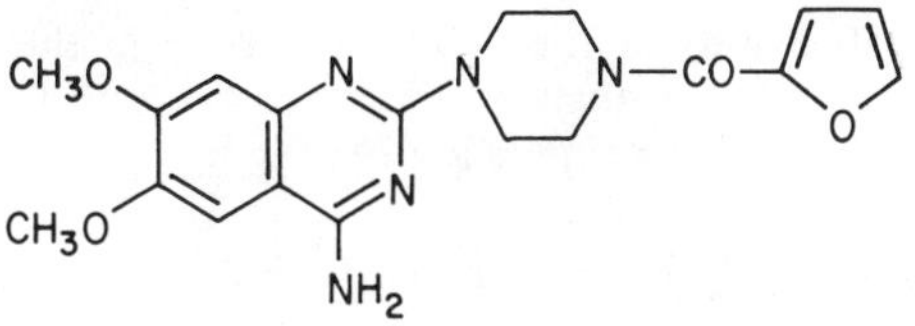

CH_3O N N N—CO O

CH_3O N

NH_2

PHARMACOLOGY

The exact mechanisms by which this drug produces its effects on the cardiovascular system are unknown. Probably its main action is that it blocks postjunctional α-adrenoceptors (α_1) while having little effect on presynaptic α-adrenoceptors (α_2). It is also a powerful phosphodiesterase inhibitor, being about 20 times as potent as theophylline. Despite the fall in peripheral resistance there is relatively little increase in cardiac output or tachycardia. It has been suggested that prazosin impairs the baroreceptor reflex possibly by an action on the carotid sinus impairing the afferent pathway response. Another suggestion is that it enhances the effects of the vagus by raising cardiac cyclic guanosine monophosphate (GMP) levels. This it does by inhibiting the phosphodiesterase responsible for the breakdown of cyclic GMP. Cyclic GMP is a 'second messenger' involved in the cardiac effects of acetylcholine. Prazosin differs from hydrallazine, another vasodilator, in that it appears to be less likely to produce tolerance and it does not raise renin levels. Unlike diazoxide, it enhances sodium excretion.

Fate in the body. Prazosin is metabolized by the liver and there is a noticeable first-pass effect. Some of its metabolites also produce a fall in blood pressure and this may be why, in spite of its relatively short half-life, ($t_{½}$ about 4 hours), twice daily administration is usually sufficient.

DOSAGE AND ADMINISTRATION

For antihypertensive therapy the dosage range is 0.5–20 mg daily. The initial starting dose should be 0.5 mg three times a day, slowly increasing on the basis of the patient's blood pressure response.

PRECAUTIONS AND SIDE EFFECTS

Orthostatic hypotension occurs infrequently. Headache, dry mouth, blurred vision, nasal congestion, pruritus, and impotence have been reported but are infrequent or mild. In some patients high initial doses (2 mg) can precipitate a severe fall in blood pressure and collapse. This is more likely to occur in patients treated with β-adrenoceptor blocking agents or sodium-depleted patients following diuretic therapy. Such reactions usually occur within 2 hours of the initial dose. It is thus advisable to monitor the effects of the first dose for at least this period.

Indoramin probably has a similar selectivity for α_1-adrenoceptors. It causes sedation in a high percentage of patients. Dosage is 100–200 mg daily.

Agents inhibiting noradrenaline release

These drugs interfere with the release of noradrenaline from stores in the adrenergic nerve axons, and so block nerve impulse transmission. They include reserpine, guanethidine, bethanidine, and bretylium (which is no longer used as tolerance to it may suddenly develop).

MAO inhibitors, such as pargyline, inhibit the intraneuronal metabolism of noradrenaline, and probably produce their action by causing a persistent depolarization of the adrenoceptor.

These drugs are used in the treatment of hypertension. They may be used alone or in combination with diuretics.

Bethanidine sulphate

Bethanidine sulphate (*BP*)
Chemical name: 1-benzyl-2,3-dimethylguanidine sulphate

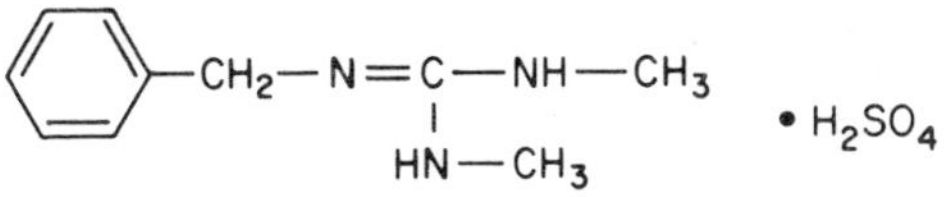

$$C_6H_5-CH_2-N{=}C(-NH-CH_3)(-HN-CH_3) \cdot H_2SO_4$$

PHARMACOLOGY

Bethanidine is a benzylguanidine compound related chemically to bretylium and guanethidine. It has a powerful hypotensive action due to vasodilatation of both resistance and capacitance vessels brought about by the inhibition of noradrenaline release from adrenergic nerve fibres. The response of treated patients to circulating catecholamines is increased but that to tyramine is decreased. The actions of bethanidine are rapidly reversed by indirectly acting sympathomimetic amines. After intravenous injection in animals, there is a short-lived pressor response due to noradrenaline release, which precedes the onset of hypotension. This is not seen after oral administration.

Bethanidine differs from guanethidine in that noradrenaline stores are not depleted so readily and its duration of action is considerably shorter. Tolerance is not a problem although dosage may have to be increased with the duration of treatment.

Side effects include orthostatic hypotension, which is worse on exercise. There may be some stuffiness in the nose but diarrhoea, which is common with some members of this group, is rare.

The drug is well absorbed after oral administration. Its action reaches its peak in 4–5 hours and lasts about 12 hours. It is mostly excreted in the urine within 12 hours.

INDICATIONS

Bethanidine is used in the treatment of hypertension, either alone or in conjunction with other antihypertensive drugs, or diuretics such as chlorothiazide.

DOSAGE AND ADMINISTRATION

Treatment is commenced by giving 5 mg three times daily; the daily dose is then increased by 10–20 mg until hypertension is controlled. This will require 30–250 mg or more in divided doses two or three times a day.

PRECAUTIONS

It is contraindicated in phaeochromocytoma.

Guanethidine monosulphate

Guanethidine monosulphate (*BP* and *USP*)
Chemical name: 1-[2-(perhydroazocin-1-yl)ethyl] guanidine monosulphate

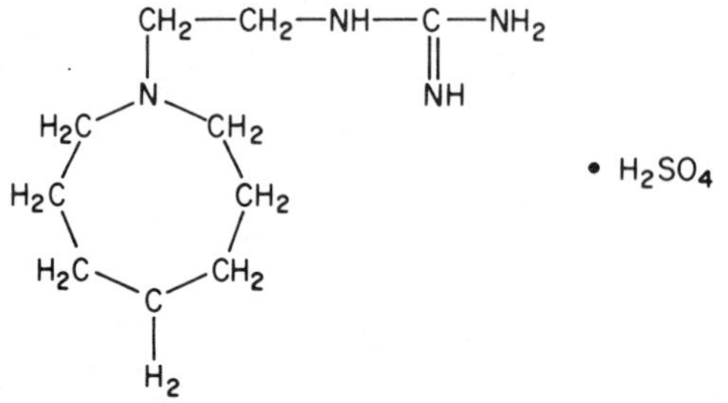

```
     CH2—CH2—NH—C—NH2
     |          ||
     N          NH
 H2C   CH2
H2C     CH2              • H2SO4
 H2C   CH2
     C
     |
     H2
```

PHARMACOLOGY

Guanethidine is a hypotensive agent with a similar but not identical action to that of bretylium tosylate.

In experimental animals it has been shown to deplete the catecholamine store in the spleen, heart, and blood vessels but not in the brain or adrenal glands. In some respects, therefore, it resembles reserpine, but the latter drug depletes the catecholamines stored in the brain as well. Its chief peripheral action is the prevention of release of noradrenaline by nerve impulses from its storage sites in adrenergic nerves, thus leading to vasodilatation. Pooling of blood in capacitance vessels results in a fall in cardiac output, or a failure to raise cardiac output on exercise, and thus causes hypotension. On intravenous administration there is an initial rise in blood pressure before the onset of hypotension; this rise may be due to the release of transmitter from labile stores and this is not seen after oral administration. As a late effect of oral administration, the nerve terminal storage granules become depleted of noradrenaline, but the onset of the hypotension precedes this action. These effects could be explained by a persistent depolarization of the nerve terminal region, but this has not been demonstrated. There is certainly no effect on transmission in the remainder of the sympathetic nerve.

Guanethidine is taken up into the noradrenaline storage sites, and this uptake is prevented by reserpine, amphetamine, and tricyclic antidepressants such as imipramine. Amphetamine, and other indirectly acting amines which are not themselves metabolized by MAO, will also reverse its action. Adrenoceptors are unaffected. They behave as though denervated and are consequently considerably more sensitive to sympathomimetic substances whose action would normally be terminated by re-uptake into the nerve terminal. There is no action on the parasympathetic system, but the reduction in sympathetic activity may cause parasympathetic preponderance with over-activity of the bowel and consequent diarrhoea. Tolerance can occur but develops much less readily than with bretylium, and its duration of action is much longer. When the drug is withdrawn several days may elapse before the blood pressure returns to its pretreatment level. Side effects are mainly due to postural hypotension. Myalgia, muscle weakness, and blurring of vision have also been reported.

INDICATIONS

Guanethidine is used in the treatment of hypertension, either alone or in combination with diuretics such as chlorothiazide.

DOSAGE AND ADMINISTRATION

Guanethidine is given by mouth. It has a slow onset of action but its effects are prolonged. Treatment is commenced with a small dose of 10 mg/day in divided doses for the first week, increasing by 10 mg/day each week until 60 mg/day are given in the sixth week, by which time the majority of patients are under control. The drug does not appear toxic even in doses up to 500 mg/day, but with doses over 60 mg/day there is an increased likelihood of side effects and hypotension may become excessive. On a constant effective dose the blood pressure often falls progressively for about a week and then remains stable at the lower level unless the dose is changed. It can be given with a ganglion-blocking drug such as pempidine, especially if diarrhoea is troublesome, and with chlorothiazide and its derivatives. Guanethidine eye-drops 5 per cent are used in the treatment of glaucoma.

PRECAUTIONS

Guanethidine is contraindicated in phaeochromocytoma as it increases the sensitivity of blood vessels to adrenaline and noradrenaline. It should be used with caution in coronary and severe renal disease. The blood pressure of patients who are under treatment with guanethidine may become markedly labile during anaesthesia. Excessive falls may arise from summation or even potentiation of the effects of treatment by the effect of anaesthesia. Acute rises in blood pressure may be due to hypersensitivity to circulating catecholamines released in response to a surgical stimulus. Premedication with atropine is advisable to prevent the potential risk of cardiac arrest. Stopping the drug the day before operation has little effect as its action lasts for more than a week. Excessive hypotension due to overdose can usually be controlled by keeping the patient recumbent. If pressor agents are required minimal doses should be used.

Guanoxan sulphate and **guanoclor sulphate** are drugs with peripheral actions similar to guanethidine. Guanoxan is contraindicated in patients with a previous history of liver disease, as some patients on treatment have developed jaundice. Initial dose is 10 mg daily increasing gradually to a maximum of 120 mg daily, if necessary.

Guanoclor, like guanoxan, has been shown to cause central as well as peripheral amine depletion. Initial dose is 20 mg daily rising gradually to 200 mg daily, if necessary.

Debrisoquine sulphate is another drug whose main action is the prevention of release of noradrenaline from storage granules. There is no depletion of noradrenaline stores on oral administration. Early reports suggest that side effects are less troublesome but its chief advantage is its rapid onset and short duration of action, making it practicable to vary the intensity of dosage throughout the day and to minimize the inevitable orthostatic hypotension. Doses start at 15 mg/day, increasing gradually to 100–150 mg/day.

Reserpine

Reserpine (*BP* and *USP*)
Constitution: an alkaloid obtained from certain *Rauwolfia* species, or prepared synthetically.

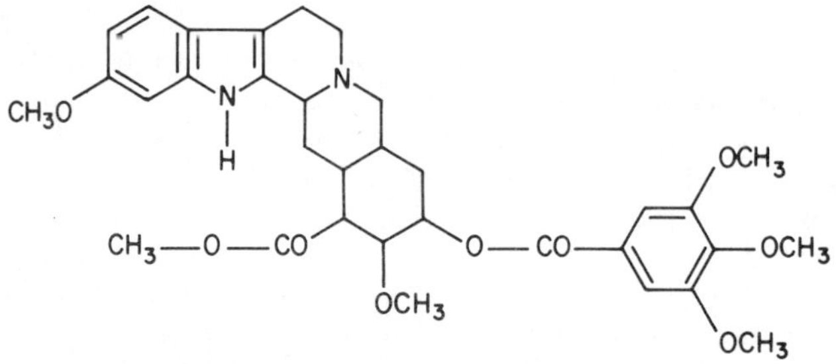

PHARMACOLOGY

Reserpine depletes stores of 5-hydroxytryptamine and catecholamines in many organs, including the brain and adrenal medulla. The actions on the CNS produce depression in some individuals but do not appear to play an important role in the reduction in sympathetic nerve effects. There may even be an increase in sympathetic outflow. The hypotensive effect can be attributed to its action in depleting the stores of noradrenaline in adrenergic nerve fibre terminals. The capacity to take up noradrenaline is also reduced.

Central nervous system. Reserpine produces a prolonged sedative action, even in small doses. This may proceed to nightmares and psychic depression and the drug should not be administered to patients with a history of depressive episodes. Large doses cause extrapyramidal side effects.

Cardiovascular system. Reserpine causes a slowly developing fall in blood pressure, frequently associated with bradycardia. There may be a decrease in peripheral resistance, which is most marked in the skin. There is usually a reduction in cardiac output. On acute intravenous administration these changes are preceded by a transient sympathomimetic effect. It has a greater effect on hypertensive than normal subjects.

Gastrointestinal tract. There is increased peristalsis and secretion of acid by the stomach and quiescent peptic ulcers may be activated. Diarrhoea may occur but can be antagonized by atropine.

Other effects. The most frequently observed side effects are nasal congestion, gain in weight, and diarrhoea.

Absorption and fate in the body. Reserpine takes about 2 hours to act after intravenous injection, and there is a latent period of several days before its has full effect when it is given by mouth, although it is well absorbed by the gastrointestinal tract. The slow development of its action is probably because stores of noradrenaline in the nerve terminal have to be depleted to about 5 per cent of the normal content before its action is clinically apparent.

INDICATIONS

Reserpine has been used in the treatment of hypertension, usually in conjunction with ganglion-blocking or other hypotensive drugs. The newer more powerful hypotensive agents, however, are now more commonly used. It is useful in mild anxiety states and in chronic psychoses.

DOSAGE AND ADMINISTRATION

In the treatment of hypertension, 0.5–2.0 mg is given by mouth daily in divided doses. In psychiatry small doses are used where possible to avoid depression, but in severely agitated patients as much as 10 mg intramuscularly may be given for a few days after which the dose is reduced and oral treatment instituted.

PRECAUTIONS

Reserpine is contraindicated in peptic ulcer and in colitis. Mild side effects such as anorexia, headache, nausea and vomiting, or nightmares are usually controllable with a reduction in dosage. Any suicidal tendency with severe depression is an indication for withdrawal of the drug.

Direct-acting vasodilators

All of the drug groups mentioned above produce vasodilatation by their action on the vasomotor nervous mechanism at various levels. Other drugs act directly on the smooth muscle of the arterioles, independently of its innervation. They include nitrites and nitrates, sodium nitroprusside, xanthines, papaverine, diazoxide, and nicotinic acid. Amyl nitrite, octyl nitrite, and glyceryl trinitrate are used in the relief of the pain of angina pectoris, theophylline as a bronchodilator and coronary dilator, and sodium nitroprusside as a short-acting hypotensive agent in anaesthesia, and in hypertensive crises. The xanthines by their central stimulant action tend to produce vasoconstriction in the splanchnic area, but where the tissue or organ has a poor vasoconstrictor supply, as in the coronary arteries, kidney, and brain, the peripheral vasodilator effect predominates.

Nicotinic acid dilates the vessels of the skin and pia arachnoid, and is used when this action is desired, but nicotinamide is used preferably when only vitamin action is required, because it has little or no vasodilator effect. Histamine dilates capillaries and increases their permeability; it also dilates arterioles in man but in some animals causes constriction of these vessels. The drugs in this group may therefore be used to dilate blood vessels in a localized area, or to lower blood pressure by general vasodilatation.

Nitrites and nitrates

Nitrites were introduced into medicine in 1860, amyl nitrite and glyceryl trinitrate both being used for angina pectoris. The pain was thought to be due to paroxysmal increases in blood pressure which was reversed by the nitrites. This theory, although false, led to their use in the treatment of hypertension before ganglion-blocking agents and other more suitable drugs became available.

Nitrites relax smooth muscle with an intensity that varies markedly according to the organ, and the route by which they are administered. Postarteriolar blood vessels are affected, but the greatest effect is probably on the venous side of the circulation resulting in a fall in venous return. The muscle of the biliary tract may be strongly relaxed, but that of the bronchial tree, ureters, and gastrointestinal tract is less responsive. The basis for their efficacy in angina pectoris is that they produce peripheral vasodilatation and a fall in venous return, thus reducing the work of the heart. Sodium nitrite is the most effective, but it is also the most toxic; it is rarely used now as its action is too short, it is too toxic for repeated use, and nitrites can produce headache.

Certain organic nitrates such as glyceryl trinitrate and pentaerythritol tetranitrate, with amyl and octyl nitrites and some others, exhibit the 'nitrite' type of action in the body. Amyl and octyl nitrites are given by inhalation and glyceryl trinitrate by absorption sublingually. Orally administered nitrates (glyceryl trinitrate and isosorbide dinitrate) are too slow and uncertain for acute therapy and have given inconsistent results as prophylactic agents against angina. This is because they undergo extensive but variable 'first-pass' metabolism in the liver. The major metabolite of isosorbide dinitrate is the mononitrate, and this is in fact the haemodynamically active agent. Isosorbide mononitrate is now available for oral administration and is claimed to provide a powerful and consistent antianginal activity with a duration of action allowing three times daily administration. The dose is 20–40 mg.

All nitrites tend to cause methaemoglobinaemia but this does not occur to any extent except with sodium nitrite, or with excessive doses of glyceryl trinitrate used over a long period. In acute cases of methaemoglobinaemia, methylene blue 1 mg/kg can be given intravenously together with the administration of oxygen. In the chronic condition 300 mg/day by mouth and full doses of ascorbic acid are given.

Nitrites in the treatment of cyanide poisoning

In cyanide poisoning, the induction of methaemoglobinaemia by sodium nitrite can, if given in time, be a life-saving measure. Methaemoglobin forms cyanmethaemoglobin and renders the cyanide ion less toxic by combination. This gradually dissociates, but by giving sodium thiosulphate, the cyanide ion is converted into thiocyanate. The dose of sodium nitrite for adults is 0.3–0.5 g dissolved in 10–15 ml of water, given by slow intravenous injection. While the solution is being prepared, amyl nitrite can be inhaled for 30 seconds every 2 minutes. After the injection of nitrite, but not with it, sodium thiosulphate 12.5 g in 50 ml of water should be given slowly intravenously, taking about 10 minutes over the injection. This procedure can be repeated if necessary with half doses of each drug. The administration of hydroxocobalamin (5 mg) has also been recommended for the treatment of cyanide poisoning (*see* page 359).

If the fall in blood pressure is too profound, a pressor drug should be used. Oxygen and a blood transfusion may also be required.

Diazoxide

Diazoxide (*BP* and *USP*)
Chemical name: 7-chloro-3-methyl-2*H*-1,2,4-benzothiadiazine 1,1-dioxide

CH_3 N NH Cl S O O

PHARMACOLOGY

Diazoxide is structurally closely related to chlorothiazide. Unlike that compound, it has no diuretic activity, but actually causes renal retention of sodium and water, probably by stimulating antidiuretic hormone secretion. Intravenous administration does, however, have a profound hypotensive effect which is due to direct vasodilator action on arteriolar smooth muscle. Neither α- nor β-adrenoceptor blockade can antagonize this action. At a cellular level the drug interferes with the responses to Ca^{2+}, either by blocking the release of bound intracellular calcium or by blocking calcium receptors.

The fall in peripheral resistance is accompanied by reflex tachycardia and a rise in cardiac output. These effects can be blocked by β-adrenoceptor blocking drugs. The reflex β-effects also reveal themselves in an increase in plasma free fatty acids.

Diazoxide also relaxes other smooth muscle so that when used in eclampsia or pre-eclampsia, delay in the second stage of labour may occur. This can be reversed by oxytocic drugs.

Diazoxide also causes a rise in blood sugar. This is due not only to a rise in circulatory catecholamine levels, but also to a direct inhibitory action on the β-cells of the pancreas, blocking insulin release. This can be reversed by oral hypoglycaemic agents.

Diazoxide crosses the placenta.

INDICATIONS

Diazoxide is a drug of choice in the immediate management of hypertensive crisis associated with encephalopathy, congestive heart failure, eclampsia, and acute glomerular nephritis. It has also been recommended as a means of limiting haemorrhage in hypertensive patients undergoing renal biopsy or arteriography.

Its hyperglycaemic effects have been utilized in the management of inoperable islet cell tumours, some of the glycogen storage diseases, and in postgastrectomy hypoglycaemia.

DOSAGE AND ADMINISTRATION

For the control of severe hypertension, diazoxide is given by rapid intravenous injection with the patient recumbent. The normal adult dose is 300 mg, but in the obese 5 mg/kg may be taken as a guide. The response should occur within 5 minutes and lasts for several hours. The dose may be repeated up to four times in 24 hours but conventional antihypertensive therapy should normally be substituted as soon as possible. For its hyperglycaemic effects diazoxide is given by mouth, 5 mg/kg/24 h initially, increasing according to the blood sugar response. Doses as high as 1 g/day may be necessary in islet cell tumours.

PRECAUTIONS

The solution is highly alkaline and care must be taken to avoid extravenous leakage. It must *not* be given intramuscularly. Increasing sodium retention can be controlled with diuretics; in patients already on diuretics, the hypotensive action of diazoxide may be intensified. Delay in the second stage of labour may occur. Following oral therapy in pregnancy alopecia in the newborn has been reported. With each injection there is a rise in blood sugar of about 1.5 mmol/ℓ (10 mg per cent). Prolonged oral therapy can cause hypertrichosis and a parkinsonian syndrome.

Glyceryl trinitrate

Glyceryl trinitrate (*BP*) and Nitroglycerin (*USP*)
Chemical name: propane-1,2,3-triol trinitrate

$$
\begin{array}{l}
CH_2-O-NO_2 \\
| \\
CH-O-NO_2 \\
| \\
CH_2-O-NO_2
\end{array}
$$

PHARMACOLOGY

Glyceryl trinitrate (GTN) relaxes vascular muscle by direct action and is claimed to have a greater effect on capacitance vessels than on arterioles. Dilatation of postcapillary vessels, including large veins, results in peripheral pooling, reduced venous return, and a fall in cardiac output. It is thus particularly of value in left ventricular failure, reducing preload rather than afterload.

Systemic vascular resistance, pulmonary vascular resistance, and arterial pressure are all reduced: left ventricular end-diastolic volumes and pressures are reduced as well as myocardial wall tension and oxygen consumption. There may be an improvement in coronary blood flow: redistribution from normal to ischaemic cardiac muscle has been demonstrated.

The effects of GTN are apparent within 2–3 minutes of starting an intravenous infusion and are reversed within 5–10 minutes of discontinuing it. The metabolites are considerably less toxic in overdose than those from sodium nitroprusside, but this apart, the drugs are very similar. Both drugs increase intracranial pressure.

INDICATIONS

GTN can be used for the rapid control of hypertension during cardiac surgery or for inducing and maintaining controlled hypotension during anaesthesia. It has also been used to reduce preload in patients with unresponsive congestive cardiac failure, secondary to acute myocardial infarction.

DOSAGE AND ADMINISTRATION

The drug is commercially available as a solution of 0.5 mg/ml, stabilized in 10 per cent alcohol, lactose, and potassium monophosphate. It may be given by syringe pump or be diluted in an infusion of 5 per cent dextrose or isotonic saline. The recommended final concentration is 100 mg/ℓ (100 μg/ml). The dose required to produce adequate control of blood pressure generally lies between 25 and 200 μg/min, but may reach twice this amount.

PRECAUTIONS

The solution is incompatible with PVC and should be administered after dilution only from glass or rigid polyethylene containers.

Side effects of nitrates include nausea and retching, headache, restlessness, muscle twitching, palpitations, and dizziness. Overdose leads to hypotension which should be treated by elevating the legs, discontinuing the infusion or, if severe, by administering α-adrenoceptor stimulators such as methoxamine or phenylephrine.

Hydralazine hydrochloride

Hydralazine hydrochloride (*BAN*) and Hydralazine hydrochloride (*USP*)
Chemical name: 1-hydrazinophthalazine hydrochloride

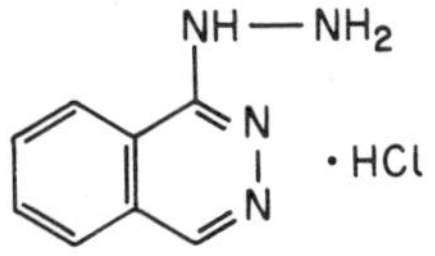

PHARMACOLOGY

Hydralazine is a hypotensive agent which produces peripheral vasodilatation mainly by a direct action; it also has a mild α-adrenoceptor blocking action. Cardiac output and rate are reflexly increased by central sympathetic action. There are a number of side effects – headache, tachycardia, dizziness, nausea and vomiting. Renal blood flow is increased.

INDICATIONS, DOSAGE AND ADMINISTRATION

It is used in the treatment of hypertension, often in conjunction with other drugs such as β-blocking agents or thiazide diuretics. It is of value in the treatment of hypertensive crises when 10–40 mg may be given intravenously. Otherwise the usual commencing dose is 10 mg 4-hourly by mouth increasing up to 200 mg daily if necessary. Tolerance may occur. A serious toxic effect which can occur with prolonged use and large doses is a condition resembling systemic lupus erythematosus. Note, there are fast and slow acetylators of hydralazine.

Sodium nitroprusside

Sodium nitroprusside (*BP* and *USP*) and Sterile sodium nitroprusside (*USP*)
Chemical formula: $Na_2[Fe(CN)_5NO]\cdot 2H_2O$

PHARMACOLOGY

Sodium nitroprusside was first described in 1849 and its hypotensive action in 1929. It has a direct vasodilator action on the smooth muscle of the vessel wall, proportional to the blood concentration, and this action is independent of autonomic innervation. It thus causes a fall in peripheral resistance and an increase in venous capacity. Cardiac output, however, falls only when the pressure is lowered unduly. There is a marked increase in coronary blood flow with moderate falls in mean arterial pressure. Hypotension is more marked in elderly and hypertensive subjects, and is potentiated by ganglion-blocking drugs. There is usually a moderate compensatory tachycardia; on discontinuing the infusion the blood pressure rapidly returns to normal, usually within 2–5 minutes. Renal blood flow decreases, as expected, as the mean arterial pressure falls and there is a release of renin. Pulmonary artery pressure also falls, presumably due to dilatation of pulmonary vessels. Dilatation of systemic capacitance vessels is responsible for a fall in right atrial pressure. The effect on blood flow in other organs is uncertain.

Fate in the body. Nitroprusside is rapidly broken down by haemoglobin non-enzymatically; electron transfer from haemoglobin (Fe^{2+}) yields methaemoglobin (Fe^{3+}) and an unstable nitroprusside which quickly breaks down to yield five cyanide ions. One of these then reacts with the methaemoglobin to form cyanmethaemoglobin. The remaining cyanide ions are converted into thiocyanate by an enzyme rhodanese, principally in the liver, but also in the kidney. Any cyanide not so inactivated causes biochemical toxicity by inactivating essential enzymes such as cytochrome oxidase. In sufficient doses this will result in cyanide poisoning. This syndrome has been reported clinically with large doses of nitroprusside and leads to a base deficit, indicating anaerobic metabolism.

INDICATIONS

Sodium nitroprusside is used as an alternative to trimetaphan for the induction of hypotension during surgery. Its advantage over that drug is an absence of tachyphylaxis. However, it does share the tendency to be associated with compensatory tachycardia. This may be controlled with a β_1-adrenoceptor blocking drug. It has also been used in the control of hypertension during the removal of a phaeochromocytoma. Disadvantages would seem to be a potential difficulty in reversing any overdose, the production of cyanmethaemoglobin and potential cyanide poisoning.

DOSAGE AND ADMINISTRATION

Although it can be given orally, sodium nitroprusside is now given only as a continuous intravenous infusion; the strength of infusion may need to be varied according to the subject. In older subjects the infusion is usually 50 mg/ℓ, or even 20 mg/ℓ, but young subjects are rather resistant and the infusion strength should be increased to 100 mg/ℓ. The total dose administered is related to the development of toxicity and should not normally exceed 3.5 mg/kg; 7 mg/kg is a lethal dose.

PRECAUTIONS

Toxicity is associated with increases in the blood concentration of both thiocyanate and cyanide but, for various reasons, neither is a reliable guide to the extent of toxicity. Evidence of increased anaerobic metabolism (rise in base deficit, elevated lactate and lactate/pyruvate ratios) is the most reliable indication of the onset of toxicity. Traditional treatment for cyanide poisoning has been the administration of nitrites to augment the antidotal effects of thiosulphate which was thought to have too slow an onset. In the context of the metabolism of sodium nitroprusside this may not be true and Krapez and his colleagues (1981) have shown that dogs pretreated with thiosulphate, 75 mg/kg, maintained low cyanide concentrations even with high doses. They suggest that thiosulphate should be given prophylactically whenever doses of nitroprusside close to the toxic limit are likely to be used. Vitamin B_{12a} (hydroxocobalamin) is also a cyanide neutralizer, but only in very high doses. Reasonable doses undoubtedly have some beneficial effects but there is disagreement as to whether these are synergistic with thiosulphate.

Sodium nitroprusside solutions are normally browny-pink; a change to blue indicates deterioration.

Krapez, J. R., Vesey, C. J., Adams, L. and Cole, P. V. (1981) Effects of cyanide antidotes used with sodium nitroprusside infusions; sodium thiosulphate and hydroxocobalamin given prophylactically to dogs. *British Journal of Anaesthesia*, **53**, 793

13

Drugs affecting cardiac force, rhythm and rate

Inotropic agents

Inotropic agents alter the force of the heartbeat: those that increase it are used therapeutically or act physiologically and are generally beneficial, while those that decrease the force of the heart have not hitherto been much employed, as it is not often desirable to reduce cardiac output. However, β-adrenoceptor blocking agents are being used to decrease myocardial work and oxygen consumption in angina pectoris. Use is also made of the fact that some of these, the antidysrhythmic drugs, at the same time as reducing the force of contraction also lessen the excitability of the myocardium. All anaesthetics cause progressive myocardial depression although their effects may be masked by sympathetic over-activity.

In the normal heart, control in exercise is effected by the release of adrenaline and noradrenaline which increase both the rate and force of contraction and produce a considerable increase in cardiac output. The opposite, or occurrence of excessive parasympathetic activity, occurs in the state of neurogenic shock when there is marked slowing of the heart through vagal stimulation and the cardiac output per minute is greatly reduced. Initially the output per beat is not much affected until vasopressin is liberated from the posterior pituitary gland; this causes vasoconstriction of the coronary arteries, which, with the slowing, cause a profound drop in blood pressure leading to fainting and unconsciousness.

Drugs that stimulate myocardial contraction shorten the refractory period of cardiac muscle and increase its excitability, thus tending to promote irregular rhythm which may predispose to ventricular fibrillation. When they are administered, the object is to employ them at a dose level that will give the desired therapeutic effect without running this risk. Thus, it is dangerous to inject adrenaline intravenously unless it is given diluted and very slowly; endogenous adrenaline and noradrenaline may be liberated in amounts sufficient to cause cardiac irregularities under conditions of stress and during anaesthesia. This can be particularly dangerous in the presence of vagal stimulation, because as the heart slows it also becomes more excitable.

The sympathomimetic amines are the drugs that have been most widely employed for the production of a positive inotropic effect. Their potency depends on the extent to which the drug stimulates β_1(cardiac)-adrenoceptors (*see* page 319). The effect on the blood pressure is, however, modified by the drug's action on other adrenoceptors. Stimulation of β_2-adrenoceptors causes vasodilatation whereas stimulation of α-adrenoceptors causes vasoconstriction. The effects on force of contraction and blood pressure can thus be predicted if the pattern of receptor activation is known. For example, isoprenaline and dopamine are more powerful inotropic agents than noradrenaline.

A notable action of inotropic agents is to increase the intracellular concentration of cyclic AMP, an important energy substrate. Sympathomimetic agents such as the catecholamines do so by stimulating the enzyme adenyl cyclase, which converts ATP into cyclic AMP (*Figure 13.1*). The concentration of cyclic AMP can also be increased by inhibition of the enzyme phosphodiesterase, the enzyme responsible for the inactivation of cyclic AMP to 5′-AMP. The methylxanthines such as aminophylline are inhibitors of phosphodiesterase and probably owe their inotropism to this mechanism. However, there is some evidence that, in the case of the catecholamines, stimulation of adenyl cyclase and positive inotropism are separate effects and so this aspect of their actions is still controversial.

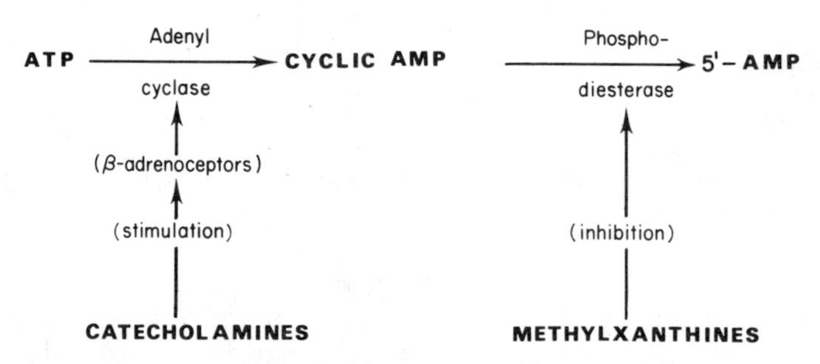

Figure 13.1 Influence of inotropic agents on cyclic AMP

Inotropic effects can also be produced by drugs that affect ion movements in myocardial cells. The most important group of drugs with this effect are the cardiac glycosides and strophanthin. They are most effective in congestive heart failure, in hypertensive and ischaemic heart disease involving the left ventricle, when the failure is mainly muscular, and when contractility is unimpeded by obstructed or incompetent valves. They are often ineffective in severe aortic valvular disease, certain types of cor pulmonale, and anaemic heart failure.

The xanthines, such as aminophylline, exhibit positive inotropism by an intracellular action which involves increasing the concentrations of cyclic AMP and also affecting calcium fluxes (*see* page 389). These effects are additive to those of β-adrenoceptor agonists which increase cyclic AMP by a different mechanism. The effects of the xanthines are associated with an increase in the duration of the action potential in cardiac muscle.

Glucagon, the hormone secreted by the α-cells of the islets of Langerhans, also exerts positive inotropic effects. These are not blocked by β-adrenoceptor blockade. However, it increases adenyl cyclase activity which in turn increases intracellular cyclic AMP levels.

Calcium ions play a crucial role in excitation–contraction coupling in muscle and all these drugs may fundamentally act by facilitating calcium transport across the cell membrane. Calcium ions are also, therefore, inotropic agents.

Muscle contraction

Although it was approximately 100 years ago that Sydney Ringer noted that the isolated heart would only contract if calcium was present in the medium, it is only relatively recently that the basis for this observation has been elucidated. Contraction depends on an interaction between two proteins, actin and myosin, which in the highly purified state contract in the presence of ATP and magnesium without requiring calcium ions. Normally, however, contraction is regulated by the presence of two regulating proteins, troponin and tropomyosin. Calcium interacts with troponin and prevents it from inhibiting the actin–myosin interaction (*Figure 13.2*). In cardiac muscle the calcium ions necessary to produce contraction may

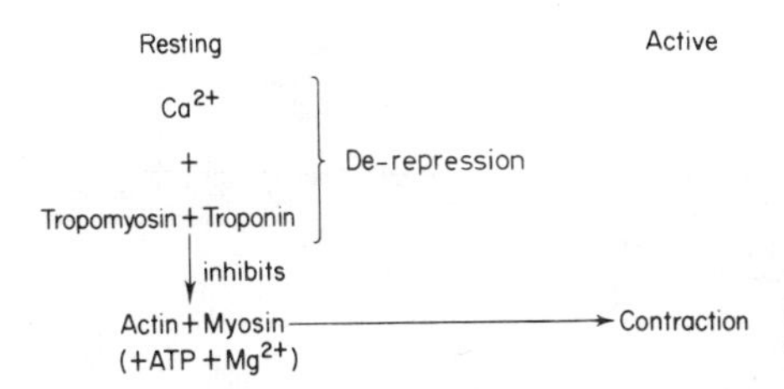

Figure 13.2 Effect of calcium ion on contractile processes. Ca^{2+} removes inhibition of actin–myosin complex

come from calcium bound to the sarcoplasmic reticulum, or from mitochondrial stores. In contrast to skeletal muscle, cardiac muscle has a small calcium pool bound to the sarcoplasmic reticulum and therefore influx of extracellular calcium is probably indispensable, even under normal conditions, to maintain cardiac muscle contraction.

The cardiac electrical cycle

This is dependent on ionic movements of sodium, potassium, and calcium; consider *Figure 13.3*. Prior to excitation the resting potential is −80 mV; permeability of the cell membrane to the sodium ion is low but permeability to the potassium ion is high. On excitation there is a large increase in sodium permeability and sodium moves into the cell. The decrease in the external sodium concentration initiates calcium ion movement and calcium moves inwards. At this plateau stage sodium permeability decreases. These calcium ions react with inhibitors (for example troponin) on the myofilaments. The removal of the inhibitor results in de-repression so contraction can occur. The rate of force developed is proportional to the rate at which calcium ions are delivered to the myofilament. The duration of action is related to the time the calcium ions remain in contact with the myofilament. Calcium is removed from the myofilament into the mitochondria, possibly by means of a calcium pump. It is also extruded from the cell, the sodium–potassium ATPase pump also being involved.

Cardiac action potentials

The heart is made up of a syncytium of cardiac cells. Cells that are part of a syncytium usually exhibit threshold behaviour. The cell membrane potential may vary in the absence of external stimuli and action potentials can arise spontaneously. The form and characteristics of the action potential can vary from place to place and this certainly occurs in the heart (*see* below).

A hypothetical action potential is shown in *Figure 13.4*. There is a spontaneous depolarization (called phase 4) which proceeds until a threshold transmembrane

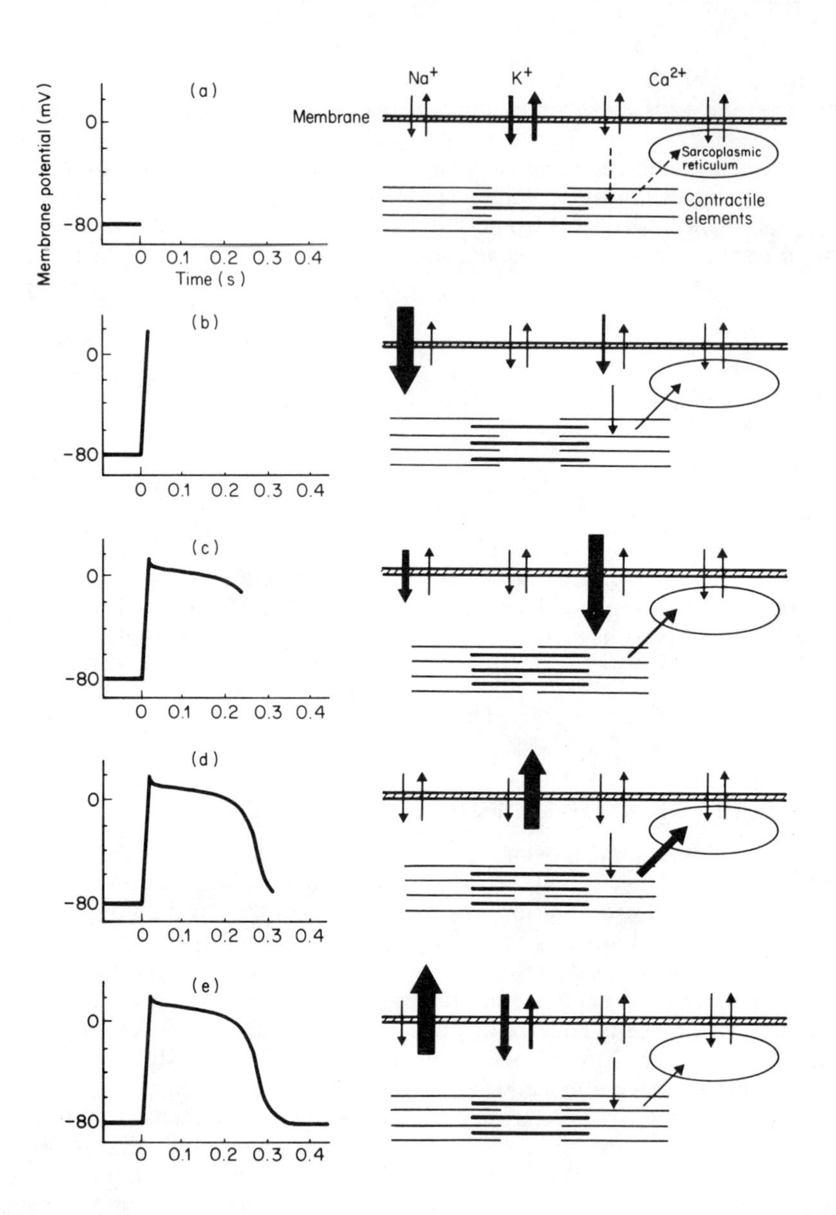

Figure 13.3 Ionic movements during the cardiac action potential.
(a) At rest, sodium permeability is low, potassium permeability is relatively high, and there is little calcium movement.
(b) The rapid depolarization phase of the action potential is due to a large increase in sodium permeability. This reduces the potassium permeability and allows calcium entry to increase.
(c) In the plateau phase, sodium permeability falls and massive calcium influx occurs, stimulating the contractile process.
(d) Repolarization begins as the potassium permeability rises and sodium permeability falls towards the resting level. Calcium influx stops and sequestration of calcium leads to relaxation of the contractile elements.
(e) At the end of the repolarization phase, passive permeabilities have fallen to resting levels, but active extrusion of sodium and uptake of potassium restores the ionic concentration gradients

potential of about −70 mV is reached, at which point a rapid depolarization is triggered (phase 0) and this institutes the action potential. This is followed by an effective refractory period (ERP), which includes not only the absolute refractory period but a period during which the membrane is excitable but impulse propagation does not occur. Towards the end of phase 3 there is a relative refractory period when impulses can be transmitted at reduced velocity.

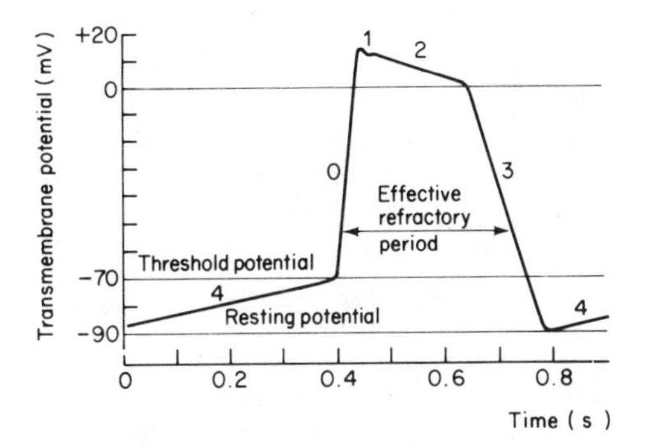

Figure 13.4 Transmembrane potential of a spontaneously firing Purkinje fibre (hypothetical)

Normally, excitation starts in the sinoatrial (S-A) node and an excitation wave is spread three-dimensionally over the surface of both atria and channelled into the atrioventricular (A-V) node. Here a dramatic slowing occurs. The wave then proceeds through the Purkinje fibres in the bundle of His and is distributed to the endocardial surface of both ventricles.

Sinoatrial node

This consists of a group of cells with special characteristics which are anatomically situated in the wall of the right atrium near the opening of the superior vena cava. Normally these cells are responsible for initiation of the cardiac excitatory process. They act as the pacemaker for the heart and receive both sympathetic and parasympathetic nerve supplies.

A peculiarity of these cells is that they exhibit slow diastolic depolarization called the pacemaker potential. The pacemaker potential rises to a threshold and when this is reached the next action potential is fired off. The resting membrane potential, defined as maximum polarization between action potentials, is lower

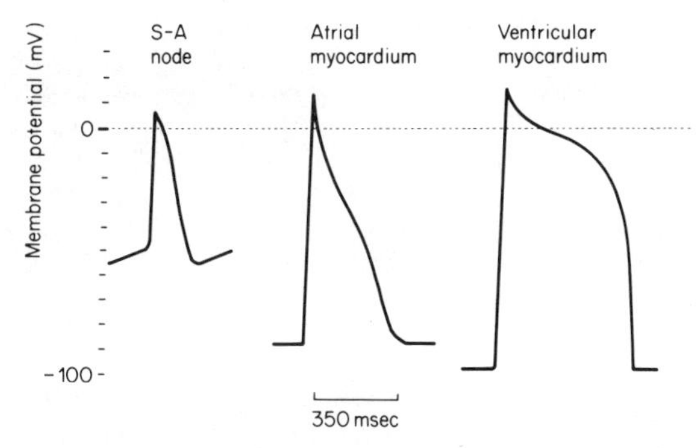

Figure 13.5 Comparison of cardiac action potentials of the S-A node, atrial myocardium and ventricular myocardium

than in other parts of the heart (*see Figure 13.5*). It is approximately −65 mV. In contrast, the atrial myocardium has a stable resting potential of approximately −85 mV. The action potential also has a different configuration, the downstroke being slow in comparison to the rising phase.

Atrioventricular node

The A-V node is innervated by both the sympathetic and the parasympathetic parts of the autonomic nervous system. Anatomically, it is found on the right septum wall. It is the origin of the specialized conducting cells, the Purkinje cells, whose fibres transmit the excitation wave from the atria into the ventricles. The A-V node has a similar pattern of activity to the S-A node. For instance, it shows slow diastolic depolarization and has a low resting membrane potential.

It normally acts as a filter to limit the frequency with which impulses are conducted from the atria to the ventricles but it can take over from the S-A node and function as a pacemaker.

Bundle of His

This consists of Purkinje fibres which originate in the A-V node. The bundle crosses the fibrous tissue which demarcates the atria from the ventricles and enters the ventricular septum. There it splits into two branches which ramify to the endocardial surface of each ventricle. Conduction through the bundle of His occurs at a faster rate (2.5 m/s) than anywhere else in the heart.

Table 13.1 Effect of stimulation of cardiac autonomic nerves. β-Adrenoceptor agonists will simulate effects of sympathetic nerve stimulation, and muscarinic agonists that of vagal stimulation.

Cardiac site	*Effects of sympathetic nerve stimulation*	*Effects of vagal nerve stimulation*
S-A node	Heart rate increases. Pacemaker potential slope steepens, thus interval between action potentials decreases.	Heart rate slows. Pacemaker potential slope becomes shallower, thus interval between action potentials increases.
Atrial myocardium	Force of contraction is increased: decreased refractory period and increased conduction velocity.	Force of contraction decreased. Note: due to reduction in action potential duration, there is also a decreased refractory period and an increased velocity.
A-V node	Quicker transmission due to decreased refractory period and increased conduction velocity.	Slower transmission due to increased refractory period and increased conduction velocity. A-V block can occur if parasympathetic stimulation is very marked.
Purkinje fibres	Marked stimulation can initiate pacemaker activity.	Marked stimulation leading to A-V block may be followed by initiation of pacemaker activity. Basis of vagal escape phenomenon.
Ventricular myocardium	Increases force of contraction.	No vagal innervation but force of contraction depressed by acetylcholine.

Ventricular myocardium

This has a resting membrane potential of about −90 to −100 mV and the resting membrane potential remains stable between action potentials. The shape of the action potential is shown in *Figure 13.5*. The action potential shape in the Purkinje fibre is similar but has a faster conduction velocity.

The effects of sympathetic and vagal nerve stimulation on the heart are shown in *Table 13.1*.

Positive cardiac inotropic agents

These increase the force of the heart. The heart may be visualized as a pump and that pump requires energy to do its work. To increase output the pump can be provided with more energy. Sympathomimetic drugs such as isoprenaline will raise the levels of intracellular cyclic AMP. This substance in turn can activate cardiac lipase which is responsible for breaking down triglyerides to free fatty acids, thus providing additional energy for the heart. Alternatively, energy available may be better utilized. Digoxin, by affecting calcium movements in the failing heart, allows better energy utilization.

Digoxin and digitoxin

Digoxin (*BP* and *USP*)
Digitoxin (*BP* and *USP*)
Prepared digitalis (*BP*) and Powdered digitalis (*USP*)

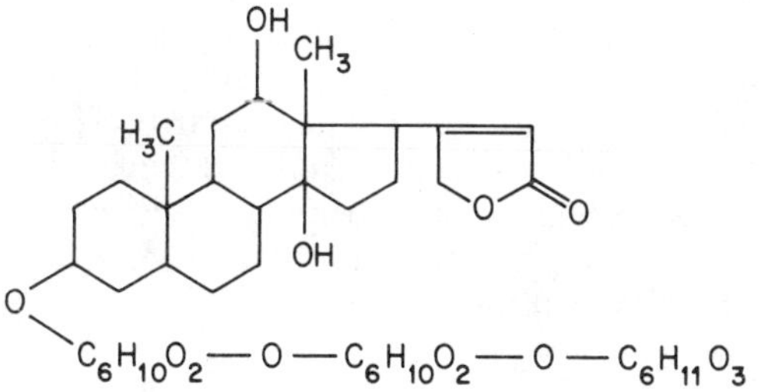

OH CH_3 H_3C O O OH O

$C_6H_{10}O_2—O—C_6H_{10}O_2—O—C_6H_{11}O_3$

Digoxin

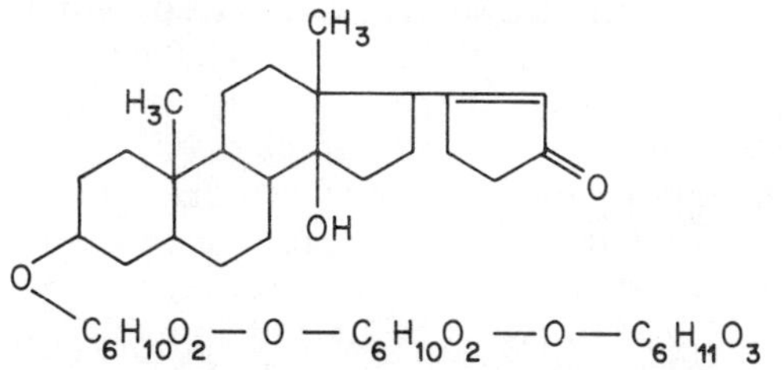

CH_3 H_3C O OH O

$C_6H_{10}O_2—O—C_6H_{10}O_2—O—C_6H_{11}O_3$

Digitoxin

The main active principle of the powdered leaf of the purple foxglove (*Digitalis purpurea*) is the glycoside digitoxin but this preparation, Prepared digitalis (*BP*), is now only of historical interest. Digoxin from *Digitalis lanata* is the most commonly used glycoside and all such preparations, used therapeutically, are loosely referred to as digitalis. The most important of these glycosides are digoxin, digitoxin, ouabain (from *Strophanthus gratus*), lanatoside C, and proscillaridin A.

Digitalis

Digitalis was first used by William Withering in 1775, having noted that it was a constituent of an old family recipe recommended for dropsy. He was unaware of its cardiac action.

Chemistry of digitalis glycosides

The basic structure of the glycosides is that of the steroid cyclopentenophenanthrene nucleus and they are chemically related to the bile acids and the sex hormones. They consist of two parts, a glycone and an aglycone portion. The glycone is a sugar, often glucose, but closely related sugars such as digitoxose are also found. They have no cardiac action in themselves, but make the glycoside more soluble, help transport and are essential for fixation to cardiac muscle, without which the drug has little action. In the aglycone portions reside the digitalis-like activity, but their actions alone are more transient and less potent as they do not remain fixed in the muscle; their power to cause toxic effects such as vomiting equals that of the glycosides. The intrinsic activity of these drugs resides in the double bond in the unsaturated lactone ring, and opening the ring or saturating the double bond causes loss of both therapeutic activity and toxic effects.

PHARMACOLOGY

Central nervous system. Neurological effects are commonly seen early in cases of digitalis intoxication. Headaches, drowsiness, and an ill-defined malaise are frequently encountered. Visual disturbances and facial neuralgia may also occur on rare occasions.

Digitalis slowing occurs when congestive cardiac failure is treated with this drug, and results largely from the improvement in cardiac output. The slowing is mediated mainly through the vagus and hence can be abolished by the use of atropine. In the absence of cardiac failure, and in the presence of normal rhythm, some slowing occurs partly because of central stimulation and partly from depression of the S-A node. In atrial fibrillation, digitalization causes slowing as a result of A-V conduction block, and this is not reversible by atropine. Thus, when cardiac failure occurs with atrial fibrillation, slowing results because of at least two different mechanisms, one of which is reversible with atropine.

Cardiovascular system. Digitalis has practically no effect on the normal heart. There is a marginal slowing effect and the heart size is slightly reduced with a proportional reduction in output, but in congestive heart failure when the heart is dilated and contracting feebly its action is marked. Its main action is direct stimulation of the heart muscle independent of catecholamine stimulation, which leads to greater force of contraction, diminution in the size of the heart, and an increase in cardiac output. A reduction in atrial and venous pressure follows. The excitant effect of the drug on heart muscle shortens the refractory period and the rate of a fibrillating atrium will be increased, and in cases of flutter the irregularity changes to fibrillation, although on withdrawal of the drug normal rhythm may be resumed. Digitalis also acts on the A-V bundle of His – initially due to vagal inhibition – which results in the slower conduction of impulses from atrium to ventricle, and is reflected in the prolonged P-R interval in the ECG. This effect is greatest in patients who have atrial fibrillation with a rapid ventricular rate. Later, due to direct block of conducting tissues, the effect of slowing becomes more marked, and can be controlled by adjusting the dose of digitalis given.

Mechanism of cardiac action. If oxygen consumption is taken as a measure of the total metabolic energy liberated then there is evidence from both animal and human studies that cardiac glycosides do not significantly change oxygen consumption. Digoxin and related compounds probably act by increasing free intracellular calcium ion concentrations in the cell. One theory on how such substances may function is shown in *Figure 13.6*. Cardiac glycosides inhibit the membrane sodium–potassium pump, thus producing an increase in sodium on the internal side of the membrane. In turn this increases the influx of calcium in the region of the myofilament which increases myocardial force.

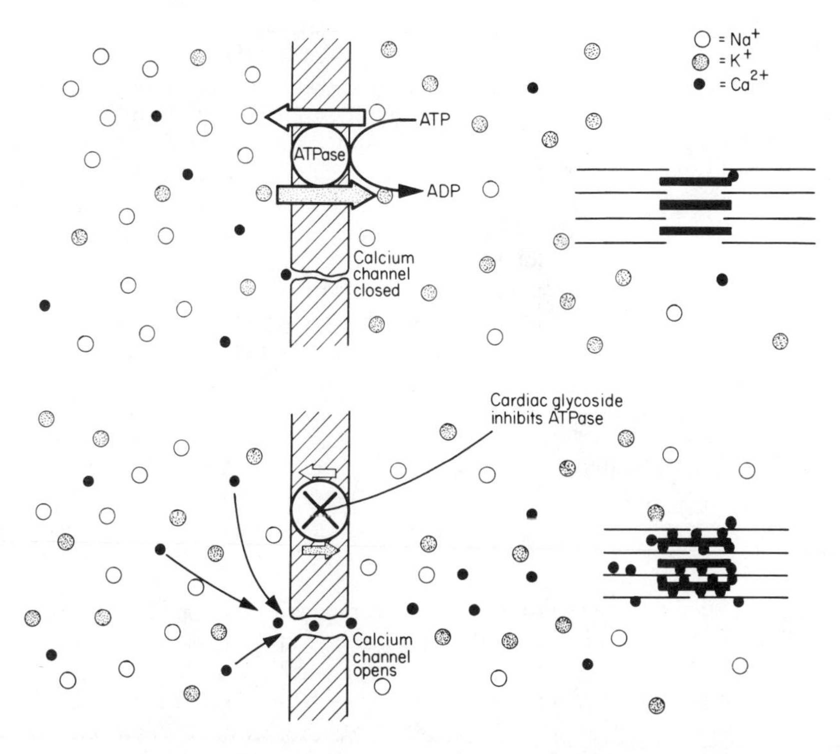

Figure 13.6 When Na^+ pumping is reduced because the membrane ATPase is inhibited by the cardiac glycoside, Na^+ accumulates within the cardiac cell. This induces the calcium channel to open, allowing Ca^{2+} influx and activation of the contractile mechanism

Diuretic action. Although digitalis can directly inhibit the ion transport system in the proximal renal tubule, high doses are necessary, and it is unlikely that this direct action plays a significant role in the diuresis that accompanies the use of digitalis in congestive cardiac failure. This is almost entirely due to its effects on cardiac output and the consequent improvement in glomerular filtration pressure. A marked improvement in urinary output and reduction in oedema will usually follow full digitalization, but many cases will also require a diuretic such as chlorothiazide.

Gastrointestinal tract. Digoxin is less irritant orally than the natural powdered leaf. Nausea and vomiting may follow overdosage, and anorexia may be the first sign that full digitalization is being approached; diarrhoea may also be present. Digoxin can be given intravenously if the drug is not well tolerated by mouth, or for a more rapid effect.

Absorption and fate in the body. Digitalis is given only by mouth or as a pure glycoside by intravenous injection. Owing to its irritant nature, the injection by subcutaneous or intramuscular routes has been abandoned; apart from pain and discomfort, absorption of the drug from these sites is irregular.

Absorption of different cardiac glycosides varies considerably, digoxin being almost totally absorbed if bioavailability is good. Because of problems of bioavailability, a new specification for Digoxin Tablets (*BP*) was introduced by the British Pharmacopoeia Commission on October 1st, 1975. All tablets from that date are required to undergo not less than 75 per cent dissolution in 1 hour. Such tablets are liable to be more potent than unbranded tablets previously available.

A single dose of digitoxin takes 6–8 hours to produce its full effect and its action lasts several days. Digoxin acts in 1–3 hours and lasts 1–2 days. Digitoxin acts as quickly by mouth as by intravenous injection, but digoxin is more rapidly effective by the intravenous route. The delayed action of these drugs is due mainly to the time taken for them to be fixed in cardiac muscle; protein binding with serum albumin also plays a part. Digitalis glycosides are not selectively retained by heart muscle which does not keep them longer than other tissues.

Digitalis glycosides are excreted by the kidney; digoxin, the most important one in the series, is excreted only by glomerular filtration and its accumulation in renal insufficiency makes dose reduction essential in this situation. The action of lanatoside C is due to its metabolic conversion to digoxin. About 40 per cent of a dose of digitoxin is excreted within 48 hours, smaller amounts being excreted for several weeks.

INDICATIONS

The prime indication for the use of digitalis is in congestive cardiac failure. Its effect is more dramatic in cases of atrial fibrillation, but its tonic action on heart muscle is the most important effect, and this is why the drug can be equally useful in cases of failure with normal rhythm. A less important use is in cases of atrial flutter. This is changed to fibrillation, which may persist on withdrawal of the drug but an adequate A-V conduction block reduces the ventricular rate.

DOSAGE AND ADMINISTRATION

Digoxin is the drug most commonly employed as it is shorter acting and its effect is more controllable. Full digitalization by digoxin requires an oral dose of 1.5–3 mg according to the weight of the patient. This is usually given as an initial dose of 0.5–0.75 mg followed by 0.25 mg at 6-hourly intervals until the total estimated dose has been given or signs of toxicity occur. If more rapid digitalization is necessary, half of the total estimated dose can be given initially followed by the remainder in 24 hours at 6-hourly intervals, or the drug can be given intravenously commencing with a dose of 0.5–1 mg followed by 0.5 mg 6-hourly. The usual maintenance dose is 0.25–0.75 mg daily. Digitoxin is as rapidly effective by mouth as by injection; it is rarely used now. Digitalization with digitoxin requires 1–1.5 mg in divided doses and the maintenance dose is 0.05–0.2 mg. Lanatoside C is another cardiac glycoside which is similar to digoxin but is excreted more rapidly. It is given in a dose of 0.25 mg three times a day.

Whenever digitalis is to be given it is of the greatest importance to ascertain whether the patient has previously been given any digitalis or strophanthin preparation during the preceding 2 weeks in order to avoid overdosage.

The possibility of varying potency should always be borne in mind, particularly in the case of children, the elderly, and others with impaired renal function, whenever patients are changed from one brand to another.

PRECAUTIONS

Digitalis should be given cautiously in angina pectoris, myocardial infarction, or ventricular tachycardia, or if heart block is only partial. Digoxin is usually contraindicated soon after a myocardial infarction, as it may cause conduction block and has a tendency to excite the myocardium. It is definitely harmful in hypertrophic obstructive cardiomyopathy and should be used in atrial fibrillation only if control of the ventricular rate is required. Where there is peripheral circulatory failure in shock or during the course of an acute infection it may aggravate the condition by further decreasing cardiac output. Thus, if congestive heart failure occurs in diphtheria, smaller doses than usual should be given. Digitalis must be given with caution to patients with impaired renal function.

It is dangerous to give calcium during digitalis therapy, as it excites heart muscle, and the effect of the two drugs is synergistic. The effect of potassium depletion is similar. This is particularly important if potassium-depleting diuretics are being given together with digitalis, and potassium supplementation will be necessary.

Digitalis intoxication

It is important to monitor the patient carefully during digitalization, especially when large doses are given to induce this state quickly. Being cumulative, it can be given safely only if the effects of overdose are immediately recognized and the drug is withdrawn until they subside. The margin between adequate therapeutic effect and overdose is small, the former being about 60 per cent of the latter. Signs of toxicity include anorexia, headache, nausea, vomiting, diarrhoea, bradycardia (more marked in the presence of atrial fibrillation), and prolongation of the P-R interval in the ECG. Extrasystoles with atrial tachycardia and incomplete heart block, any form of supraventricular tachycardia, the occurrence of regular rhythm with loss of the usual ECG pattern and coupling in sinus rhythm are all signs of serious intoxication.

Plasma levels of digoxin may now be measured and are useful both in maintaining a satisfactory clinical control and in the diagnosis of intoxication. Therapeutic levels lie in the range 1–2 ng/ml (1.3–2.6 nmol/ℓ). Levels of 3 ng/ml (4 nmol/ℓ) or more are usually toxic.

TREATMENT

Gastric lavage may be necessary if a recent dose of digitalis is still likely to be in the stomach. General supportive measures should be instituted, and serum electrolytes estimated. Potassium depletion is likely, although the level in the myocardial cells may not be reflected by that of the serum. If renal function is normal a small intravenous dose of 2–5 mEq may be given slowly regardless of the serum potassium. Potassium should not be given in the presence of A-V block as it increases the ERP of the A-V node and enhances the block.

Drug treatment of a life-threatening dysrhythmia depends on the nature of the disorder. If potassium is ineffective the most effective drug is phenytoin, which will suppress digitalis-induced ventricular tachycardia as well as supraventricular dysrhythmias. It also diminishes S-A and A-V nodal block by decreasing the conduction time at these sites. The recommended dose is 100 mg infused slowly every 5 minutes until the dysrhythmia is reverted or ECG evidence of toxicity is noted. Lignocaine can also suppress ventricular tachycardia but is less effective than phenytoin against supraventricular dysrhythmias. β-Adrenoceptor blocking agents are effective in combating extrasystoles and tachycardia of both ventricular and supraventricular origin. They are, however, liable to depress myocardial contractility and are contraindicated in the presence of A-V block because of the further decrease in nodal conduction velocity which they produce. Atropine can also be of value when there is a sinus bradycardia or vagal inhibition of a nodal pacemaker.

Medigoxin (methylated digoxin) is claimed to have some advantages over digoxin. Its bioavailability is 100 per cent (compared with 75 per cent for digoxin); therefore, not only are oral and intravenous dose regimens the same, but the onset of action after oral administration is quicker than after digoxin. The proportion eliminated in 24 hours by the kidney is the same as for digoxin. Medigoxin 0.3 mg is equivalent in potency to digoxin 0.5 mg.

Ouabain

Ouabain (*USP*)

There are two strophanthus glycosides – strophanthin-K obtained from the seed of *Strophanthus kombé*, and strophanthin-G (ouabain), from *Strophanthus gratus*. The latter is twice as potent as the former.

PHARMACOLOGY

The strophanthus glycosides resemble those of digitalis chemically, having a similar cyclopentenophenanthrene nucleus, and in their cardiac actions and toxic effects, but contain different sugars in their glycone portions. Their glycosides are much more readily destroyed in the gastrointestinal tract than those of digitalis. Ouabain is not absorbed from the gastrointestinal tract and in East Africa it is used as an arrow poison. The rate of excretion of strophanthus glycosides is slightly faster and their duration of action is consequently shorter.

INDICATIONS

Ouabain may be used whenever a rapid effect is required both for the control of congestive failure and reduction of pulse rate in uncontrolled atrial fibrillation. Once under control, therapy should be continued using a longer acting digitalis preparation.

DOSAGE AND ADMINISTRATION

Ouabain is given intravenously in a dose of 120–250 μg, in increments of 25–50 μg. It is desirable to dilute this drug for intravenous use. The total dose should not exceed 1 mg in 24 hours. It is important to ascertain whether the patient has received digitalis during the previous 2 weeks in order to avoid overdosage.

The same precautions should be observed as for digitalis. Calcium salts should not be given concurrently.

Cardiogenic shock

Acute myocardial infarction is the commonest cause of cardiogenic shock although the syndrome can develop as a consequence of any procedure that produces dysrhythmias, leading to impairment of myocardial function. Systolic arterial blood pressure can fall precipitously and associated with this fall there is reflex tachycardia which can enhance the dysrhythmia. Peripheral vasoconstriction occurs and the skin becomes pale and cold. Renal blood flow can be decreased. In many patients vomiting, decreased fluid intake, and diuretics all contribute to hypovolaemia. Therapy is directed towards treating any dysrhythmia with appropriate drugs (or by electrical pacing), replacing fluid loss, and administration of oxygen if hypoxaemia is present.

Noradrenaline, isoprenaline, and glucagon have been used to stimulate cardiac activity and raise the blood pressure. However, noradrenaline enhances peripheral vasoconstriction with the risk of kidney damage and isoprenaline markedly increases myocardial oxygen consumption. Tachyphylaxis to glucagon can occur and, at least experimentally, it can produce lung damage. For these reasons the usage of these drugs has declined and dopamine and dobutamine are now tending to be more frequently used.

Dopamine

Dopamine hydrochloride (*BAN* and *USAN*)
Chemical name: 4-(2-aminoethyl)benzene-1,2-diol hydrochloride

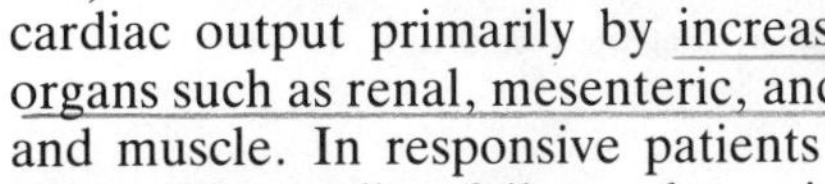

$(HO)_2C_6H_3-CH_2-CH_2-NH_2 \cdot HCl$

PHARMACOLOGY

Dopamine is a naturally occurring precursor of noradrenaline to which it is converted by the enzyme dopamine β-oxidase at various adrenergic sites (*see* page 320). It is the natural transmitter at some synapses in the CNS. Dopamine increases cardiac output primarily by increasing stroke volume: it dilates vessels to vital organs such as renal, mesenteric, and splenic beds, but constricts vessels in the skin and muscle. In responsive patients with the shock syndrome or with refractory congestive cardiac failure, dopamine improves the efficiency of the heart and increases cardiac output at lower cost in terms of excess myocardial oxygen consumption. In addition, it has specific non-adrenergic effects on renal function and natriuresis.

Dopamine has dual effects on the heart. There is a direct action via β-adrenoceptors and an indirect effect through the release of noradrenaline from myocardial storage sites. Both these effects are blocked by β-blocking agents. In the isolated heart there is little difference between inotropic and chronotropic effects. However, in the intact animal dopamine exerts a positive inotropic effect without changing the rate up to a certain dosage at which point the rate rises (*Figure 13.7*). This is probably related to the peripheral effects of dopamine. Dopamine has little effect on peripheral resistance, so that reflex tachycardia is not marked. In addition, unlike isoprenaline, it has a presynaptic effect reducing noradrenaline release.

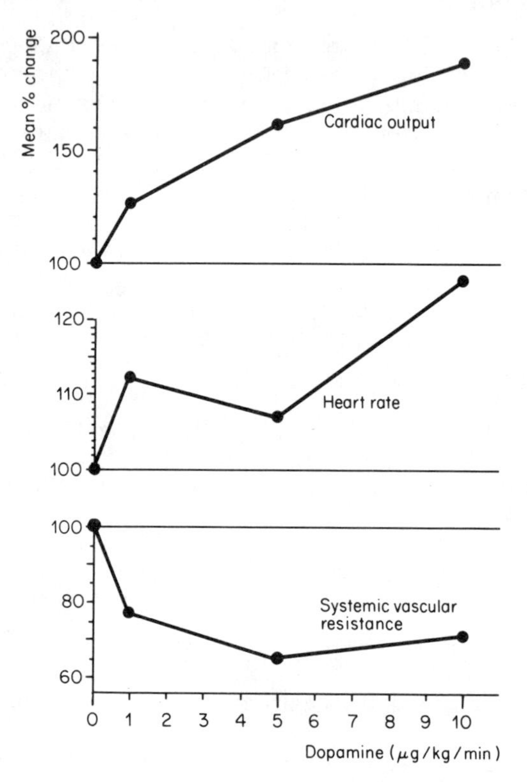

Figure 13.7 Mean percentage change in cardiac output, heart rate, and systemic vascular resistance produced by *in vivo* infusion of dopamine. Note that between 1 and 5 μg/kg/min there is a rise in cardiac output but heart rate is relatively unaffected

It can be started as an infusion soon after the onset of shock and as soon as hypotension or decreased urine flow become manifest (*Figure 13.8*). Adequate blood volume expansion is essential before dopamine therapy is initiated. Dopamine has been combined with a peripheral vasodilator such as nitroprusside or glyceryl trinitrate to reduce afterload on the heart.

INDICATIONS

Dopamine may be used as an adjunct to general supportive therapy in the treatment of haemodynamic disturbance associated with myocardial infarction, open heart surgery, traumatic shock, endotoxin shock, renal failure, cardiac failure, and circulatory decompensation. It may be of some value in improving perfusion of vital organs and in reversing hypotension due to inadequate cardiac output.

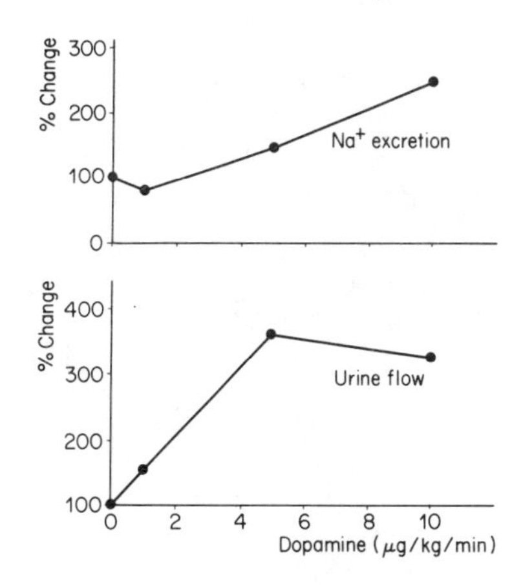

Figure 13.8 Mean percentage change in urine flow and sodium excretion produced by intravenous infusion of dopamine. Note the rise in urine flow and in sodium excretion

DOSAGE AND ADMINISTRATION

Dopamine is available for intravenous use as an aqueous solution in 5-ml ampoules containing 40 mg/ml; 5 ml (200 mg) may be added to 250 or 500 ml of isotonic saline, 5 per cent dextrose, or similar intravenous fluids. These dilutions give 800 and 400 μg/ml, respectively. The solutions are given by intravenous infusion at rates of up to 50 μg/kg/min, commencing at a rate of 2 μg/kg/min. The effect must be closely monitored and the infusion rate increased or decreased accordingly. Rates greater than 50 μg/kg/min have been used safely in advanced circulatory decompensation. However, doses exceeding 2.5 mg/kg/min can cause dysrhythmias.

PRECAUTIONS

Dopamine should be administered via a central vein where possible, as extravasation may cause local ischaemia.

If any extravasation is noted, the area should be infiltrated immediately with 10–15 ml of saline containing 5–10 mg of phentolamine to prevent sloughing and necrosis. Overdose not responding to withdrawal of the infusion should be treated with phentolamine or another α-adrenoceptor blocking agent. Smaller doses and special care are necessary in patients who have recently been treated with monoamine oxidase inhibitors.

Dopamine should not be given to patients with phaeochromocytoma or uncorrected cardiac dysrhythmias. The use of cyclopropane or halogenated hydrocarbon anaesthetics is also contraindicated. Dopamine should not be added to sodium bicarbonate or other alkaline intravenous solutions.

Dobutamine resembles dopamine chemically. It acts directly on β-adrenoceptors with some selectivity for β_1-adrenoceptors. Its other actions are slight. It therefore increases the force of cardiac contraction with a lesser effect on rate. Unlike dopamine it does not produce renal vasodilatation and it does not cause release of noradrenaline. It also has some α-adrenoceptor activity such as increasing peripheral vascular tone, an effect that can be demonstrated by giving an infusion of the drug in the presence of a non-specific β-blocking agent.

The drug is ineffective by mouth and has to be given as a constant intravenous infusion. The half-life is about 2 minutes due to rapid metabolism by the liver to inactive conjugates. Dobutamine can produce dysrhythmias, but the incidence is lower than with isoprenaline. It also raises the heart rate and blood pressure in a dose-dependent fashion if given at too high a rate of administration.

Dobutamine is used to produce a dose-dependent increase in cardiac output in patients with congestive cardiac failure. It appears to be of value in patients who have had cardiopulmonary bypass surgery. It has also been used to improve cardiac output in patients with acute myocardial infarction with congestive cardiac failure. It is given as an infusion at a rate of 2.5–15 μg/kg/min.

Prenalterol is a relatively selective agonist for β_1-adrenoceptors as compared with β_2-adrenoceptors. Thus it can increase cardiac force at doses that have little effect on bronchial smooth muscle or skeletal muscle blood vessels. Like dopamine, at certain doses it can increase myocardial contraction while having little effect on heart rate. The drug has been used to treat septic shock caused by Gram-negative organisms, shock caused by myocardial infarction, and following open heart surgery. It can increase urine flow in shocked patients. Prenalterol is administered as a slow intravenous infusion at a rate of 0.5 mg/min. Its actions are antagonized by β-blocking drugs and it can be used to counteract the effects of excessive β-blockade of the heart.

Antidysrhythmic agents

The genesis of the cardiac action potential was discussed on page 363. Antidysrhythmic drugs generally prolong the ERP as a proportion of the total action potential duration and they may suppress ectopic foci, either by reducing the rate of spontaneous depolarization (phase 4) but also by raising the threshold potential. Quinidine and procainamide, for example, exhibit all three properties. Lignocaine and phenytoin do not lengthen the ERP but depress phase 4 depolarization in S-A cells, and particularly in Purkinje tissue. This action is particularly striking in digitalis-intoxicated hearts.

Antidysrhythmic drugs may also act by decreasing the conduction velocity, which is related to the maximum rate of depolarization during phase 0. β-Adrenoceptor blocking drugs have this action and are effective in reducing digitalis toxicity by the same mechanisms as phenytoin and lignocaine.

Disorders of impulse generation include extrasystoles arising in abnormal foci in atria or ventricles, supraventricular tachycardia, atrial flutter and fibrillation, and ventricular tachycardia and fibrillation. Despite many attempts, no common physiological mechanism has been assigned to these disorders and two different mechanisms, at least, must be considered.

1. Repetitive ectopic rhythms can occur when an extranodal site undergoes spontaneous (phase 4) depolarization at an intrinsic frequency greater than that of the normal pacemaker. It may also arise when there is an 'entrance' block due, for example, to complete A-V block; this may possibly occur as a local block due to disease, thus allowing extrasystoles to occur at any time during the non-refractory phase.

2. Re-entry due to a circus movement is commonly invoked to explain atrial flutter and fibrillation. It is believed that if impulse transmission is blocked in a particular direction by a refractory tissue, the impulse makes a circuit around the obstacle. If the circuit is long enough, or the ERP short enough, the impulse will return to find the refractory tissue now responsive. This mechanism is probably also responsible for many cases of paroxysmal supraventricular tachycardia.

Re-entry may also be a functional disorder due to local disease. When an impulse meets a block, the action potential and ERP of the fibres immediately proximal to the block are very brief. Pathological Purkinje fibres may conduct very slowly, and slow conduction accompanied by a brief ERP may allow very short circuit lengths between two mutually activating foci.

Cardiac dysrhythmias

Drugs used to reverse cardiac dysrhythmias can be divided into a number of groups (Vaughan Williams, 1975). Subdivisions based on Vaughan Williams' classification are:

1. Drugs that interfere with depolarization, reducing both spontaneous (phase 4) depolarization and the maximum rate of depolarization in the spike (phase 0).
2. Drugs that block sympathetic transmission such as:
   (*a*) β-adrenoceptor blocking drugs, even though they possess no quinidine-like action;
   (*b*) adrenergic neurone blocking drugs.
3. Drugs that prolong the action potential of myocardial cells by increasing the ERP.
4. Drugs that block calcium movement from the membrane into the contractile system.
5. Cardiac glycosides.
6. Drugs that increase or induce vagal tone directly or indirectly in supraventricular tachycardia.

Examples of drugs with these actions are given in *Table 13.2* on page 378.

Procainamide hydrochloride

Procainamide hydrochloride (*BP* and *USP*)
Chemical name: 4-amino-*N*-(2-diethylaminoethyl)benzamide hydrochloride

Procainamide is a compound closely related to procaine, the —CO·O— ester grouping being replaced by —CO·NH—. It has many properties in common with procaine: peripheral blood vessels are dilated and, when given intravenously, hypotension occurs. The effect on the myocardium is greater and more sustained and approaches that of quinidine. Its analgesic action, however, is weak, and there is less danger of cerebral stimulation. The replacement of the ester link by an amide link renders the drug resistant to the action of cholinesterase and the majority is excreted unchanged in the urine.

Procainamide was at one time used for the treatment of ventricular dysrhythmias, atrial flutter and atrial fibrillation but has been replaced by new agents. Like quinidine, it impairs sodium conductance.

Table 13.2 Classification of antidysrhythmic drugs

Class 1	*Class 2*	*Class 3*	*Class 4*	*Class 5*	*Class 6*
(Slows rate of rise in phase 4 and phase 0)	(Antisympathetic)	(Prolongs EFR)	(Calcium antagonists)	(Cardiac glycosides)	(Increases vagal tone)
Quinidine	β-Adrenoceptor blocking agents	Quinidine	Verapamil	Digoxin	Methoxamine
Procainamide	Adrenergic neurone blocking agents (e.g. bretylium)	Procainamide	Methoxyverapamil	Digitoxin	Edrophonium
Lignocaine		Adrenergic neurone blocking agents (e.g. bretylium)			
Mexiletine		Amiodarone			
Phenytoin		β-Adrenoceptor blocking agents			
β-Blockers with quinidine-like action (e.g. propranolol)		Oxyfedrine			
Disopyramide					
Perhexilene					
Imipramine					
Prenylamine					

It should be noted that some drugs fall into several of the classes. For instance, propranolol is a membrane stabilizer, it will diminish the slope of the pacemaker potential, but it is also a competitive antagonist of noradrenaline at β-adrenoceptors.

Based on Vaughan Williams, E. M. (1975) Classification of antidysrhythmic drugs. *Pharmacology and Therapeutics*, **1**, 115

Quinidine salts

Quinidine sulphate and bisulphate (*BP*) and Quinidine sulfate and gluconate (*USP*)
Chemical name: (8*R*,9*S*)-6′-methoxycinchonan-9-ol sulphate

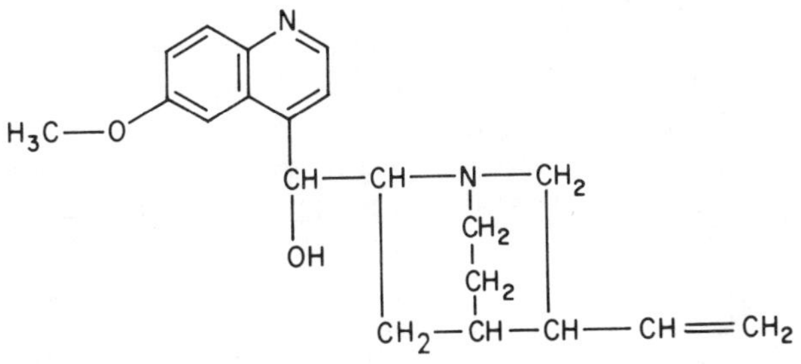

Quinidine is an isomer of the alkaloid quinine. It has a potent antidysrythmic action and has been used for the control of cardiac dysrhythmias for many years.

Its actions are complex. It directly depresses cardiac muscle with consequent decrease in irritability, lengthening of refractory period, and slowing of transmission. It also depresses transmission in the A-V node and bundle of His and decreases vagal tone. Usually the heart rate is decreased, but if vagal depression is marked it may rise.

INDICATIONS
Quinidine is used in the treatment of some cardiac dysrhythmias, such as extrasystoles and ventricular paroxysmal tachycardia. For many years it was used to convert certain recent cases of atrial fibrillation into sinus rhythm but d.c. shock conversion is now preferred.

DOSAGE AND ADMINISTRATION
In atrial fibrillation, the patient should first be digitalized and a maintenance dose continued throughout treatment to prevent an increase in ventricular rate and also to prevent the occurrence of a 1:1 ventricular response when the fibrillating atria slow below 200/min.

In a successful case a maintenance dose of 300 mg three times a day may be continued for 1 month following conversion, and digitalis is discontinued. Similar doses are given for the treatment of paroxysmal tachycardia, but the daily dose is gradually reduced after the first week. Quinidine is of limited usefulness as it can only be given orally. It is rapidly cleared from the body; to extend its effectiveness delayed absorption preparations are often employed.

PRECAUTIONS
Quinidine is a potentially dangerous agent. It can cause sudden cardiovascular collapse in high doses. Partly because of this tendency and partly because of its unreliability, its use in converting atrial fibrillation into sinus rhythm has been given up in favour of d.c. conversion. Cinchonism is another side effect of quinidine therapy; symptoms include nausea and vomiting, blurred vision, headache, tinnitus, and diarrhoea. Thrombocytopenia has also been fairly frequently reported.

β-Adrenoceptor blocking agents

Dichloroisoprenaline was the first drug found to antagonize the actions of catecholamines at β-adrenoceptor sites effectively but it was not used therapeutically because it was a partial agonist. Another derivative of isoprenaline – pronethalol – became available but was found to be carcinogenic to mice and was abandoned in favour of propranolol.

The therapeutic success of this agent has been followed by the introduction of numerous β-blocking agents. Many have been claimed to have advantages and it is important to remember that the structural and pharmacological differences between these drugs are slight and the therapeutic distinctions between them somewhat inconsequential. Before describing the detailed effects of these drugs it would be convenient to discuss briefly the differences which exist between the different members of the group.

1. Cardioselectivity

Some β-blockers are, to a greater or lesser extent, cardioselective and have a greater effect on the β_1-adrenoceptors of the heart than the β_2-adrenoceptors of the bronchi. They are, therefore, safer to administer to patients with respiratory diseases in whom bronchoconstriction would be hazardous. Unfortunately, the most selective of the drugs, practolol, cannot be used in chronic therapy because of its toxic effects, but acebutolol and some others are substantially safer than their non-selective alternatives; *see Table 13.3*, which is based on the classification of Fitzgerald (1972). It is important to remember that cardioselectivity is not complete; asthmatic patients, for example, are extremely sensitive to any adverse effect on their bronchi and even the highly cardioselective blockers may exert just enough influence to precipitate an asthmatic attack.

Table 13.3 Specificity of β-adrenoceptor blocking drugs

Selectivity	*Group I* MSA + ISA*	*Group II* MSA	*Group III* ISA	*Group IV* Neither MSA nor ISA
Non-selective	Alprenolol Oxprenolol Toliprolol	Propranolol Sotalol Timolol	Pindolol	Nadolol
Cardioselective		Acebutolol	Practolol	Atenolol

* MSA = membrane-stabilizing activity
ISA = intrinsic sympathomimetic activity

2. Intrinsic sympathomimetic activity (ISA) [partial agonist activity]

Some β-blockers, for example propranolol, reduce the heart rate during exercise and also at rest. The bradycardia may be extreme and associated with a great fall in cardiac output. Not all β-blockers, however, have the same effect in the resting subject although they all inhibit the tachycardia of exercise. *Table 13.3* also shows how some of these drugs can be divided on this basis. Experimentally, this effect can be shown to be a stimulant activity rather than incomplete blockade because these drugs produce a rise in pulse rate in reserpinized animals; such drugs are partial agonists. These drugs offer some slight advantage in patients whose heart rate is already slow or who are liable to heart failure.

3. Other cardiac actions

Some members of this group are particularly potent as antidysrhythmic agents because of a local anaesthetic or membrane-stabilizing activity. This action is only slight and may be of little importance by comparison with the pronounced antidysrhythmic properties conferred by their β-blocking action. It is, however, of interest that the drugs which produce the greatest bradycardia and a tendency to heart failure are those with the most obvious local anaesthetic-like action.

4. Metabolism

Drugs that are rapidly metabolized, such as oxprenolol and propranolol, need to be given three times daily. Atenolol, however, is eliminated so slowly that once daily administration is sufficient.

5. Toxic effects

Most of the toxic effects are a consequence of their primary pharmacological action. Bradycardia and heart failure may be made worse, as may conduction block. Severe hypotension and fainting may also occur; there is the obvious risk of precipitating bronchoconstriction in asthmatic patients and of hypoglycaemia in diabetics.

Some other effects are, fortunately, rare although serious. A dry form of conjunctivitis involving the cornea which may result in corneal ulceration has been frequently described. Fortunately, these effects regress on stopping drug administration. Other reactions affect the inner ear or the skin, or both. The most serious reaction, however, is the induction of sclerosing peritonitis by practolol. This is a sterile inflammation of the peritoneum, resulting in widespread fibrosis and intestinal obstruction. It does not regress spontaneously. This reaction was only recognized after several years of usage of the drug and so far none of the other newer drugs has been reported to cause similar effects. Practolol is no longer available for routine use but is available as an injection for the immediate treatment of dysrhythmias.

Therapeutic uses of β-blockers

Angina pectoris

Propranolol has been used effectively for many years for the treatment of angina. The beneficial effect results from a reduction in the work of the heart and blockade of the sympathetic nervous system drive. The effect is most marked on exercise-induced angina when both pain and ECG signs are prevented. Any β-blocker is usually equally effective and results in improved exercise tolerance and reduction in the consumption of glyceryl trinitrate tablets. This improvement is associated with a reduction in the rate at which ventricular muscle contracts.

Hypertension

The antihypertensive effect of β-blockers is associated initially with a fall in cardiac output. In many patients peripheral resistance remains unchanged but in some it falls. In some patients β-blockade results in a reduction in circulating renin activity, although there is no close relationship between initial renin levels and the responses to β-blocking therapy. The antihypertensive action, therefore, remains at least partly unexplained although as our understanding of the central effects of such agents increases we may be nearer a solution. Some investigators have found that β-blockers lower blood pressure when injected into the cerebral ventricles of animals. Of interest is the finding that β-adrenoceptor blocking agents are not as selective as was once imagined. Many are potent inhibitors of 5-HT, both centrally and peripherally. The combination of a β-blocker with a thiazide diuretic provides probably the best antihypertensive therapy available. It results in few unwanted effects such as postural hypotension. Labetolol has been promoted on the basis that it blocks peripheral α-adrenoceptors, thus lowering peripheral resistance, and at the same time has sufficient β-blockade to block excessive reflex cardiac stimulation induced by the vasodilatation. However, it seems likely that it is predominantly the β-blockade which is therapeutic. The potency ratio of α- to β-effect is about 1:5. The half-lives are respectively about 30 minutes and 90 minutes. Thus the α-effect is not only very much weaker but more evanescent. At present, in terms of long-term efficiency, there appears to be little to choose between various β-blockers in the treatment of hypertension.

Cardiac dysrhythmias

Dysrhythmias that are most dependent on sympathetic activity are the most responsive. These include supraventricular tachycardias, atrial fibrillation, and ventricular ectopic rhythms. Dysrhythmias associated with myocardial infarction or digitalis overdose respond less well and conduction abnormalities are usually made worse. Following infarction β-blockers are usually contraindicated because of the dual risks of conduction block and heart failure. On occasions, however, when excessive anxiety and sympathetic drive are responsible for ectopic beats, patients may benefit from β-blockers.

The efficacy of these drugs is due to their intrinsic β-blocking action, although in addition in some cases membrane stabilizing properties may also be useful. The D-isomer of propranolol has membrane-stabilizing actions but no β-adrenoceptor blocking action and is relatively ineffective. Practolol, on the other hand, has no membrane stabilizing action but is very effective in the treatment of supraventricular tachycardias and has also been found to be effective in dysrhythmias following myocardial infarction.

Ventricular outflow obstruction

In conditions such as Fallot's tetralogy and hypertrophic cardiomyopathy, β-blockers are often beneficial since the degree of outflow tract obstruction is exacerbated by sympathetic over-activity.

Other uses

Propanolol has been shown to exert a sedative effect in anxiety. Its mode of action is obscure. Propranolol has also been used to reduce the effects of thyrotoxicosis and the stimulant effect of thyroid hormones in the treatment of myxoedema. β-blockers are used in combination with α-Blockers to antagonize catecholamines before and during surgery for phaeochromocytoma. They also reduce intraocular tension and the tremor of parkinsonism. They are not drugs of first choice in the last two conditions at present.

β-Blocking drugs in the treatment of cardiac dysrhythmias during anaesthesia

Extrapolation of data obtained from conscious volunteers to patients under general anaesthesia is not always valid, as the whole autonomic balance is disturbed. The anaesthetized patient may be in a normal haemodynamic state in spite of direct myocardial depression because catecholamine release is being stimulated by the anaesthetic agent or in response to hypercapnia. The negative inotropic effects of β-adrenergic block could in such circumstances cause a marked deterioration in myocardial function. Considerable care must therefore be used if these drugs are to be given, or if the patient is receiving them preoperatively. Drugs with intrinsic stimulant activity (*see Table 13.3*) are safer in this respect than propranolol.

Surgical stimulation is known to cause sympathetic over-activity in lightly anaesthetized patients although such stimulation is rarely, if ever, of any great importance. Hypercapnia also causes release of catecholamines, thus explaining its association with cardiac dysrhythmias. It is in the field of cardiac dysrhythmias occurring during anaesthesia that β-blocking drugs are most frequently employed by anaesthetists.

Dysrhythmias occurring during cardiac surgery or in response to the injection of adrenaline should be regarded as potentially dangerous. Whether dysrhythmias occurring in the course of otherwise uncomplicated anaesthesia should be so regarded is debatable. Although they often cause concern, the majority disappear spontaneously or respond to a moderate increase in ventilation. It is undeniable that wider employment of continuous ECG monitoring has revealed the presence of more dysrhythmias than had been previously suspected, and if they were dangerous it is surprising that more patients have not developed ventricular fibrillation or asystole.

Fitzgerald, J. D. (1972) Beta adrenergic blocking drugs. Present position and future developments. *Acta Cardiologica*, Suppl. 15, 199

Oxprenolol hydrochloride

Oxprenolol hydrochloride (*BP* and *USAN*)
Chemical name: (±)-1-(2-allyloxyphenoxy)-3-isopropylaminopropan-2-ol hydrochloride

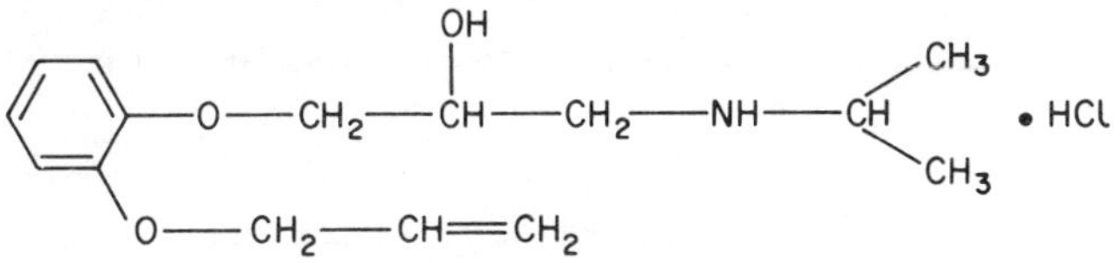

OH
CH_3
—O—CH_2—CH—CH_2—NH—CH • HCl
CH_3
O—CH_2—CH=CH_2

PHARMACOLOGY

Oxprenolol is a competitive β-adrenoceptor blocking agent. Its action is comparable to that of propranolol at cardiac receptor sites, but that at extracardiac sites is considerably less and approaches that of practolol. It has mild sympathomimetic action and a membrane-stabilizing effect on cardiac muscle, both at rest and during exercise.

Heart rate is slowed to much the same extent as by practolol, but is associated with a reduction in cardiac output with no change in stroke volume. Under anaesthesia with nitrous oxide and halothane the main haemodynamic effects in dogs are a fall in cardiac output, heart rate, stroke volume, and stroke work index, and an increase in central venous pressure. These changes are more marked with practolol than with oxprenolol. There is usually some reduction in blood pressure, but as with practolol there is considerable variation in its degree. Oxprenolol controls dysrhythmias as effectively as practolol, and angina is alleviated to a comparable extent.

The action of oxprenolol on bronchial musculature is less than that of propranolol, but appears to be somewhat greater than practolol. Nevertheless, there is a slight risk of precipitating bronchospasm in asthmatics and chronic bronchitics.

Unwanted effects are similar to those which may occur with practolol.

Fate in the body. Oxprenolol is rapidly absorbed by mouth. Metabolic degradation is mainly by conjugation with glyeuronic acid. This and other metabolites are excreted in the urine.

INDICATIONS

Oxprenolol may be used in the treatment and control of angina and in cardiac dysrhythmias including those due to atrial fibrillation, flutter, digitalis intoxication, hyperthyroidism, cardiac infarction, and also those occurring during anaesthesia.

DOSAGE AND ADMINISTRATION

Oxprenolol is normally given by mouth, 20 mg two to three times daily for the treatment of dysrhythmias, 40 mg two to three times daily in cases of angina, increasing to 120–200 mg a day or more if necessary.

PRECAUTIONS

Precautions are similar to those necessary with practolol. Special caution, however, is necessary in the treatment of asthmatics and bronchitics as there is a slightly greater danger of producing bronchial constriction. Bradycardia and hypotension may occur with effective β-blockade in patients with recent myocardial infarction. Oxprenolol is contraindicated with deep ether, chloroform, or cyclopropane anaesthesia in the presence of metabolic acidosis or incipient heart failure.

Alprenolol is another β-adrenoceptor blocking agent which has very similar actions to oxprenolol, both as regards those on cardiac function and bronchial musculature, and may be used for similar purposes. Alprenolol is normally given by mouth in a dose of 200–400 mg daily in the treatment of angina. It has no particular advantages over oxprenolol.

Nadolol is a non-selective β-blocking drug which has been used to treat angina and hypertension. It may have an advantage over some other β-blocking drugs in that it can increase renal blood flow. It is available as a once-a-day preparation.

Practolol

Practolol (*BP* and *USAN*)
Chemical name: (±)-4-(2-hydroxy-3-isopropylaminopropoxy)-acetanilide

$NH—CO—CH_3$

$O—CH_2—CH(OH)—CH_2—NH—CH(CH_3)_2$

PHARMACOLOGY

Practolol is a competitive antagonist of catecholamines at β-adrenoceptor sites with a marked selectivity for those of the myocardium, that is β_1-adrenoceptors. It is approximately two and a half times less active than propranolol at cardiac sites, and 140–150 times less active on the bronchial tree and peripheral vasculature. It possesses intrinsic sympathomimetic activity, but is virtually devoid of local anaesthetic effect or membrane-stabilizing action.

Practolol is no longer available for oral administration following the discovery that it induces a sclerosing peritonitis which is not reversible on stopping the therapy. It continues to be available for parental use in hospital. Dysrhythmias due to thyrotoxicosis, respiratory acidosis, and phaeochromocytoma during anaesthesia are abolished. It has also been effective in supraventricular dysrhythmias, such as atrial fibrillation, by increasing the A-V block, and may be superior to lignocaine for this purpose.

The effect of practolol on bronchial musculature is minimal and there is little change in airway resistance. Even in patients with bronchitis and asthma clinically important increases in airway resistance do not occur.

The half-life of practolol is about 10–12 hours, which is five times longer than that of propranolol. About 90 per cent is excreted unchanged in the urine, the remainder as metabolites, the majority within the first 24 hours.

INDICATIONS

Practolol is used in the control of all types of cardiac dysrhythmias. It has been found useful in the treatment of dysrhythmias of ventricular origin following cardiac infarction but disopyramide and mexiletine are likely to displace it.

It is of value in the treatment of dysrhythmias occurring during anaesthesia due to respiratory acidosis, phaeochromocytoma, thyrotoxicosis, and adrenaline, whether endogenous or exogenous.

DOSAGE AND ADMINISTRATION

Practolol is now only available for parenteral administration; the normal initial dose is 4–6 mg repeated at 5-minute intervals as required.

PRECAUTIONS

Overdosage leading to bradycardia or hypotension should be reversed with atropine. Alternatively, isoprenaline may be given slowly intravenously (5 μg/min) or orciprenaline up to 0.5 mg.

Propranolol hydrochloride

Propranolol hydrochloride (*BP* and *USP*)
Chemical name: (±)-1-isopropylamino-3-(1-naphthyloxy)propan-2-ol hydrochloride

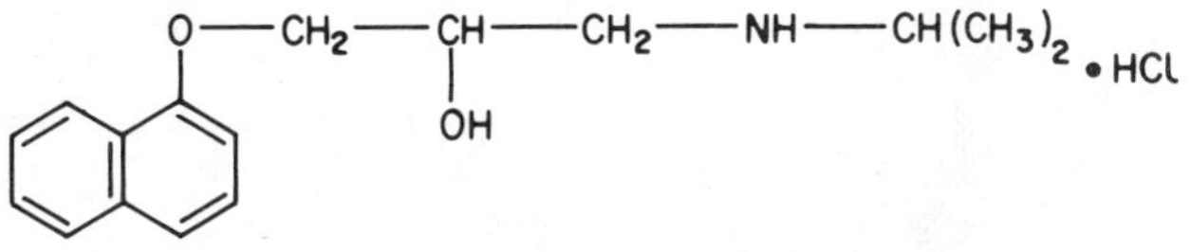

O—CH_2—CH(OH)—CH_2—NH—$CH(CH_3)_2$ • HCl

Propranolol was the first effective β-adrenoceptor blocking agent to stand the test of prolonged clinical use, and experience with it extends more widely than with any other member of this group. It blocks all β-adrenoceptors indiscriminately. By blockade of β_1-adrenoceptors it effectively slows the heart rate. This effect may be pronounced in mitral valve disease, atrial fibrillation, and phaeochromocytoma. The block is competitive and can be overcome by an adequate dose of isoprenaline. If vagal receptors are also blocked by atropine the heart rate increases, which indicates that the reduced rate produced by propranolol alone is due to blocking of normal sympathetic drive. Cardiac output is reduced in normal patients and those with cardiac impairment. By opposing the haemodynamic response to stress and exercise in ischaemic heart disease it has an 'oxygen sparing' effect and this is of benefit to patients suffering from angina of effort, but in cardiac insufficiency inhibition of normal sympathetic drive may induce failure.

In hypertensive patients there may be some reduction in blood pressure after prolonged treatment. Its mechanism of action in lowering the blood pressure of hypertensive patients is still uncertain. Besides its effects on the cardiovascular system it inhibits renin release from the kidney. Propranolol also has central effects which may be important.

Propranolol slows the ventricular rate in atrial fibrillation, but does not correct the dysrhythmia. In flutter it may slow the ventricular rate or convert the irregularity to fibrillation. In both atrial and ventricular tachycardia the ventricular rate is usually reduced and extrasystoles are either abolished or their frequency reduced, and it is of special value in the management of digitalis intoxication. Its effect on forearm blood flow is variable. Although it abolishes the vasodilator action of adrenergic β_2-fibres, reports suggest that the blood flow may be unchanged or reduced. Electron microscope studies suggest that propranolol, in common with other β-adrenoceptor blocking drugs, affects the ionic permeability of the muscle membrane to potassium.

During anaesthesia it abolishes dysrhythmias occurring in patients with thyrotoxicosis, respiratory acidosis, and phaeochromocytoma, and will prevent those which might be precipitated if catecholamines are infiltrated to reduce peripheral bleeding under halothane or cyclopropane anaesthesia. Blood pressure and pulse rate are also reduced, but these effects are abolished by atropine.

During chloroform or ether anaesthesia sympathetic over-activity is believed to maintain cardiac output, and propranolol might therefore be expected to cause hypotension or cardiac failure. As these agents produce this effect largely by the release of catecholamines into the circulation rather than by direct action on the sympathetic nervous system, propranolol in small doses has usually only a moderate effect on blood pressure during anaesthesia with these agents in adequately atropinized patients. Propranolol has likewise been used without incident in atropinized patients receiving cyclopropane. However, deep anaesthesia might well cause cardiac embarrassment. Atropine premedication is advisable to avoid vagal hyperactivity.

Fate in the body. Propranolol is rapidly absorbed after oral administration. Metabolic degradation is through two pathways: (1) hydroxylation followed by conjugation with D-glucuronic acid; (2) side chain oxidation. The metabolites are excreted in the urine.

INDICATIONS

Propranolol may be used to control cardiac dysrhythmias, such as those associated with digitalis intoxication and those that occur during anaesthesia whether induced by adrenaline (endogenous or exogenous) or respiratory acidosis. It may also be used in the control of tachycardia in the management of phaeochromocytoma before and during operation, and the tachycardia that is induced by ganglion-blockers when employed in controlled hypotension and when the ventricular rate in atrial fibrillation is not adequately controlled by digitalis alone. It is of value in the treatment of angina and to control the β-adrenoceptor stimulating effects of thyroid medication if they hamper adequate therapy in the management of myxoedema. Its use may well be superseded by the more selective β-adrenoceptor blocking drugs, such as oxprenolol or alprenolol, which cause less cardiac depression and bronchial constriction. Propranolol can control the tremor in cases of parkinsonism, in which emotional stress and adrenaline aggravate the condition.

DOSAGE AND ADMINISTRATION

Propranolol is normally given by mouth, but it can also be given intravenously. For the treatment of dysrhythmias, 10–30 mg may be given three to four times a day. Larger doses are usually required for the treatment of angina, which may require up to 80 mg four times a day. When a rapid effect is required, 0.5–5 mg may be given slowly intravenously at a rate not exceeding 1 mg/min.

PRECAUTIONS

Propranolol should be used with the greatest caution in the presence of incipient cardiac failure and metabolic acidosis, and it should not be given to asthmatics or those subject to bronchospasm. It should also be used cautiously during chloroform and ether anaesthesia and only after atropine premedication.

When given intravenously propranolol must be administered very slowly with pauses so that its full effect can be ascertained. Should marked bradycardia or hypotension occur, atropine 0.5–1 mg should be given intravenously.

Chronotropic agents

Chronotropic agents influence the rate of the heart, which may be increased or decreased. They can be divided into two main groups, those that act directly on the heart and those that act indirectly. The two aspects of cardiac function, the force of the muscular contraction and the rate, are closely connected, and when the drug is one that acts directly on the heart the force is often influenced as well.

For example, adrenaline increases both force of contraction and rate, whereas noradrenaline has less effect on force and the rate may be unaffected or even slowed. The reason for this is that the reflex slowing from the rise in blood pressure produced by vasoconstriction tends to overcome the feebler action of noradrenaline on the heart, whereas with adrenaline the reverse occurs. It is seldom necessary to alter the rate alone except in conditions such as paroxysmal tachycardia, or hypotension due to bradycardia.

The rate of the heart is controlled through the vagus, which is inhibitor, and the sympathetic, which is accelerator. The influence of drugs on the heart rate through indirect action is complex, and many that act on the CNS, such as atropine, halothane, and digitalis, cause slowing. Those that have a stimulant action also usually cause liberation of adrenaline and noradrenaline from the adrenal medulla so that a biphasic effect may be seen, the central effect preceding the release effect. Vasodilator drugs which cause a fall in blood pressure by a peripheral action give rise to a compensatory increase in cardiac rate.

The main reflex involved (Marey's) is the depressor reflex with its afferent impulses from the baroreceptors of the carotid sinuses and the aortic arch. Other important receptors are in the lungs and the chemoreceptors of the carotid bodies.

In addition to blood pressure, further factors affecting heart rate include the oxygen tension of the blood, intracranial pressure, muscular exertion, and internal secretions. Changes in rate can also be caused by drugs affecting the rate of conduction or refractory period of the myocardium in the presence of abnormal rhythms, or by acting directly on the pacemaker of the heart by intracellular mechanisms that are neither sympathomimetic nor parasympathomimetic, such as digitalis and quinidine.

The heart is slowed by parasympathomimetic agents such as carbachol, methacholine, and the anticholinesterases. Certain anaesthetic agents such as halothane also cause bradycardia through a central vagal action. Acceleration of the heart by sympathomimetic action is produced by drugs which include adenaline, ephedrine, isoprenaline, and cocaine. Drugs that block parasympathetic or sympathetic action will have the opposite effects. Atropine-like drugs will increase the heart rate by blocking vagal transmission and blockade of adrenergic β-receptor fibres will decrease it. Atropine, when given subcutaneously and in low concentration, will initially cause slowing. This is due to a central stimulatory effect preceding its peripheral blocking action, which only develops later when blood levels are higher. The same effect occurs with hyoscine but larger doses than are normally given are required to produce a peripheral effect and a consequent increase in heart rate.

Drugs that have chronotropic effects associated with their action on conduction or refractory period of the myocardium or pacemaker, or on intracellular metabolism, include procainamide, the cardiac glycosides (digitalis and ouabain), some xanthines (theophylline and caffeine), and catecholamines (adrenaline and isoprenaline). Their effects are complex and are described in their individual monographs.

Atropine is used to antagonize or prevent the bradycardia produced by halothane and neostigmine, and conversely neostigmine can be used in the treatment of paroxysmal tachycardia.

Drugs affecting coronary blood vessels

A number of drugs can cause coronary blood vessels to constrict. Among these are angiotensin II, vasopressin, 5-HT, histamine, and some prostaglandins. *In vivo* their effects can be modified by their other pharmacological actions. For instance, angiotensin II may increase coronary flow: although it constricts coronary vessels, it is less potent on such vessels than on arterioles elsewhere in the body and thus coronary perfusion pressure rises.

Bradykinin, adenine nucleotides, adenosine, and prostacyclin dilate coronary vessels. Catecholamines like dopamine have a biphasic action, α-adrenoceptor stimulation causing constriction and β-adrenoceptor stimulation causing dilatation.

Coronary vasodilator drugs possibly act by depriving the contractile mechanism of the cell of calcium ions. This can be achieved in three ways:

1. By raising cyclic AMP concentrations the concentration of free intracellular calcium ions is reduced; inhibitors of phosphodiesterase, such as papaverine, or activators of adenyl cyclase, such as isoprenaline, can produce such effects.
2. Drugs may block calcium ion transport into the smooth muscle vascular cell; verapamil, methoxyverapamil, and nifedipine have such actions.
3. The active transport into cardiac cells of adenosine, a potent vasodilator, can be inhibited by dipyridamole, lidoflazine, and dilazep.

It is important to appreciate that drugs that increase total coronary flow are not necessarily useful drugs for the treatment of angina. The coronary vessels in some patients with angina are atherosclerotic and thus unable to dilate in response to vasodilator drugs. Moreover, in the ischaemic area beyond the obstruction, the arterioles may be already dilated to their maximum capacity due to accumulation of vasodilator metabolites and reflex inhibition of sympathetic tone. Under such conditions vasodilator drugs may increase blood flow to other parts of the heart and actually divert flow away from the ischaemic area, the so-called 'coronary steal' phenomenon.

Disopyramide

Disopyramide (*BP*) and Disopyramide phosphate (*BP* and *USP*)
Chemical name: 4-di-isopropylamino-2-phenyl-2-(2-pyridyl)butyramide

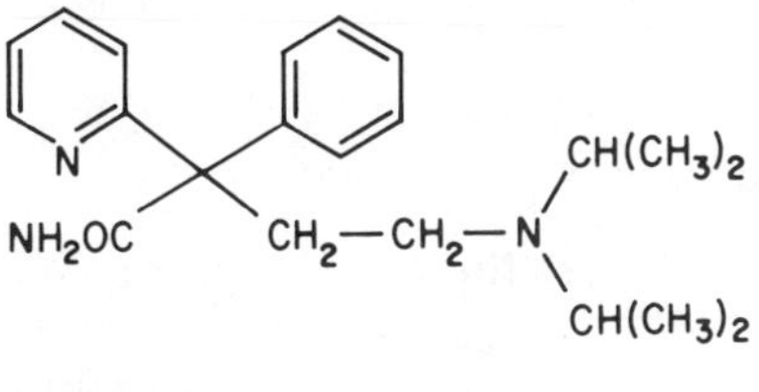

N
$CH(CH_3)_2$
NH_2OC $CH_2—CH_2—N$
$CH(CH_3)_2$

PHARMACOLOGY

This class 1 antiarrhythmic drug has quinidine-like actions. It appears to be more potent in producing atrial or ventricular refractoriness and less potent on the Purkinje system. Therapeutic concentrations will decrease the slope of phase 4 depolarization in Purkinje fibres and decrease their spontaneous firing rate. The drug has a direct effect on the sinus node, slowing its rate of discharge. It also has antimuscarinic activity.

The drug is well absorbed following oral administration, and first-pass metabolism is not marked. About 50 per cent of a dose is excreted unchanged through the kidney; the elimination half-life is approximately 7 hours.

INDICATIONS AND DOSAGE

Disopyramide is used for the treatment of ventricular or atrial dysrhythmias and the usual oral dose is 100–200 mg four times a day.

PRECAUTIONS

The drug can produce anticholinergic effects, such as a dry mouth, blurred vision, and urinary retention. It will reduce cardiac output and this effect appears more pronounced in patients with pre-existing ventricular failure. Great care should be taken if such patients are exposed to the drug or if patients are on β-blockers.

Dipyridamole decreases coronary vascular resistance and increases coronary flow and oxygen tension in coronary sinus blood. It has little effect on vascular resistance in ischaemic areas of the heart where small vessels are already maximally dilated, since adenosine, which is released from a hypoxic myocardium, is a coronary vasodilator. Dipyridamole can inhibit adenosine uptake into cells and this in part could account for its action. In therapeutic doses it does not usually cause marked changes in systemic blood pressure or peripheral blood flow but in large doses it can produce hypotension. In can produce nausea, vomiting or diarrhoea, and occasionally headache or vertigo. It also has an effect on platelets. This may be due to a potentiation of prostacyclin which in turn inhibits platelet function, or to an increase in platelet cyclic AMP by inhibition of platelet phosphodiesterase. It is used in the prophylaxis of thromboembolism in patients with prosthetic heart valves.

Mexiletine also has quinidine-like actions. It has been used to treat dysrhythmias produced by cardiac glycosides and ventricular dysrhythmias after myocardial infarction. A dose of 200 mg orally is given three times daily for at least a week. It is several days, usually, before a therapeutic effect is observed. The dose is then reduced weekly to a maintenance dose of 200 mg daily or on alternate days. Following the cessation of treatment, antidysrhythmic effects persist for about 4 weeks. It may produce a bradycardia and a fall in blood pressure and can produce cerebellar toxicity, for example nystagmus and ataxia. There is also an intravenous formulation of the drug.

Calcium antagonists

Calcium antagonists are being used for the treatment of angina pectoris. They lower myocardial oxygen requirement by at least three mechanisms:

1. Reduction of contractile force of the heart.
2. Reduction of blood pressure and therefore myocardial work.
3. Relaxation of veins thereby reducing venous return.

They are else effective in Prinzmetal's variant angina. In this condition the pain is thought to be due to coronary spasm. Some are also being tried in hypertensive states and in cardiac dysrhythmias.

Calcium ions are known to be involved in excitation–contraction coupling in skeletal, smooth, and cardiac muscle. This ion also plays an important part in stimulus–secretion coupling in endocrine and exocrine glands and in transmitter release from neurones. Thus it can be seen that drugs which can modify calcium-dependent processes can have a wide spectrum of activity. Calcium antagonists are used as local anaesthetics, anticonvulsants, antidysrhythmic agents, coronary vasodilators, and skeletal muscle relaxants.

Calcium-dependent processes can be altered by increasing or inhibiting the influx or efflux of extracellular calcium, or by encouraging or preventing binding of calcium to specific intracellular sites. Calcium antagonists can be classified on the basis of whether they block the influx of extracellular calcium or interfere with mobilization of intracellular calcium. *Table 13.4* lists some calcium antagonists according to the above classification. The selectivity of these compounds varies; for instance, local anaesthetics interfere with the influx of both sodium and calcium, whereas verapamil and nifedipine inhibit the transmembrane calcium influx (slow channel) without affecting sodium movement (fast channel).

Table 13.4 Agents modifying calcium-dependent processes

Agents that block influx of extracellular calcium	*Agents that interfere with mobilization of intracellular calcium*
Local anaesthetics	Sodium nitroprusside
Phenytoin	Diazoxide
Barbiturates	Alkyl-3,4,5,5-trimethoxybenzoates (TMB compounds)
Fendiline	2-Substituted 3-dimethyl-amino-5,6-methylenedioxyindines (MOI compounds)
Perhexilene	
Prenylamine	
Verapamil	
Methoxyverapamil	
Nifedipine	
Diltiazem	
3 α-amino-2β-hydroxy-5α-androstan-17-one (Org 6001)	
Morphine	
Methadone	
Pentazocine	
Dantrolene	
Nitrites	
Alcohol	
Aminoglycoside antibiotics	
Flunarizine	
Cinnarizine	
Lanthanum	

Calcium antagonists as antidysrhymic agents

Several drugs with this basic mode of action are discussed elsewhere according to their main therapeutic use, for example local anaesthetics such as lignocaine and procainamide (pages 219 and 377). Propranolol and other β-adrenoceptor antagonists (pages 383–387) may at least in part owe their antidysrhythmic effects to inhibition of calcium influx. Nifedipine, verapamil, methoxyverapamil, and diltiazem all block slow channel calcium entry and have been used clinically. These drugs reduce myocardial oxygen consumption in electrically stimulated heart tissue and this effect may prove of value in the treatment of angina.

Verapamil

Verapamil hydrochloride (*BP*)
Chemical name: 5-[*N*-(3-4-dimethoxyphenethyl)-*N*-methylamino]-2-(3,4-dimethoxyphenyl)-2-isopropylvaleronitrile hydrochloride

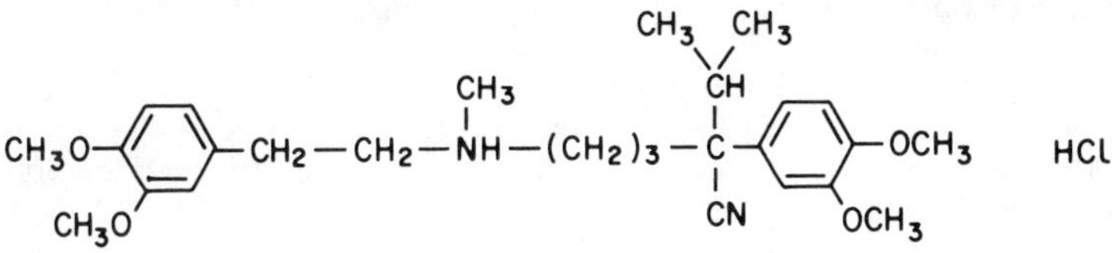

CH3 CH3
CH
CH3
CH3O—C6H3—CH2—CH2—NH—(CH2)3—C—C6H3—OCH3 HCl
CH3O CN OCH3

PHARMACOLOGY

Verapamil inhibits the influx of calcium ions into cardiac cells and is used in the treatment of angina and in the control of cardiac dysrhythmias.

INDICATIONS

The drug appears of particular use in the treatment of supraventricular tachycardias since it reduces A-V node conduction. Many supraventricular tachycardias, for example Wolff-Parkinson-White syndrome, are maintained by re-entry through the A-V node. The drug has also been used successfully in the treatment of dysrhythmias occurring during halothane anaesthesia.

DOSAGE AND ADMINISTRATION

Verapamil can be given orally and doses of up to 120 mg three times a day have been used in the prophylaxis of angina. Supraventricular tachycardias and ventricular dysrythmias during anaesthesia can be controlled by 20 mg intravenously. After intravenous injection of therapeutic doses the effect lasts about half an hour.

PRECAUTIONS

Verapamil can cause nausea and dizziness, and after intravenous injection flushing can occur. If verapamil is given to patients who are already receiving β-blocking drugs there is an increased risk of bradycardia, fall in blood pressure, and cardiac arrest. It should be used with great caution in patients with heart block.

Nifedipine and **diltiazem** are two other calcium antagonists that are used in the treatment of angina of effort. The pharmacological profile for nifedipine differs from verapamil (*Table 13.5*). Nifedipine is more potent on smooth muscle than cardiac muscle; the converse applies to verapamil.

Table 13.5 Pharmacological actions of verapamil and nifedipine

Drug	*Cardiac muscle contraction*	*Tissue A-V node conduction*	*Smooth muscle contraction*
Nifedipine	+	–	+++
Verapamil	++	++	+

+++ Marked effect → + slight effect

Other drugs exhibiting calcium antagonism

Sodium nitroprusside, which has a relaxant effect on smooth muscle, is believed to produce its antihypertensive effect by affecting intracellular calcium mobilization. There is evidence that diazoxide and hydralazine also act by interfering with calcium movement. Calcium antagonists have also been used in the treatment of peripheral vascular disease. Cinnarizine, a calcium antagonist which also blocks 5-HT and histamine receptors, has been reported to improve patients with intermittent claudication, as does a related drug, flunarizine. Both these drugs also produce sedation.

Amiodarone

Chemical name: 2-butylbenzofuran-3-yl 4-(2-diethylaminoethoxy)-3,5-di-iodophenyl ketone

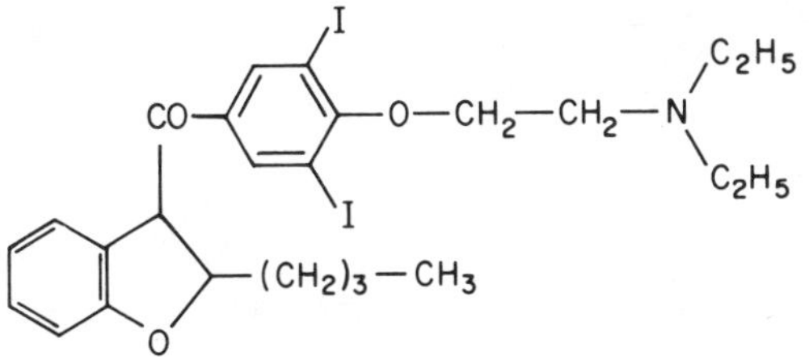

PHARMACOLOGY

This is a class 3 antidysrhythmic drug whose main effect is to delay repolarization (*see* page 377). It increases the duration of the action potential of myocardial tissue and thus increases the refractory period of atrial, nodal, and ventricular tissue. The drug can cause a mild sinus bradycardia.

It is an iodinated compound and some iodine is released when it is metabolized. It has an elimination half-life of about 4 weeks. The drug is stored in muscle (including cardiac muscle) and fat. Cumulation can occur.

INDICATIONS

The drug has been used in the treatment of supraventricular and ventricular dysrhythmias and has proved beneficial in patients with the Wolff-Parkinson-White syndrome.

DOSAGE AND ADMINISTRATION

Initial treatment is with 200 mg three times a day until full response is achieved, which is usually about a week, thereafter reducing to about 200 mg daily.

PRECAUTIONS

It is contraindicated in patients with advanced A-V block or with S-A block. It should be used with special caution in patients who are receiving β-blockers. The drug can cause micro-deposits of lipofuscin in the cornea of some patients. While not an indication to withdraw the drug immediately, such patients should be carefully watched and the dose reduced if visual haloes or photophobia occur. The corneal deposits can disappear a few months after stopping the treatment. Thyroid metabolism can also be disturbed. Iodine released from the drug can interfere with the protein-bound iodine test. Photosensitivity of the skin and blue pigmentation of it has been reported. Nightmares and vivid dreams can occur. Peripheral neuropathy, pulmonary fibrosis, and hepatitis have been reported. The drug increases free plasma digoxin concentration and maintenance doses of digoxin may need to be halved. It will also potentiate the action of warfarin.

14

Diuretics

The composition of the body fluids, especially the blood, would vary widely unless the excretory mechanisms of the kidneys and lungs kept them in a constant state. The kidneys maintain the volume and composition of the extracellular fluid by excreting variable amounts of water and selectively eliminating Na, K, Cl, HPO_4 and SO_4 ions. Plasma concentrations of non-electrolytes such as urea, glucose, and creatinine are also controlled, and waste products, drugs, and toxic substances which enter the body are excreted.

With the assistance of the lungs, which eliminate volatile acid as carbon dioxide, the kidneys maintain the hydrogen ion concentration of the blood by the excretion of non-volatile acid (HPO_4) in the urine. By this mechanism they can normally dispose of 50 mEq of hydrogen ions a day. Renal tubular cells are also capable of synthesizing ammonia; this combines with hydrogen ions in the tubular fluid to form ammonium ions and, in conditions of persistent severe acidosis, can account for over 300 mEq of hydrogen ions a day.

Structure of the nephron

The kidney consists of units called nephrons which are composed of three functionally different parts, as follows.

The malpighian corpuscle, consisting of Bowman's capsule and the glomerulus, which acts as a filter.

The renal tubule, down which the filtrate passes, and which consists of three histologically different segments; the proximal tubule, the loop of Henle, and the distal tubule.

The collecting tubule, which leads into larger ducts and thence into the pyramids.

The kidneys receive sympathetic innervation which is mainly distributed to the afferent arterioles in the cortex. No parasympathetic supply has been demonstrated.

The cortex is the site of production of renin, which is an essential component of the renin–angiotensin system which is concerned with sodium and water homeostasis (*see* page 418). Renin is formed in the cells of the juxtaglomerular apparatus and is secreted whenever the perfusion pressure in the afferent arteriole falls and the arteriolar wall is not stretched.

The *macula densa* cells are well placed to sense the sodium and potassium content of the tubular fluid in the proximal end of the distal tubule and are thought to provide additional local input to the juxtaglomerular cells. The juxtaglomerular cells are also innervated by β-adrenergic sympathetic postganglionic fibres.

The blood flow to the cortex remains unchanged over a range of arterial blood pressure from 80–180 mmHg (10.7–24.0 kPa) in man. The much smaller flow to the medulla varies directly with perfusion pressure.

The glomerular filtrate

The renal blood flow, which under normal circumstances hardly varies, is considerable, and at about 1300 ml/min may take as much as 25 per cent of the cardiac output. Plasma flow is in the region of 700 ml/min and the glomerular filtrate is formed at a rate of about 120 ml/min. The greater part of this large blood flow is required for the formation of urine; provided that the blood flow is not less than one fifth of the normal (200–300 ml/min) the oxygen requirements of the renal parenchyma are satisfied.

The glomerular filtrate has the same composition as the plasma except that substances with a molecular weight greater than 67 000 are retained, so that in health minute amounts of serum albumin and no globulin are present. The volume of glomerular filtrate is dependent on the net effective filtration pressure. This is the difference between the positive hydrostatic pressure in the glomerular capillaries minus the sum of the oncotic pressure of the plasma proteins and the intratubular pressure. The intratubular pressure is 15–20 mmHg (2.0–2.7 kPa) in man and for glomerular filtration to occur a net filtration pressure of approximately 55 mmHg (7.3 kPa) is necessary.

The effect of anaesthesia on various aspects of renal function is inconsistent; there is considerable variation both above and below control values, the most variable of all being the urinary output. In the postoperative period the usual finding is oliguria and this is due to the release of antidiuretic hormone by the posterior pituitary gland.

Modification of the glomerular filtrate

During its passage down the tubules the greater part of the filtrate is reabsorbed. Of the 170 litres produced in 24 hours, only 1.5 litres are excreted as urine. In order to excrete excess of acid from the body, carbonic acid in the tubular cell dissociates and the hydrogen ions are exchanged for sodium in the tubules and the sodium bicarbonate thus formed is returned to the blood; in states of alkalosis, however, large amounts of bicarbonate may be excreted. The glomerular filtrate, pH 7.4, resembles blood as it contains mainly dibasic sodium phosphate, but through the action of carbonic anhydrase hydrogen ions are exchanged for sodium and the urine thus becomes more acid as the amount of acid phosphate increases and, for every hydrogen ion excreted a bicarbonate ion is generated and reabsorbed.

The kidney reduces the acidity of the blood both by the conversion of basic to acid phosphate and by forming ammonia from amino acids, which combines with chloride ions in the tubules and is excreted as ammonium chloride in the urine.

The pH of urine depends therefore on the pH of blood, which is controlled by the carbon dioxide: bicarbonate ratio, and this in turn is governed by the carbon dioxide tension in blood which regulates the rate of carbonic acid formation by carbonic anhydrase.

The proximal and distal tubules differ widely in their functions. About 80 per cent of the filtered sodium is reabsorbed actively (that is, against an electrochemical gradient) in the proximal tubule; chloride ions are also actively absorbed. Water is passively reabsorbed as a result of removal of these ions from the tubular fluid. Ten per cent of the sodium is reabsorbed in the loops of Henle, and the remainder in the distal tubules and collecting ducts. The distal tubule effects an ion-exchange mechanism, sodium being exchanged for potassium and hydrogen ions. When there is a need to conserve sodium this distal mechanism is so effective that the urine is virtually sodium-free.

The passive reabsorption of 80 per cent of the filtered water is obligatory and occurs whatever the state of hydration of the patient. The isotonic fluid in the loops of Henle becomes hypotonic as a result of active reabsorption of sodium and chloride without water in the first part of the distal tubule, which is not permeable to water. If pituitary antidiuretic hormone is not acting on the distal tubules and collecting ducts, no further water is reabsorbed and hypotonic urine will result.

The action of antidiuretic hormone is to make the cells of the distal convoluted tubules and of the collecting ducts permeable to water. These parts of the nephron normally separate hypotonic tubular fluid from relatively hypertonic interstitial fluid; they behave as a waterproof membrane which is made temporarily permeable to water by the action of antidiuretic hormone. Extraction of water beyond that necessary to render urine iso-osmotic with plasma occurs in the collecting ducts which pass into the medulla. Medullary interstitial fluid is hypertonic due to accumulation of sodium and chloride derived by active transport from tubular fluid in the loops of Henle.

The control of the renal handling of the body's principal osmotically effective electrolytes, sodium and potassium, is to a great extent exerted by the adrenal corticosteroid hormone, aldosterone. Numerous factors influence the release of this hormone – posture, the potassium content of the body, circulatory haemodynamics, and the sodium concentration of the blood perfusing the adrenal glands are among them. Aldosterone production and secretion are also stimulated by angiotensin, the level of which is determined by renin output from the juxtaglomerular cells. This mechanism is probably the most important controlling factor. Aldosterone has powerful sodium-retaining and potassium-excreting effects on renal tubular cells of the distal tubule. The daily output averages 200 μg and over 90 per cent of this is rapidly inactivated by the normal liver, the remainder appearing as a conjugate in the urine.

Action of diuretics

Diuretics are drugs that cause an increase in the output of urine. They are mainly employed in the treatment of hypertension and to reduce oedema and ascites in renal and congestive heart failure.

They can produce a diuresis in five different ways:

1. By increasing the blood supply to the kidney.
2. By preventing tubular reabsorption of water by osmotic action.
3. By preventing the tubular reabsorption of sodium and, as a secondary effect of this, of chloride or bicarbonate ions which carry water with them.

4. By inhibiting the action of the hormones that play a part in the control of normal urine volume.
5. By inhibiting the production of aldosterone and cortisone by the adrenal cortex.

The commonly employed clinically useful diuretics all act at one or more of the sites where sodium is removed from the lumen of the nephron.

If the normal mechanism of urine formation, as outlined above, is studied it will be seen that little increase in output is possible by increasing blood flow, as it takes more than 100 ml of glomerular filtrate to produce 1 ml of urine. When the blood supply to the kidneys is impaired, however, as in congestive heart failure, a diuresis can often be produced by the use of digitalis alone. Aminophylline also produces a good diuresis under these circumstances, but despite its vasodilator action and depressant effect on tubular reabsorption, it is normally only a weak diuretic when used alone.

Various salts and crystalloids can produce an osmotic diuresis by retaining water in the distal tubules and collecting ducts. These include urea, glucose, sucrose, mannitol, potassium nitrate, and sodium sulphate. Present practice is confined to the use of mannitol, which is an undissociated crystalloid and is given intravenously. It can be given in sufficiently high concentration to cause a net water loss from the body. Such an osmotic diuresis can be induced despite the maximal operation of pituitary antidiuretic hormone and mannitol will therefore produce large volumes of urine during and immediately after surgery. This type of diuresis is characterized by a high concentration and rate of excretion of the loading solute associated with a decrease in concentration of other solutes (chiefly sodium and potassium). However, the fall in concentration is more than offset by the increase in urine flow-rate, so that other solutes tend to be lost from the body in slightly greater total amounts than would otherwise occur.

To be effective as an osmotic diuretic a substance should be rapidly and completely excreted in the glomeruli and not reabsorbed at all in the rest of the nephron. The smaller its molecular weight the more effective it will be: substances such as dextran 40 (1 mosmol = 40 g) cannot exert any significant osmotic effect even in very high urinary concentrations. It is also desirable that such a substance should be inert and not penetrate the body cells.

Osmotic diuretics are given in very hypertonic concentrations and therefore will cause extensive tissue necrosis if they leak extravascularly. They cause a rapid expansion of the extracellular space with intracellular water, and therefore increase the plasma volume. They should not be used when this would be undesirable and with the important exception of the use of mannitol to determine if intrinsic renal damage has occurred (*see* below) they should also be avoided whenever there is any doubt that the kidneys can excrete them.

The volume of water extracted from the body by these agents depends on many factors, but the urine osmolality resulting from their use is generally about twice that of plasma, that is, 500–700 mosmol/ℓ. In practice, the use of 100 g of mannitol in an adult who is normally hydrated will result in the excretion of approximately 1 litre of water more than would otherwise have been expected.

Certain salts, such as ammonium chloride and potassium citrate, which alter the pH of the urine and produce a mild diuresis, are no longer employed for this purpose, and they may be dangerous in the absence of efficient kidney function. However, they may be useful adjuvants to antibacterial therapy when dealing with simple urinary infections, and ammonium chloride will supply chloride ions which are depleted following the use of mersalyl.

The most important group of diuretics is that which interferes with tubular reabsorption of sodium, chloride, and bicarbonate ions. They belong to unrelated chemical groups and act at various sites in the tubular part of the nephron. They include mersalyl, acetazolamide, thiazides, loop diuretics, and potassium-sparing diuretics. Of these, three groups are in general use:

1. The thiazides and other medium efficacy diuretics which act principally on the cortical diluting segment of the distal convoluted tubule causing a natriuresis equivalent to between 5 and 10 per cent of the sodium that is normally filtered.
2. The 'loop' diuretics, frusemide, bumetanide, and ethacrynic acid, which act principally on the ascending loop of Henle and have a high peak effect, equivalent to 30 per cent filtered sodium.
3. The potassium-sparing diuretics, spironolactone, amiloride, and triamterene, which act on the distal renal tubule.

There are also the saline diuretics or salts which alter the pH of the urine either to the acidic or the alkaline side. In each case there is a slight diuresis accompanying this change. The sodium salts of acetates, tartrates, and citrates, which are oxidized in the body to bicarbonates, raise the pH of the urine. The chlorides of ammonia and calcium increase the acidity of the urine. By means of these drugs the pH of the urine can be altered over a range from pH 5–8.5.

Although not used for the purpose, renal function can be affected by blocking the production of aldosterone and cortisone by the adrenal cortex with metyrapone.

An important side effect of all diuretic drugs is the alteration they produce in the renal excretion of potassium. The normal driving force for potassium secretion by the distal tubule is the transtubular electrical potential difference created by sodium reabsorption. Most diuretics allow higher concentrations of sodium to reach the distal tubule and this increased sodium reabsorption stimulates secretion of potassium. Thiazide diuretics cause a small loss of potassium; in terms of whole body potassium this loss is not important and serum potassium concentrations although reduced, rarely fall below 3.0 mmol/ℓ. Hypertensive patients tend to lose more potassium than patients in cardiac failure, in whom it might be clinically more significant. Unless there are reasons for avoiding even mild hypokalaemia, there is no reason to give simultaneous oral potassium supplements. Spironolactone, amiloride, and triamterene when added to a thiazide diuretic reduce the potassium loss to a considerable extent. Given alone they are thus associated with only a slightly lower loss of potassium than other diuretics. However, when other sodium-losing diuretics are given simultaneously, or when potassium loss is associated with increased aldosterone activity, the reduction in potassium loss is marked. The administration of potassium as Slow-K tablets (32 mEq, or four tablets daily) will reverse any deficits.

Acetazolamide

Acetazolamide (*BP* and *USP*)
Chemical name: *N*-(5-sulphamoyl-1,3,4-thiadiazol-2-yl)acetamide

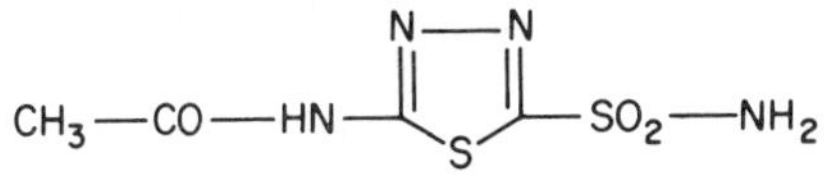

$$CH_3—CO—HN—C_2N_2S—SO_2—NH_2$$

PHARMACOLOGY

Acetazolamide is an inhibitor of carbonic anhydrase. This results in diminished production of hydrogen ions by the tubules, which are therefore not available for exchange with sodium ions in the distal tubular fluid; there is an inverse association between hydrogen and potassium ion excretion in the distal tubules so that potassium is excreted in greater amounts together with bicarbonate ions.

The net result is a metabolic acidosis with retention of chloride ions. This is the opposite effect to that resulting from mercurial diuretics; consequently the two drugs were often given alternately.

INDICATIONS

It used to be given in conjunction with organic mercurial diuretics in the treatment of oedema associated with congestive heart failure; it is used in the treatment of glaucoma.

DOSAGE AND ADMINISTRATION

Acetazolamide is given orally or intravenously, 250 mg–1 g per 24 hours. As its action lasts about 12 hours it is best given in the morning. The dose should be carefully calculated as overdosage may cause drowsiness or paraesthesia.

Thiazides

PHARMACOLOGY

Chlorothiazide was the first of a number of benzothiadiazine derivatives which have similar properties. Subsequently a number of other thiazide analogues have been introduced but in optimal dosage they all have a similar effect on sodium excretion. Bendrofluazide, cyclopenthiazide, and hydroflumethiazide are now the most commonly prescribed drugs in this group now on the market, largely on cost grounds. Other drugs with similar properties include chlorthalidone, clorexolone, clopamide, quinethazone, mefruside, metolazone, indapamide, and xipamide. These drugs all act on the cortical diluting segment of the distal convoluted tubule causing a natriuresis of up to 10 per cent of the filtered sodium. They also have a weak inhibitory effect on carbonic anhydrase; this increases the bicarbonate and potassium excretion into the distal tubular fluid in the same manner as does acetazolamide.

The loss of potassium that occurs does not normally require a supplement to make up for the deficiency although the serum level is usually reduced. However, relative to the body as a whole, the loss is not a major one. The loss of sodium and chloride results in an increase in urinary volume. Recently it has become recognized that thiazide diuretics reduce arterial blood pressure by a direct action independent of the long-recognized effects of sodium depletion and the resultant fall in circulating blood volume. This is thought to be due to a direct effect on peripheral circulatory tone. In consequence they may be sufficient to control moderate hypertension, particularly in the elderly. The dose necessary to produce this hypotensive effect is smaller than that required for the relief of oedema and does not usually result in potassium depletion.

Thiazide diuretics have a paradoxical effect on patients suffering from diabetes insipidus in whom they effectively reduce the urine volume. They reduce free water clearance and thus tend to lower serum osmolarity. It is thought that the effect of this is to lessen the sensation of thirst and so reduce the water intake.

Diabetes mellitus may be provoked by prolonged treatment with thiazide drugs in patients who are latent diabetics. These drugs may also provoke a rise in serum uric acid and precipitate gout.

Absorption and excretion. After oral administration, maximum effect is obtained in about 4 hours, with onset of action within 2 hours, and these drugs are rapidly eliminated by the kidney. The duration of action varies between 12 and 72 hours but all have the desired therapeutic action with once-a-day administration.

INDICATIONS

Thiazide diuretics are used widely in hypertension and for the relief of oedema in mild cardiac failure; they are used less often in other oedamatous states, for nephrogenic diabetes insipidus, and for prophylaxis against renal stones.

DOSAGE AND ADMINISTRATION

These drugs are usually given daily. The various drugs differ on a weight-for-weight basis but as there is no significant difference between them, there is no reason not to give the cheapest. At the time of writing this is bendrofluazide. The relative potencies are as follows:

Bendrofluazide	2.5–5 mg
Chlorothiazide	0.5–1 g
Chlorthalidone	50–100 mg
Clopamide	20–40 mg
Clorexolone	10–25 mg
Cyclopenthiazide	0.25–1 mg
Hydrochlorothiazide	50–100 mg
Hydroflumethiazide	25–50 mg
Indapamide	2.5 mg
Mefruside	25–50 mg
Methylclothiazide	2.5–5 mg
Metolazone	5–10 mg
Quinethazone	50–100 mg
Xipamide	20–40 mg

Potassium loss can be reduced by combining thiazide and spironolactone therapy.

PRECAUTIONS

Side effects are infrequent, nausea being the commonest, and this can usually be overcome by taking the drug after food. Rarely a skin rash or purpura may be seen.

Thiazides, in common with other antihypertensives, may cause impotence. They tend to potentiate the action of digitalis, and the dose of digitalis may therefore need to be reduced should anorexia, nausea, vomiting, of bradycardia occur. Metabolic abnormalities, hypokalaemia, hyperuricaemia, glucose intolerance, hypercalcaemia, raised serum cholesterol levels, and reduction in high density lipoproteins have been cited as potentially prognostically adverse, but so far the benefits of treatment seem to outweigh these theoretical hazards.

In cases of hypertension, not only the actions of ganglion-blocking agents, but also those of reserpine, hydralazine, and veratrum alkaloids are potentiated. The dose of these hypotensive drugs can often be reduced by 25–50 per cent. While routine administration of potassium supplements is no longer regarded as necessary, it is important to identify patients in whom even moderate reductions may prove a hazard. These include those with dysrhythmias, myocardial infarction, severe ischaemic heart disease, or chronic liver disease, and patients on a poor diet, or taking digoxin, corticosteroids, carbenoxolone, or drugs that interfere with ventricular repolarization, such as tricyclic antidepressants and phenothiazines. Oral potassium may not be sufficient in these circumstances and combination with a potassium-sparing diuretic is to be preferred. Loss of potassium may cause malaise, apathy, weakness, and loss of deep tendon reflexes.

Frusemide

Frusemide (*BP*) and Furosemide (*USP*)
Chemical name: 4-chloro-2-furfurylamino-5-sulphamoylbenzoic acid

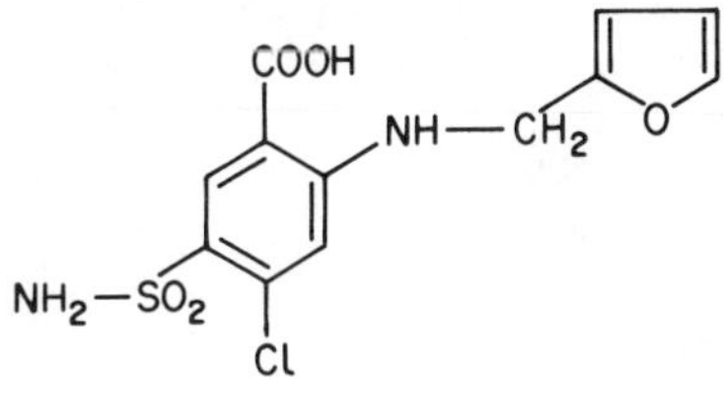

PHARMACOLOGY

Frusemide, although a sulphonamide derivative and thus having certain structural similarities to the thiazides, does not resemble them closely either chemically or pharmacologically. Its action is to prevent sodium and chloride reabsorption in the proximal and first part of the distal tubule and in the ascending limb of the loop of Henle. An important consequence of this is that the osmolarity of the renal medulla is reduced. Thus free water clearance is almost always increased and unlike the thiazides it produces a hypotonic urine in which the sodium ion concentration is lower than that of the plasma. There is, therefore, less stimulus to the induction of hyperaldosteronism. It is unaffected by disturbances of acid–base balance, and in large doses will tend to produce a hypochloraemic alkalosis. The ion-exchange mechanism in the distal tubule is not affected and therefore potassium loss is increased although to a lesser extent than with the thiazides; the natriuresis may be enhanced and the potassium loss diminished by the addition of spironolactone.

There is no inhibition of carbonic anhydrase and since sodium bicarbonate reabsorption is either normal or increased with these diuretics, the addition of acetazolamide, by decreasing the availability of hydrogen ions for exchange with sodium, will augment the diuresis.

The response to frusemide is proportional to the glomerular filtration rate (GFR) over a wide range, while the reponse to the thiazides is unaltered for GFR over 20 ml/min. The GFR is transiently raised in cases of poor renal function by the former. Larger doses may, therefore, need to be given in the presence of low GFR, and large doses may be used in the diagnosis of suspected renal failure. The plasma uric acid level is increased and although it has been claimed that frusemide does not impair glucose tolerance, a few cases of diabetes have presented following therapy.

A mild hypotensive effect similar to that of the thiazides, affecting both supine and standing blood pressures, has occasionally been noted. Addition of ethacrynic acid to frusemide or the converse does not enhance the diuresis; but the addition of either of these two drugs will augment the diuresis resulting from thiazide administration.

Absorption and excretion. The onset of action following intravenous injection occurs within 2–3 minutes, while oral therapy produces a peak diuresis in 1 hour with a total duration of 4–6 hours. Excretion occurs rapidly by filtration and tubular secretion.

INDICATIONS

Frusemide is particularly of value by intravenous injection in the emergency treatment of acute pulmonary oedema, and in the preparation of patients with congestive cardiac failure for surgery. In view of its potency it is otherwise usually reserved for cases resistant to milder diuretics. It is effective in all forms of refractory oedema, whether of cardiac, renal, or hepatic origin. It is of limited value in cases with poor renal function.

DOSAGE AND ADMINISTRATION

The initial dose is usually 40–80 mg given orally on alternate days or on 3 consecutive days a week. This may be increased to 120 mg daily. In cases very resistant to treatment attempts have been made to produce a diuresis with amounts of up to 500 mg daily. The danger of electrolyte disturbances with low dosage is not marked although in patients likely to be sensitive to even mild hypokalaemia potassium chloride supplements and biochemical control are essential. The addition of spironolactone has resulted in a satisfactory diuresis in cases previously resistant to frusemide alone. As in the treatment of all cases of oedema, some restriction of sodium intake is important if benefit is to be gained.

For immediate response 40 mg may be given intravenously or intramuscularly and repeated in 20 minutes.

PRECAUTIONS

Apart from the occurrence of transient diarrhoea and the rare reports of reversible thrombocytopenia and leucopenia, the only side effects have resulted from electrolyte disorders. These can be severe: the potency of this drug is such that 40 per cent of the glomerular filtrate can be excreted as urine, and severe water and electrolyte disturbances can occur. Contraindications include anuria, hepatic coma, and electrolyte deficiencies. It should only be used in early pregnancy with great caution.

Ethacrynic acid, although chemically unrelated to any other diuretic, has pharmacological actions closely resembling those of frusemide. It was originally thought that its cellular mechanism of action was a combination with sulphydryl groups in the kidney, blocking sodium transport. This, however, would not explain the inhibition of chloride absorption or the fact that frusemide and bumetanide do not share this property.

The indications and precautions are the same as for frusemide. The dose of ethacrynic acid is 50–200 mg daily, usually on 3 days of the week. The addition of a potassium-sparing diuretic or spironolactone will reduce potassium loss. In emergencies, 50 mg may be given by intravenous injection.

Bumetanide is another powerful 'loop' diuretic, chemically unrelated to any other diuretic. Its site of action is also on the proximal convoluted tubule, ascending limb of the loop of Henle, and the first part of the distal convoluted tubule, where active sodium and chloride absorption is inhibited. It thus closely resembles frusemide in its actions, differing only in its milligram potency, 1 mg being equivalent to 40 mg of frusemide.

Mannitol

Mannitol (*BP* and *USP*)

$$
\begin{array}{ccccccccccc}
 & & H & & H & & OH & & OH & & \\
 & & | & & | & & | & & | & & \\
CH_2OH & - & C & - & C & - & C & - & C & - & CH_2OH \\
 & & | & & | & & | & & | & & \\
 & & OH & & OH & & H & & H & &
\end{array}
$$

Mannitol is an undissociated crystalloid and is an effective osmotic diuretic. It is completely filtered at the glomerulus and none is reabsorbed; it is inert in the body and does not penetrate the cells.

INDICATIONS

Mannitol is used to increase the excretion of drugs such as salicylates and phenobarbitone, to reduce the brain volume in cerebral oedema, and in the prevention of acute renal failure, for which purpose its use is now well established. It is also believed to protect the kidneys against damage by certain nephrotoxins. Thus, it is indicated in mismatched blood transfusions and in poisoning with carbon tetrachloride and ethylene glycol.

DOSAGE AND ADMINISTRATION

Mannitol is normally given intravenously in 10 or 20 per cent solutions in a dose of 0.5–1 g/kg. A 25 per cent supersaturated solution can be prepared but there is little to be gained by using this as it has to be kept above room temperature to remain in solution. Its use in forced diuresis in the management of phenobarbitone and salicylate overdose is discussed on page 105. The above dose of mannitol may be given during surgical operations to all cases in whom the risk of acute renal failure is known to be high. The most common instance of this is in operations for the relief of severe obstructive jaundice when mannitol should always be given.

Suspected intrinsic renal failure. One of the most difficult problems in intensive care units is to determine when extrarenal causes of oliguria have caused intrinsic renal damage. When the urine volume is less than 20 ml/h and the provoking incident has occurred less than 48 hours beforehand the following regimen may be employed. Three doses of 100 ml of 20 per cent mannitol are given, each dose being given in 10–20 minutes and at 2-hourly intervals. If a urine volume of at least 50 ml/h is established the oliguria is unlikely to recur; if no diuresis results fluids must be restricted to 400–500 ml/day plus measured losses and no more mannitol given.

PRECAUTIONS

As with all hypertonic solutions, care must be taken to ensure that there is no extravascular leakage. Giving sets should either be flushed with isotonic saline or changed when mannitol is followed by blood. Mannitol should not be given more rapidly than 3 g/min.

Urea is an undissociated crystalloid and is an effective osmotic diuretic although it has certain disadvantages: it is highly diffusible and has a small molecule so that over 60 per cent of urea filtered at the glomerulus is reabsorbed in the remainder of the nephron. Urea therefore recirculates and gradually penetrates the cells to equilibrate across the cell membrane. For this reason its use is declining in favour of mannitol, which is without these disadvantages.

It can be used to hasten the excretion of drugs such as salicylates and barbiturates in cases of overdose, and in the treatment of cerebral oedema.

It can be given intravenously as a 30 per cent solution in a dose of 0.5–1 g/kg, administered over a period of at least 20 minutes.

A 30 per cent solution of urea must not be given too rapidly as it will cause a considerable rise in blood pressure. Haemolysis may also occur; rates in excess of 2 g/min should therefore be avoided and giving sets should be flushed with isotonic saline or changed if blood is to follow its use. As it is highly irritant, care must be taken to ensure that it does not leak subcutaneously. Urea should not be given when renal function is likely to be impaired.

Mersalyl acid is usually given as the sodium salt in the form of Mersalyl injection (*BP*), which is a sterile solution of 10 per cent w/v of mersalyl sodium and 5 per cent w/v of theophylline, pH 7.6–8.2. The theophylline promotes absorption and reduces reaction in the tissues locally. It increases the free water clearance and the amount present in mersalyl injection has been shown to produce a diuretic effect greater than that of the mercurial alone.

Mersalyl probably acts at several sites in the nephron and, by inhibiting intracellular enzyme systems, interferes with transport processes. Reabsorption of sodium and chloride is reduced. This leads to a greater loss of chloride than bicarbonate in the urine and tends to produce a hypochloraemic alkalosis. If this develops, mersalyl may become ineffective through shortage of chloride ions. This can be counteracted by giving ammonium chloride.

The diuretic response, which may be considerable, is governed by the electrolyte balance at the time. It usually takes about 2 hours before this is apparent; the maximum effect occurs between 6 and 9 hours and may last for 12–24 hours. The usual dose is 50–200 mg intramuscularly at intervals of 3–4 days.

Since the introduction of more efficient diuretics which are active by mouth, mersalyl has fallen into disuse.

Spironolactone

Spironolactone (*BP* and *USP*)
Chemical name: 7α-acetylthio-3-oxo-17α-pregn-4-ene-21,17β-carbolactone acid γ-lactone

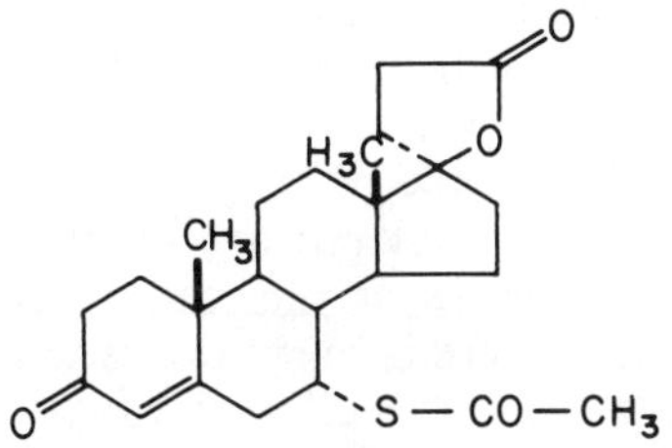

PHARMACOLOGY

Spironolactone blocks the action of aldosterone on the distal tubule and prevents the reabsorption of sodium and accompanying chloride at this site. Reabsorption of potassium is increased. It is not a powerful diuretic when used alone but acts synergistically with other diuretics. It is most active when aldosterone is present in excess. When used with diuretics that cause excessive loss of potassium, potassium supplements are usually unnecessary.

INDICATIONS

Spironolactone is used in oedematous conditions associated with congestive cardiac failure, ascites, and the nephrotic syndrome. It is also used in the treatment of hypertension. It is especially useful in the management of secondary aldosteronism.

DOSAGE AND ADMINISTRATION

Spironolactone is readily absorbed from the intestinal tract. It is normally given in tablet form, 25 mg four times a day. Larger doses are occasionally required. It has a cumulative action and may take several days to exert its full effect. It is usually given in conjunction with another diuretic.

PRECAUTIONS

Side effects are infrequent. Drowsiness, mental confusion, and erythematous skin eruptions have been reported on rare occasions. It should be used with caution in patients whose serum potassium levels are raised.

Triamterene

Triamterene (*BP* and *USP*)
Chemical name: 6-phenylpteridine-2,4,7-triamine

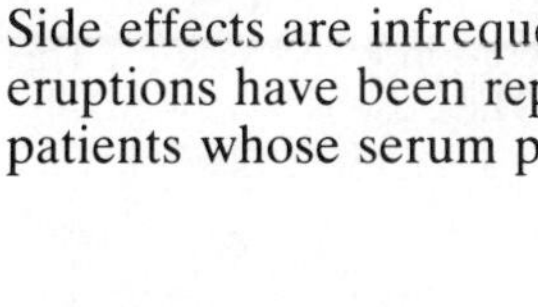

Triamterene is a pteridine derivative and is chemically unrelated to other diuretics. It increases the excretion of sodium and depresses that of potassium by a direct action on the distal tubule where it diminishes sodium absorption. Bicarbonate excretion is increased and the pH of the urine is raised. Uric acid excretion is also increased. Further evidence that it acts in a different way to the thiazides or spironolactone is provided by the fact that when it is given with these drugs together in full doses its effect is additive. Triamterene has a weaker natriuretic action than the thiazides, but it can be usefully employed with them when it will mitigate the extent of the potassium loss which would otherwise occur.

The potassium-sparing action is probably an indirect one: the driving force for potassium secretion by the distal tubule is the transtubular electrical potential difference created by the sodium reabsorption which occurs at this site. This sodium reabsorption is inhibited by triamterene but the effect is magnified when larger quantities of sodium are reaching the distal tubule as a consequence of diuretic action elsewhere in the nephron. It cannot, however, wholly prevent some potassium loss when potent loop diuretics such as frusemide are employed. Toxic effects appear to be minimal, but diarrhoea may occur following large doses. Nausea and vomiting have also been reported.

ABSORPTION AND EXCRETION

Triamterene is well absorbed after oral administration and can be detected in the urine in 15–20 minutes. It is excreted partly unchanged and partly in the form of metabolites. Excretion reaches a peak in 6–8 hours.

INDICATIONS

Triamterene may be used in the treatment of oedema associated with congestive heart failure, cirrhosis of the liver, nephrotic syndrome, and idiopathic and drug-induced oedema. It is more commonly used with a thiazide diuretic as it is less effective when used alone.

DOSAGE AND ADMINISTRATION

Triamterene 50 mg in capsule form twice daily is usually sufficient, but up to 200 mg a day may be required.

Amiloride is another potassium-sparing diuretic, whose actions closely resemble those of triamterene. It causes a small increase in excretion of sodium and chloride (and also hydrogen ion) accompanied by only a small or no increase in secretion of potassium. This effect is most striking when it is given with other saluretic agents. The dose is 5–10 mg daily, given with other diuretics.

15

Uterine stimulants

Uterine muscle

Uterine muscle shows spontaneous intermittent activity throughout reproductive life. Unlike the heart there is no pacemaker and the contraction process spreads from one cell to another at a rate of 1–3 cm/s, usually starting in the cornual regions. A and B types of contraction have been designated, the former occurring frequently and with low amplitude and the latter being of higher amplitude and more infrequent. B waves are usually called Braxton Hicks contractions and become more frequent as pregnancy advances. The contractions of labour result in a peak of intrauterine pressure during the first stage contractions of 40–60 mmHg (5.3–8 kPa), rising to 60–80 mmHg (8–10.7 kPa) in the second stage. The resting uterine pressure in labour is approximately 10 mmHg (1.3 kPa). The cervix has some muscle in it but takes no part in the expulsive contractions.

Uterine stimulants

Uterine stimulants may be classified as general and specific. Of the general uterine stimulants the local hormones predominate, including bradykinin, histamine, acetylcholine, noradrenaline, and 5-hydroxytryptamine. The depolarizing relaxants have no demonstrable action on the uterine muscle.

The specific uterine stimulants are the ergot alkaloids, oxytocin, and synthetic derivative prostaglandins E_2 and $F_{2\alpha}$.

Uterine inhibitors

Drugs stimulating uterine β-adrenoceptors relax the uterus and salbutamol is now used therapeutically to prevent premature labour in the first trimester. Other drugs used for this purpose are orciprenaline, isoxsuprine, terbutaline, and ritodrine. All have β_2-receptor agonist activity. Since they can stimulate β_2-adrenoceptors at sites other than the uterus they can produce a dose-dependent maternal tachycardia and a fall in blood pressure. The general anaesthetics, particularly halothane, also relax the uterus as does the narcotic diamorphine. Papaverine and amyl nitrite inhibit the muscle of the cervix, as does general surgical anaesthesia. Spinal and epidural analgesia and paracervical block have only a transient inhibitory action on the uterine contractions in established labour.

Ergometrine maleate

Ergometrine maleate (*BP*) and Ergonovine maleate (*USP*)
Chemical constitution: originally obtained from ergot (*Claviceps purpurea*), this alkaloidal derivative of the indole compound lysergic acid is now produced synthetically.
Chemical name: *N*-(2-hydroxy-1-methylethyl)-(+)-lysergamide hydrogen maleate

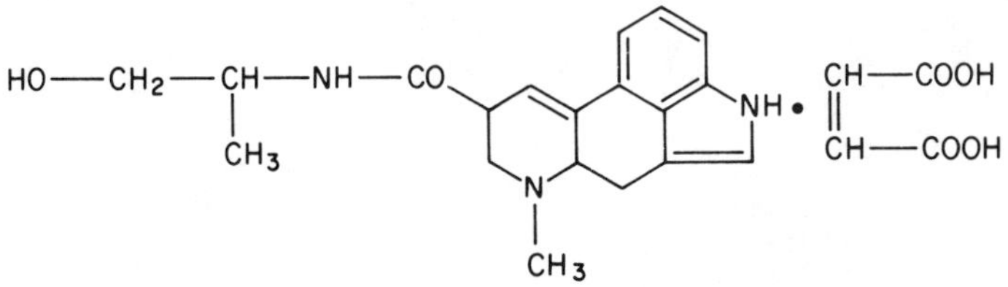

PHARMACOLOGY

Ergometrine is the most effective oxytocic of the ergot alkaloids. Its action is rapid, stimulating contractions within 2–4 minutes by intramuscular injection and within 30–45 seconds by intravenous injection. If given in the first stage of labour, violent, abnormal contractions occur which might lead to uterine tetany, with resultant marked reduction in placental blood flow and fetal hypoxia. In the third stage, ergometrine produces sustained uterine contraction with superimposed irregular contractions. In doses of 0.25 or 0.5 mg, intravenous injection causes a rise in arterial blood pressure due to an increase in systemic vascular resistance, and this may persist for several hours. It also produces vomiting, probably by a direct action on the vomiting centre.

Absorption and fate. Its fate has not been elucidated, but it is probably inactivated in the liver, and a small proportion excreted unchanged in the urine.

INDICATIONS

Ergometrine is used to contract the uterine muscle in the third stage of labour, either before or after delivery of the placenta. In this situation its routine use has dramatically reduced the volume of postpartum haemorrhage. Unlike oxytocin, ergometrine is equally effective in early pregnancy. It should be used with caution in patients with pre-eclamptic toxaemia, hypertension, or in the presence of other vasopressors.

DOSAGE AND ADMINISTRATION

In obstetrics it is usually given in a dose of 0.2–1 mg intramuscularly or 0.25–0.5 mg intravenously. It may be given directly into the uterine muscle at caesarean section.

Ergotamine tartrate

Ergotamine tartrate (*BP* and *USP*)
Chemical constitution: the tartrate of an alkaloid, ergotamine, obtained from certain ergot species.

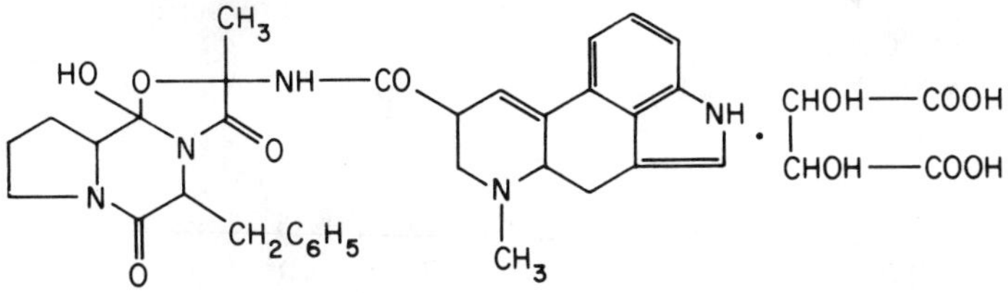

PHARMACOLOGY
Ergotamine is much less effective as an oxytocic than ergometrine. It increases uterine contractions but tends to cause spasm. Like ergotoxine it causes vasoconstriction by a direct action on the plain muscle of arterioles and can reverse or abolish the constrictor effects of adrenaline and of sympathetic nerve stimulation. Dihydroergotamine has less pressor and oxytocic effects, but is a better sympathetic antagonist, and has less side effects. Both ergotamine and ergotoxine are toxic substances and may give rise to gangrenous ergotism.

INDICATIONS
The main use of ergotamine tartrate is in migraine where it constricts dilated vessels and reduces the pulsations in the temporal artery. Other types of headache are not improved and may be aggravated.

DOSAGE AND ADMINISTRATION
Ergotamine is given as a single dose of 1–2 mg orally or 0.25–0.5 mg subcutaneously or intramuscularly.

PRECAUTIONS
The use of ergotamine tartrate is contraindicated in pregnancy, occlusive vascular and cardiovascular diseases, and in the presence of sepsis.

Oxytocin

Oxytocin injection (*BP* and *USP*), Oxytocin tablets (*BP*)
Chemical constitution: this hormone is an octapeptide with a five-membered ring and a tripeptide tail. The cystine molecules are connected by a sulphur bridge. It can be produced synthetically.
Chemical name: 3-isoleucine-8-leucine-vasopressin

```
Glutamine—Asparagine—Cystine—Proline—Leucine—Glycinamide
 (NH2)      (NH2)       |                        (NH2)
   |                    S
   |                    |
Isoleucine — Tyrosine — Cystine
```

PHYSIOLOGICAL ROLE

Oxytocin is synthesized in nerve cell bodies in the paraventricular nuclei of the hypothalamus. It travels in secretory granules along the axons to the posterior pituitary gland where it is stored. It can be released abruptly and independently of antidiuretic hormone (ADH, vasopressin). Oxytocin has a physiological role in lactation. Following stimulation of the nipple by suckling there is an immediate release of oxytocin which, by virtue of its smooth muscle-contracting effect, transports milk along the ducts; this is the so-called milk 'let down'. Oxytocin may have a physiological role in initiating and maintaining labour but its presence is not essential.

PHARMACOLOGY

The posterior pituitary secretes the hormones oxytocin and ADH whose release is triggered by different stimuli. The early oxytocic preparations contained ADH as a contaminant, and therein confusion arose because both hormones stimulated the uterus and contracted smooth muscle, including the muscle of blood vessels. This action on smooth muscle and in particular coronary vessels is more marked in the case of ADH, and may have been the mechanism of 'pituitary shock' feared by earlier obstetricians when giving oxytocin in what was relatively high dosage. The synthetic preparation of oxytocin now used is syntocinon, which contains no ADH. A bolus injection causes a transient fall in arterial blood pressure and peripheral resistance with an increase in central venous pressure, while infusions have little cardiovascular effect. Oxytocin acts mainly on the gravid uterine muscle, causing it to contract rhythmically, and may induce spasm in high dosage, but is insufficient by itself to produce complete abortion. The sensitivity of uterine muscle to oxytocin progressively increases as pregnancy advances, so that the oxytocic dose in early pregnancy is some 10-fold that in later pregnancy. This is due to changes in hormonal balance in early pregnancy.

Fate in the body. Oxytocin is readily absorbed orally and inactivated by chymotrypsin in the plasma, liver, and kidney. During pregnancy, a specific enzyme exists for its degradation, called oxytocinase, which is present in high concentration in the uterus and placenta.

INDICATIONS

Oxytocin can be used to induce abortion in early pregnancy (although it is rarely effective), to induce labour at term, and to contract the uterus in postpartum haemorrhage. Contraindications include fetal distress and disproportion, hypertonic uterine inertia, and placenta praevia.

DOSAGE AND ADMINISTRATION

By the oral route oxytocin tablets (100–200 units) sucked sublingually to a total daily dose of 2000–4000 units have been used to induce labour at term. Because of the variable rate of absorption and a tendency to produce uterine spasm this method has been largely abandoned.

Oxytocin 2–5 units are given by intramuscular injection for postpartum haemorrhage. To stimulate abortion 10–20 units are given intravenously in a dextrose infusion in the first hour, increasing by 20 units/h up to a maximum of 100 units/h. For induction of labour at term the use of an oxytocin intravenous infusion must be supervised carefully, and the dose quantified by accurate volumetric syringe or infusion with direct or indirect tocography of uterine muscle to safeguard against uterine spasm or rupture. The dose required is very much smaller and ranges from 0.1–8 units/h.

A combined injection of 5 units of oxytocin and 0.5 mg of ergometrine in one ampoule is available. This can be used in the third stage of labour or after delivery of the placenta. It is contraindicated if the patient has liver or kidney dysfunction. It contains the maximum recommended dose of each drug and if given intravenously may produce marked hypertension with severe headache.

Prostaglandins

Chemical structure: prostaglandin is a generic term for a group of polyunsaturated fatty acids (*Figure 15.1*). The molecule contains a cyclopentane ring and two side chains. The configuration of the five-membered ring (in dotted box) determines the group; subscript numbers (for example E_2, F_1) indicate progressive degrees of unsaturation of the fatty acid side chain (1 = least, and so on). There are six major groups, designated E, F, A, B, C, and D. Their synthesis from phospholipids is described on page 414.

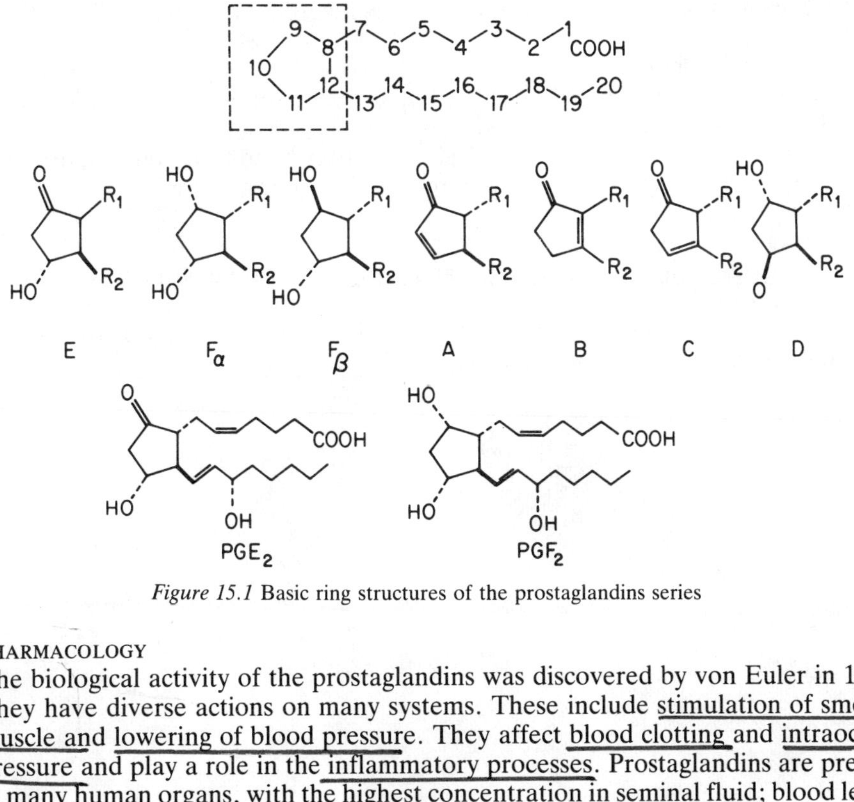

Figure 15.1 Basic ring structures of the prostaglandins series

PHARMACOLOGY

The biological activity of the prostaglandins was discovered by von Euler in 1936. They have diverse actions on many systems. These include stimulation of smooth muscle and lowering of blood pressure. They affect blood clotting and intraocular pressure and play a role in the inflammatory processes. Prostaglandins are present in many human organs, with the highest concentration in seminal fluid; blood levels are very low. They are estimated by bioassay but immunoassay for certain members of the group is now available and is more sensitive and specific. They can also be identified using the mass spectrometer.

PGE_2 and $PGF_{2\alpha}$ are now used clinically for their stimulant action on the uterus. As with oxytocin, the uterus in early pregnancy is less sensitive than at term. PGE_2 appears to be superior to $PGF_{2\alpha}$ as a stimulant throughout pregnancy, and has less side effects.

Intrauterine administration has been used for induction of abortion without significant side effects and in greatly reduced dosage.

Ninety per cent of prostaglandins are believed to be inactivated in passage through the pulmonary circulation and this is the reason for the higher doses needed by the intravenous route.

INDICATIONS

PGE_2 and $PGF_{2\alpha}$ are used for the induction of abortion and for the induction of labour.

DOSAGE AND ADMINISTRATION

They may be given by the oral, intravenous, or intrauterine routes. The intrauterine is the most effective and the oral the least effective route.

Labour may be induced at term by a single oral dose of 0.5 mg of PGE_2 or 5 mg of $PGF_{2\alpha}$. Contractions are stimulated in 5–15 minutes and continue for 2–3 hours. In early pregnancy the oral route is ineffective in inducing abortion without significant side effects.

Labour can be induced by intravenous infusion of 0.5–2 μg/min of PGE_2 or $PGF_{2\alpha}$ up to a dose of 600 μg. In early pregnancy doses of 2–5 μg/min up to a total dose of 2500–4000 μg may be needed.

By the intrauterine route, smaller doses have been used to produce abortion in early pregnancy. This route is not used to induce labour at term.

TOXIC EFFECTS

Significant nausea, diarrhoea, vomiting and fever, which are dose dependent, have been noted with $PGF_{2\alpha}$, and this limits its use in early pregnancy by the oral or intravenous route. Phlebitis has been noted in a high proportion of patients receiving intravenous infusions of PGE_2.

16

Chemical transmitters and enzymes

Chemical transmitters

To a considerable extent the functions of cells and tissue are controlled by a large variety of specifically adapted chemicals. Those that are secreted by specialized organs and exert their effects on various remote tissues are called hormones and are discussed fully in Chapter 17.

Much voluntary and reflex activity is controlled by the release of chemical substances in response to nerve impulses at nerve endings both within the nervous system and at blood vessels. The commonest of these are acetylcholine and noradrenaline, which are discussed in Chapters 10 and 12, but within the CNS other agents such as γ-aminobutyric acid, dopamine, 5-hydroxytryptamine (5-HT), and probably many others function as transmitters at certain synapses.

Autacoids

An important group of chemical transmitters consists of those substances that act locally at the site of liberation in inflammatory or allergic reactions, and via the circulation may reach distant sites where they can also have important actions. A substance in this category is histamine which acts locally at its site of liberation in allergic reactions, and can reach the circulation and act at a distance to increase gastric secretion. When histamine is liberated by tissue injury, by drugs, or by chemical transmitters such as adrenaline, heparin which increases the clotting time of blood is often also released. Histamine and its antagonists at various sites are considered in Chapter 8.

Histamine is an example of an autacoid (Greek, *autos* – self, and *akos* – medicine) or local hormone. Other substances that also have intense pharmacological actions at the site of release include the prostaglandins, 5-HT, angiotensin, and the various kinins.

Prostaglandins

Prostaglandins are a group of long-chain fatty acids derived from a 20-carbon compound, prostanoic acid: their basic ring structures are shown in *Figure 15.1*, page 411. These substances are present in most mammalian tissues which have the capacity to synthesize them from precursors. They have numerous and diverse effects and the pattern of their actions varies widely between the different members of the group. Generally they are potent vasodilators although $PGF_{2\alpha}$ is a vasoconstrictor of pulmonary arteries and veins. Capillary permeability is always increased. Prostaglandins have effects on most other types of smooth muscle. For example, PGFs contract bronchial and tracheal muscle in man, particularly in asthmatics. However, PGEs are potent bronchodilators with a potency greater than that of isoprenaline when given by aerosol. Their actions on uterine muscle are discussed in Chapter 15.

Gastric, pancreatic, and intestinal secretions are inhibited by PGEs and PGA, probably by a direct effect on the secretory cells. This may prove to be of therapeutic use.

Prostaglandins are released by a wide variety of physicochemical insults; their role in chronic inflammation, particularly in the eye and in arthritis, is well established. The ability of aspirin-type drugs to block the synthesis of prostaglandins seems to be crucial to their effectiveness as anti-inflammatory agents.

Prostaglandins are synthesized from 20-carbon polyunsaturated fatty acids present in the phospholipids of cell membranes. Their main precursor is arachidonic acid. Arachidonic acid in cell membrane is derived from linoleic acid found in vegetables, or from arachidonic acid found in meat. Other precursors of prostaglandins are dihomo-γ-linolenic acid and eicosapentaenoic acid (*Table 16.1*).

Table 16.1 Fatty acid precursors of prostaglandins

Precursor	*Prostaglandin*	
Dihomo-γ-linolenic acid	PGE_1	PGF_1
Arachidonic acid	PGE_2	PGF_2
Eicosapentaenoic acid	PGE_3	PGF_3

A key enzyme in arachidonic acid metabolism is phospholipase A_2. Chemical or mechanical stimulation of cell membranes activates this enzyme, which then releases arachidonic acid from membrane phospholipids. Arachidonic acid can then be converted via two distinct pathways (*Figure 16.1*). Lipoxygenases, which have been found in platelets, lungs, and white cells, can attack it, resulting in hydroperoxy-arachidonic acids. These are unstable compounds. In the other pathway, cyclo-oxygenase (present in cell membranes), catalyses the formation of an unstable cyclic endoperoxide, PGG_2. PGG_2 is converted rapidly into PGH_2 which in turn is converted to more stable prostaglandins PGE_2, PGF_2 and PGD_2. The half-life of both PGG_2 and PGH_2 is about 5 minutes at 37°C. The prostaglandin endoperoxides are also transformed by other enzymes, prostacyclin synthetase and thromboxane synthetase, into prostacyclin (PGI_2) and thromboxane A_2 respectively. These in turn are converted to 6-oxo-$PGF_{1\alpha}$ and thromboxane B_2.

Platelet aggregation

Thromboxane A_2 is a potent aggregator of platelets, whereas prostacyclin is a potent anti-aggregator of platelets. The explanation may lie in the fact that thromboxane A_2 reduces the concentration of cyclic AMP inside platelets, thereby increasing platelet adhesiveness while prostacyclin increases cyclic AMP concentration.

Aspirin and related non-narcotic analgesics inhibit cyclo-oxygenase and thereby should theoretically reduce both prostacyclin and thromboxane A_2 levels. Indeed,

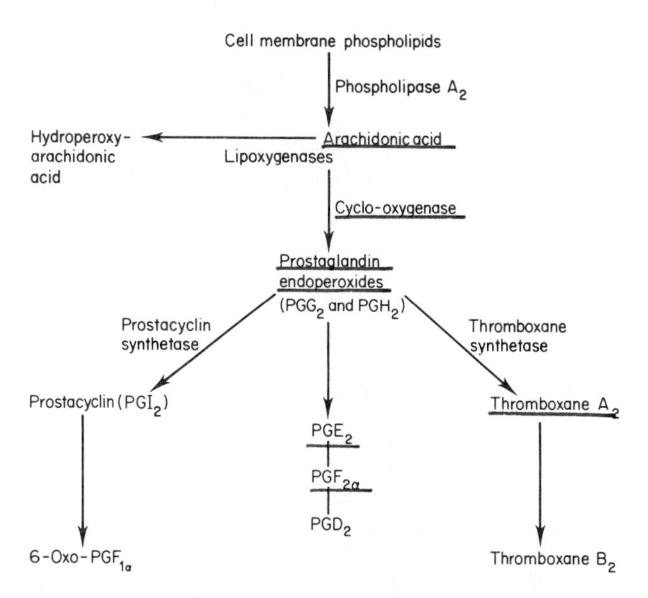

Figure 16.1 Arachidonic acid metabolism

aspirin has been reported to reduce platelet thromboxane A_2 levels and prostacyclin formation in arterial intima. However, the dose required for each inhibition is different. Thus in theory selective depression of thromboxane A_2 formation is possible and this could have therapeutic potential in the prevention of thromboembolic disease. Another possible approach to this problem is the use of specific thromboxane synthetase inhibitors such as imidazole. However, this drug is too toxic and not sufficiently specific; more specific and less toxic substances may appear in the next few years.

An alternative approach which is being used therapeutically already is to use prostacyclin or a derivative. Moncada and Vane (1978, 1979) have suggested that prostacyclin is crucial to maintaining the integrity of the vascular endothelium. They postulate that the arterial intima normally synthesizes prostacyclin and this inhibits platelet aggregation. Platelets near the intimal wall may be a source of prostaglandin endoperoxide which the endothelial cells use to generate prostacyclin. When the intima is damaged less prostacyclin is produced since the concentration of prostaglandin synthetase decreases as one moves from the intima to the adventitia. This would leave the prostaglandin endoperoxides available for conversion to thromboxane A_2 leading to aggregation (*Figure 16.2*). This local control of platelet aggregability could explain why thrombosis occurs in artificial grafts unless they become coated with endothelium, which secretes prostacyclin. Lipid peroxides are known to inhibit prostacyclin synthetase and this might explain why thrombosis occurs on atheromatous plaques. Dipyridamole's antiplatelet activity may be due to its ability to inhibit platelet phosphodiesterase, thereby raising platelet cyclic AMP.

Prostacyclin

Prostacyclin is also synthesized by the lung and released into the circulation. This may be a mechanism for the dispersion of aggregated platelets trapped in fine vessels in the lung. Prostacyclin is a powerful vasodilator; it causes a fall in blood

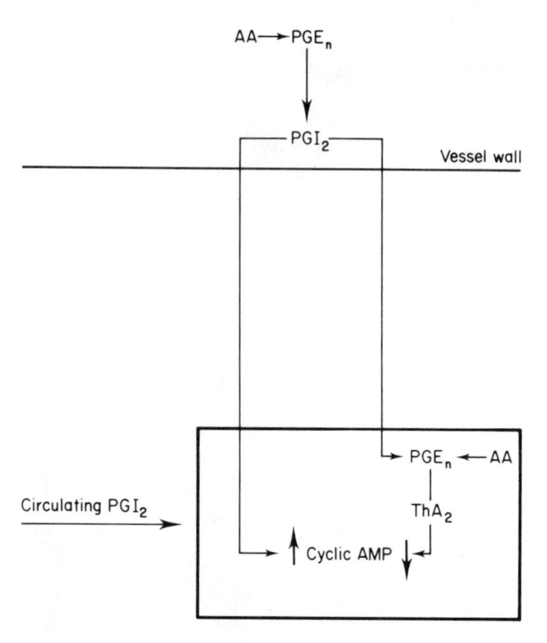

Figure 16.2 Regulation of platelet cyclic AMP. AA = arachidonic acid; PGE_n = prostaglandin endoperoxide; ThA_2 = thromboxane A_2; PGI_2 = prostacyclin

pressure and dilates coronary vessels. Following prostacyclin infusion in man at rates of 20 μg/kg, there is a fall in diastolic pressure and a rise in heart rate. Prostacyclin also reduces the acid secretion which is induced by pentagastrin. Among the therapeutic uses being considered for prostacyclin are to replace heparin in dialysis, cardiopulmonary bypass, and charcoal haemoperfusion, and in the treatment of arteriosclerosis obliterans, crescendo angina, and incipient myocardial infarction (Shaw, 1980).

Slow-reacting substance

As well as being the precursor of the prostaglandins and thromboxanes, arachidonic acid can be converted to substances known as leukotrienes (*Figure 16.3*). Their existence has been known since Feldberg and Kellaway in 1938 described a factor which appeared in the perfusate of guinea-pig lung treated with cobra venom and which they named slow-reacting substance (SRS). In anaphylactic

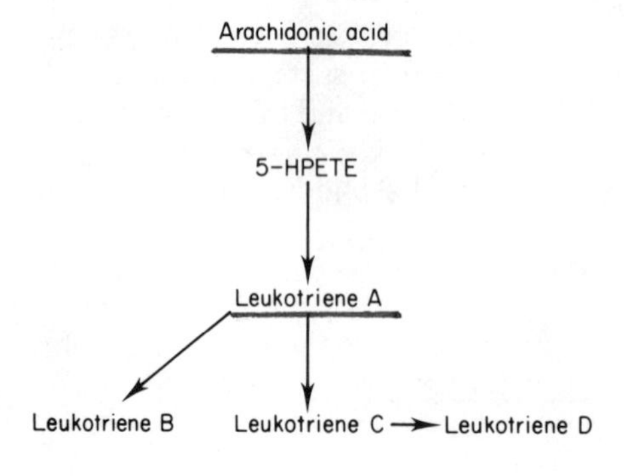

Figure 16.3 Formation of leukotrienes (5-HPETE is 5-hydroperoxy-eicosatetraenoic acid)

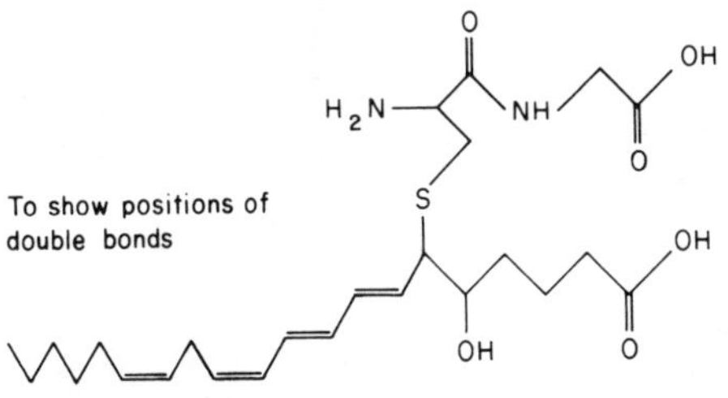

Figure 16.4 Reported structure for SRS-A from guinea-pig lung (from Morris *et al.*, 1980, reproduced by courtesy of the authors and publisher).

conditions and allergic states, SRS is immunologically released from mast cells and is usually referred to as SRS-A. Leukotrienes such as LTC (leukotriene C) and LTD (leukotriene D) also possess SRS-A activity. The structure of SRS-A obtained from guinea-pig lung is shown in *Figure 16.4* (Morris *et al.*, 1980; Samuelsson, 1980).

5-Hydroxytryptamine

5-Hydroxytryptamine (serotonin, enteramine) occurs widely in the body, particularly in the chromaffin cells of the gastrointestinal tract, and in the spleen, platelets, and brain. Large amounts are found in carcinoid tumours of the intestine, ovary, testis, and bronchus, and may be released from mast cells along with histamine in allergic conditions. Morphine and reserpine cause its release in animals, and the tissues in which it is found become depleted. It is synthesized in the body from tryptophan, broken down by monoamine oxidase, and excreted in the urine as 5-hydroxyindoleacetic acid (*Figure 16.5*).

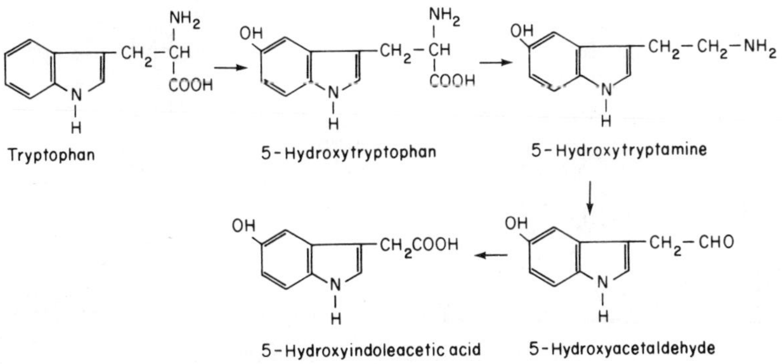

Figure 16.5 Synthesis and metabolism of 5-hydroxytryptamine (5-HT). 5-HT is converted to 5-hydroxyacetaldehyde by monoamine oxidase

Although its physiological significance is not yet known, it is believed to have some action on the CNS as its antagonists cause mental aberrations. It has been suggested that it might be important in the control of sleep. It may also have a role in the maintenance of cardiovascular tone and intestinal gland activity. Although it is released from the platelets when blood clots, it has no action on the clotting process but may shorten the bleeding time as a consequence of its vasoconstrictor action. Its vascular response when injected depends upon the dose administered, the state of vasomotor tone, and whether or not an anaesthetic is employed. The response also varies with different species. Often there is a transient fall in blood pressure, followed by a more prolonged rise. The fall is probably due to vagal reflex action as it can be abolished by atropine and similar drugs. The rise is due to vasoconstriction, and will still take place in the presence of ganglion-blocking drugs. Other actions include hyperpnoea, antidiuresis, and diarrhoea.

Carcinoid tumours may be of importance to anaesthetists; such patients may present preoperatively with cyanosis, raised jugular venous pressure, oedema, wheezing, and right-sided heart murmurs and thus mimic heart failure. An estimation of urinary 5-hydroxyindoleacetic acid will confirm the diagnosis. Carcinoid tumours may also give rise to sudden and transient episodes of hypertension and skin blanching, alternating with hypotension during anaesthesia.

Many substances antagonize the action of 5-hydroxytryptamine. Two types of 5-HT receptors have been postulated: the M receptor (so-called because morphine antagonizes the action of 5-HT on such receptors) and the D receptor because Dibenyline (phenoxybenzamine) antagonizes the action of 5-HT on the receptors. M receptors were said to be present on autonomic ganglia; D receptors were said to be present in smooth muscle. 5-HT contraction of intestine, bronchioles, blood vessels, and uterus were thought to be mediated via D receptors. Aminophylline is an effective antagonist, both to 5-HT and to histamine, and is said to be an effective antidote to the bronchospasm found in the carcinoid syndrome. Two D receptor antagonists which are available are methysergide, a congener of lysergic acid diethylamide (LSD), and cyproheptadine. Methysergide has been used chiefly as a prophylactic against migrainous headache. Cyproheptadine is of interest in that it is also a very potent antihistamine, and is of use in various allergic diseases. It is also a non-hormonal appetite stimulant both in animals and in man, although its therapeutic value is somewhat questionable. The D and M receptor theory is now being superseded. Recent studies on the CNS have suggested that there are three types of 5-HT receptors. These have been called 5-HT_1, 5-HT_2 and 5-HT_3 receptors. Antidepressant drugs have been found to increase the sensitivity of 5-HT_1 and 5-HT_2 receptors for 5-HT. There are 5-HT receptors in the spinal cord which are involved in the analgesic effect of morphine. These receptors may be 5-HT_3 receptors, or a different type altogether (Haigler, 1981).

Angiotensin

This compound, which is formed *in vivo*, is the most powerful pressor agent known. It exists in the plasma as an inactive precursor, angiotensinogen, which is converted by renin into angiotensin I, a decapeptide which is also relatively inactive (renin is secreted by special juxtaglomerular cells in the kidney, located in the walls of the afferent arterioles as they enter the glomeruli). Angiotensin I is converted into the active angiotensin II, an octapeptide, by converting enzymes found in all tissues, but principally in the lung. Angiotensin II is rapidly inactivated by peptidases. Angiotensin acts on receptors in smooth muscle independently of those reacting to noradrenaline. It depolarizes chromaffin cells in the adrenal medulla to release adrenaline; it selectively increases the synthesis and secretion of aldosterone from the adrenal cortex with little effect on other steroid hormone production.

The functions of the renin–angiotensin system are those of water and electrolyte balance: factors that tend to lower the blood volume, the perfusion pressure of the kidney, or plasma sodium concentration stimulate the system to conserve sodium and water. Excessive secretion of renin is also a factor in the pathogenesis of some cases of hypertension.

Preparations of angiotensin amide are available and have been used for their pressor properties. Angiotensin has less tendency to provoke dysrhythmias and does not cause venospasm or tissue necrosis. It does not, however, constrict capacitance vessels, and has no inotropic effect on cardiac muscle. Angiotensin antagonists such as captopril are now becoming available and these may develop into important therapeutic agents.

Plasma kinins

There are two plasma kinins, a decapeptide called kallidin and a nonapeptide called bradykinin. Both are formed from an inactive precursor, kininogen, which is an α_2-globulin. This conversion is achieved by a variety of enzymes, including kallikreins, trypsin, plasmin, and proteolytic enzymes in snake and insect venoms. Of these, plasma kallikrein and the venoms produce bradykinin, whereas glandular kallikreins (in saliva, pancreatic juice, and so on) produce kallidin. It is notable that all of the ingredients for the production of kinins are present in the plasma. However, the kallikrein is present as an inactive precursor, prekallikrein. Its conversion into kallikrein is initiated by many of the same factors as initiate clotting, for example factor VII, the Hageman factor, and contact with glass and damaged tissues, and the process involves a 'cascade' of enzymatic reactions reminiscent of that which initiates coagulation. The half-life of kinins in plasma is less than 1 minute, being enzymatically degraded by peptidases and proteinases.

Like other autacoids, the plasma kinins are highly active, causing vasodilatation, increased capillary permeability and pain. They relax vascular smooth muscle and a fall in blood pressure can occur by this mechanism. However, they contract the smooth muscle of the bronchioles, the uterus, and the intestine. They have no therapeutic applications at present. The kinins have been implicated in the pathogenesis of gout, acute inflammatory responses, hypersensitivity reactions, and traumatic shock. Unfortunately there are no specific antagonists comparable to the antihistamines. However, there are inhibitors of kallikrein activation such as aprotinin which may be of benefit in certain situations (*see* below).

Substance P

This was discovered in 1931 and was first isolated as a powder, hence called substance P. It is now known to be an undecapeptide. Substance P and related undecapeptides have been called tachykinins. Substance P contracts gastro-intestinal smooth muscle. In contrast to bradykinin it has a fast onset of action but it has similar actions on smooth muscle, contracting bronchial smooth muscle and relaxing vascular smooth muscle. Its physiological role may be as a local hormone controlling peristalsis. It is also found in sensory nerves, in the brain, for example, in the substantia nigra, and in the spinal cord, especially the posterior roots and columns. It thus may also be of importance in the control of pain pathways.

Enzymes

Another large class of specialized chemicals is the enzymes.

Enzymes are formed by body cells. They may remain within the cell or be secreted by it. Those secreted may circulate in extracellular fluids or be discharged externally such as into the alimentary tract. Their action is to break down, activate, or inactivate other chemical substances in body tissues or the digestive system, and this may be brought about by oxidation, hydrolysis, deamination, or more complex processes. Thus, acetylcholine is hydrolysed by cholinesterase, adrenaline is oxidized by amine oxidase and catechol-*O*-methyl transferase, and proteins, carbohydrates, and fats are converted into simpler products in the alimentary tract.

Although other substances play a part in their actions, those enzymes that have been purified are all of a protein nature. The proteins are composed of peptide chains and enzymes are globular, not fibrous, proteins. They can be composed either of single or multiple peptide chains. Ribonuclease has only a single chain of 124 amino acid residues; insulin is composed of two peptide chains, one of 21 and the other 30 amino acid residues.

The activity of an enzyme is thought to reside in a certain part of it which is called an active or catalytic site. This site probably consists of a small area of amino acid residues arranged in a very specific manner in such a way that it enhances the particular type of chemical reaction that the enzyme catalyses. It probably has also a geometrical arrangement of active groups which is complementary to that of the substrate on which it acts so that only those substrates or compounds of a very similar structure can combine with the enzyme at its site of activity.

For an enzyme to act quickly in a particular reaction it must form, temporarily, an unstable complex with its substrate. Frequently the enzyme cannot act on the substrate alone and it requires a coenzyme to be present. Many of the vitamins play an important role, biologically, by acting in this manner.

It may be that most drugs act by accelerating or slowing some enzyme process, but until more is known about their action, not only on individual cells or organs but also on some of the vital contents of the cell, little will be understood about the mechanisms involved.

Amine oxidases

There are at least two distinct types of amine oxidases – monoamine oxidase and diamine oxidase. The former is rather non-specific in that it is responsible for catalysing the destructive deamination of many different types of amine. These include adrenaline, many other sympathomimetic amines, and 5-hydroxytryptamine. It affects tyramine, phenylethylamine, and phenylephrine, but ephedrine, amphetamine, and mescaline are resistant to its action. It is also ineffective against histamine, which can be broken down by diamine oxidase. It is, however, responsible for the second stage of the major metabolic degradation of histamine, converting methylhistamine into methylimidazoleacetic acid.

Although they are inhibitors of this enzyme, amphetamine and ephedrine owe their sympathomimetic action to their ability to liberate noradrenaline from nerve terminals.

A physiological role of monoamine oxidase is the intraneuronal conversion to inactive metabolites of any noradrenaline that leaks from storage granules.

It is a mitochrondrial enzyme which is present in the brain, kidney, lung, liver, and intestine. The largest amount is found in the liver and it may be primarily concerned with the breakdown of certain amines formed by bacterial action in the gut. Monoamine oxidase inhibitors are rapidly active against the enzyme in the liver but have less effect on the brain enzyme. There are two iso-enzymes; monoamine oxidase A which is present in peripheral tissues, and monoamine oxidase B which is present in the brain. Selegiline, a type B monoamine oxidase inhibitor, has been claimed to enhance the activity of levodopa in patients with Parkinson's disease. Monoamine oxidase A inhibitors include iproniazid, isocarboxazid, phenelzine, tranylcypromine, and pargyline; this last substance has been used in the treatment of hypertension, while the remainder are employed in the treatment of certain forms of depression. Their usage, toxic effects, and important interactions with certain foods and drugs are discussed on page 227.

It has been demonstrated that there is an enzyme in certain tissues which is capable of destroying histamine. This enzyme is diamine oxidase, commonly called histaminase. Experimentally it is effective, particularly with weak solutions of this substance. Histamine absorbed from the intestine may be inactivated in the intestinal mucosa where, together with the kidney, the enzyme is present in greatest amount.

Diamine oxidase plays a secondary role in the normal breakdown of histamine, 25–35 per cent of an injected dose appearing as metabolites attributable to its action. The remainder is methylated by imidazole-*N*-methyl transferase. The majority of the methylhistamine so formed is then oxidized by monoamine oxidase.

There is a marked increase in histaminolytic activity of plasma during normal pregnancy, which may be attributable to an increase in enzyme elaborated in the placenta. This increase begins at about the third month, reaches a maximum at the sixth and continues until term. After delivery it drops abruptly. Retained placental tissue is associated with a continuing high level. The significance of this rise is not known.

Carbonic anhydrase

Carbonic anhydrase catalyses the reaction $H_2O+CO_2 \rightleftharpoons H_2CO_3$. It is a natural enzyme, a zinc-protein compound found in the erythrocytes, whose function it is to accelerate the transfer of carbon dioxide from the tissues to the red cells in the capillaries, and from the red cells in the lung capillaries to the alveolar air. Without the action of this enzyme the transfer of carbon dioxide would be too slow to be effective.

It has been shown that in the stomach the enzyme is localized in the oxyntic cells and that they contain five to six times as much enzyme as the red corpuscles. Under appropriate experimental conditions it is possible to block secretion of gastric acid by enzyme inhibition, but these secretory processes are insensitive *in vivo* to ordinary doses of carbonic anhydrase inhibitors and this effect has no therapeutic use. The enzyme is present in the eye where it probably plays a role in the secretion of the aqueous humour. Inhibitors are of value, therefore, in the treatment of glaucoma.

Carbonic anhydrase inhibitors affect renal tubular function (*see* page 399) but more than 99 per cent of the enzyme in the kidney must be inhibited before the effects become apparent. An inhibitor of carbonic anhydrase, dichlorphenamide, has also been used in the treatment of chronic respiratory failure. The mechanism of action is not clear, but it may be central, and due to a local increase in carbon dioxide tension in the brain affecting respiratory drive. The lowering of arterial P_{CO_2} brought about is usually not striking.

Cholinesterases

There are two main enzymes; acetylcholinesterase, also known as true cholinesterase, and plasma cholinesterase, often referred to as pseudo-cholinesterase.

Acetylcholinesterase

Acetylcholinesterase is widely distributed in the body and is found in erythrocytes and in the region of synapses and nerve endings wherever acetylcholine is the chemical transmitter. Inhibitors of this enzyme are important therapeutic substances; they are widely employed as insecticides and some are known to be the most toxic human poisons ever developed. The behaviour of the enzyme and its inhibitors is discussed in Chapter 10.

Plasma cholinesterase

This enzyme is elaborated in the liver, and the serum level closely parallels that of serum albumin, except in albumin-losing nephritis. The esteratic site does not seem to be closely related to an effective anionic site, and the enzyme readily hydrolyses other esters, including benzoylcholine, suxamethonium, propanidid, and procaine. Its physiological role is not known. Complete absence of the enzyme has been reported and was compatible with normal health. The serum level of enzyme may be low in advanced liver disease and malnutrition, and is depressed by many cholinesterase inhibitors. These include therapeutic agents such as ecothiopate eye drops, tacrine, hexafluorenium, some anti-cancer agents, and organophosphate poisons, including many insecticides and the nerve gases. Prosthetic inhibitors of acetylcholinesterase have comparatively less action on plasma cholinesterase, although the relative effects in the body depend on additional factors such as lipid solubility. For example, hexafluorenium is a potent acetylcholinesterase inhibitor *in vitro*, but has no such action *in vivo*, and is used as an inhibitor of plasma cholinesterase.

The importance of this enzyme depends on its essential role in the breakdown of suxamethonium, and procaine-like esters. In practice, the action of suxamethonium is not clinically prolonged until the enzyme has been about 80 per cent inhibited.

Atypical enzymes, genetically determined, have been identified which have a limited capacity to metabolize suxamethonium. These atypical enzymes are resistant to the action of various inhibitors. The 'usual' enzyme has been designated E_1^u, meaning that the 'usual' enzyme is found at the first esterase locus. An individual with the genotype $E_1^uE_1^u$ is homozygous for the usual gene, elaborating the usual enzyme. Genes E_1^a and E_1^f have been identified using 10^{-5}M dibucaine and 10^{-5}M fluoride as inhibitors. E_1^s is a silent gene which does not elaborate any enzyme.

The pattern of inheritance is consistent with the view that plasma cholinesterase elaboration is largely under the influence of a pair of allelomorphic non-dominant autosomal genes. A second locus has, however, been identified, and has been named the C_5 variant on the basis of its electrophoretic separation. Those who possess this additional activity (a small minority) do not show 'resistance' to suxamethonium.

Choline acetylase

This enzyme catalyses the final step in the synthesis of acetylcholine. In the initial steps of this synthesis phosphoro-transacetylase catalyses the formation of adenyl acetate from acetate and adenosine triphosphate (ATP) and then the transfer of the acetate moiety from this compound to coenzyme A (CoA). Choline acetylase now catalyses the reaction between CoA acetate and choline with the formation of acetylcholine.

Choline acetylase is found in the nervous system in any location in which cholinesterase and acetylcholine are also present, and is essential for the normal function of the acetylcholine mechanism. Hemicholinium prevents acetylcholine synthesis and its configuration suggests that it inhibits choline acetylase by acting as a false substrate in place of choline.

Hyaluronidase

The accidental finding that aqueous extracts of normal testicle, when added to vaccinia virus and injected intradermally, produced unusually widespread lesions, led to the suggestion of the presence of a 'spreading factor'. This factor was later obtained from many sources, as widely diverse as streptococci and snake venom. Subsequent investigation showed that this spreading factor was an enzyme. It was named hyaluronidase as it was demonstrated that its specific substrate was hyaluronic acid. It depolymerizes hyaluronic acid which is a mucopolysaccharide containing glycuronic acid and *N*-acetylglucosamine and is now regarded as the tissue cement or ground substance of the mesenchyme. Hyaluronidase is non-toxic and will produce a reversible reduction in the viscosity of the intercellular matrix. It also has mucolytic properties when applied topically to mucous surfaces.

Hyaluronidase is used with local analgesics to spread their effect and increase the area of analgesia. It is advisable, however, to use adrenaline to delay absorption which would otherwise be accelerated. It may also be useful in the reduction of inflammatory swellings due to trauma, and in the dispersal of irritant substances such as thiopentone inadvertently injected into subcutaneous tissues. When it is impossible to administer fluids by intravenous or other routes, hyaluronidase may be used as an aid to hypodermoclysis. Its effect seems to be dependent upon the state of the subcutaneous tissue. When these tissues are loosely constructed, the rate of absorption of fluid is increased two-fold, but where the subcutaneous tissue turgor is high the rate of fluid administration can be increased to a much greater extent.

DOSAGE AND ADMINISTRATION

For use with local analgesics various strengths have been recommended. The addition of 1000 iu to 20 ml of the analgesic solution is common practice and gives satisfactory results. To aid in the dispersal of thiopentone injected perivenously 1500 iu may be dissolved in 5–10 ml of sterile water and injected into the surrounding tissues. For hypodermoclysis 1500 iu are effective when mixed with 500–1000 ml of infusion fluid. As hyaluronidase is non-toxic and free from side effects, accurate measurement of dose is not essential.

Proteinases

Proteinases are enzymes that break down protein. They include trypsin, chymotrypsin, plasmin, thromboplastin activators, and carboxypeptidases. Trypsin and chymotrypsin are important digestive enzymes produced in the pancreas; thromboplastin activators and plasmin, also referred to as fibrinolysin, are proteinases which are essential in the formation and removal of fibrin, processes which in health are normally in dynamic equilibrium.

Proteinases obtained from microbial and fungal sources have been used to dissolve clot, both in closed cavities and intravascularly to unblock haemodialysis shunts and dissolve emboli. They are discussed in Chapter 18.

Inhibitors of proteinases are multivalent and can inhibit kallikrein activation. Proteinase inhibition may thus be useful therapeutically. A naturally occurring inhibitor, aprotinin, and a synthetic inhibitor, ε-aminocaproic acid (EACA), are available. They form a reversible complex with proteinases and are, therefore, competitive enzyme inhibitors.

The main indications for proteinase inhibitor therapy are acute pancreatitis and certain cases of pathological bleeding. In acute pancreatitis, proteolytic and lipolytic enzymes escape from the pancreas and give rise to much of the systemic illness; present evidence suggests that the administration of proteinase inhibitors may be beneficial in alleviating pain and hypotension. Kallikrein inactivation has been recommended for the control of pathological bleeding, when, it is sugggested, natural inhibitors are overwhelmed by a great increase in proteolytic enzyme activation (*see* Chapter 18).

Haigler, H. J. (1981) Serotonergic receptors in the central nervous system. In *Neurotransmitter Receptors, Part 2 – Biogenic Amines*, p. 1, Eds. Yamamura, H. I. and Enna, S. J. London: Chapman Hall

Moncada, S. and Vane, J. R. (1978) Unstable metabolites of arachidonic acid and their role in haemostasis and thrombosis. *British Medical Bulletin,* **34,** 129

Moncada, S. and Vane, J. R. (1979) Arachidonic acid metabolites and the interaction between platelets and blood vessel walls. *New England Journal of Medicine,* **300**, 1142

Morris, H. R., Taylor, G. W., Piper, J. Priscilla and Tippins, J. R. (1980) Structure of slow-reacting substance of anaphylaxis from guinea-pig lung. *Nature,* **285,** 104

Samuelsson, B. (1980) The leukotrienes: a new group of biologically active compounds including SRS-A. *Trends in Pharmacological Science,* **1,** 227

Shaw, J. F. L. (1980) Prostacyclin: potential therapeutic roles. *Hospital Update,* **6,** 301

17

Hormones

The nature of hormones and endocrine disease makes it necessary to consider aspects of endocrine disease and the physiological roles of hormones, as well as the use of hormones in a strictly pharmacological sense. Endocrine disorders are unusual in human disease in several ways. Many of them are characterized by deviations from normal which, in mild cases, lie only just outside the range of normal physiology. More severe disease is characterized by changes that are recognizable as increases or decreases in physiological functions although sometimes, of course, frankly pathological changes supervene.

Endocrine glands are particularly liable to undergo neoplastic change, usually benign, and often the tumour retains the capacity to synthesize the hormone produced by the parent tissue. The hormone output from most endocrine glands is controlled physiologically by a system of feedback modulation but most hormone-secreting tumours escape from this control and excess secretion results.

Nearly all hormones are available for therapeutic use and usually have applications, in larger doses, which are essentially pharmacological as opposed to their physiological use in replacement therapy. The anaesthetist may wish to employ hormones in either way but will, in addition, encounter patients in whom hormone excess or deficiency, either spontaneous or induced, influences anaesthesia.

Precautions

A particular hazard arises in the administration of an anaesthetic to a patient with an unsuspected endocrine disorder. If this is only, for example, some minor gonadal defect, there is no material danger, but if the patient has Addison's disease the consequences could be serious. It is important that the possibility of unrecognized disease be borne in mind and superficial explanations for changes such as weight loss should not necessarily be accepted. Some simple observations should be made and the following points will be helpful.

1. If the patient's weight has not changed much and the pulse rate is normal, cryptic thyroid disease is unlikely, although mild hypothyroidism in the young or middle-aged patient is easily missed. Diabetes mellitus and adrenal insufficiency are also improbable. A goitre should be sought as this may impede intubation.
2. If there is no glycosuria, significant diabetes is excluded. A history of polyuria or polydipsia should also be sought.

3. If the blood pressure is normal and there is no vomiting, weight loss or pigmentation, adrenal insufficiency is unlikely.
4. If the blood pressure is normal and there is no history of hypertension or paroxysmal headache, phaeochromocytoma is unlikely.
5. If the menses are normal or, in the male, the external genitalia, a major pituitary defect is most unlikely. In the older patient, however, the clinical detection of hypopituitarism is much more difficult.
6. If previous corticosteroid therapy has been discontinued for 3 months or more, a reduced adrenal response is unlikely (but *see* below).

It follows that if the patient's weight is steady, the appetite, sexual function, pulse, and blood pressure are all normal, and there is no glycosuria or recent medication, then cryptic endocrine disease is improbable.

Effects of anaesthesia

The responses of the endocrine system to anaesthesia are variable, complex, and of uncertain significance. In man it is difficult to obtain information that distinguishes between the effects of anaesthesia and the effects of surgery, because there is the ethical problem of giving anaesthetics without operation. Also, changes in plasma levels alone may be misleading because of simultaneous and unrecognized changes in protein binding and/or hormone turnover. Thus, the introduction of relatively simple methods of assay for most hormones has been of only limited value so far, and a large area remains to be explored.

Many of the reports on the endocrine responses to anaesthetic agents are based on small numbers of observations and are not consistent.

Any stress can be expected to diminish carbohydrate tolerance by reducing insulin release but the effect of anaesthetic agents alone, although distinct (Stoelting, 1980), is small (Houghton *et al.*, 1978). Recent evidence indicates no particular effect of halothane (Aarimaa, Syvalahti and Ovaska, 1978). Similarly, an adrenocortical response to stress is to be expected but anaesthesia causes little change in plasma cortisol (Oyama *et al.*, 1979a). Vasopressin is a stress hormone also but again anaesthesia alone has little effect. The choice of drug modifies the response during operation in that there is a greater response with halothane than with morphine (Philbin and Coggins, 1978).

Animal experiments indicate a major effect of anaesthesia on the renin–angiotensin–aldosterone system (Pettinger, 1978) and in man the rise in plasma aldosterone is related to the particular anaesthetic employed, with increasing effects of methoxyflurane, halothane, enflurane, and ether in that order (Oyama *et al.*, 1979b).

Plasma levels of the thyroid hormones show little change although the evidence is conflicting (Halevy *et al.*, 1978; Oyama *et al.*, 1979b). The same is true of the sex hormones and gonadotrophins (Soules *et al.*, 1980).

As Millar (1974) has pointed out, 'It is difficult to comment on the possible functional significance of endocrine responses to anaesthetic agents in relation to the general welfare of the surgical patient'. There is always the possibility that the endocrine responses may be beneficial rather than otherwise and much additional information is required before it can be asserted that one anaesthetic agent is superior to another in this respect.

Aarimaa, M., Syvalahti, E. and Ovaska, J. (1978) Does adrenergic activity suppress insulin secretion during surgery? *Annals of Surgery,* **187,** 68

Halevy, S., Lui-Barnett, M., Ross, P. L. and Roginsky, M. S. (1978) Serum thyroid hormone changes in patients undergoing Caesarean section under general or regional anaesthesia. *British Journal of Anaesthesia,* **50,** 1053

Houghton, A., Hickey, J. B., Ross, S. A. and Dupre, J. (1978) Glucose tolerance during anaesthesia and surgery. Comparison of general and extradural anaesthesia. *British Journal of Anaesthesia,* **50,** 495

Millar, R. A. (1974) Anaesthesia and endocrine secretion. In *Scientific Foundation of Anaesthesia,* 2nd Edn. Eds Scurr, C. and Feldman, S., p. 304. London: Heinemann

Oyama, T.,Taniguchi, K., Ishihari, H., Matsuki, A., Maeda, A., Murakawa, T. and Kudo, T. (1979a) Effects of enflurane anaesthesia and surgery on endocrine function in man. *British Journal of Anaesthesia,* **51,** 141

Oyama, T., Taniguchi, K., Jin, T., Satone, T. and Kudo, T. (1979b) Effects of anaesthesia and surgery on plasma aldosterone concentrations and renin activity in man. *British Journal of Anaesthesia,* **51,** 747

Pettinger, W. A. (1978) Anaesthetics and the renin–angiotensin–aldosterone axis. *Anesthesiology,* **49,** 393

Philbin, D. M. and Coggins, C. H. (1978) Plasma anti-diuretic hormone levels in cardiac surgical patients during morphine and halothane anesthesia. *Anesthesiology,* **49,** 95

Soules, M. R., Sutton, G. P., Hammond, C. B. and Haney, A. F. (1980) Endocrine changes at operation under general anaesthesia; reproductive hormone fluctuations in young women. *Fertility and Sterility,* **33,** 364

Stoelting, R. K. (1980) Metabolic effects of anesthesia. In *International Anesthesiology Clinics,* **18,**(3), Ed. Owens, W. D., p. 53. Boston: Little, Brown & Co.

Pituitary gland (hypophysis) and hypothalamus

The pituitary gland, with its multiple controlling functions, is also the site of functional interaction between the CNS and the endocrine system.

The hypothalamic control of the anterior pituitary is exercised by the secretion of releasing or inhibiting hormones which reach the gland via the portal venous system of the pituitary stalk. The four releasing hormones for thyrotrophin, corticotrophin, growth hormone and both gonadotrophins have been characterized. The release-inhibiting hormone for growth hormone is somatostatin and that for prolactin is dopamine; other inhibitors have been postulated. Feedback modulation of anterior pituitary secretion appears to be mediated either by variation in the sensitivity of the pituitary cells to the hypothalamic hormones or by the rate of secretion of those hormones. Thyrotrophin-releasing hormone and gonadotrophin-releasing hormone are useful in endocrine function testing and the latter now has a place in therapy.

The posterior pituitary hormones, oxytocin and vasopressin (antidiuretic hormone), are synthesized in the hypothalamus and pass down into the gland from where they are released. After surgical ablation of the gland, normal control of water-balance is usually soon restored spontaneously so that it must be presumed that when necessary these hormones can be released into the circulation directly from the hypothalamus.

Hypopituitarism

Hypopituitarism may occur either as a general loss of pituitary function with deficiencies of all the hormones (panhypopituitarism) or as a partial hypopituitarism with a variable degree of deficiency of one or several hormones individually.

The commonest causes of hypopituitarism are surgical ablation, irradiation, trauma, thrombosis, pressure from a tumour inside or close to the pituitary fossa, infection, granulomatous disease, and postpartum necrosis (Sheehan's syndrome).

The clinical features of panhypopituitarism are due largely to a combination of hypothyroidism, hypogonadism and adrenocortical insufficiency, plus growth failure in children. The patient is likely to be unduly sensitive to all drugs and anaesthetic agents and to have a reduced or absent adrenocortical response to stress. As panhypopituritarism in the elderly patient may not be readily apparent, an unexpected anaesthetic hazard may arise and emergency steroid therapy may be needed. In the treated patient on full replacement therapy with thyroxine and corticosteroids no particular anaesthetic difficulty is to be expected although additional corticosteroids will be required, as described below for Addison's disease.

Partial hypopituitarism may occur without obvious pathology, presumably due to subtle changes in hypothalamic–pituitary function leading in some patients to short stature, infertility, menstrual disorder, or eunuchoidism. Rare examples of isolated thyrotrophin or corticotrophin deficiency have been reported; these are significant in the present context because they may present as hypothyroidism or Addison's disease. Deficiencies of the other pituitary hormones do not appear to present any anaesthetic hazard.

Diabetes insipidus

Diabetes insipidus is due to a lack of antidiuretic hormone (vasopressin) which is secreted by the posterior pituitary and hypothalamus. The dominant clinical feature of a large diuresis only becomes prominent if there is an adequate level of circulating corticosteroids, and therefore in complete pituitary destruction diuresis may not be present and will appear when corticosteroids are given.

In treated diabetes insipidus, no particular anaesthetic difficulty should arise. Probably the patient will be receiving desmopressin (a long-acting analogue of vasopressin) by nasal spray and this should be given as usual on the day of operation and continued as necessary (usually twice a day only) during the postoperative period. If the patient is not able to co-operate in taking the spray, desmopressin may be given by intramuscular or intravenous injection in a dose of 1–4 μg daily, as necessary, to control the urine volume.

Alternatively, thiazide diuretics have a paradoxical action in diabetes insipidus and reduce urine flow. Chlorpropamide and tolbutamide may help in the patient with partial loss of vasopressin secretion; carbamazepine may be effective also. If patients with diabetes insipidus are being maintained on these drugs, it is preferable to discontinue them and rely on vasopressin or desmopressin during and following major surgery.

Hypophysectomy

For therapeutic reasons, the pituitary may be attacked by external irradiation, the implantation of radioactive seeds, or open surgery. It is the latter which poses anaesthetic problems. The operation is now relatively common and is carried out for the removal of pituitary tumours or microadenomas, often with the intention of leaving behind a functioning pituitary remnant. If there is much suprasellar extension of the tumour, particularly if the optic nerves are compressed, operation from above by a transcranial route is necessary. Otherwise, a trans-sphenoidal approach is favoured because it is a less traumatic procedure.

The preoperative situation is variable; if the tumour has produced hypopituitarism, the patient may already be taking replacement hormones.

The essential feature of hormonal management is to give sufficient hydrocortisone to prevent an addisonian crisis. Opinions differ as to the optimal dose. One scheme is to give hydrocortisone in the intravenous infusion fluids at a rate of 200 mg in the first day, 100 mg in the second day, and thereafter oral hydrocortisone in reducing dosage to reach 20–30 mg/day after 5 days. Mineralocorticoid treatment is not required.

The turnover of thyroxine in the circulation is so slow (*see* Thyroid) that doses can safely be omitted for several days. In patients with previously normal thyroid function there is a choice. Some authorities think it is best to assume that thyroid-stimulating hormone (TSH) secretion will fail and start thyroxine replacement treatment in full doses (150 μg/day in a single dose by mouth) a few days after operation. Alternatively, thyroxine treatment may be withheld and given only if found to be necessary by monitoring the level of plasma thyroxine – the author favours this latter approach as it avoids unnecessary therapy.

The loss of the other pituitary hormones has no immediate implications except that if the patient is diabetic the sensitivity to insulin will be much increased, so this drug should be given with extreme caution. Immediately after operation a diuresis begins and this may be substantial so that careful fluid replacement is needed to avoid dehydration. Desmopressin can be used freely to control urine volume if necessary, the intranasal dose being 10–20 μg once or twice a day. Alternatively, 1–4 μg may be given daily by intravenous or intramuscular injection. After pituitary surgery about half the patients need desmopressin and some degree of diabetes insipidus may persist for several weeks, but it is most unusual for this defect to be permanent.

Whether by chance or design, in some patients hypophysectomy is incomplete. Sufficient pituitary tissue remains or regenerates to assume normal functions so that some or all replacement therapy may be withdrawn, although stress response may still be inadequate. In a few patients, even menstruation and normal unaided pregnancy has occurred.

Further reading

Abboud, C. F. and Laws, E. R. (1979) Clinical endocrinological approach to hypothalamic–pituitary disease. *Journal of Neurosurgery*, **51**, 271

Corticotrophin

Corticotrophin injection (*BP*), Corticotrophin gelatin injection (*BP*), Corticotrophin zinc injection (*BP*) and Tetracosactrin acetate (*BP*). A depot preparation of tetracosactrin is available.

Synonyms: adrenocorticotrophic hormone, ACTH.

Chemical constitution: corticotrophin is a polypeptide containing 39 amino acids. The series of acids numbered 1–24 are common to all species and this portion of the whole polypeptide contains all the hormonal activity. The region numbered 25–33 contains the species differences and immunological specificity. The amino acid sequence 1–24 of natural corticotrophin is available as a synthetic product termed tetracosactrin.

PHYSIOLOGY

Corticotrophin stimulates the adrenal cortex, particularly the zona reticularis and fasciculata, leading to the formation and release of various corticosteroids but particularly cortisol and dehydroepiandrosterone (DHA). Corticotrophin is released from the anterior pituitary under the influence of the corticotrophin-releasing hormone. The release varies in a cyclical fashion over a 24-hour period and this is responsible for the diurnal rhythm of plasma cortisol level. In addition, the release of corticotrophin is controlled by a feedback system involving the level of plasma cortisol. The synthetic corticosteroids are active in this respect also.

INDICATIONS

Corticotrophin stimulates the adrenal cortex and is of most value in adrenal function tests. It can be used also to produce the pharmacological effects of increased levels of cortisol via endogenous production in any situation where systemic corticosteroids are indicated. The response varies, so dosage is somewhat uncertain. It has been suggested that corticotrophin is superior to corticosteroids in the treatment of some diseases, but this is unproved. Adrenal atrophy is prevented but hypothalamic–pituitary–adrenocortical responsiveness is nevertheless depressed.

The action of the aqueous preparations of corticotrophin and tetracosactrin lasts only a few hours; the other preparations are all 'slow release' and act for at least 24 hours. Tetracosactrin depot often has an even longer effect. Tetracosactrin is probably the superior preparation because of its purity, reliability of potency, and reduced likelihood of producing allergic reactions.

DOSAGE AND ADMINISTRATION

Corticotrophin and tetracosactrin have to be injected. Aqueous tetracosactrin in a dose of 0.25 mg by intramuscular injection may be used for an adrenal stimulation test. Tetracosactrin depot by intramuscular injection is usually given in a dose of 0.5–1.0 mg every day or less frequently as necessary. The dose of corticotrophin is usually in the range of 20–120 u/day.

PRECAUTIONS

Corticotrophin leads to suppression of the pituitary–adrenal response to stress and therefore its use calls for the same precautions as the use of corticosteroids (*see* page 437).

Vasopressin

Vasopressin injection (*BP* and *USP*), lypressin injection (*BP*) (lysine vasopressin), desmopressin (*BAN*)

Chemical constitution: As shown below. Lysine vasopressin is identical to vasopressin except for the substitution of lysine for arginine. Desmopressin is 1-desamino-8-D-arginine vasopressin, that is, it has lost an amino group from part of cystine at the 1 position and has D-arginine instead of L-arginine at the 8 position. Oxytocin has other amino acids at positions 3 and 8. The conventional numbering of the positions in the molecule is confusing because although vasopressin is an octapeptide, cystine, containing a disulphide bridge, is accorded two positions for its two halves (1 and 6) and thus there are nine positions in all.

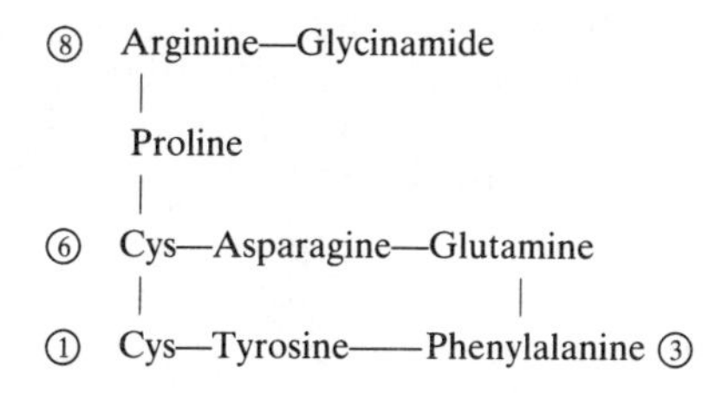

PHYSIOLOGY

Despite its name, and the fact that it can be shown to contract smooth muscle and act as a pressor agent, a major physiological role of vasopressin in man is as the 'antidiuretic hormone'. Vasopressin acts on the distal tubule and collecting duct of the nephron to increase their permeability to water, thus increasing the concentration and reducing the volume of the urine. Vasopressin release is controlled by changes in osmotic pressure of the plasma and constitutes the major control system for body water and urine volume (*see* page 396 for a more detailed account of the role of vasopressin in the physiological control of water balance).

INDICATIONS

The analogues of vasopressin are used in the treatment of diabetes insipidus. Vasopressin and its analogues are not used as pressor agents.

DOSAGE AND ADMINISTRATION

The analogue desmopressin is recommended because of its prolonged action. It may be given by intramuscular or intravenous injection in a dose of 1–4 μg once a day, or as a nasal spray of 10–20 μg once or twice a day. Lysine vasopressin may bc used as a nasal spray but more frequent doses are needed.

PRECAUTIONS

Vasopressin analogues may cause vasoconstriction at the site of injection and nasal administration may cause mucosal damage. Nausea and intestinal colic may occur. Because of their constrictive effect on the coronary arteries, vasopressin analogues should be avoided or used sparingly in the elderly and in persons with ischaemic heart disease (*see* management of diabetes insipidus, above).

Oxytocin

Although oxytocin is a pituitary hormone, its use is mainly as a uterine stimulant and it is therefore considered in Chapter 15.

Thyrotrophin-releasing hormone

Chemical constitution: L-pyroglutamyl-L-histidyl-L-prolinamide

Thyrotrophin-releasing hormone (TRH) is a synthetic tripetide which causes an immediate release of TSH and prolactin from the anterior pituitary gland with a consequent rise in the serum levels.

INDICATIONS

TRH is used to test pituitary function and to aid the diagnosis of thyroid disease. The level of plasma TSH is measured before and up to 60 minutes after the administration of TRH. An absent or impaired response may indicate pituitary disease, whereas a delayed response implicates the hypothalamus. In primary hyperthyroidism there is no response in TSH. A lack of response may be observed also in patients with thyroid eye disease but apparently normal thyroid function.

DOSAGE AND ADMINISTRATION

TRH is given as an intravenous bolus of 200 μg.

PRECAUTIONS

There do not appear to be any absolute contraindications to TRH administration, but as it has been suspected of causing smooth muscle contraction it should be administered with caution to patients with bronchial asthma, obstructive airway disease, or myocardial ischaemia.

Adrenal cortex

All of the steroid hormones have the same primary molecular framework, sometimes called the steroid nucleus (*see Figure 17.1*). The structures of both rings and side chains can be modified in many ways; slight changes can cause major differences in biological activity. Many corticosteroids have been isolated or synthesized and some aspects of the physiology of the adrenal cortex are complex. However, in man only three corticosteroids are released into the circulation in significant amounts and only two of these are of major physiological importance.

Cortisol

The most important hormone produced by the adrenal cortex is cortisol (hydrocortisone) which is released at the rate of about 30–60 μmol/day. In the circulation about 90 per cent of cortisol is carried bound to a specific globulin called transcortin. The half-life of cortisol in the plasma is about 90 minutes. Cortisol is predominantly glucocorticoid in its actions with some mineralocorticoid activity (*see Table 17.1*, page 434). Cortisol is synthesized in the zona fasciculata and reticularis of the adrenal cortex under the influence of corticotrophin; the resulting level of plasma cortisol controls corticotrophin secretion through a system of feedback modulation involving the hypothalamus and corticotrophin-releasing hormone. The synthetic corticosteroids used in therapy also suppress corticotrophin secretion but the other corticosteroids released physiologically by the adrenal cortex do not.

Aldosterone

Aldosterone is synthesized by the zona glomerulosa (or outer layer) of the adrenal cortex and released at the rate of about 150–400 nmol/day. Synthesis and release are not dependent on corticotrophin but are apparently caused by angiotensin II. The renin–angiotensin system is of great theoretical interest, but its practical importance remains to be determined (*see* page 312). Aldosterone is a powerful mineralocorticoid and accounts for about 75 per cent of the total mineralocorticoid activity produced by the adrenal hormones.

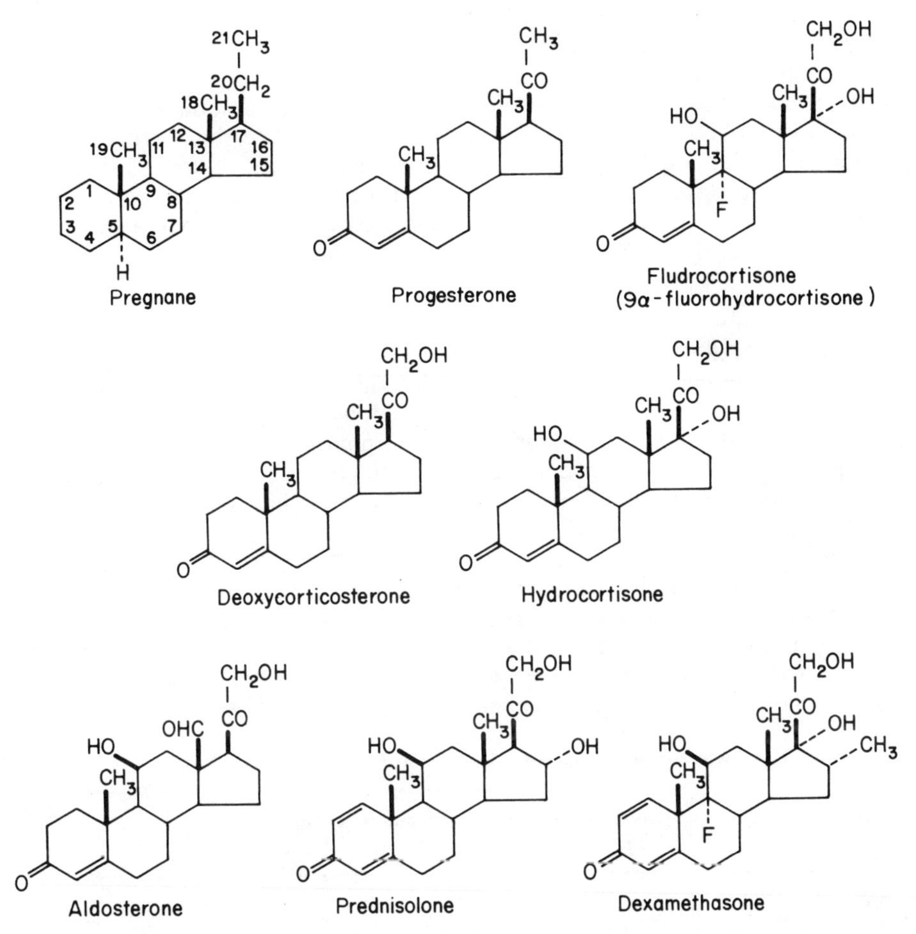

Figure 17.1 The steroid nucleus and structures of some common steroid hormones

Dehydroepiandrosterone

This compound is produced by the same tissue as produces cortisol and is similarly corticotrophin dependent. It has weak androgenic and anabolic properties but although it is released in quantities comparable to cortisol it does not seem to have any physiological role, and after total adrenalectomy normal health can be maintained without DHA being replaced.

Metabolism

Small amounts of free cortisol and free aldosterone are lost in the urine but most of the corticosteroids are metabolized by the liver to a variety of derivatives of low biological activity. These are conjugated with glucuronic, phosphoric, or sulphuric acid and the resulting compounds, without biological activity, are excreted in the urine. With improved methods of estimating plasma corticosteroids, measurement of urinary corticosteroids except for the free hormones is now little used in routine practice.

Actions of corticosteroids

The actions of corticosteroids are classified broadly as mineralocorticoid or glucocorticoid. The mineralocorticoid effect is on the distal renal tubule, to cause the reabsorption of sodium in exchange for potassium. The glucocorticoid effect is generalized and complex. It includes maintenance of blood glucose, anti-inflammatory action, and increased fat synthesis. The mineralocorticoid and glucocorticoid effects can be exercised almost completely independently and this has been exploited in the development of many synthetic compounds.

Synthetic corticosteroids

It has been possible to develop synthetic compounds with almost exclusively glucocorticoid or mineralocorticoid activity (*Table 17.1*). Unfortunately, all the synthetic glucocorticoids, when used in pharmacological doses as anti-inflammatory agents, produce undesirable effects such as weight gain, muscle wasting, osteoporosis, and suppression of the hypothalamic–pituitary–adreno-cortical axis.

It follows that there is little to choose between the various alternatives and usually a selection can be made on the grounds of price, which at present favours prednisone and prednisolone. The exception to this generalization is 9α-fluorohydrocortisone, which is a potent mineralocorticoid with little glucocorticoid activity, which is used to replace aldosterone. It is rather confusing that this material has the pharmacopoeial name of fludrocortisone.

Table 17.1 Relative potencies of corticosteroids in common use

Steroid	*Anti-inflammatory effects**	*Salt retention*
Hydrocortisone	1	++
Cortisone	1	++
Prednisolone	5	+
Prednisone	5	+
Betamethasone	30	±
Dexamethasone	30	±
Fludrocortisone	15	++++

* These values should be taken as an approximate guide only.

Use of corticosteroids

Physiological replacement

For physiological replacement, oral hydrocortisone is preferred although oral cortisone acetate has been used. Hydrocortisone 20 mg in the morning and 10 mg in the evening is a satisfactory regimen and mimics the normal diurnal rhythm to some extent. Parenteral hydrocortisone is suitable for short-term use. In hypopituitarism, aldosterone production is preserved and hydrocortisone is the only replacement corticosteroid required. However, in Addison's disease or after total adrenalectomy most patients require additional mineralocorticoid, and fludrocortisone 100 μg once a day by mouth is suitable.

Pharmacological uses
For use as an anti-inflammatory agent, either prednisone or prednisolone can be recommended as their low mineralocorticoid activity reduces the risk of water retention and hypertension. Despite published statements indicating differences in potency, in clinical practice they appear to be interchangeable at the same dose. The more potent synthetic corticosteroids are particularly valuable in various endocrine function tests, but do not appear to have any advantages for ordinary therapeutic use.

Corticosteroids are of benefit in a variety of inflammatory conditions, such as active rheumatoid arthritis, some types of nephrotic syndrome, systemic lupus erythematosus, bronchial asthma, and ulcerative colitis. Doses vary with the condition from the equivalent of 5 mg to 60 mg of prednisone per day. They are also used topically for ulcerative colitis, in the eye for such conditions as uveitis and iritis, and for various skin disorders. Suitable preparations can also be injected into joints and soft tissues. Corticosteroids are helpful in reducing cerebral oedema associated with acute head injuries, cerebral tumours, and craniotomy. The administration of massive doses of corticosteroids in shock has been recommended by various authors, mainly on anecdotal evidence, and by analogy with shock preparations in the dog. While it is not impossible that they may have some pressor effects in large doses, there is no satisfactory body of fact on which to recommend either for or against them.

Diseases of the adrenal cortex

Cushing's syndrome
Cushing's syndrome is due to prolonged hypersecretion of cortisol either from an adrenal tumour or from adrenal glands rendered hyperplastic by excessive corticotrophin stimulation. This may be released from a malignant tumour of non-endocrine origin or, more typically, from an anterior pituitary gland which is the site of an adenoma.

In the case of an adrenal tumour, the correct and obvious treatment is its surgical removal. The preoperative management will depend on the severity of the condition. In the average case no special precautions are needed, but if there has been severe long-standing Cushing's syndrome, potassium depletion is to be expected and potassium replacement should be attempted. Adrenal-suppressing drugs such as metyrapone may be used. It must be assumed that the remaining normal adrenal will be atrophic, and that following removal of the tumour there will be no capacity for corticosteroid synthesis and full doses must therefore be administered. These must meet not only the basal requirements but also the increased stress of surgery. Also, the patient's tissues will have become habituated to high cortisol levels and replacement must be withdrawn slowly.

During the operation, hydrocortisone 100 mg is given and this may be continued as 100 mg 8-hourly intramuscularly or intravenously for 2 days. Thereafter, it is better to change to treatment by mouth if possible, in a dose of 60 mg 6-hourly at first, diminishing over 2 weeks to about 40 mg/day. Any further reduction of dosage depends on circumstances. Injections of corticotrophin may aid adrenal recovery but will not help the restoration of normal pituitary–adrenal responsiveness and some cortisone replacement may be required for a long time. During the postoperative period the patient is particularly liable to cardiovascular collapse with hypotension, and sepsis. While it is important to administer adequate amounts of corticosteroid, it is wrong to suppose that every set-back should be treated by more of this remedy. To do so may make the Cushing's syndrome steadily worse and distract from more appropriate methods of resuscitation, such as transfusion, pressor agents, and antibiotics, when indicated.

For adrenal hyperplasia (except in patients with ectopic corticotrophin production) treatment in the past has been total bilateral adrenalectomy. The management is similar to that for an adrenal tumour, but with two important differences: mineralocorticoid activity must be provided from the outset in the form of fludrocortisone, in a dose of 100 μg twice a day reducing to 100 μg daily, and replacement doses of cortisone and fludrocortisone must be given for the remainder of the patient's life. However, pituitary ablation may be a better form of treatment.

Addison's disease

The patient with undiscovered Addison's disease faces a severe risk of circulatory collapse during surgery, but this should be treatable with hydrocortisone and salt replacement. In the patient with known Addison's disease or in patients following adrenalectomy, no particular anaesthetic problems should arise provided that the obvious precautions are taken. Replacement therapy should aim to mimic the physiological pituitary–adrenal response which the patient is denied. Normal doses of corticosteroids should be continued until the evening before surgery. Preoperatively, hydrocortisone 100 mg should be given intramuscularly and then further similar doses 8-hourly for 24 hours. This is replaced as soon as possible by oral treatment, 60 mg 6-hourly, diminishing rapidly over 3 days to normal replacement levels. The administration of fludrocortisone should be resumed as soon as possible after surgery. These doses are appropriate for major surgery. For minor procedures lower doses will suffice. For a review and differing recommendations *see* Kehlet (1975).

Conn's syndrome

Conn's syndrome is a rare condition due to an aldosterone-secreting tumour or hyperplasia of the adrenal cortex and is treated by surgical excision.

Congenital adrenal hyperplasia

This rare condition occurs in various forms but all are due to specific enzyme defects in the adrenal which interfere at some stage with the synthesis of cortisol and sometimes aldosterone. Usually there is a concomitant excess production of adrenal androgen. Physiologically the patients should be considered to have Addison's disease because of the cortisol lack, and are treated with replacement therapy as for Addison's disease. If they require intercurrent surgery, the management of their steroid dosage is the same as for Addison's disease.

Previous treatment with corticosteroids

Perhaps the commonest problem that anaesthetists meet in relation to hormone treatment is intercurrent surgery in patients who are having or have had treatment with corticosteroids. Four circumstances may be encountered, as follows.

Patients receiving replacement doses of corticosteroids

These will be patients with hypopituitarism, Addison's disease, or congenital adrenal hyperplasia. Their management is straightforward and has already been discussed.

Patients receiving pharmacological doses of corticosteroids
These are the patients having treatment with doses in excess of replacement requirements for pharmacological (as opposed to physiological) effects. Usually, one of the synthetic steroids, for example prednisone, will have been used. All of the synthetic corticosteroids suppress the release of corticotrophin and when used in pharmacological doses will suppress it completely. This suppression lasts as long as the drug is administered and continues for some time after the drug has been discontinued (*see* below). During the administration of the corticosteroids the capacity of the pituitary–adrenal system to respond to stress is reduced or abolished. If the administration of corticosteroids has been prolonged, the adrenal cortex will be hypotrophic so that the response to corticotrophin will be reduced and slow. Consequently, the patient receiving pharmacological doses of corticosteroids has in effect paralysis of the pituitary–adrenal system and must be dealt with as if he had Addison's disease, using the routine described above. After the short period of increased dose the patient should be returned as soon as possible to his previous regimen.

Patients receiving corticotrophin
These individuals will have raised levels of plasma cortisol and these should be maintained by continuing the corticotrophin injections throughout the period of surgery. For minor surgery, maintenance on the same dose is sufficient. However, the raised levels of cortisol will have paralysed the pituitary–adrenal response to stress just as effectively as treatment with synthetic corticosteroids and therefore the normal corticosteroid response to surgical stress will be diminished or absent. For major surgery additional circulating corticosteroid will be required and this could possibly be achieved by doubling the corticotrophin dose for 3 days and then reverting to the previous regimen. Unfortunately, there is considerable individual variation in the adrenal response to corticotrophin and it is more reliable to add exogenous corticosteroid. It is unlikely that large doses will be required and the addition of hydrocortisone 60 mg, 8-hourly for 3 days by mouth, or by injection when necessary, should suffice. The corticotrophin should be continued unchanged and additional corticosteroid during surgery, if needed, may be given as intravenous hydrocortisone.

Patients who have had treatment with corticosteroids or corticotrophin in the past
The management of these patients is a vexed question and opinions differ. The problem arises because even where treatment with corticosteroids or corticotrophin has been withdrawn carefully, there follows a period of time during which the normal responsiveness of the system to stress is absent or defective, even though the system is able to maintain normal levels of plasma cortisol under basal conditions. Thus there is a danger than an apparently normal person not currently treated with corticosteroids may collapse from acute adrenal insufficiency under surgical stress. Unfortunately, the duration of this danger is variable and unpredictable, although it is likely to be longer following heavy and prolonged corticosteroid treatment.

Within 3 months of ending substantial corticosteroid treatment is is wise to give corticosteroid cover for major surgery with a dosage scale as recommended above (page 436) for Addison's disease. After 3 months, no corticosteroid cover need be given unless the patient has received heavy doses of corticosteroids, for example over 20 mg of prednisone per day for several years, in which case up to 6 months might be considered to be a danger period. If there is the opportunity, the level of plasma cortisol during an intravenous insulin stress test may give evidence as to whether a normal response to surgery is to be expected. In all patients who have received corticosteroids the possibility of adrenal failure should be borne in mind so that rapid treatment with intravenous hydrocortisone may be given if necessary.

Kehlet, H. (1975) A rational approach to dosage and preparation of parenteral therapy during surgical procedures. *Acta Anaesthesiologica Scandinavica,* **19**, 260

Further reading

Nelson, D. H. (1980) *The Adrenal Cortex: Physiological Function and Disease.* Eastbourne: W. D. Saunders

Prednisone and Prednisolone

Prednisone (*BP* and *USP*), Prednisolone (*BP* and *USP*), Prednisolone acetate (*USP*), Prednisolone pivalate (*BP*), Prednisolone sodium phosphate (*BP* and *USP*), Prednisolone sodium succinate for injection (*USP*), Prednisolone succinate (*USP*) and Prednisolone tebutate (*USP*)
Chemical constitution: these synthetic compounds are similar. They are derived from cortisone and hydrocortisone respectively by the single change of inserting a double bond between carbons 1 and 2 (*see Figure 17.1*). The two parent compounds differ in having an =O (cortisone) and an —OH (hydrocortisone) group at the C-11 position.

Related preparations
Derivatives and preparations for intra-articular injection, rectal application, eye drops, and enteric-coated tablets are available in addition to the usual oral preparations.

PHARMACOLOGY
Prednisone and prednisolone normally have an identical therapeutic effect, prednisone being converted into prednisolone by the healthy liver. These compounds are more potent in glucocorticoid action than cortisol, but have only weak sodium-retaining power (*see Table 17.1*).

INDICATIONS
These compounds are the standard preparations for use when the pharmacological effect of steroid therapy is required as they are cheap and less likely to produce troublesome sodium retention and hypertension than cortisone. The indications for corticosteroid treatment both systemically and locally are numerous; the commonest conditions in which it is used are rheumatoid arthritis, asthma, ulcerative colitis, and some skin diseases.

DOSAGE AND ADMINISTRATION
For systemic use the dose of prednisone is usually in the range of 10–60 mg/day in three doses. Maintenance doses of less than 10 mg/day may be useful in some conditions. An enema containing 20 mg is available. The intra-articular dose of a suitable preparation is 25–100 mg. The oral route is usually satisfactory but

intramuscular injections may be used. Some authorities recommend the use of enteric-coated tablets as less likely to cause gastric irritation.

There are other synthetic corticosteroids with similar properties; they tend to be more expensive but some have virtually no sodium-retaining effect, which may be advantageous in some patients.

PRECAUTIONS

All patients receiving systemic corticosteroids (or corticotrophin) should carry a special card indicating the dose and other relevant details. Systemic corticosteroid therapy of any kind produces Cushing's syndrome if the dose is high enough and suppression of pituitary–adrenal responsiveness to stress is likely to occur (*see* page 437). However, local and rectal applications of corticosteroids are unlikely to lead to sufficient systemic absorption to cause significant physiological derangement.

Particular care must be exercised in using corticosteroids in the treatment of patients with peptic ulceration, hypertension, osteoporosis, infections, diabetes mellitus, and pregnancy.

Hydrocortisone

Hydrocortisone (*BP* and *USP*), Hydrocortisone acetate (*BP* and *USP*), Hydrocortisone sodium succinate (*BP* and *USP*)
Chemical name: 11β,17α,21-trihydroxypregn-4-ene-3,20-dione
For structural formula *see Figure 17.1*, p. 433

PHARMACOLOGY

Hydrocortisone is a naturally occurring adrenal hormone, with predominantly glucocorticoid actions. These include maintenance of blood glucose, fat synthesis, and anti-inflammatory effects. It also has some mineralocorticoid actions.

INDICATIONS

Hydrocortisone may be used for physiological replacement when the endogenous supply is inadequate because of disease or suppression of the anterior pituitary or adrenal cortex. Pharmacological doses are used in severe bronchial asthma, in severe illness to improve the resistance to stress, and in particular to maintain blood pressure. It may be used to provide additional hormone at times of surgical stress when the ability of the adrenal gland to respond is believed to be impaired.

DOSAGE AND ADMINISTRATION

Hydrocortisone tablets by mouth are given in a dose of 20 mg each morning and 10 mg each night as a replacement treatment. In some patients variations on this routine seem to be helpful. Hydrocortisone for injection (intravenously or intramuscularly) is given as the sodium phosphate or sodium succinate salts. The usual dose is 50 or 100 mg, which may be repeated every few hours or given as a continuous infusion.

PRECAUTIONS

Replacement treatment with hydrocortisone may need adjustment to the needs of the individual. Replacement doses do not, contrary to common belief, involve the hazards such as osteoporosis associated with the long-term use of corticosteroids in pharmacological doses.

Short-term use of systemic hydrocortisone in large doses is virtually free from obvious side effects and this leads to a tendency to give unnecessarily large amounts. Such therapy may have deleterious effects on wound healing and resistance to infection.

Adrenal medulla

The chromaffin tissue of the adrenal medulla shares with the brain and sympathetic nerve endings the capacity to synthesize the catecholamines (*see* page 317). Chromaffin tissue occurs also in the organ of Zuckerkandl and in 'rests' of neural crest tissue so that the destruction or removal of the adrenal medulla does not normally lead to any consequences from catecholamine deficiency. There are three principal catecholamines: dopamine, noradrenaline, and adrenaline. The first is involved mainly in brain metabolism but the latter two have important peripheral effects.

Phaeochromocytoma

The only disease of the adrenal medulla known with certainty is the phaeochromocytoma. This is a tumour which is bilateral in perhaps 10 per cent of cases and secretes catecholamines. Usually the tumours are benign but malignancy is not rare. As chromaffin tissue is widely distributed it is not surprising that phaeochromocytoma may arise also outside the adrenal medulla but almost always in the paraspinal area.

The patients present with hypertension which is typically intermittent and accompanied by some other features, such as headache, palpitations, and sweating. Confirmation of the diagnosis is obtained by demonstrating raised levels of catecholamines in the plasma or urine, or of their metabolites in the urine. Radiology can locate the tumour in most instances.

Treatment

The anaesthetist has the difficult task of trying to normalize the blood pressure before, during, and after the surgical procedure. Phaeochromocytomas produce a mixture of adrenaline and noradrenaline but the ratio of the two varies considerably between different tumours. This implies corresponding variations in management so a flexible approach is essential.

Blockade of adrenoceptors is the essential feature with the principal aims of lowering the blood pressure and diminishing venous tone. Chronic stimulation of capacitance vessels by catecholamines leads to a reduction in blood volume; preoperative treatment with a long-acting α-adrenoceptor blocking agent such as phenoxybenzamine, combined with fluid replacement, restore the blood volume and help to minimize the hypotension which may result when the tumour is removed. β-Adrenoceptor blockade is useful in lowering heart rate but if used alone may block vasodilator nerve fibres to the muscles and then unrestrained α-adrenoceptor stimulation will cause blood pressure to rise even further. A suitable regimen would entail giving phenoxybenzamine 4 days before surgery in a dose of 1 mg/kg intravenously in 200 ml of fluid. The next day the dose is repeated or doubled, if necessary, to achieve a normal blood pressure. Further infusions are given daily and then a rather smaller dose on the day of operation. β-Blockade may be instituted if necessary to control tachycardia.

For the operation, enflurane is recommended but whatever technique is employed close monitoring is essential. Short-acting α-blockers such as phentolamine may be helpful during operation for fine control of the blood pressure. There is some virtue in having rather less than complete β-blockade so that if the surgeon handles tissue suspected of containing the tumour a hypertensive response may still be observed, thus helping to verify its identity. An ample supply of blood should be available as the tumours are extremely vascular.

As soon as the tumour has been removed, pressor drugs may be required. Postoperatively, there may still be difficulty in maintaining the blood pressure and expansion of blood volume may be needed.

Alternative techniques are discussed by Pratilos and Pratila (1979). The pharmacological use of the catecholamines, adrenaline and noradrenaline, with further details concerning α- and β-adrenoceptor blocking drugs, are given in Chapters 12 and 13.

Pratilos, V. and Pratila, M. G. (1979) Anaesthetic management of phaeochromocytoma. *Canadian Anaesthetic Society Journal,* **26,** 253

Thyroid

There are two principal thyroid hormones – L-thyroxine (T_4) and L-tri-iodothyronine (T_3). Both are released from the thyroid gland but some T_4 is converted into T_3 in the tissues. Normal daily disposal rates for the two hormones are approximately 100 nmol (T_4) and 45 nmol (T_3). The half-life of T_4 in the circulation is about 6 days and that of T_3 is only about 12 hours, so that the plasma level of T_4 (50–150 nmol/ℓ) is much higher than that of T_3 (1.5–3.5 nmol/ℓ). Due probably to its faster metabolism T_3 has a faster onset of action than T_4. In addition, T_3 is thought to be several times more potent on a molar basis than T_4.

The result of these differences is that approximately half the biological action of the thyroid hormones in man is exerted by T_3 although nearly all the circulating hormone is T_4.

Anaesthesia and thyroid disease

Goitre

In the management of thyroid disease it is necessary to consider both the size of the gland and its level of function, as these may be independent.

The presence of a goitre, its size, and particularly its position may present mechanical problems for the anaesthetist and should be considered beforehand. It is the retrosternal goitre which is more likely to cause unexpected tracheal obstruction or distortion, but a plain radiograph will clarify the situation.

Hyperthyroidism

Thyroid surgery in the untreated hyperthyroid patient is dangerous and, therefore, the preparation of the patient is of unusual importance. The routine in general use is to render the patient euthyroid with antithyroid drugs. The preparations most commonly employed are the thionamides, of which carbimazole is preferred in the UK and methimazole in the USA. They act by preventing the incorporation of iodine into tyrosine radicals to form mono- and diiodotyrosine, and also inhibit the combination of two diiodotyrosine molecules to form L-thyroxine. Propylthiouracil is an alternative. Potassium perchlorate, which inhibits the concentration of iodine by the gland, may be used if sensitivity occurs to other drugs, but the risk of toxicity is greater so it is not a drug of choice. Normal initial doses of these drugs are given in *Table 17.2*.

The main disadvantage of this therapy in the present context is its slowness as it may take 2 months or more before the patient becomes euthyroid. Usually, this does not matter but if pressure symptoms are troublesome, the delay may be unacceptable. Also, antithyroid drugs may cause an increase in the size and vascularity of the goitre. With a view to making surgery easier, some surgeons prefer to stop the antithyroid drugs 2 weeks before operation and treat the patient with iodine which temporarily inhibits the release of thyroid hormones and causes some reduction in the vascularity of the gland. The *British National Formulary* recommends aqueous iodine solution (Lugol's solution) in a dose of 0.5 ml three times a day. Potassium iodide tablets (60 mg once a day) are more convenient but unstable on storage.

Table 17.2 Initial doses of antithyroid agents

Drug	*Starting dose,* mg/day
Carbimazole	30
Propylthiouracil	300
Potassium perchlorate	600

One of the problems in thyroid disease is how to tell when a patient has in fact reached a euthyroid state. A test measuring tissue function such as the basal metabolic rate or reflex relaxation time might be helpful but such tests are either not available or unreliable. Measurement of plasma thyroxine is of some value but the results have to be interpreted with caution because during treatment with thionamides the level may fall well below normal without clinical hypothyroidism. Consequently clinical judgement is important. Considering the patient's symptoms or lack of them, restoration of usual weight and normal pulse rate gives a reasonably accurate guide and is adequate in practice.

An alternative method of preparation is with β-adrenoceptor blockade, which usually will quickly control many of the features of hyperthyroidism, particularly the tachycardia and tendency to dysrhythmias. This scheme is particularly useful if operation is urgent or if thyroid suppression by antithyroid drugs or iodine is incomplete. Atrial fibrillation if present should be dealt with in the usual way (*see* Chapter 13).

Premedication is important, particularly if anxiety is a prominent feature. Except in the presence of airway obstruction, any of the usual agents can be used. The choice of anaesthetic agent is wide and in the well-prepared patient can be made on general grounds.

During the operation, the anaesthetist should give particular care to the patient's eyes. If exophthalmos is present, an undue degree of drying of the cornea may take place and this should be prevented by protective drops (such as hypromellose) and, if necessary, securing the eyelids in the closed position.

Postoperatively, difficulties may also arise if the parathyroid glands have been damaged or removed; hypoparathyroidism leads to a falling level of plasma calcium. This never happens abruptly but may be significant after 12 hours or so and, as the larynx is particularly sensitive to hypocalcaemia, laryngeal spasm and stridor may be the first indication of this complication. Intravenous calcium gluconate is immediately effective and as this is safe if given slowly, it should be used freely if spasm is suspected.

Thyrotoxic crisis (thyroid storm)
This serious condition is caused by the sudden release into the circulation of excess thyroid hormone. It may occur postoperatively if the patient has not been properly prepared but is rare in current practice. It is manifested at first by a rising temperature and pulse rate. After recovery from anaesthesia other features appear, including sweating, restlessness, pulmonary oedema, and hypotension. Treatment must be immediate and vigorous with intravenous fluids and hydrocortisone. If they have not already been given, large doses of carbimazole by nasogastric tube and intravenous iodine are indicated. Full β-adrenoceptor blockade has been recommended.

Hypothyroidism
Patients with reduced thyroid function may present a problem when they come to surgery for an unrelated condition. If the hypothyroidism is known, and has been adequately treated, no particular difficulties need be anticipated. The standard drug is L-thyroxine sodium and the maintenance dose is almost always between 100 and 200 μg per day. For convenience this may be taken as a single dose. The anaesthetist may wish to enquire as to whether an adequate dose is being taken.

If the patient has been well and is at his usual weight, it is likely that replacement therapy has been adequate. If time permits, this may be confirmed by the demonstration that the patient's plasma thyroxine and thyrotrophin are in the normal range.

The intercurrent disease for which the patient requires surgery may have interfered with the taking of regular treatment. If only a few days' medication has been missed, the slow turnover of thyroxine will ensure that an adequate blood level remains and no trouble should arise. However, a long illness may have led to the patient slipping back almost imperceptibly into hypothyroidism.

When patients present for surgery in a hypothyroid state they are at a considerable risk. If time permits, L-triiodothyronine, 20 μg intravenously, may be given for rapid action but the effect will be small and larger doses are dangerous. Premedication and doses of anaesthetic agents must be kept to a minimum because the patient will be unduly sensitive to them. There may be a tendency to hypothermia and also hypotension because adrenal function may be depressed by the lack of thyroxine. Hydrocortisone may be needed. Postoperatively, replacement therapy should be commenced as soon as possible but again it is dangerous, particularly in the elderly, to give a large dose immediately because of the risk of cardiac dysrhythmia; in the previously untreated patient, L-thyroxine 50 μg/day is the most that should be given at first.

Further reading

Clinics in Endocrinology and Metabolism. Thyrotoxicosis (1978) **7,** (1); Hypothyroidism and goitre (1979) **8,** (1); Pathology and management of thyroid disease (1981) **10,**(2)

Hoffenberg, R. (1980) Thyroid emergencies. *Clinics in Endocrinology and Metabolism,* **9,** 503

Kim, J. M. and Hackman, L. (1977) Anesthesia for untreated hypothyroidism. *Anesthesia and Analgesia,* **56,** 299
Werner, S. C. (Ed) (1978) *The Thyroid: A Fundamental and Clinical Text,* 4th Edn. London: Harper Row
Zonzein, J., Santangelo, R. P., Mackin, J. F., Lee, T. C., Caffey, R. J. and Canary, J. J. (1979) Propranolol therapy in thyrotoxicosis. *American Journal of Medicine,* **66,** 411

Thyroid hormones

I Thyroxine sodium (*BP*) and Levothyroxine sodium (*USP*)
Chemical name: sodium 4-*O*-(4-hydroxy-3,5-di-iodophenyl)-3,5-di-iodo-L -tyrosinate

II Liothyronine sodium (*BP* and *USP*)
Synonym: L-tri-iodothyronine sodium
Chemical name: sodium 4-*O*-(4-hydroxy-3-iodophenyl)-3,5-di-iodo-L-tyrosinate

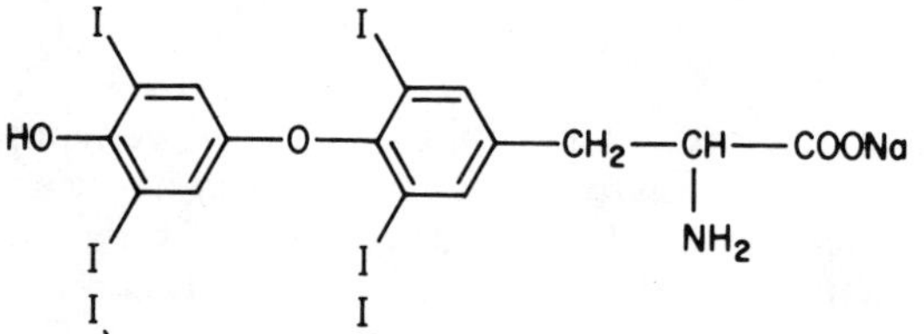

I I
HO—⟨ring⟩—O—⟨ring⟩—CH_2—CH—COONa I
I I NH_2

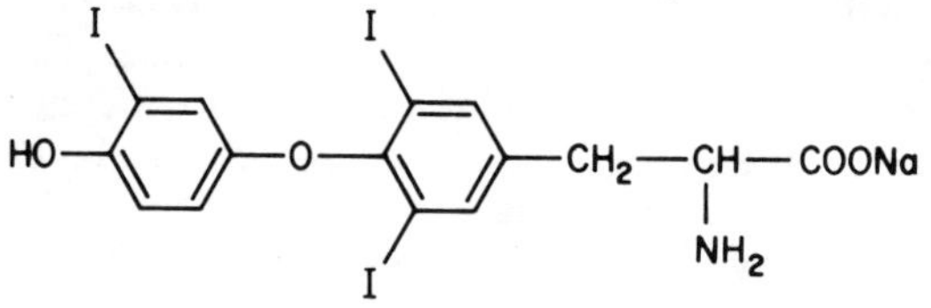

I I
HO—⟨ring⟩—O—⟨ring⟩—CH_2—CH—COONa II
I NH_2

PHYSIOLOGY

The action of the thyroid hormones, to which most tissues are responsive, is to increase metabolism and to promote growth in the young. As noted above, T_3 acts more rapidly and more intensely than T_4, but this difference is of little significance for therapy.

INDICATIONS

Thyroid hormones are employed in the treatment of hypothyroidism and occasionally in thyroid function tests.

DOSAGE AND ADMINISTRATION

Thyroxine sodium is the standard preparation and is given by mouth in a single daily dose. Injections are not available. The starting dose should not be greater than 50 μg/day and in the elderly patient 25 μg/day is safer. Thereafter the dose may be increased to 50 μg/day after a week, then by a further 50 μg/day each week until 150 μg/day is reached. It is then best to maintain that dose for at least a month before deciding whether the patient is euthyroid or not. Tablets of 25, 50, and

100 μg are available. They look much the same and this may be a source of confusion if there is doubt as to what dose a patient is taking.

Liothyronine sodium has been used in hypothyroid coma and also to achieve rapid treatment of hypothyroidism before surgery but its advantages have not been established.

PRECAUTIONS

Whole thyroid preparations should not be used. Caution should be exercised in treating patients who may have coronary insufficiency, and initial doses should be small.

In 1980 a change in formulation of thyroxine tablets resulted in an 11 per cent increase in potency although the designation and apparent strength is unchanged. It is unlikely that this alteration need cause any change in practice, but should accentuate the trend of recent years towards the use of lower doses of thyroxine sodium.

Parathyroids

Parathyroid hormone has three principal modes of action, all tending to raise the level of calcium in the plasma. By its action on bone, the hormone stimulates the activity of the osteoclasts which leads to the dissolution of bone crystal and the release of calcium with phosphate. On the kidney, the action is to stimulate the tubular reabsorption of calcium to the glomerular filtrate. In the small intestine, the hormone, possibly via vitamin D metabolism, promotes the absorption of calcium. In addition, the action on the kidney diminishes the tubular reabsorption of phosphate and hence lowers the plasma phosphate. It would seem that parathyroid hormone should lower the urine calcium, but in practice primary hyperparathyroidism is associated with a normal or raised urine calcium. This occurs because the level of urine calcium is determined more by the plasma level than by renal tubular activity and therefore the raised plasma level has the predominant effect.

Hyperparathyroidism is classified into three types:

1. *Primary* – due to a parathyroid tumour (usually a benign adenoma) or hyperplasia of unknown cause.
2. *Secondary* – due to a parathyroid hyperplasia in response to a low plasma calcium, for example in uraemia.
3. *Tertiary* – in which an autonomous adenoma arises in a gland made hyperplastic by secondary hyperparathyroidism.

Primary hyperparathyroidism is characterized by a raised level of plasma calcium, whereas in secondary hyperparathyroidism the plasma calcium is by definition below normal. Biochemically, tertiary hyperparathyroidism resembles the primary form.

The advent of biochemical profiles with ready and reliable measurement of plasma calcium has led to a change in the usual clinical pattern of primary hyperparathyroidism. It is now recognized as a common condition and most patients are asymptomatic or have non-specific symptoms. Some patients present with renal calculi, but osteitis fibrosa (the bone disease of primary hyperparathyroidism) is now rare.

Parathyroidectomy

Because of early diagnosis most patients who present nowadays for an excision of a parathyroid adenoma are in good general condition with only moderate elevation of plasma calcium, that is, under 3.0 mmol/ℓ. Such patients need no particular preoperative care and there are no particular considerations in the selection of premedication or anaesthetic agents.

Patients with levels of plasma calcium much above 3.0 mmol/ℓ, however, may be gravely ill. Vomiting and polyuria may have led to dehydration; there may be uraemia and hypertension due to renal damage. Careful preoperative preparation is essential. The first step is to correct the dehydration with oral fluids, but in the more severely ill patient intravenous isotonic saline will be needed. Rehydration will lower the level of plasma calcium and may be all that is required.

There are other measures that can be used to lower plasma calcium further. The most reliable and safe method is to give oral sodium acid phosphate in a dose equivalent to 500 mg of elemental phosphorus three to six times a day. It is convenient to use Phosphate-Sandoz tablets, each of which constitutes a single dose. Phosphate treatment is effective and will virtually normalize the plasma calcium in a few days. Uraemia is not a contraindication. Prolonged treatment carries a risk of ectopic calcification. Intravenous phosphate has been used but is now thought to be dangerous. Corticosteroids cannot be expected to lower the plasma calcium in hyperparathyroidism but calcitonin is being evaluated.

During operation the main problem is likely to be finding the tumour. Preoperative palpation and radiography are rarely helpful and radioscanning has so far been disappointing. Some degree of preoperative localization may have been achieved by differential venous sampling in the neck with measurement of parathyroid hormone. The anaesthetist must be prepared for a prolonged search with repeated frozen sections being necessary. Occasionally, the surgeon will wish to divide the sternum to explore the superior mediastinum. A modest elevation of plasma calcium does not increase the risk of cardiac arrhythmia (Gunst and Drop, 1980).

Postoperatively some fall in plasma calcium should be found the next day but the minimum level may not be reached for several days. Tetany is unusual before the second day but should be sought frequently by attempting to elicit Chvostek's sign. If the plasma calcium falls sharply or if any tetany appears, 20 ml of 10 per cent calcium gluconate should be given slowly over 10 minutes. If tetany persists, 10 g of calcium gluconate in an intravenous infusion over 10 hours should prove effective. Oral calcium supplements should be started and considerable amounts are needed. Cows' milk can be useful as it contains about 1.0 g of calcium per litre. The preparation Sandocal is convenient, each effervescent tablet containing 400 mg of calcium; the dose is 3–5 tablets a day. Care is needed in renal failure as each of these tablets also contains 6.6 mEq of sodium and 4.5 mEq of potassium. Calcium-Sandoz syrup, which contains no sodium or potassium, is an alternative.

If the hypocalcaemia is severe and prolonged, as it may be if hyperparathyroid bone disease is present, calciferol should be given in a dose of 2.5 mg (100 000 units)/day by mouth or 7.5 mg/day by injection. Calciferol toxicity can be induced easily so that frequent measurement of plasma calcium is essential and the treatment should be withdrawn as soon as possible. The metabolites of calciferol (*see* below) may be superior for immediate use.

Gunst, M. A. and Drop, L. J. (1980) Chronic hypercalcaemia secondary to hyperthyroidism: a risk factor during anaesthesia? *British Journal of Anaesthesia,* **52,** 507

Vitamin D

Ergocalciferol (*BP* and *USP*)
Synonyms: calciferol, vitamin D_2
Chemical name: (5*Z*,7*E*,22*E*)-9,10-secoergosta-5,7,10(19),22-tetraen-3β-ol

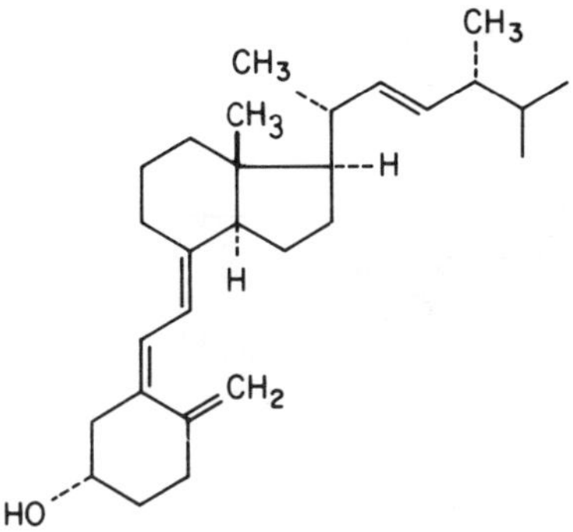

PHYSIOLOGY

The metabolism of the calciferols is complex and still not fully understood. Cholecalciferol (vitamin D_3) is synthesized in the skin by the action of ultraviolet light, but only the shorter wavelengths are effective. Ergocalciferol (vitamin D_2) is the form which is usually used in therapy. Cholecalciferol (and presumably ergocalciferol) has to be metabolized before it is biologically active. In the liver it is hydroxylated at the 25-position to 25-hydroxycholecalciferol (calcifediol, 25-OHD_3). This compound is then hydroxylated at the 1-position in the kidney to form 1,25-dihydroxycholecalciferol (1,25$(OH)_2D_3$) which is the active substance. In a healthy person, the combination of small amounts of dietary vitamin D, some synthesis in the skin, and probably some control of vitamin D metabolism ensures appropriate absorption of calcium from the intestine.

PHARMACOLOGY

Large amounts of vitamin D, that is 50–100 times the physiological requirements, override the control system and lead to excessive absorption of calcium and hypercalcaemia. The derivatives 1-α-OHD_3 (alfacalcidol) and 1-α,25$(OH)_2D_3$ (calcitriol) are available. They are highly potent and only 1 or 2 μg a day are required. Because they are already hydroxylated they do not require metabolism by the kidney and may therefore be useful in treating some patients with renal disease. It is claimed that the rapidity of action permits faster and easier control of the plasma calcium but their superiority over ergocalciferol for routine use has not been established.

INDICATIONS

The toxic effects of vitamin D can be used to advantage in correcting the hypocalcaemia of hypoparathyroidism (transient or permanent) and in chronic renal disease or severe malabsorption. Low dose vitamin D supplements are used in the prophylaxis of nutritional rickets.

DOSAGE AND ADMINISTRATION

High dose: Ergocalciferol in a dose of 2.5 mg (100 000 units)/day is appropriate for starting treatment in most patients, but in severe hypocalcaemia this dose can be doubled. Intramuscular injections can be used. For long-term maintenance the dose usually lies between 1.25 mg and 2.5 mg/day.

Low dose: For prophylaxis of rickets 50 μg (1000 units)/day is appropriate.

PRECAUTIONS

Ergocalciferol is slow acting so that plasma calcium may rise or fall slowly over many weeks. Hypercalcaemia is a continual hazard so that frequent monitoring of the plasma calcium is essential and the long time scale must be taken into account when adjusting dosage.

Confusion may occur between various preparations and care is needed:

Calcium with Vitamin D Tablets → 12.5 μg ergocalciferol
Calciferol Tablets, High Strength → 250 μg ergocalciferol
Calciferol Tablets, Strong → 1.25 mg ergocalciferol.

Pancreas

Nearly all the pancreas is concerned with its non-endocrine function, and the islets of Langerhans constitute only about 1 per cent of the total mass. The islet has complex internal structural relationships which may have functional significance. The central mass consists of B cells which secrete insulin while the outer layer of A cells secrete glucagon; the D cells secrete somatostatin. Other hormone-producing cells are present also.

Insulin acts mainly on the liver, muscle, and adipose tissue by reacting with specific receptors on cell membranes. The major result of insulin action is to enable glucose to enter cells, but in addition the intracellular phosphorylation of glucose and protein synthesis are accelerated while lipolysis is reduced. Severe insulin lack is followed by fat catabolism leading to a rise in plasma ketones causing acidosis and consequent symptoms.

The main action of glucagon is to produce hyperglycaemia by promoting glycogenolysis in the liver but its place in physiology is uncertain.

Diabetus mellitus

It is difficult to generalize about this enormously variable disease so the anaesthetist's therapeutic response must be suitably flexible. The classification of diabetes is unsatisfactory but there is some advantage in recognizing two main types. *Type I diabetes* (also called early onset or juvenile onset) begins usually in juveniles or young adults. It is characterized by a substantial or total failure of insulin secretion which leads to severe symptoms, weight loss, and ketosis. Treatment with insulin is essential. *Type II diabetes* (also called late onset or adult onset) presents in later life and most of the patients are obese. The amount of insulin secreted is normal or raised, but there is a resistance to its action due perhaps to a lack of insulin receptors in adipose tissue. Symptoms are less severe and there is no ketosis. This type of diabetes can be controlled usually by weight reduction, calorie/carbohydrate restriction, and oral hypoglycaemic drugs. Nevertheless, some Type II patients need eventually to be treated with insulin, particularly on a temporary basis after stress. In practice, appropriate treatment has to be designed for the individual patient rather than using preconceived schemes.

Diabetic complications occur in all forms of the disease and are related more to the duration of the diabetes than its immediate severity. Complications are not likely to present any particular anaesthetic hazard although it is important to be aware of the increased incidence of cardiac, vascular, and renal disease and that the neuropathy may impair cardiovascular reflexes.

Treatment
All diabetics need to modify their diet. The most important changes are regulation of calorie intake (for example, for weight loss in obesity) and reduction of the intake of refined carbohydrate. For the patient on insulin the timing of food intake is important.

Oral hypoglycaemic drugs
The sulphonylureas are the most commonly employed. They act by increasing the release of insulin from the pancreas. Some patients do not respond to them and increasing the dose above the recommended level is ineffective. Tolbutamide is used in a daily dose of 0.5–3.0 g which must be given in two or three doses as the drug is excreted quickly. Chlorpropamide (100–500 mg/day) and glibenclamide (2.5–20 mg/day) are metabolized slowly so a single morning dose will suffice, but they do carry the slight but definite risk of nocturnal hypoglycaemia. The biguanide drug, metformin, may be useful in the obese patient despite the remote risk of lactic acidosis.

Insulin
This is the mainstay of treatment in the more severe diabetic. There are now many commercial varieties of insulin available but they all fall into three main categories in terms of the timing of their action (*see* below). An insulin regimen has to be designed individually for each patient and there are many possible variations. A total insulin dose in the range 20–60 units is usual but any stress such as infection, trauma, surgery, or fever will increase requirements, even as much as two-fold.

Anaesthesia
For induction, thiopentone and methohexitone are satisfactory. Ketamine may have some sympathetic stimulant action which might be undesirable but information about other agents is lacking. In general, all anaesthetic agents tend to casue a reduction in carbohydrate tolerance with consequent hyperglycaemia. It has been claimed that fentanyl is better than halothane in this respect (Hall *et al.*, 1978). Anoxia tends to raise plasma glucose and should be avoided. Muscle relaxants and analgesics have been safely employed. Regional analgesia may be indicated in emergency surgery of a poorly controlled diabetic (for example, amputation of a gangrenous leg). Postoperative hyperglycaemia is usual but is related to the stress of surgery rather than to the anaesthetic.

Management
This will depend on the severity of the diabetes, previous treatment, and the extent of the intended surgery. Urine testing is still conventional and may be useful in detecting ketosis but measurements of blood glucose are more valuable. This can be done rapidly and cheaply in any ward or theatre using the test-stick methods and meters now available.

If the diabetes has been controlled satisfactorily by diet, no particular preparations are needed but after operation blood glucose should be monitored.

Up to 15 mmol/ℓ with no more than slight ketosis (due to starvation) is acceptable but higher levels should be controlled by small doses of soluble insulin – this is rarely necessary.

If the patient has been well controlled on oral hypoglycaemic agents and the surgical procedures planned are of only moderate severity, no difficulty need be expected. Normal doses of the drugs are given the day before operation, none on the day of operation, and then the normal dose again the next day. Blood glucose monitoring will indicate any need for more vigorous treatment. However, if diabetic control has been poor, particularly if there is any ketosis or if extensive surgery is planned, it is best to treat the patient with insulin instead of oral hypoglycaemics for several days before operation and afterwards as necessary. Soluble insulin should be used and small doses (for example 8–16 units twice a day) should suffice. It is easier and safer to use a fixed dose and accept some hyperglycaemia, providing there is little or no ketosis.

An insulin-dependent diabetic coming to surgery needs careful supervision. For the patient who is well controlled on a single daily dose of long-acting insulin, and in whom only minor surgery is planned, it is satisfactory to simply omit food and insulin on the day of operation. Postoperative monitoring of blood glucose will indicate whether a small dose of soluble insulin is necessary or not and the next day the usual regimen can be resumed.

For anything more than minor surgery, more is required. The general principle of management depends on the fact that moderate doses of insulin, although too low to normalize the level of blood glucose, will nevertheless almost always prevent serious ketosis, while continuous intravenous glucose will prevent serious hypoglycaemia. Moderate hyperglycaemia is acceptable but excessive amounts of intravenous glucose must not be given because of the danger of producing a hyperosmolar state.

On the day of operation, nothing is given by mouth. An intravenous infusion of 5 per cent dextrose is started and continued at the rate of about 500 ml in 4 hours (25 g dextrose) until the patient can take fluids by mouth. When the infusion is begun a subcutaneous injection of *soluble* insulin is given in a unit dose which is half of the patient's usual morning requirement. It is unlikely that any further insulin will be needed during the operation. Any suspicion of hypoglycaemia should be managed by increasing the rate of dextrose infusion at once and measuring the blood glucose.

For extensive surgery or when diabetes is unstable it is best to transfer the patient from long-acting insulins to soluble insulin. The total daily dose should be reduced by about 20 per cent and then the appropriate amount of soluble insulin given in two approximately equal doses before breakfast and the evening meal. If this dosage does not achieve good control, postponement of the operation to allow for adjustment of dose is desirable. It is, of course, impossible to generalize; if there is a rising ketosis, only urgent surgery should be undertaken without a further period of stabilization because anaesthesia in uncontrolled ketosis is particularly hazardous. The same danger is present in the less common non-ketotic hyperosmolar diabetic coma.

After operation any delay in the regaining of consciousness, abnormal sweating, or tachycardia should raise the possibility of hypoglycaemia which should be treated and investigated promptly. A few hours after operation a decision should be reached as to whether to give a further dose of insulin. The dose given before operation will serve as a guide; it is unlikely that a larger dose than that will be needed and if the blood glucose is below 10 mmol/ℓ none need be given. The following day a half dose should be given in the morning and then a reversion should be made to the usual dose as soon as the patient returns to a normal diet.

If for any reason there has to be a longer period before normal food intake can be resumed, intravenous dextrose should be continued and soluble insulin given every 8 or 12 hours. When the postoperative course is stormy the diabetes is likely to be unstable. Soluble insulin should be given every 6 or 8 hours. The use of a predetermined 'sliding scale' of insulin dosage cannot be recommended. There is no satisfactory alternative to frequent determinations of the blood glucose and consequent alterations of insulin dose. If necessary, every dose of insulin should be prescribed separately. A return to regular diet and insulin dose schedule should be made as soon as possible.

Emergency treatment

Diabetic ketoacidosis (coma or pre-coma)

General principles of treatment include the control of hyperglycaemia and ketosis with soluble insulin, the restoration of fluid and electrolyte balance, and the treatment of any precipitating cause.

Soluble insulin is given by continuous intravenous injection from a pump in a dose of 3–6 units/h. Blood glucose can be expected to reach normal levels in a few hours. Frequent intramuscular injections of small doses of soluble insulin (for example, 5 units every 30 minutes) are successful also. Adding insulin to large volumes of infusion fluids is not satisfactory because of losses onto the walls of containers and tubing and the difficulty of controlling dosage. Frequent monitoring of blood glucose is necessary in particular to avoid overshoot into hypoglycaemia.

After a few hours of treatment the level of plasma potassium should be measured and if necessary potassium chloride can be added to the infusion fluid at the rate of 20 mmol/ℓ to correct hypokalaemia. The use of bicarbonate is debatable. It should be given only if severe acidosis persists after initial treatment. Moderate amounts such as 100 mmol in an hour (that is, 250 ml of 3 per cent sodium bicarbonate solution) may be given intravenously and the biochemical tests repeated.

Hyperosmolar non-ketotic diabetic coma or pre-coma

This is a less common form of diabetic coma which tends to arise in older and previously undiagnosed diabetics. The initial treatment is the same as for ketoacidosis but after a few hours less insulin is needed and half-strength saline is given. Bicarbonate is not required.

Hypoglycaemia

The effects of insulin overdose are due to hypoglycaemia and a consequent increased output of adrenaline. They include sweating, salivation, hunger, difficulty in focusing, faintness, unsteadiness, palpitations, tremors, giddiness, confusion leading to coma, convulsions, and even death. The blood sugar must be raised as quickly as possible since irreversible brain damage may occur. The methods available are to give sugar (sucrose) or dextrose in solution by mouth if the patient can still swallow, or up to 50 ml of a 50 per cent solution of dextrose intravenously. The dose of dextrose may have to be repeated more than once, particularly in the case of coma due to depot insulin which comes on more insidiously, and at a lower blood glucose level. Glucagon 0.5–1 mg can be given subcutaneously or intramuscularly and causes an increase in blood sugar by increasing the conversion of liver glycogen to glucose.

Insulinoma

Insulinoma is a rare tumour of the pancreatic islet cells which secretes insulin and leads to intermittent hypoglycaemia. Operation to remove the tumour may prove difficult and prolonged. Preoperatively an intravenous infusion of dextrose is given for several hours and the infusion may be continued during the operation. As soon as the tumour is removed hyperglycaemia occurs and may continue for up to 2 weeks, but ketosis is rare and treatment with insulin is not often needed.

Hall, G. M., Young, C., Holdcroft, A. and Alaghband-Zaden, J. (1978) Substrate mobilisation during surgery. *Anaesthesia,* **33,** 924

Further reading

Alberti, K. G. M. M. and Thomas, D. J. B. (1979) The management of diabetes during surgery. *British Journal of Anaesthesia,* **51,** 693

Barnett, A. H., Robinson, M., Harrison, J. and Watkins, P. (1980) Mini-pump: method of diabetic control during minor surgery under general anaesthesia. *British Medical Journal,* **1,** 78

Clinics in Endocrinology and Metabolism. New aspects of diabetes (1982) **11,** 2

Insulin

Chemical constitution: Insulin consists of two polypeptide chains containing 21 (A) and 30 (B) amino acids, respectively, and linked by two disulphide bridges. Commercial insulin is produced from ox and pig pancreas and the constitutions of the animal insulins differ from each other and from the human form. This does not affect their biological activity in man but can have immunological consequences. Synthetic human insulin is now available and looks likely to become the standard preparation within a few years.

There are only three formulations of insulin in common use (*Table 17.3*) but there are now a bewildering array of commercial preparations available. Some of them are mixtures but most of them are made with insulin that has been purified to a greater or lesser degree. Although the purified insulins are now in general use their advantage has not been firmly established. However, the use of the older acid-soluble insulin is not recommended.

Table 17.3 Preparations of insulin

Name	*Comments*	*Approximate duration of action,* hours
Neutral Insulin Injection	Also called soluble or regular	6–8
Isophane Insulin Injection	Also called NPH (neutral protamine Hagedorn)	12–18
Insulin Zinc Suspension	Also called lente, a mixture of 30% amorphous and 70% crystalline zinc insulin	18–24

PHYSICAL CHARACTERISTICS

Soluble insulin is a clear solution while all of the longer acting preparations are cloudy. Insulins are labelled with their animal sources.

INDICATIONS

The treatment of diabetes mellitus is the only major use for insulin, but it may be employed to produce deliberate hypoglycaemia to test anterior pituitary responsiveness in respect of growth hormone and corticotrophin.

DOSAGE AND ADMINISTRATION

Insulin is available in strengths of 20, 40, 80 and 100 units/ml. By mid-1984 all diabetics in the UK will have been changed onto 100 units/ml preparations and the other strengths will be withdrawn, but their use will continue in some other countries. It is essential that the graduations on the syringe match the insulin strength employed. All insulin is given by injection. This is usually subcutaneous but intramuscular injection is possible. Soluble insulin may be given intravenously. Dosage must be determined for the individual patient. Mixtures of long- and short-acting insulins may be used.

PRECAUTIONS

Cloudy suspensions must be shaken before being drawn into the syringe. With insulin therapy, hypoglycaemia is an ever-present hazard.

Glucagon

Glucagon (*BP* and *USP*) and Glucagon injection (*BP*)
Chemical structure: a straight-chain polypeptide of 29 amino acid residues; molecular weight 3483. It is extracted from pancreatic tissue during the manufacture of insulin.

PHYSIOLOGY

Glucagon is secreted by the A cells of the islets of Langerhans in response to a fall in the level of blood glucose. In the normal person, glucagon stimulates the secretion of insulin; the balance of the two hormones tends to normalize the blood glucose and ensures a regular supply of other metabolic substrates. One action of glucagon that is involved in this role is its effect of raising blood glucose by hepatic glycogenolysis. This is the basis of its therapeutic use.

INDICATIONS

Glucagon may be used instead of glucose to raise the blood sugar in patients with hypoglycaemia. It has the advantage that it can be given subcutaneously or intramuscularly and its use avoids the irritant effect of concentrated dextrose solutions on veins.

DOSAGE AND ADMINISTRATION

Doses of 0.5–1 mg may be given by subcutaneous or intramuscular injection.

PRECAUTIONS

Being an animal protein, glucagon can provoke allergic hypersensitivity, but this is rare.

Further general reading

Clinics in Endocrinology and Metabolism — a continuing series
DeGroot, L. J. *et al* (Eds) (1979) *Endocrinology* (3 vols). New York: Grune and Stratton
Hall, R., Anderson, J., Smart, G. A. and Besser, M. (1980) *Fundamentals of Clinical Endocrinology*, 3rd Edn. Tunbridge Wells: Pitman
White, V. A. (1979) Pre-operative endocrine and metabolic considerations. *Medical Clinics of North America,* **63** (6), 1321
Williams, R. H. (Ed.) (1981) *Textbook of Endocrinology,* 6th Edn. Philadelphia: W. B. Saunders

18

Anticoagulants, antithrombotic, thrombolytic and haemostatic agents

Anticoagulants delay or prevent the clotting of blood or plasma. There are several stages at which they can exert this action, both directly and indirectly. Anticoagulants, however, have no effect on thrombus once it has been formed. Antithrombotic agents influence the natural incidence of thrombus formation, usually by an effect on platelet function; some are therapeutically effective. Substances that have fibrinolytic activity, or that enhance the body's fibrinolytic system are thrombolytic agents. Haemostatic agents enhance platelet adhesiveness or strengthen capillary cement substance by enhancing resistance to lytic agents.

To understand the mechanism of action of these agents, it is necessary to appreciate the normal clotting process and the means by which the fluidity of blood is maintained.

The normal clotting process

There are two theories concerning the coagulation mechanism. The 'cascade' theory has been the one most acceptable to clinicians, although there is no direct evidence in support of the postulated early stages. Although the alternative theory by Seegers (1969) is experimentally based, its terminology and concepts are difficult to interpret in the clinical setting and it will not be discussed here. The

Table 18.1 Blood clotting factors

Factors	*Synonyms*
I	Fibrinogen
II	Prothrombin
III	Thromboplastin
IV	Calcium ions
V	Accelerator globulin (AcG)
VII	Proconvertin
VIII	Antihaemophilic globulin (AHG)
IX	Christmas factor
X	Stuart–Prower factor
XI	Plasma thromboplastin antecedent (PTA)
XII	Hageman factor
XIII	Fibrin-stabilizing factor

Note: Factor VI is no longer considered to be a separate entity cascade theory postulates that following 'activation' by either intrinsic or extrinsic factors, a series of proenzymes are converted into active enzymes in turn, each enzyme activating the next proenzyme in the chain. One supposed benefit of such a system is that at each stage one molecule of enzyme would activate several molecules of the next precursor, thus producing a progressive multiplying effect. The recognized factors are listed in *Table 18.1*. A simplified outline of the process is shown in *Figure 18.1*. The early stages of coagulation are not given in detail since the evidence for them is uncertain. The well-established stages are the conversion of prothrombin to thrombin, and its activation of the conversion of fibrinogen to fibrin.

Sites of action of anticoagulants

In the light of *Figure 18.1* the sites of action of these drugs can be outlined.

The *coumarin drugs* reduce or prevent the production by the liver of prothrombin and at least three other factors (VII, IX and X) which require vitamin K for their elaboration. They have no effect on clotting if added to whole blood, but must be absorbed and metabolized by the liver. They are discussed in greater detail below.

Heparin (and protamine if given alone) acts at several stages. It inhibits factors that are involved in the conversion of prothrombin to thrombin, particularly factors IX, X,XI and XII. Thus, prevention of the formation of thrombin is probably its primary effect. In addition, it interacts with any thrombin present to prevent it catalysing the conversion of fibrinogen to fibrin. A full monograph is given on page 462.

Inhibition of platelet aggregation can be achieved by aspirin, which prolongs the bleeding time. It is being employed in the prevention of coronary and cerebral artery thrombosis in high-risk groups; it is not likely to be of great value in the prophylaxis of venous thrombosis. Dextran, which also interferes with the function and aggregation of platelets has, however, been shown to be an effective prophylactic against venous thrombosis. This may be because it also coats erythrocytes and forms complexes with plasma proteins, thereby preventing rouleaux formation and sludging, both of which may contribute to the antithrombotic effect (*see* page 522).

Tissue factors that inhibit platelet aggregation include prostaglandin (PG)X. This has been identified in arterial walls, where it is synthesized by microsomal enzymes from prostaglandins G_2 and H_2. PGX has a powerful action against platelet aggregation as well as possessing smooth muscle relaxing properties which have given rise to hopes that it may be a useful hypotensive agent. It is postulated that PGG_2 and PGH_2 are released from platelet aggregates deposited on vessel walls to generate PGX, so preventing the build-up of a platelet thrombus. This has not yet been developed as a therapeutic tool.

Arvin is extracted from the Malayan pit viper and has been used to produce a different kind of anticoagulant effect, namely defibrination. Arvin breaks down fibrin which is rapidly phagocytized by macrophages. All circulating fibrinogen is consumed in this way.

Calcium ion chelating agents, such as citrate, oxalate, and ion-exchange resins, interfere with coagulation at several key points; they are suitable only for *in vitro* usage. For storage of blood that is to be transfused, the chelating agent must not be toxic. Oxalate is thus ruled out but citrate is safe within limits.

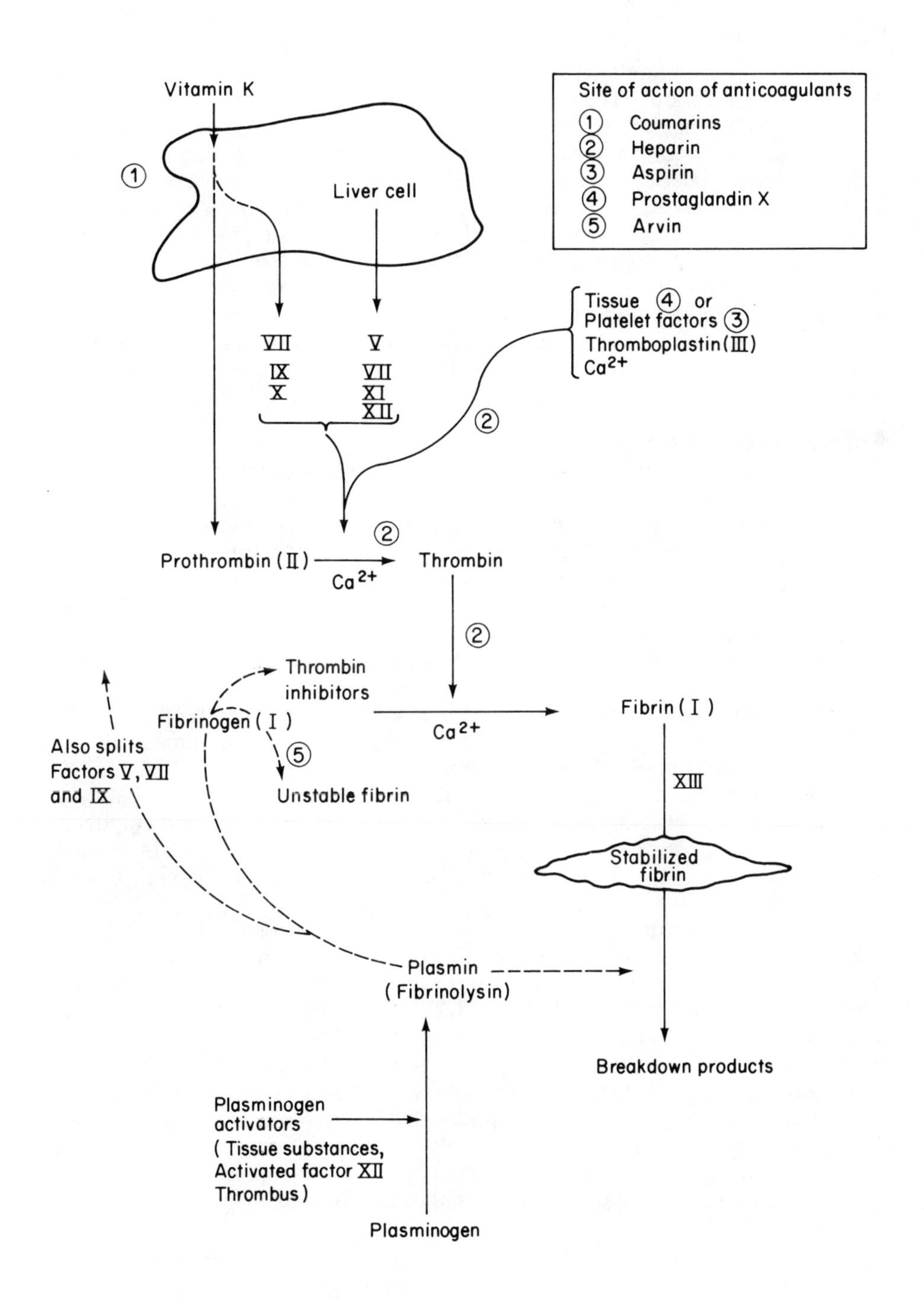

Figure 18.1 Schematic representation of clotting and fibrinolysis

Fibrinolysis

Fibrinolysis is a continuous natural function which ensures the continuing fluidity of the circulating blood. The main component of the fibrinolytic system is plasminogen, an inactive precursor which can be converted into the proteolytic enzyme plasmin (fibrinolysin) by a variety of endogenous activators. Other activators have been obtained from bacteria, moulds, and plants; of these the most important is streptokinase. It can be used by intravenous and intra-arterial infusion in the treatment of acute thromboembolic episodes to hasten the lysis of clot. An initial dose of 600 000 units is given over 30 minutes and is followed by 100 000 units hourly for 3–7 days. It has also been used as a single dose of 50 000 units to unblock clotted haemodialysis shunts. Overdose can be reversed with one of the fibrinolysin inhibitors discussed below. Streptodornase is a similar enzyme, and mixtures of streptokinase and streptodornase have been used to dissolve clot within closed cavities.

Antifibrinolytic therapy

An important regulatory mechanism of intravascular clotting is the presence of inhibitors of proteolytic enzymes. In some pathological states excessive production of these enzymes may result in the inhibitors being overwhelmed. Under these conditions the unrestrained activity of plasmin may cause not only excess fibrinolysis, but breakdown of other proteins such as factors V and VIII. Proteinase inhibition may thus be useful therapeutically. A naturally occurring inhibitor aprotinin and a synthetic inhibitor ε-aminocaproic acid (EACA) are available. They form a reversible complex with proteinases and are, therefore, competitive enzyme inhibitors. An effective inhibitor is one that has a much greater affinity for proteinase than does protein. This is so for aprotinin, but less marked for EACA, which therefore has to be given in large quantities. Natural proteinase inhibitors have a wide spectrum of action, and inhibit many other enzymes also.

The main indications for proteinase inhibitor therapy are acute pancreatitis and certain cases of pathological bleeding. In acute pancreatitis, proteolytic and lipolytic enzymes escape from the pancreas and give rise to much of the systemic illness, and proteinase inhibitors may be beneficial in alleviating pain and hypotension.

At least two syndromes of pathological bleeding are recognized as being due to imbalance between proteinases and their inhibitors, although unfortunately it is rarely possible to distinguish between these conditions quickly by clinical or laboratory methods. One such syndrome is hypofibrinogenaemia. This, it is suggested, arises when excess thromboplastic material from damaged tissue enters the circulation and causes widespread fibrin deposition. This causes over-activation of plasmin, which not only lyses the fibrin, but also attacks fibrinogen itself, converting them both into fibrinopeptides. This syndrome has also been called consumption coagulopathy, and is the likely pathology of excessive bleeding when tissues containing large amounts of thromboplastin are damaged. This occurs in many obstetric emergencies such as retroplacental haemorrhage, dead fetus, and amniotic fluid embolism.

Alternatively, the fibrinolytic system may be primarily activated, and this may occur as a result of severe stress and some shock states.

Therapy of these conditions with proteinase inhibitors is based on inhibition of both groups of activators. It is advisable to give fibrinogen concurrently, in case there has been excessive consumption of fibrin and fibrinogen.

Several other indications for fibrinolytic therapy have been suggested. In haemophilia, when there is deficient formation of fibrin, inhibition of fibrinolysis may permit adequate haemostasis, and treatment with EACA will reduce bleeding after extraction of teeth in haemophilia.

Inhibition of fibrinolysis has been shown to reduce menstrual flow in menorrhagia; it will reduce the incidence of blood loss after prostatectomy although it does not affect the incidence of thromboembolic complications unless heparin is given concurrently.

Aprotinin is best administered by continuous intravenous infusion after an initial dose of 50 000–100 000 kiu (kallikrein inactivator units). To keep a constant level it is necessary to give about 7 per cent of the initial dose per hour. It is excreted through the kidney in an inactive form. EACA is also best given as a continuous infusion of 3g/h or may be given at a rate of 0.2 g/kg 4-hourly by mouth. The half-life in the plasma of a single intravenous injection is about 2 hours and it is excreted unchanged almost entirely by the kidney within 12 hours.

Oral anticoagulants

Sweet clover disease in cattle was shown in 1921–22 to be the cause of serious, even fatal, bleeding in cattle following trauma or surgical operations.

From spoiled sweet clover hay a substance was subsequently isolated and named dicoumarol which was found to prolong coagulation time and reduce the plasma prothrombin level. This substance is slowly absorbed from the gastrointestinal tract and slowly metabolized. Since its introduction several other chemically related compounds have been produced which differ mainly in their duration of action. These compounds are of two chemical groupings, those related to dicoumarol and a newer group related to indanedione, the commonest being phenindione. In both cases they bear a chemical relationship to vitamin K and are thought to act as alternative substrates for the enzyme system, and by displacing it prevent the synthesis of prothrombin (factor II) as well as factors VII, IX, and X by the liver.

Table 18.2 Duration of action and dosage of oral anticoagulants

Drug	*Time of peak effect*	*Duration after discontinuing dose*	*Initial dose*	*Maintenance dose*
	hours	days	mg	mg
Warfarin	36–72	5–6	50	2–15
Ethyl biscoumacetate	18–36	2–3	1200 1st day, 600–900 2nd day	300–600
Dicoumarol	36–48	5–6	300 1st day, 200 2nd day	25–150
Nicoumalone	36–48	1.5–2	16 1st day, 12 2nd day	2–10
Phenindione	24–48	1–4	200 1st day, 100 2nd day	25–100

The usage of phenindione is now much reduced. While it has a more rapid onset and a shorter duration of action and is said to be much easier to control, these advantages have been outweighed by the serious nature of some of the toxic effects that have been reported, particularly agranulocytosis. Severe allergic reactions involving the skin and kidney have also been reported. This drug should therefore be reserved for patients who have demonstrated sensitivity to other oral anticoagulants. The dose and other characteristics are given in *Table 18.2*.

Excessive doses of this group of drugs cause haemorrhages, particularly from mucous membranes, skin, and the gastrointestinal and genitourinary tracts. Haematuria is probably the commonest manifestation, but uterine bleeding, ecchymosis, and epistaxis can all occur and anaemia may be severe. It is important, therefore, that prothrombin levels should be estimated daily until they are stabilized. Overdose can be controlled by the administration of phytomenadione (vitamin K_1), 5–20 mg intravenously.

Interactions between oral anticoagulants and other drugs

A large number of commonly prescribed drugs can give rise to dangerous interactions during anticoagulant therapy by a variety of mechanisms.

Drugs that diminish the reponse

A wide variety of sedatives, tranquillizers, and antidepressants stimulate the proliferation of liver microsomal enzymes, which are responsible for inactivating many other drugs, including the oral anticoagulants. Thus, a patient on one of these enzyme-inducing drugs will require a higher dose of anticoagulant to maintain the prothrombin time in the therapeutic range. If the sedative drug is stopped, there is an increase in anticoagulant effect and it may take weeks before the half-life of the anticoagulant returns to normal.

Diminution of effect would also be caused by the administration of vitamin K or by inhibition of absorption of the anticoagulant. Clofibrate and griseofulvin have been implicated in such a mechanism but the clinical relevance is slight.

Drugs that enhance the response

Drugs of the coumarin–indanedione group are highly bound to plasma proteins and can be displaced by other highly protein-bound acidic drugs such as phenylbutazone, salicylates, indomethacin, nalidixic acid, sulphonamide, clofibrate, and ethacrynic acid. Although this mechanism is well established, such enhancement is usually only very temporary. Displacement makes more drug available for biotransformation, the half-life is shortened, and a new steady state is soon reached. However, serious haemorrhage has resulted when this possible complication has been overlooked.

Simultaneous interference with anticoagulant metabolism would, of course, make displacement from binding a much more serious problem; chloramphenicol, some monoamine oxidase inhibitors, and possibly other drugs may inhibit the hydroxylation of warfarin. Salicylates have an enhancing effect which may work through several mechanisms including the production of gastric erosions, inhibition of platelet function, and a hypoprothrombinaemic effect. Broad-spectrum antibiotics or liquid paraffin may interfere with vitamin K absorption, but the effect is slight unless there is a deficient dietary intake of the vitamin.

There are many other miscellaneous interactions. Large doses of glucagon increase the effect of warfarin, although the mechanism has not been elucidated. Steroids can produce two opposing types of interaction: they cause enzyme induction but also compete for the same enzyme systems. In the case of the anabolic steroids the predominant effect is to reduce warfarin requirements. Alcohol is also a potent enzyme inducer, but again a contrary effect has been reported, the suggestion being that either cholestasis leads to malabsorption of vitamin K or that defective secretion of bile salts inhibits the microsomal enzymes.

It is important, too, to remember that the initiation of anticoagulant therapy in a patient who is stabilized on some other chronic medication may lead to serious problems due to drug interactions. The coumarins inhibit the metabolism of tolbutamide, chlorpropamade, and phenytoin, and may thus produce hypoglycaemia in diabetics or phenytoin intoxication in epileptics. Phenindione does not have this effect. A full list of drugs that potentiate or antagonize coumarin anticoagulants, as well as drugs whose metabolism is affected by the anticoagulant, has been published by an expert committee (Standing Advisory Committee for Haematology of the Royal College of Pathologists, 1982).

Seegers, W. H. (1969) Blood clotting mechanisms; three basic reactions. *Annual Review of Physiology*, **31**, 269

Standing Advisory Committee for Haematology of the Royal College of Pathologists (1982) Drug interactions with coumarin derivative anticoagulants. *British Medical Journal*, **2**, 274

Ethamsylate

Chemical name: diethylammonium 2,5,-dihydroxybenzene sulphonate

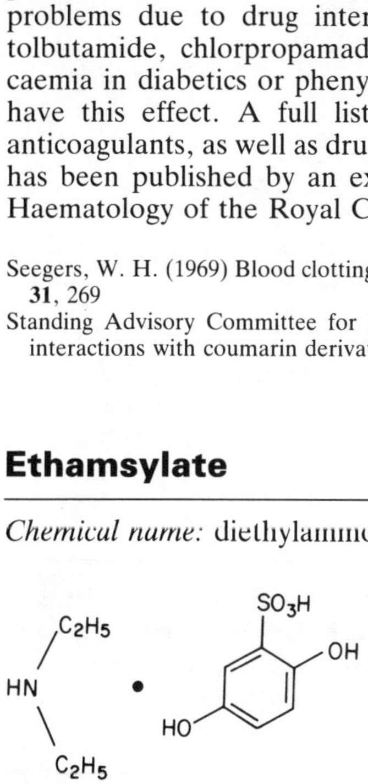

$$HN(C_2H_5)_2 \cdot C_6H_3(OH)_2SO_3H$$

PHARMACOLOGY

Ethamsylate significantly reduces the bleeding time without any effect on the prothrombin time, clotting time, or fibrinolysis. It acts principally on the capillary wall causing a demonstrable increase in capillary strength. It is believed to be due to an enhanced resistance to the effect of bradykinin on the cement substance between capillary endothelial cells. It also seems to enhance platelet adhesiveness thus maintaining the integrity of the capillary wall by platelet occlusion.

INDICATIONS

Ethamsylate has been recommended in a variety of situations in which capillary haemorrhage may be a problem. It has been shown to be effective in controlled trials in reducing haemorrhage associated with tonsillectomy and prostatectomy (Symes *et al.*, 1975).

DOSAGE AND ADMINISTRATION

Ethamsylate is effective both orally and parenterally. Initial dosage should be between 0.75 and 1.0 g intravenously or intramuscularly. For prophylaxis or maintenance therapy, 500 mg should be given every 4–6 hours.

PRECAUTIONS AND SIDE EFFECTS

There are no known contraindications although there has been one report of an increase in experimentally detectable deep vein thrombosis. Transient falls in blood pressure have been reported after intravenous administration. Oral administration may cause nausea.

Symes, J. M., Offen, D. M., Lyttle, J. A., Blandy, J. P. and Chaput de Santonge, D. M. (1975) The effects of Dicynene on blood loss during and after transurethral resection of the prostate. *British Journal of Urology,* **47**, 203

Heparin

Heparin (*BP*) and Heparin sodium (*BP* and *USP*)
Constitution: The sodium salt of a complex organic acid obtained from mammalian tissue which has the characteristic property of delaying the clotting of shed blood.

Heparin is prepared from lung and liver of domestic animals. The *BP* preparation is the sodium salt and must contain at least 110 units/mg of anticoagulant activity. The *USP* preparation must contain 120 units/mg. A unit is that amount which will prevent 1.0 ml of citrated sheep plasma clotting for 1 hour after addition of 0.2 ml of a 1:100 CaCl solution. Injection of heparin *BP* is a sterile solution in water for injections, pH 5–8.

PHARMACOLOGY

Heparin was first isolated by McLean in 1916 from heart and liver tissue. It is a complex polysaccharide containing several sulphuric acid residues combined with mucoitin, and is probably a mixture of closely related compounds. It is strongly acidic. It occurs widely throughout the body and is found in the granules of mast cells of connective tissue surrounding blood vessels.

The physiological functions of heparin, if any, are a matter of debate. It is possible that its most important function is to bind amines such as 5-hydroxytryptamine, noradrenaline, and histamine in mast cells, which it does exceedingly well by virtue of its negative charges. It is also a precursor of lipoprotein lipase, which appears to play a role in clearing lipid droplets from the blood, possibly by facilitating transport of triglyceride fatty acids through the vessel wall. It is released with histamine in anaphylactic and peptone shock.

The anticoagulant property of heparin probably depends on the fact that it has a strong electronegative charge. Its action can be antagonized by substances with a strong positive charge, such as protamine sulphate, or by a basic dye such as toluidine blue O (tolonium chloride). This suggests that its mode of action is on the enzymes that take part in the clotting mechanism of blood. Heparin forms a reversible combination with proteins and, although the exact mechanism of its anticoagulant effect is not understood, this heparin–protein complex inhibits the conversion of prothrombin to thrombin and also interferes with the action of thrombin on fibrinogen. Although clotting time is prolonged, bleeding time is unaffected. Bleeding from small abrasions is therefore not a hazard.

Fate in the body. After intravenous injection of large doses the heparin concentration of plasma falls rapidly. Duration of effect is brief. A single dose will cause up to a five-fold increase in clotting time within 10 minutes and its effect lasts for 1–4 hours. A portion is metabolized to an inactive material, uroheparin, by depolymerization; a little appears in the urine in an active form, and the remainder is destroyed in the body by the enzyme heparinase.

INDICATIONS

The chief uses of heparin are in the treatment of arterial and venous thrombosis and in vascular and cardiac surgery where an anticoagulant is required and when blood is circulating extracorporeally for any reason. Postoperatively it can be given by a low-dose subcutaneous regimen as a prophylaxis against deep vein thrombosis and embolism. Although it is not used as an anticoagulant for stored blood, it can be added to blood that has been anticoagulated with acid–citrate–dextrose (ACD) or citrate–phosphate–dextrose (CPD). The calcium content can then be safely restored, thus eliminating at least one of the disadvantages associated with the transfusion of large quantities of stored blood. Heparin may be added to fat emulsion to reduce the liability to venous thrombosis and is the *only* drug that can be safely added to such preparations. It is also used at the commencement of treatment with oral anticoagulants, such as phenindione, and discontinued after 36–48 hours when the slower acting drug has reached its full effect.

DOSAGE AND ADMINISTRATION

Owing to its rapid but transient action, heparin must be given by intermittent intravenous injection every 4–6 hours or by continuous infusion, the object being to keep the clotting time at about three times the pretreatment figure. Although it is commonly said that 1 mg of heparin is equivalent to 100 units, it should not be prescribed in milligrams. Preparations are standardized by a biological assay, and this equivalence is not guaranteed; the actual dry preparation may be considerably more active and is suitably diluted to give a solution of stated activity in units. It is customary to give about 12 000 units initially, followed by repeated doses of 10 000 units. If given by intravenous infusion 20 000–30 000 units may be added to 1 litre of Hartmann's solution or isotonic saline and administered over 24 hours. For prophylaxis in surgical patients, subcutaneous heparin is given in doses of 5000 units in 0.2 ml 8-hourly, the first dose being given immediately postoperatively. Heparin can be given intramuscularly but larger doses are necessary and the response is slower. The injections are painful and haematomas may occur at the site of injection.

PRECAUTIONS

Solutions lose their stability if kept below pH 6, and should not be mixed with dextrose solutions which are usually acidic. Heparin is incompatible with drugs containing methyl groups such as streptomycin and cetrimide. It is incompatible with hydrocortisone hemisuccinate, ristocetin, and vancomycin and should, therefore, not be used in infusions containing these substances.

In therapeutic doses heparin rarely produces toxic effects. Occasionally haematuria or bleeding from mucous membranes may occur and, rarely, haemothorax has been reported. In hypersensitive patients, allergic reactions have been observed.

Heparin is contraindicated if a patient has a known tendency to bleed, in cases of subacute bacterial endocarditis, in peptic ulcer, in malignant disease, and in threatened abortion or advanced renal or hepatic disease.

Withdrawal of the drug alone may be sufficient in cases of heparin overdosage, or its effect can be neutralized immediately by an injection of protamine sulphate. This may be given intramuscularly or intravenously in a dose of 1 mg for every 100 units of heparin previously administered.

Protamine sulphate

Protamine sulphate injection (*BP*) and Protamine sulfate for injection (*USP*)
Constitution: the sulphate of protamine, a protein from the sperm or mature testes of fish of the genera *Oncorhynchus, Salmo* or *Trutta*

PHARMACOLOGY

Protamine sulphate is a simple protein with basic properties. Although it has anticoagulant properties, it is only used as an antagonist to heparin where its strongly positive charge can neutralize the negatively charged heparin molecule to form a complex which is rapidly deposited, probably on vascular endothelial cells.

DOSAGE AND ADMINISTRATION

It is given intravenously in a 1 per cent solution and should be administered slowly over a period of several minutes, otherwise a serious fall in blood pressure may be encountered.

The amount of protamine sulphate required is 1 mg for each 100 units of heparin injected. If more than 15 minutes has elapsed since the injection of the heparin, proportionately less is required, particularly as protamine sulphate is itself an anticoagulant. Not more than 50 mg should be injected at any one time.

Warfarin sodium

Warfarin sodium (*BP* and *USP*)
Chemical name: sodium 4-hydroxy-3-(3-oxo-1-phenylbutyl) coumarin

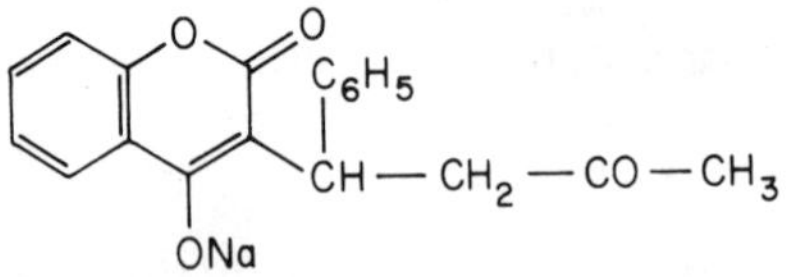

O
C_6H_5
$CH—CH_2—CO—CH_3$
ONa

PHARMACOLOGY

Warfarin inhibits the hepatic synthesis of the vitamin K-dependent clotting factors by substrate competition with vitamin K in their synthetic pathway. It is therefore not active *in vitro* and there is a delay in onset after administration of 12–24 hours until the existing circulating clotting factors disappear. While the major effect is to inhibit the synthesis of prothrombin (factor II) the plasma concentrations of factors VII, IX and X also decline.

Fate in the body. Warfarin is readily and completely absorbed after oral administration and this is a most important advantage over other coumarin-type anticoagulants. It is 97 per cent bound to albumin and this contributes to its negligible urinary excretion and long half-life of about 48 hours. Individual variation in half-life has been attributed to genetic factors. It is hydroxylated in the liver, the metabolites appearing in the urine. Warfarin crosses the placental barrier and is secreted in milk, but does not appear in the CSF.

INDICATIONS

Warfarin is used in the treatment of thromboembolic disorders, particularly those of venous origin, and for prophylaxis against further thromboses and pulmonary embolism. After a considerable vogue, the usage of coumarin anticoagulants in myocardial infarction has been progressively reduced. It is sometimes employed to minimize embolism associated with rheumatic heart disease.

DOSAGE AND ADMINISTRATION

An initial dose of 50 mg by mouth is followed by doses between 2 and 15 mg daily according to prothrombin time. Satisfactory results can also be obtained with a daily dose of 10–15 mg for 3–5 days without an initial loading dose. Smaller doses are advisable in the elderly. This regimen has the advantage of minimizing the risk of haemorrhage if the patient is unduly sensitive to the drug.

CONTROL OF THERAPY

The dose of warfarin is adjusted by measuring the 'prothrombin time' by Quick's one-stage test. In this, a tissue extract (rabbit brain) and a solution of calcium chloride are added to an oxalated sample of patient's plasma, and the time taken for the clot to form is measured. It is customary to aim at a prolongation of prothrombin time by a factor of two to three.

After the initial dose of oral anticoagulant it takes 24–36 hours before its anticoagulant effect can be assessed. The prothrombin time should therefore be measured on the morning before the third dose and then daily, adjusting the dose as required. When the patient is stabilized the frequency of estimation can be reduced to once every few weeks.

PRECAUTIONS

All coumarin-type anticoagulants can be the subject of numerous drug interactions (*see* page 460). Not only must changes in warfarin dose be monitored by prothrombin time estimations, therefore, but also all other drug regimen alterations. Warfarin is antagonized by phytomenadione (vitamin K_1); a dose of 10 mg is usually sufficient to reduce the prothrombin time to a safe level, but higher doses up to 150 mg may be required and are not toxic.

Dicoumarol was the earliest coumarin derivative but is now rarely employed in the UK. Absorption after oral administration is slower and more erratic than that of warfarin and the half-life is only 10–30 hours, depending on dose. Apart from these differences, the mechanism of action, metabolism, toxic effects, and precautions required are the same as for warfarin. It is susceptible to the same drug interactions. The recommended dose schedule for these and other similar compounds are given in *Table 18.2* (page 459).

19

Antimicrobial agents

History

The first antimicrobial compound to be introduced into clinical practice was compound 606, introduced by Ehrlich in 1909 and named by him Salvarsan because this compound, being active against the spirochaete of syphilis, was for him about to prove to be the saviour of the human race. He looked forward to the day when other compounds could be tailored to kill micro-organisms and yet leave mammalian tissues unharmed. However, several factors, such as the toxicity of the then used antiseptics and the active and fruitful studies in progress on the immunological defence mechanisms against infective diseases, combined to delay the next advance in antimicrobial agents for 25 years.

Much has been written concerning the excitements and counterclaims surrounding the discovery and development of penicillin and two publications by Hare (1970) and by Abraham (1971) have given more details of the eventful years up to 1942. Less has been heard about the early development of sulphonamides but these compounds also had a tortuous early course, with a cautious introduction by Domagk in 1935 and argument about the nature of the active principle which *in vivo* produced dramatic clinical effects.

The discovery of the effectiveness of these two compounds created areas of research that have produced a series of compounds which more than any other group of medicines has changed the pattern of clinical medicine. Taking benzylpenicillin as a model, many other micro-organisms have been examined to detect and extract antibiotic substances, many of which have clinical importance. Biochemical reactions have also been widely used to modify existing antimicrobials and produce valuable new compounds. In the 1940s and 1950s the screening of fungi yielded many new agents such as tetracycline, chloramphenicol, and streptomycin, whereas chemical modifications of the sulphonamide nucleus produced useful pharmacological changes in behaviour and reduced toxicity, although they failed to produce any broadening of the antimicrobial spectrum.

By 1960 antibiotic resistance particularly among staphylococci created a need for new antibiotics, and biochemical modifications of the benzylpenicillin nucleus led to a further advance. Using an amidase produced by *Escherichia coli* it was possible to split off the side chain from penicillin, yielding the nucleus 6-aminopenicillanic acid to which different side chains could be added to give compounds which were acid-stable (phenethicillin), broader spectrum (ampicillin, carbenicillin), or resistant to staphylococcal penicillinase (methicillin, cloxacillin). This type of biochemical rearrangement has also produced many new cephalosporins, using the

Table 19.1 Classification of antimicrobial agents

Group 1: *Active against Gram-positive bacteria and Gram-negative cocci*	*Group 2:* *Active mainly against Gram-negative bacilli*	*Group 3:* *Broad-spectrum antibiotics*	*Group 4:* *Specific antibacterials*	*Group 5:* *Antifungal, antiviral agents*
Standard penicillins Benzylpenicillin Phenoxymethylpenicillin Other oral penicillins	*2a. For systemic infections* Penicillins Aminopenicillins Carboxypenicillins Acylureidopenicillins Amidinopenicillins	Sulphonamides	*4a. Anaerobic organisms* Lincomycin (clindamycin)	*5a. Antifungal agents* Nystatin
Antistaphylococcal penicillins Methicillin Cloxacillin Flucloxacillin	Temocillin	Co-trimoxazole	Metronidazole	Amphotericin
Erythromycin and other macrolides	Monobactams	Cephalosporins	*4b. Tuberculosis* Streptomycin	Clotrimazole
Lincomycin Clindamycin	Aminoglycosides	Thienamycin	PAS	Griseofulvin
Rifampicin	Polymyxins	Beta-lactamase inhibitors Clavulanic acid Sulbactam	Isoniazid	*5b. Antiviral agents* Idoxuridine
Vancomycin	*2b. For urinary tract infections* Nitrofurantoin	Tetracycline Oxytetracycline etc.	Rifampicin	Amantadine
Bacitracin	Nalidixic acid Cinoxacin	Chloramphenicol	Ethionamide	Arabinosides
			Pyrazinamide	Acycloguanides
			Ethambutol	
			Cycloserine	

nucleus 7-aminocephalosporanic acid, the rifamycins and lincomycins and, more recently, trimethoprim. This latter compound is one of a series of dihydrofolate reductase inhibitors which show maximal effect on bacterial enzymes but minimal effect on mammalian enzymes. It also demonstrates an important synergistic action with sulphonamides.

New compounds have continued to appear as a result of the screening of fungi: more aminoglycosides (kanamycin, gentamicin, tobramycin, sissomicin, amikacin), polymyxins, and fusidic acid. New agents have appeared for the treatment of drug-resistant tubercule bacilli, for systemic fungal infections, and as antiviral agents.

Table 19.1 shows a classification of antimicrobial agents which is based on the antimicrobial spectrum of the compounds.

Intravenous administration of antibiotics

In order to produce rapid results, antibiotics are frequently given intravenously, particularly in shocked patients and in operating theatres where intravenous therapy provides a convenient route. On occasions the antibiotic is added to the bottle containing intravenous fluids and allowed to infuse continuously but, apart from highly irritant antibiotics, such as amphotericin, when a large volume of fluid may be necessary, this practice should be avoided and the antibiotics given by bolus injection.

The problems of mixing and administering intravenous drugs are discussed in detail in Chapter 20, but are of special relevance to the administration of antibiotics. Inactivation of antibiotics by some intravenous fluids has been reported; the penicillins are the most unstable, especially when put into dextrose solutions of low pH. This destruction of penicillins progresses more slowly in saline solutions but these solutions cannot be transfused indefinitely into a patient. There is little information available on the antibiotic levels following slow intravenous infusion of small amounts but if 500 mg of a penicillin are added to 500 ml of solution which is transfused over an 8-hour period, only 1 mg/min is being administered to the patient; conversely, fatal overdosage of some compounds, such as tetracycline, has occurred because of the ease with which an excessive dose can be given. Intravenous infusions are unreliable in their rate of flow and can stop; leakage of antibiotics into the subcutaneous tissues can cause marked inflammatory reactions. Incompatible mixtures, such as hydrocortisone and amphotericin, or gentamicin and carbenicillin, may be mixed and allowed to inactivate one another in the bottle. Finally, the dangers of introducing infected material into the bottle are not lessened by the fact that the additive is an antibiotic.

Because of these disadvantages, many people prefer to use a bolus injection technique, giving the whole intravenous dose of the antibiotic directly into the vein or venous line. In this way one can be assured of a high blood level, that the whole dose has been given, that the antibiotic is still active, and that the subcutaneous tissues will not be irritated.

Neuromuscular blockade by antibiotics

Some antibiotics have the ability to produce neuromuscular blockade in high dosage. They have a similar effect to curare but are much less potent, the effect of polymyxins being 0.5 per cent of that of curare and that of aminoglycosides about

0.1 per cent. However, the doses of antibiotics are much larger than those of curare-like substances and cases of paralysis have been recorded from polymyxins in patients with renal failure, and cases of apnoea have occurred following intraperitoneal administration of large doses of neomycin. Lincomycin has also been reported to produce a similar effect and has been shown *in vitro* to produce neuromuscular blockade. It is not uncommon to see neuromuscular blockade in patients who are also receiving muscle relaxants or anaesthetics. The mechanism is described in more detail in Chapter 9.

Sulphonamides

This group of antimicrobial agents was discovered during the investigation of dye-stuffs in experimental animal infections. One such dye, prontosil rubrum, was found to be highly active in streptococcal infection in mice although inactive *in vitro*. The revelation that the activity of this compound was due to the conversion in the body of this substance to the simpler compound *p*-aminobenzenesulphonamide (sulphanilamide, *p*-NH_2—C_6H_5—SO_2NH_2) gave chemists a simple molecule which has since been modified in many ways. Forty years after their introduction, new modifications continue to appear.

GENERAL PROPERTIES

Sulphonamides are poorly soluble in water but the sodium salts are readily soluble. Their acetyl derivatives (in which form they are partly excreted) are poorly soluble. They act by interfering with the utilization of *p*-aminobenzoic acid in folate metabolism in a wide range of micro-organisms. This effect does not occur in man in whom dietary folate is absorbed from the gut.

ANTIBACTERIAL ACTIVITY

The sulphonamides affect a broad spectrum of bacteria because of the wide distribution of the enzyme system which they disrupt. They are active against Gram-positive cocci (streptococci, pneumococci), Gram-negative cocci (*Neisseria gonorrhoeae* and *N. meningitidis*), Gram-negative bacilli (*E. coli, Proteus* species, some *Salmonella* and *Shigella* species) and Gram-positive bacilli (actinomyces, *Clostridium perfringens*, anthrax bacillus). Because of the purely bacteriostatic effects of sulphonamides and the greater activity of antibiotics, the latter have tended to replace many of the original indications for sulphonamide use. Sulphonamide resistance is now very common among *Salmonella* and *Shigella* species and local variations occur in the prevalence of sulphonamide resistance in *E. coli*. Another important resistance that is increasing is among strains of meningococci. There is little difference between the various sulphonamides in the degree or the range of antibacterial activity but important differences are seen in their pharmacological properties.

PHARMACOLOGY

Most sulphonamides are readily absorbed after oral administration. Succinylsulphathiazole and phthalylsulphathiazole, however, are not absorbed to any significant extent and are excreted unchanged in the faeces. They are used only for their actions on organisms in the bowel.

After absorption from the gut, sulphonamides undergo varying degrees of acetylation and binding to protein. Acetylation renders the drug inactive; the acetyl derivatives are usually more toxic than the free drug and some are poorly soluble and may give rise to crystalluria. Protein binding affects the diffusion of the drug into various compartments of the body and excretion into the urine is also delayed with highly protein-bound drugs. Because of the reversible nature of the binding, however, the drug is not rendered inactive but only released more gradually to the tissues. Sulphonamides can be displaced from their binding sites by a variety of agents such as phenylbutazone and ethyl biscoumacetate.

Sulphonamides are excreted in the urine partly unchanged and partly acetylated. The rate of excretion and the degree of acetylation vary widely between different drugs. Plasma clearance values range from less than 10 to more than 200 ml/min. Sulphafurazole has a high clearance rate and high concentrations appear rapidly in the urine. Sulphamethoxypyridazine has a low clearance rate, and therapeutic levels are maintained in the plasma for 24 hours. Highly protein-bound drugs are long acting because of the small amount that can be removed by the kidney although active tubular reabsorption may also delay the excretion of drugs with little protein binding. The effect of renal disease on excretion is unpredictable; it may allow some drugs to accumulate whereas others may be excreted more rapidly if tubular reabsorption is impaired.

The degree of protein binding influences to some extent the passage of the drug into the body compartments such as the CSF and the liquor amnii, but in general the sulphonamides are highly diffusible and reach therapeutic levels in such compartments.

For parenteral use sodium salts are used as intravenous injections in a concentration of 5–10 per cent. They are too alkaline to be added to a blood transfusion and cause severe irritation if there is any leakage into the tissues. Sodium sulphadimidine is the sulphonamide most commonly used for this purpose.

The pharmacological variations that have been described have resulted in a large number of sulphonamides being made available for therapy and the most popular ones are listed in *Table 19.2*.

Table 19.2 Sulphonamides of clinical importance

Types of compound	*Name*	*Dosage*
Poorly absorbed from gut	Succinylsulphathiazole	20 g single dose
	Phthalylsulphathiazole	10 g single dose
Rapid excretion into urine	Sulphafurazole	1 g 6-hourly
	Sulphamethizole	200 mg 6-hourly
General use compounds	Sulphadiazine	1 g 6-hourly
	Sulphadimidine	1 g 6-hourly
Blood levels maintained for 24 hours	Sulphamethoxypyridazine	0.5 g daily
Blood levels maintained for 7 days	Sulphamethoxydiazine	2 g single dose

In addition to those listed in *Table 19.2* there are several sulphonamides with special uses, such as mafenide acetate which is used topically as an application to wounds and burns where high concentrations inhibit *Pseudomonas aeruginosa*, and sulphasalazine which is used in the treatment of ulcerative colitis.

TOXICITY AND SIDE EFFECTS

The dangers of crystalluria vary between compounds. Of the commonly used compounds, sulphadiazine is most liable to precipitate in the tubules and ample fluid should be given and the urine kept alkaline when this compound is indicated. Skin reactions are usually mild, a maculopapular rash appearing after about a week's treatment. With current sulphonamides the incidence of rash is about 1 per cent and a reaction to one sulphonamide often means that a reaction will occur with others. An association between long-acting sulphonamides and the severe skin and mucous membrane necrosis known as Stevens–Johnson syndrome is difficult to prove or disprove owing to the extreme rarity of the cases. Haemolytic anaemia may occur in persons with glucose-6-phosphate dehydrogenase deficiency. Agranulocytosis is a rare complication.

Sulphonamides compete for the same protein-binding sites as bilirubin and there is a possibility of enhancement of jaundice in premature babies or those with haemolytic disease. Sulphonamides are therefore best avoided in the last 2 weeks of pregnancy and in neonates.

CLINICAL APPLICATIONS

The main uses of sulphonamides at present are:

1. Meningococcal meningitis – together with benzylpenicillin for cases; alone for treatment of carriers and close family contacts;
2. Uncomplicated urinary tract infections due to *E. coli* or *Pr. mirabilis*;
3. Suppression of the gut flora either in bacterial diarrhoea or prior to bowel surgery; there is little or no evidence of the effectiveness of this application.

Co-trimoxazole

This preparation is a fixed combination of two antibacterial substances (sulphamethoxazole and trimethoprim in a ratio of 5:1), which act in synergy on sequential stages in the metabolic pathway leading to purine synthesis. One member of this combination, sulphamethoxazole, is closely related to *p*-aminobenzoic acid and interferes with folic acid production. Folic acid is important in purine synthesis, being successively oxidized and reduced. The reducing enzyme, dihydrofolate reductase, is inhibited by trimethoprim, the second component of co-trimoxazole.

This combination therefore attacks two sequential steps in an essential biochemical process within the micro-organism. Since the process of purine synthesis is practically universal a very wide spectrum of micro-organisms is open to attack. The mammalian dihydrofolate reductases of the host are many thousands times less susceptible to trimethoprim than are the bacterial enzymes. Several preparations are available but the combination of drugs is identical in all of them.

ANTIBACTERIAL SPECTRUM

The trimethoprim component is active against Gram-positive bacteria and most Gram-negative bacilli except *Ps. aeruginosa*. The spectrum includes most organisms responsible for urinary tract infection and *Haemophilus influenzae*. The combination has a bactericidal action. Co-trimoxazole is an important advance in therapy and is widely used in many different types of infection.

Trimethoprim is now available as a single agent and may be given without sulphamethoxazole. The argument in favour of this is that the side effects of the sulphonamide are avoided. The argument against is that the antimicrobial spectrum is reduced and that emergence of resistance may be more likely to occur. Transferable antibiotic resistance to trimethoprim has been described and some hospitals have a rising incidence of strains of bacteria resistant to trimethoprim.

PHARMACOLOGY

Trimethoprim is well absorbed after oral administration and excreted relatively slowly into the urine. The plasma half-life is about 10 hours and about 40 per cent of the drug is protein bound. Sulphamethoxazole has a similar half-life to trimethoprim and was therefore chosen as the sulphonamide best able to act synergistically with trimethoprim. However, with difference in urine pH and in urine flow-rate, and with variation in renal function, the ratio of the two drugs may vary considerably in the urine. In renal failure it may be necessary to adjust the doses of the two drugs independently.

TOXICITY AND SIDE EFFECTS

The sulphonamide component is as liable to give skin rashes as other sulphonamides, and rashes are therefore seen in about 1 per cent of cases. Trimethoprim has only a very small effect on the folate system in man but some instances of a fall in haemoglobin have occurred in patients on treatment without complete evidence of a causal effect. Similarly, the response to vitamin B_{12} may be delayed in patients with pernicious anaemia if the patient is receiving trimethoprim. Accordingly, the haemoglobin level should be regularly checked in patients on co-trimoxazole or trimethoprim if they have received it for more than 2 months.

When injected in high doses into pregnant rats at a critical stage of pregnancy, trimethoprim can produce abortion; for this reason it is not recommended in early pregnancy.

DOSAGE AND INDICATIONS

The standard dose is two tablets (each containing 80 mg of trimethoprim and 400 mg of sulphamethoxazole) twice daily. Paediatric tablets have one quarter of the contents of adult tablets.

Indications for its use are:

1. Urinary tract infections associated with Gram-negtive rods (septicaemia, abdominal sepsis, febrile episodes in leukaemic patients);
2. Respiratory tract infections, particularly those associated with *H. influenzae*;
3. Enteric fever.

Penicillins

Classification

There are now many penicillins available for therapy and they are usually subdivided on the basis of their antibacterial activity although other subdivisions can be made on pharmacological properties, such as acid-stability or absorption from the gut. The four main groups are shown in *Table 19.3*.

Table 19.3 Classification of penicillins

Groups of penicillins	*Type of compound*	*Analogues, complexes and esters of similar antibacterial spectrum*
Group I Standard penicillins – highly active against cocci, both positive and negative, and against Gram-positive rods; susceptible to staphylococcal penicillinase	Penicillin G (benzylpenicillin) given by parenteral route	V analogues which are absorbed after oral administration include penicillin V Procaine penicillin and benzathine penicillin are complexes which slow down absorption from intramuscular injection sites
Group II Antistaphylococcal penicillins – penicillins that are stable to staphylococcal penicillinase	*a* Methicillin – the original parenterally administered penicillinase-stable penicillin	Analogue – nafcillin
	b Cloxacillin – acid-stable isoxazole penicillin which is absorbed after oral administration	Analogues – flucloxacillin, oxacillin, dicloxacillin
Group III Pencillins that are active against Gram-negative bacteria but susceptible to hydrolysis by Gram-negative and Gram-positive β-lactamases	*a* Aminopenicillins Ampicillin – activity similar to benzylpenicillin but additional activity against *E. coli, Proteus, Streptococcus faecalis, H. influenzae* and salmonellae	Esters of ampicillin which hydrolyse after absorption to release ampicillin include talampicillin, pivaloylampicillin (pivampicillin), and bacampicillin Closely related analogues are amoxycillin and epicillin
	b Carboxypenicillins Carbenicillin – extends the antibacterial range to include *Ps. aeruginosa* and indole-positive *Proteus* species	Esters of carbenicillin which are hydrolysed after absorption include carfecillin and indanyl carbenicillin Closely related analogue is ticarcillin which is not absorbed orally
	c Acylureidopenicillins Mezlocillin – extends the range of ampicillin to *Klebsiella* and other Gram-negative rods	No esters are available One related analogue – azlocillin – shows activity against *Ps. aeruginosa* Piperacillin has some activity against *Bacteroides fragilis* and *Ps. aeruginosa*
	d Amidinopenicillins Mecillinam – anti-Gram-negative spectrum but minimal activity against Gram-positive organisms	One ester – pivaloylmecillinam (pivmecillinam) – is absorbed after oral administration
Group IV Penicillins that are stable to Gram-negative β-lactamases	Temocillin	None

All members of the group have a dicyclic nucleus, 6-aminopenicillanic acid:

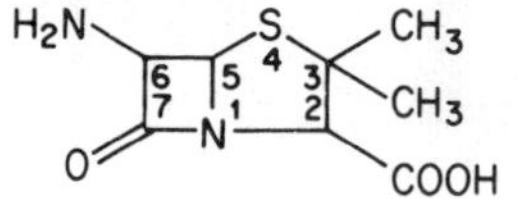

Variations in the side chains confer differences in antibacterial activity, absorption, excretion, and protein binding. The possession of a common nucleus means that a patient who is hypersensitive to one compound will be sensitive to all the others. However, reactions to substances other than the penicillin nucleus may occur and this can cause confusion (*see* Toxicity).

Benzylpenicillin was the first antibiotic to be made available and brought about dramatic effects. Although it has been joined by many other newer penicillins it has not lost its place as the first-choice antibiotic for many infections. It is remarkable that this compound, among the most active of the antibiotics, was the first to be discovered.

Benzylpenicillin and other penicillins with a similar spectrum (that is, against Gram-negative cocci and Gram-positive bacteria, excluding penicillinase-producing staphylococci) should be regarded as standard penicillins. Other standard penicillins include those resistant to attack by gastric acid. The activity of benzylpenicillin against the above organisms exceeds that of the other penicillins, which ought to be regarded as special purpose penicillins against specific pathogens rather than 'super' penicillins.

Benzylpenicillin

GENERAL PROPERTIES

The sodium and potassium salts of benzylpenicillin are white crystalline powders, highly soluble in water. They are stable when dried but the activity is slowly lost in aqueous solution. Acids and alkalis transform the molecule into penicillanic and penicilloic acids, respectively, which are microbiologically inactive. Enzymes that split the penicillin nucleus (penicillinases, β-lactamases) are widespread among Gram-negative and Gram-positive bacteria. Many different types of β-lactamase have now been described and there is evidence of transfer of β-lactamases between bacterial species. They were reported in *H. influenzae* for the first time in 1974 and in gonococci in 1976. They have an important role in resistance.

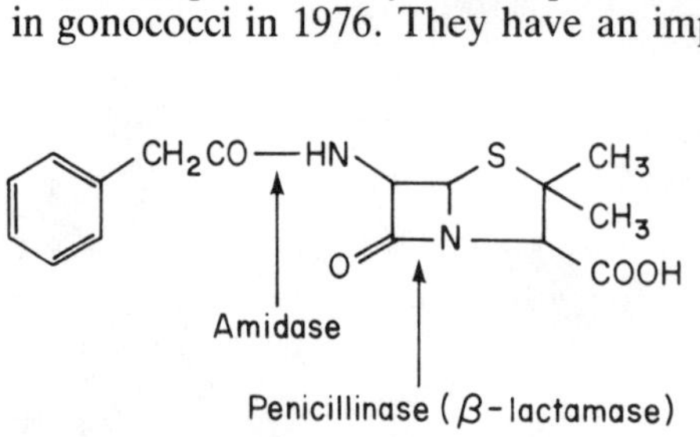

Amidase

Penicillinase (β-lactamase)

These enzymes are different from the enzyme amidase, which can split the side chain from the penicillin nucleus.

ANTIBACTERIAL ACTIVITY

The main activity of benzylpenicillin is against Gram-positive and Gram-negative cocci, pneumococci, streptococci, meningococci, gonococci, and staphylococci which do not produce penicillinase. It is also highly active against Gram-positive bacilli such as *Corynebacterium diphtheriae* and *Cl. perfringens*. It is also active against *Treponema pallidum*.

Penicillinase-producing staphylococci existed before the discovery of penicillin and have gradually become more prevalent, until at present 85 per cent of staphylococci isolated from patients in hospital and about 40 per cent of those isolated from patients in general practice are resistant to penicillin. However, those staphylococci that are sensitive to benzylpenicillin are more sensitive to this than to any other penicillin. Apart from staphylococci, some strains of gonococci and rare strains of *Str. pneumoniae*, there is no evidence of resistance developing among other cocci, Gram-positive bacilli, or treponema, and benzylpenicillin remains for them the drug of choice. Apart from the production of penicillinase, bacteria may be intrinsically resistant to penicillin and able to grow in its presence without actually destroying it. Examples of this are salmonella and *Str. faecalis*. Many Gram-negative bacilli, such as *Ps. aeruginosa, E. coli* and *Pr. mirabilis*, may have both mechanisms of resistance.

PHARMACOLOGY

Benzylpenicillin is inactivated by gastric acid and, although rapidly absorbed from the upper small intestine, a variable amount is lost in the passage through the stomach. It therefore should be given by intramuscular or intravenous injection. It is readily absorbed from muscle and diffuses into many body cavities. It passes into the fetus and into the liquor amnii, possibly by way of the fetal urine. The levels in normal CSF are low but when the meninges are inflamed it diffuses more readily. It is not necessary to give penicillin intrathecally in meningitis and it is much safer to use the intramuscular route.

Excretion occurs into the bile and into the urine. Concentrations in the bile are two to three times higher than those found in the blood, but the main excretion route is into the urine via the kidney tubules. Because absorption and excretion are so rapid, frequent doses are necessary to maintain adequate blood levels. More prolonged action can be obtained by delaying absorption by using salts of penicillin, such as procaine and benzathine penicillin which are less soluble than the sodium or potassium salts. Procaine penicillin gives a lower blood level than sodium benzylpenicillin but will maintain that level for 24 hours. Benzathine penicillin is even less soluble and can be detected in the serum for several days after injection. Procaine and benzathine penicillin should be given by intramuscular and *not* intravenous injection. Alternatively, the tubular excretion of penicillin may be delayed by giving probenecid, 1 g twice a day.

TOXICITY AND SIDE EFFECTS

Benzylpenicillin is not toxic when given parenterally. Doses of up to 30 g/day may be given with impunity, although one must remember that appreciable amounts of sodium or potassium are also being administered with these high doses and may be more toxic than the penicillin. Toxicity to the CNS occurs when the level in the CSF reaches 10 units/ml. It is difficult to reach these levels with intramuscular or intravenous therapy but easy by direct injection into the CSF. Several avoidable fatalities have occurred due to an overdose being given by this route.

There are two types of hypersensitivity reaction. The most serious reaction is anaphylactic shock, which may be rapidly fatal, but fortunately is uncommon. Clinics and other places where penicillin is injected should have adrenaline readily available and patients who give a history of a reaction to penicillin should not be given the drug. Many people claim to be 'penicillin-sensitive' with little or no evidence of hypersensitivity, but once such a history is established penicillins are contraindicated because there is no safe way of establishing that the history is incorrect. Death has on occasion followed an intracutaneous test dose of as little as 1 unit. Skin tests with penicilloyl compounds and many other tests have been used in the study of hypersensitivity but none will exclude penicillin hypersensitivity with certainty.

A more common and less serious reaction is fever accompanied by a widespread maculopapular rash developing after several days of treatment with penicillin. Some of these reactions probably indicate hypersensitivity to the compounds derived from the penicillin nucleus and, therefore, preclude further use of all penicillins. However, many of these reactions are due either to protein fractions arising as contaminants during manufacture or to polymerization of partially degraded penicillin fragments. In such cases it is likely that the patient is not hypersensitive. Much attention has been given to identifying such cases. It is an important problem because of the serious reactions that can occur should a genuinely hypersensitive person be given penicillin and because many other people are deprived of the benefits of penicillin who are not truly hypersensitive. Unfortunately, there is no clear solution to this problem at present.

CLINICAL APPLICATIONS AND DOSAGE

The main clinical uses of benzylpenicillin are as follows:

1. Upper respiratory infections – mainly due to *Str. pyogenes*;
2. Lobar pneumonia – due to *Str. pneumoniae*;
3. Meningococcal meningitis – in combination with sulphadiazine;
4. Gonorrhoea;
5. Syphilis;
6. Treatment of cases and carriers of *C. diphtheriae* – in combination with antitoxins;
7. Treatment and prophylaxis of gas gangrene and other clostridial infections;
8. Bacterial endocarditis due to streptococci – often in combination with streptomycin or gentamicin.

The dose of benzylpenicillin ranges from 300 mg units 6-hourly in minor infections to 20 g or more per day intravenously in bacterial endocarditis.

Acid-resistant penicillins

Phenoxymethylpenicillin (penicillin V) is less active than benzylpenicillin against gonococci but the difference is probably not of clinical importance. There are several acid-resistant penicillins which vary in their protein binding and absorption following oral therapy but the differences are marginal. Although benzylpenicillin is not acid-stable, some may be absorbed if large doses are given or enteric-coated capsules are used. Nevertheless, it is best kept for parenteral use. Phenoxymethyl-penicillin and phenethicillin are both acid-stable and, although patients vary in their ability to absorb them, this can be simply checked by examining the serum level of penicillin 1 hour after an oral dose. The clinical applications are identical to those of benzylpenicillin.

Penicillins resistant to staphylococcal penicillinase

The production of these valuable agents came at a crucial time for antimicrobial therapy. In the late 1950s an epidemic of severe staphylococcal infections occurred in most hospitals in Great Britain and in developed countries overseas. These strains were resistant to many of the non-toxic antibiotics then available, such as benzylpenicillin, erythromycin, tetracyclines, and streptomycin. Only compounds with severe side effects, such as vancomycin and ristocetin, were available for treatment of these conditions.

The removal of the side chain of benzylpenicillin to produce 6-aminopenicillanic acid (6-APA) was a major advance in therapy providing a nucleus on which many new side chains could be substituted.

Methicillin

Methicillin was the first compound to appear for clinical use and was made by replacing the benzyl side chain with a dimethoxybenzyl figuration. This compound was stable to staphylococcal penicillinase and, although of lesser activity than benzylpenicillin, it soon proved to be highly effective in severe infections due to staphylococci. Like benzylpenicillin it was not acid-stable and had to be given by intramuscular injection but, like all subsequent penicillins, the substance was relatively non-toxic and large amounts could be given.

Many other penicillinase-resistant penicillins were produced shortly afterwards, but the next important step was the development of isoxazole penicillins which were not only penicillinase-resistant but also acid-stable. Cloxacillin, which is more acid-stable than methicillin, was the first. This was followed by flucloxacillin, which is absorbed from the gastrointestinal tract about twice as well as cloxacillin, but has similar activity. The absorption of cloxacillin is irregular and it should be given before meals. It is being superseded as an oral agent by flucloxacillin, although some clinicians still prefer to use cloxacillin or even methicillin parenterally when a penicillinase-resistant penicillin is required. All of these penicillins are readily soluble in water but deteriorate when in solution.

Staphylococci resistant to methicillin appeared shortly after its introduction. This resistance is of the drug-tolerance type and the organisms do not produce enzymes to destroy methicillin. Organisms resistant to methicillin are also resistant to cloxacillin and flucloxacillin but as they are more readily detected in the laboratory using methicillin in the culture plates they have continued to be known as methicillin-resistant staphylococci. The incidence of these strains has remained low during the past 16 years although they have been isolated on a world-wide basis — even in places where methicillin has not been used. The incidence of resistance in staphylococci isolated in large hospitals is usually between 1 and 2 per cent, although certain units have reported a higher incidence. Measures to control the spread of infection in hospitals and to reserve antibiotics for special use have helped to prevent these organisms becoming too widespread.

CLINICAL APPLICATION AND DOSAGE

Members of the penicillinase-resistant group of penicillins should be reserved for the treatment of penicillinase-producing staphylococci. The dose need not exceed

500 mg 6-hourly in the majority of cases but larger doses may be needed in exceptional circumstances.

Aminopenicillins

The substitution of an amino group on the α-carbon atom of the side-chain produces compounds that are active against a wide range of Gram-negative bacteria.

Ampicillin

Ampicillin is α-aminobenzylpenicillin. This minor change from benzylpenicillin makes it much more active against Gram-negative bacilli. Many strains of *E. coli, Pr. mirabilis, Shigella* and *Salmonella* species are sensitive as judged by clinically orientated susceptibility guidelines. Most strains of *Klebsiella* and *Pseudomonas* are resistant. Ampicillin is susceptible to staphylococcal penicillinase, and organisms that destroy benzylpenicillin also destroy ampicillin. Strains of Gram-negative bacilli that produce penicillinase are therefore also resistant. Staphylococci that are resistant to benzylpenicillin are always resistant also to ampicillin.

Although ampicillin is only half to one quarter as active as benzylpenicillin against other Gram-positive cocci and Gram-negative cocci, this is still a high degree of activity against these organisms.

H. influenzae is also sensitive to ampicillin in concentrations of 1 mg/ℓ or less. In 1974, strains of *Haemophilus* which produced β-lactamase appeared in several countries. This created considerable therapeutic problems with *H. influenzae* meningitis. The prevalence of such capsulated strains had reached 13 per cent in England by 1981.

PHARMACOLOGY

Ampicillin is acid-resistant but absorption from the intestine is incomplete and also varies between patients. Peak levels are obtained 1.5–2 hours after an oral dose. Considerably higher blood levels can be obtained after intramuscular injection.

Excretion is mainly into the urinary tract, about 70 per cent of parenterally administered ampicillin being removed in this way. Some excretion also occurs via the bile when liver function is normal.

The passage of ampicillin into the body cavities resembles that of benzylpenicillin. In view of the actions against *H. influenzae*, much work has been done on sputum levels; these are high when the sputum is purulent and low when the sputum is mucoid. Levels sufficient to inhibit some strains of *Haemophilus* can only be obtained when high doses of the order of 4–6 g/day are given. Passage into the fetus and liquor amnii is slow when given orally but if given intramuscularly, therapeutic levels can be reached in the liquor within 6 hours.

TOXICITY AND SIDE EFFECTS

Ampicillin shares with other penicillins a freedom from toxicity. Unfortunately, ampicillin has been associated with skin rashes more frequently than any other penicillin. This reaction is delayed, appearing 7–10 days after the start of therapy and almost 10 per cent of patients have been affected. Factors such as high dosage increase the frequency of the rash, while if patients with glandular fever are given ampicillin, the incidence of rash is almost 100 per cent. It is likely that a mechanism different from true penicillin hypersensitivity is responsible for this rash. Many ampicillin rashes are due to protein impurities, and the manufacturing processes have already been modified and the incidence of rashes has been reduced although not eliminated.

CLINICAL APPLICATION AND DOSAGE

Ampicillin is often used as a substitute for benzylpenicillin in situations where benzylpenicillin is to be preferred. The two major indications for ampicillin therapy are:

1. Urinary tract infections due to *E. coli, Pr. mirabilis* or *Str. faecalis*;
2. Acute bronchitis or acute exacerbations of chronic bronchitis, which are normally due to either *H. influenzae* or *Str. pneumoniae*.

The dose is usually 250 mg 6-hourly but larger doses are often given.

Other uses include the treatment of typhoid carriers and of acute bacterial meningitis in childhood.

Other aminopenicillins

Amoxycillin is a hydroxylated ampicillin which confers upon it some microbiological and pharmacological changes. The antibacterial spectrum of amoxycillin is almost identical with that of ampicillin. Pharmacologically it is acid-stable and absorbed much more completely than ampicillin, serum levels being approximately twice those of a comparable dose of ampicillin. Urine and bile levels are also twice as high as with ampicillin and it appears in the sputum even when the sputum is mucoid.

Talampicillin is a phenyl ester of ampicillin and is better absorbed than ampicillin. Free ampicillin is released by esterases after absorption giving higher blood levels than can be reached by ampicillin alone.

Neither amoxycillin nor talampicillin is available for parenteral use although these two compounds are now frequently used as an alternative to oral ampicillin.

Carboxypenicillins

These are in the main reserved for treatment of *Ps. aeruginosa* and infections due to non-*mirabilis* strains of *Proteus*. However, they are increasingly used even for strains sensitive to ampicillin.

Carbenicillin is disodium α-carboxybenzylpenicillin. This compound shows an increase in activity against *Ps. aeruginosa*. The activity is not high; 25–50 mg/ℓ are needed for inhibition (compared with 0.03 mg/ℓ of benzylpenicillin for staphylococci) but because of their lack of toxicity sufficiently large doses of carboxypenicillins can be given to reach this level in the serum. Some strains resistant to over 1000 mg/ℓ have occurred, but these are uncommon at present except in some specialized units where they have become established. Carbenicillin is also active against most of the *Proteus* strains which are resistant to ampicillin, but not against penicillinase-producing *Klebsiella* and *Pr. mirabilis*, which are resistant. Pharmacologically, carbenicillin resembles other penicillins. It is not acid-stable and has to be given parenterally. Excretion is predominantly into the urine where extremely high levels are reached.

The very high levels of carbenicillin that are necessary may give rise to haemorrhage due to defective platelet function. The platelet count is normal but the bleeding time is prolonged.

Carfecillin is a phenyl ester of carbenicillin which undergoes similar pharmacological changes to talampicillin (*see* above). Following absorption and de-esterification, carbenicillin is excreted in the urine in amounts adequate for the treatment of urinary tract infection caused by carbenicillin-sensitive strains of bacteria.

Ticarcillin has an identical spectrum to carbenicillin with somewhat enhanced specific activity. Because it is given as the disodium salt, the electrolyte disturbance is less marked than with carbenicillin. Bleeding due to alteration of platelet function has been observed with both the carboxypenicillins, possibly related to the very high blood levels which are a result of the high doses employed.

Acylureidopenicillins

The ureidopenicillins are derived from ampicillin by substitution of the α-amino group with a heterocyclic compound. This has the effect of enhancing the antibacterial spectrum towards some micro-organisms. The effects on β-lactamase stability are marginal and all ureidopenicillins are unstable to gastric acid and have to be given parenterally. Azlocillin and mezlocillin are very similar in their activity, azlocillin being generally less active than mezlocillin except against *Ps. aeruginosa* where the activity is about four times that of carbenicillin. Apart from the activity against *Pseudomonas* and to some extent against indole-positive *Proteus* species the spectrum is very similar to that of ampicillin and they share the same susceptibility to hydrolysis by Gram-negative β-lactamases. *Ps. aeruginosa* plasmid-mediated β-lactamases do not inactivate ureidopenicillins to the same extent as they inactivate carbenicillin but the efficacy of ureidopenicillins in *Pseudomonas* infections remains to be confirmed.

Amidinopenicillins

This name is given to two penicillins, mecillinam and its pivoyl ester, pivmecillinam. They have an unusual mode of action for penicillins and readily produce *laevo*-forms in sensitive bacteria. They are much more active against Gram-negative rods than against Gram-positive organisms, in contrast to all other penicillins. This includes very high activity against *Salmonella* species.

Mecillinam can only be given parenterally but the pivoyl ester is absorbed orally and hydrolysed to mecillinam *in vivo*. The pharmacology after absorption resembles that of other penicillins. Currently it has been used primarily in the treatment of urinary tract infections but may become more widely used in the treatment of more severe forms of infection.

Temocillin

Temocillin is a new β-lactam antibiotic which is of considerable interest because it is the first penicillin that shows complete stability to hydrolysis by most Gram-negative β-lactamases.

The activity against carbenicillin-sensitive Gram-negative rods is of the same order as carbenicillin, azlocillin, and piperacillin, but against carbenicillin-resistant Gram-negative rods temocillin remains active whereas other penicillins show varying degrees of resistance. Similarly with *H. influenzae* strains that produce β-lactamase, the susceptibility is unchanged to temocillin whereas the resistance to ampicillin and carbenicillin increases four- to eight-fold. It has lowered activity against Gram-positive organisms compared with ampicillin and the ureidopenicillins.

Monobactams

Monocyclic β-lactams, or monobactams, have a spectrum of activity very similar to temocillin in that they are active against a wide range of Gram-negative bacilli regardless of whether or not they are producing β-lactamases. *Ps. aeruginosa* is relatively sensitive (minimum inhibiting concentration 4–8 mg/ℓ) but *E. coli, Proteus, Klebsiella*, and other related organisms are susceptible to 1–2 mg/ℓ. Gram-positive organisms are generally resistant.

Cephalosporins

The complexity of the products of *Cephalosporium acremonium* was such that the unravelling of the compounds produced by them required many years' study. The history extends from 1950 when Professor Brotzu first recognized that *Cephalosporium acremonium* produced antibiotic substances. Three main groups have been isolated from this mould: cephalosporin N, which is identical with penicillin N and has a nucleus of 6-aminopenicillanic acid; cephalosporin P, of which the main component is a steroid related to fusidic acid; and cephalosporin C, which has a nucleus slightly different from that of the penicillins – 7-aminocephalosporanic acid. It is upon this nucleus that the present-day cephalosporins have been built. The derivatives of cephalosporin C which are currently in use or shortly to become widely available are shown in *Table 19.4*. It will be seen that the cephalosporins show as much diversity as do the penicillins.

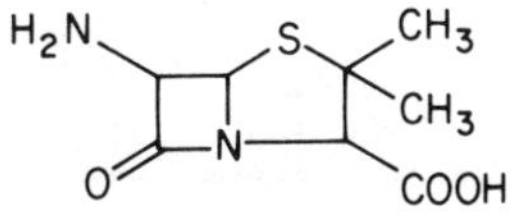

6-aminopenicillanic acid

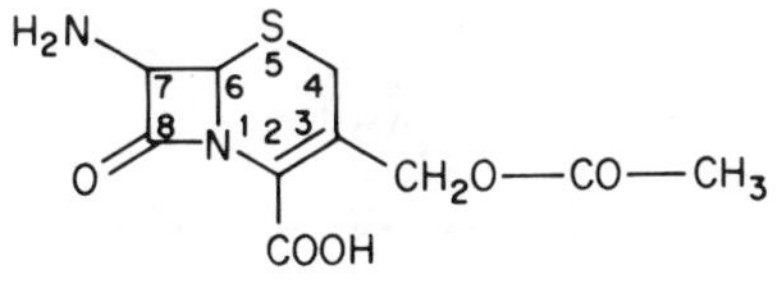

7-aminocephalosporanic acid

ANTIBACTERIAL SPECTRUM

Cephalosporins are often considered to be broad-spectrum antibiotics, but their activity against different bacterial species shows considerable variation. Activity against staphylococci is variable, being relatively low with the oral cephalosporins, but the activity of the compounds in Group II is high and their activity against penicillin-sensitive staphylococci is similar to that of benzylpenicillin. Penicillinase-producing staphylococci are also very sensitive to cephaloridine and cephalothin, but those which are resistant to methicillin are also resistant to the cephalosporins. Cephaloridine is more active than cephalothin but is also more susceptible to high concentrations of penicillinase.

Of the common Gram-negative bacilli, the cephalosporins show clinically useful activity against *E. coli, Pr. mirabilis* (including those strains resistant to ampicillin) and *Klebsiella* species. Among these species are strains resistant to some of the compounds but the newer Gram-negative β-lactamase-stable cephalosporins are active even against enzyme-producing strains. Compounds in Group III are particularly active against Gram-negative rods, including *H. influenzae*. Other *Proteus* species and *Pseudomonas* are resistant. Compounds in Group IV have useful activity against *Ps. aeruginosa*, while the cephamycins (Group V) are active

Table 19.4 Classification of cephalosporins based upon chemical structure, antibacterial activity, β-lactamase stability and metabolic stability. Cephalosporins have a wide antibacterial activity but there are significant variations in the degree of activity against groups of bacteria

Group	*Features*	
I: Oral group	Compounds that are very well absorbed after oral administration. Antibacterial activity relatively low compared with parenteral cephalosporins. Stable to Gram-positive β-lactamases and to some Gram-negative β-lactamases.	Cephalexin Cephradine Cefaclor
II: Gram-positive group	High activity against penicillinase-producing staphylococci and other Gram-positive bacteria. Activity against Gram-negative rods is relatively low. (a) are metabolically stable. (b) are desacetylated with loss of antibacterial activity.	(a) Cephaloridine Cephazolin (b) Cephalothin Cephacetrile
III: Enterobacteria group	Compounds with high activity against many aerobic Gram-negative rods and stability to many β-lactamases produced by these bacteria. (a) are metabolically stable. (b) is metabolically unstable.	(a) Cephamandole Cefuroxime (b) Cefotaxime
IV: Pseudomonas group	Compounds with high activity against *Pseudomonas* strains in addition to activity against enterobacteria. (a) are more stable than (b) to plasmid-mediated β-lactamases.	(a) Ceftazidime Cefsulodin (b) Cefoperazone Ceftriaxone
V: Cephamycins (7-α-methoxycephalosporin-s)	Compounds with high stability to β-lactamases of aerobic and anaerobic bacteria.	Cefoxitin Moxalactam Cefotetan

against anaerobic bacteria, in particular *Bacteroides fragilis*. Cephalexin is the least active oral cephalosporin, the other two compounds showing broadly similar activity. Activity against *Str. faecalis* is marginal and not of clinical value. Most cephalosporins show only marginal activity against *H. influenzae*, except for cephamandole, which shows high activity *in vitro*.

PHARMACOLOGY

With the exception of cephalexin, cephradine, and cefaclor, cephalosporins are not absorbed when given orally and parenteral administration is necessary. The three oral cephalosporins are very well absorbed. Distribution into the tissues is rapid. There is relatively rapid passage into the liquor amnii and fetus during pregnancy and into the CSF in meningitis, but not through normal meninges. A variable degree of protein binding occurs.

Excretion is mostly via the kidney but the compounds are handled differently and the effect of probenecid on the excretion of cephalosporins also differs. For example, cephaloridine is removed by glomerular filtration and tubular activity is minimal; probenecid therefore has no effect on serum levels. Cephalothin and cephalexin are removed by tubular secretion and probenecid is able to block this and prolong higher blood levels. A small amount of all the cephalosporins passes into the biliary tract.

TOXICITY AND SIDE EFFECTS

The toxicity of cephalosporins is low. Intramuscular injections may be painful and large doses are best given intravenously. The most serious toxic effects are on the kidney. High blood levels of cephaloridine cause renal tubular necrosis, especially if diuretics such as frusemide are also being administered. Patients with some degree of renal failure are those most likely to accumulate cephaloridine thus allowing blood levels to reach a dangerous level. It is therefore essential to check the blood levels in patients receiving high doses of cephaloridine, and it should not be allowed to exceed 80 mg/ℓ. High doses of cephaloridine and frusemide also cause renal damage in experimental animals but cephalothin and cephalexin do not appear to damage the kidney. Data are not available for the effects of newer cephalosporins on the human kidney.

Hypersensitivity, which is a complex matter with penicillin therapy, is even more obscure with the cephalosporins because in addition to patients with reactions to cephalosporins alone there is some evidence in other patients of cross-sensitivity to penicillin. The incidence of skin rashes with cephalosporins is lower than with ampicillin and some other penicillins. It has been estimated that 10 per cent of patients hypersensitive to penicillin are also hypersensitive to cephalosporins, but most of the evidence is based on *in vitro* tests or skin testing. The number of reported cases of severe cross-reactions is small. However, as one of the main indications for using cephalosporins is hypersensitivity to penicillins, some caution is necessary.

Other side effects reported include the development of a positive direct Coombs' test when high doses of cephalothin are given (more rarely with cephaloridine and cephalexin). This finding has not been associated with development of anaemia but can interfere with cross-matching of blood. Vulvovaginitis due to candida superinfection occurs frequently in pregnant women treated with cephalosporins.

CLINICAL APPLICATIONS AND DOSAGE

The main uses of cephalosporins at present are as substitutes for penicillins in hypersensitive patients, and caution on this was advised in the previous section. However, parenteral cephalosporins are active against a wide variety of organisms and they are often used in combination with other agents in the treatment of severe undiagnosed infections arising in hospitals. They are active against some Gram-negative bacilli not affected by ampicillin (for example, *Klebsiella*) and are also widely used in treating staphylococcal infections. The main use of cephalexin at present is in urinary tract infections when the organism is resistant to sulphonamides and the patient hypersensitive to penicillins.

The dosage of parenteral cephalosporins ranges from 1 g twice a day intramuscularly up to 12 g/day intravenously (6 g of cephaloridine) depending on the severity of the infection. Cephalexin is given orally and the usual dose is 250–500 mg 6-hourly.

Aminoglycosides

Several aminoglycosides have been produced and found a place in therapy, including streptomycin, neomycin (and framycetin), kanamycin, gentamicin, tobramycin, amikacin, sissomicin and netilmicin.

Table 19.5 Relationships of the aminoglycoside (aminocyclitol) antibiotics

Group	*Amino sugar*	*Type of compound*	*Features*	*Derivatives*
1	The central ring is streptone and the amino sugar is glucosamine	Streptomycin	Of prime importance is the activity against *Mycobacterium tuberculosis*	Dihydrostreptomycin – formed by dehydration of the free aldehyde group – has greater ototoxicity than streptomycin and is no longer used
2	The central sugar is deoxystreptone			
	2a. Pentose and glucosamine	Neomycin B C	Neomycin is a combination of two closely related compounds; too toxic for systemic use	Framycetin is neomycin B
	2b. Kanosamine	Kanamycin A B	Closely related kanamycins, of which kanamycin A is most commonly used; mainly of importance now because of its two derivatives	Amikacin is a kanamycin A derivative which has a hydroxybutyric acid substituent which confers resistance to most inactivating enzymes from Gram-negative rods Tobramycin is a kanamycin B derivative which is dehydrogenated in the 3′-position conferring resistance to many phosphorylating enzymes from *Ps. aeruginosa*
	2c. Garosamine	Gentamicin C_1 C_{1a} C_2	Active against a wide range of Gram-negative rods; gentamicin is a mixture of three related compounds derived from an actinomycete, therefore not spelled with a 'y'	Sissomicin is 4′-5″-dehydrogenated gentamicin C_{1a} and has a similar spectrum to gentamicin Netilmicin is *N*-ethyl sissomicin and this substituent is resistant to many aminoglycoside-inactivating enzymes
3	Actinamide	Spectinomycin	It only has moderate activity and its main use is against *N. gonorrhoeae* (including β-lactamase-producing strains)	

Streptomycin was one of the first antibiotics to be discovered. A systematic search of the streptomycetes for antibiotic substances was begun in 1939 by Waksman and colleagues. By 1942 they had isolated streptotricin, an antibiotic too toxic for systemic use, and this was followed in 1944 by streptomycin isolated from *Streptomyces griseus*. Its use in the treatment of tuberculosis alone has saved countless lives. Neomycin followed in 1949 isolated from *Streptomyces fradiae*. This was again too toxic for systemic use, but is used extensively as a topical preparation.

The other members in this group were isolated elsewhere: kanamycin in Japan, gentamicin and tobramycin in the USA. It is now possible to modify aminoglycosides chemically and the newer compounds are substituted gentamicins or kanamycins.

The aminoglycosides are chemically complex with three separate ring structures, two of which are substituted amino sugars. They are strongly basic and, of the salts formed, the sulphate is the most important in all cases. The sulphates are all soluble in water and are stable for long periods in solution especially if kept cold. They are strongly bactericidal, interfering with protein synthesis of micro-organisms, and all have a broad spectrum of activity.

Resistance of bacteria to aminoglycosides is often mediated by enzymes collectively known as aminoglycoside-inactivating enzymes. At least 16 different enzymes have been described, each attacking different points in the aminoglycoside nucleus, acetylating, adenylating, or phosphorylating side chains in the nucleus. The acquisition of these enzymes is by way of R-factors. The patterns of resistance and cross-resistance between aminoglycosides are complex and depend not only on the enzymes but also on the barriers to penetration of the antibodies. A wide range of aminoglycosides has been synthesized and the relationships are shown in *Table 19.5*.

Aminoglycosides are not absorbed from the gut, and their behaviour following intramuscular injection closely resembles that of streptomycin with peak blood levels 1 hour after injection and elimination primarily through the urinary tract by glomerular filtration.

Excessive serum levels of the antibiotic can cause damage to the eighth cranial nerve. All patients should have blood concentrations of kanamycin checked, and the dose adjusted so that the level is kept below that causing ototoxicity, especially if there is any doubt about renal function.

The main uses of these agents is as a primary treatment for undiagnosed severe infections, such as septicaemia arising in hospital. The main organisms in mind when treating these infections are *E. coli* and *Proteus* and *Klebsiella* species, but they are also active against most strains of staphylococci. Aminoglycosides are not usually given alone in these circumstances as this type of infection may also be caused by streptococci that are resistant to aminoglycosides, and a penicillin is therefore added.

Aminoglycosides are also used in the treatment of urinary tract infections due to strains of bacteria resistant to agents which can be given orally; these are usually found only in patients with chronic urological disease. Kanamycin was the most important of the aminoglycosides in the 1960s, but because of the lack of activity against *Ps. aeruginosa* its use has been largely superseded by analogues such as tobramycin or amikacin, and by gentamicin and its analogues.

Streptomycin

ANTIBACTERIAL ACTIVITY

The most important organism sensitive to streptomycin is *Mycobacterium tuberculosis*; strains are usually inhibited by 0.5 mg/ℓ. High activity is also shown against Gram-negative bacilli but the sensitivity cannot be predicted and laboratory tests are necessary to establish the sensitivity of the organisms, particularly in hospital. Outside hospitals most strains of *E. coli* and *Pr. mirabilis* are sensitive. All types of streptococci and clostridia are resistant to streptomycin.

Resistance in rapidly growing organisms develops quickly in laboratory experiments; development of resistance can also occur in patients on treatment, particularly in infections of the urinary tract. Resistance in new cases of clinical infection with *Myco. tuberculosis* has, however, remained at 1–2 per cent, due to careful antibiotic management by chest physicians and the use of combined chemotherapy.

PHARMACOLOGY

After oral administration, streptomycin is excreted unchanged in the faeces. After intramuscular injection serum levels are maximal after 1 hour and fall slowly. Streptomycin diffuses readily to most tissues but does not pass into cells; it passes readily into serous fluids and into the fetal circulation. Streptomycin does not enter the CSF readily and many cases of tuberculous meningitis have been treated by intrathecal installation of small doses of streptomycin; prolonged therapy of this type may, however, itself cause pleocytosis of the CSF. Most paediatricians today do not use the intrathecal route, relying on intramuscular injection to produce levels in the meninges adequate for treatment.

Excretion occurs into the urinary tract by glomerular filtration and high levels are obtained in urine; accumulation in plasma occurs if there is even a slight degree of renal impairment and blood levels should be monitored in such cases. The amount excreted into the bile is low.

TOXICITY AND SIDE EFFECTS

Streptomycin, in common with all aminoglycosides, can damage the eighth cranial nerve and/or be involved in neuromuscular blockade. Although it is possible that a few cases of eighth-nerve damage have been due to hypersensitivity, the majority are due to a direct toxic effect related to excessively high blood levels of the drug, either from the administration of too high a dosage or following a prolonged course of treatment.

Both the patient's age and renal function influence the blood level. In the presence of oliguria even short courses of treatment (for example, 1 g daily for 5 days) can cause vertigo or even total deafness. In elderly patients on prolonged therapy for tuberculosis and in patients with renal damage who require short courses of treatment, the dose should be determined with reference to measurements of the blood level of streptomycin. Although both vestibular and auditory branches of the eighth nerve can be affected, vestibular effects such as vertigo and unsteadiness are more common. Deafness was much commoner with dihydrostreptomycin.

Minor skin rashes and drug fever are common but are readily controlled. Exfoliative dermatitis has occurred on rare occasions. Nurses or doctors handling streptomycin sometimes develop skin sensitivity. Blood dyscrasias are rare.

CLINICAL APPLICATIONS AND DOSAGE

Streptomycin is of great value in tuberculosis; it is mainly used in the treatment of this disease in combination with other compounds. In combination with penicillin, a highly active bactericidal effect is obtained and this mixture was formerly widely used in treating infections arising in the course of abdominal surgery. Some surgeons still use it to provide 'cover' for clean abdominal surgery, but fortunately this practice is declining. The synergy with penicillin is useful clinically in the treatment of bacterial endocarditis. In tuberculosis 0.5–1 g/day is given, usually as a single dose intramuscularly. In systemic infections the dose is 0.5 g intramuscularly twice daily. These doses vary with the renal function of the patient.

Neomycin consists of two compounds, neomycin B and neomycin C which are of almost identical activity; as they are extracted in a mixed form during preparation they are not separated further. There is some evidence that the closely related compound framycetin is neomycin B. The sulphate is readily soluble in water and solutions are stable. Neomycin is too toxic for systemic use.

A wide spectrum of organisms are sensitive to neomycin including staphylococci, enterobacteria (except *Ps. aeruginosa*) and *Myco. tuberculosis*. Staphylococci resistant to neomycin have appeared and have become widespread in some hospitals. They are best controlled by stopping the use of neomycin sprays.

Neomycin is excreted unchanged in the faeces after oral administration. Minimal amounts may be absorbed and can accumulate if given for prolonged periods in hepatorenal failure. Absorption can also occur if neomycin is instilled into serous cavities and this should also be avoided. The main toxic effects are on the auditory branch of the eighth nerve producing total deafness. Neuromuscular block can also occur. Skin sensitization can occur with topical use.

Neomycin and framycetin are widely used topically in powders and sprays for such purposes as treating nasal carriers of *Staphylococcus aureus*, superficial pyogenic infections and, in combination with other compounds such as bacitracin and polymyxin, to prevent wound sepsis. It is also widely used for preoperative bowel 'sterilization' and to treat children with gastroenteritis due to enteropathic *E. coli* and *Shigella* species. In small children doses of 50–100 mg twice daily by mouth are used and in adults 500 mg twice daily.

Gentamicin

Gentamicin is not derived from *Streptomyces* but from the closely related micro-organism *Micromonospora purpurea*.

Gentamicin is active against both Gram-negative and Gram-positive bacteria. Its main advantage is its high activity against *Ps. aeruginosa* but strains of *Proteus* and *Klebsiella* are often sensitive to gentamicin. Strains resistant to gentamicin are resistant to the aminoglycosides previously mentioned. Gentamicin also shows slightly greater activity against streptococci than other aminoglycosides but not enough to be clinically useful.

Many of the enzymes referred to above also inactivate gentamicin. The isolation of Gram-negative rods resistant to gentamicin is now a frequent occurrence in some hospitals in the UK. During 1976 for the first time outbreaks of staphylococcal infections due to gentamicin-resistant staphylococci occurred in several areas of the UK.

PHARMACOLOGY AND TOXICITY

Gentamicin is more toxic than kanamycin to the eighth nerve, particularly the vestibular branch, and when first introduced, very low doses were given and only low blood levels were obtained. However, toxic effects have not been seen when blood levels of gentamicin are below 10 mg/ℓ and the dose has been gradually increased to give blood levels nearer this level. The renal handling of the drug is primarily by glomerular filtration without tubular reabsorption and therefore even with minor degrees of renal impairment the intervals between doses should be lengthened to prevent accumulation to toxic levels.

Gentamicin does not itself cause any renal toxicity in animal experiments. The concentrations of gentamicin in the CSF are low, and the concentrations in bile and serous fluids are about half of those found in the serum.

CLINICAL APPLICATIONS AND DOSAGE

Gentamicin has been widely used in septicaemia arising in neonatal units, intensive therapy units and following extensive surgical procedures. Patients with leukaemia or burns or whose immunological responses have been suppressed are likely candidates for pseudomonas infection and may require gentamicin therapy. In such circumstances gentamicin is often given with high-dose carbenicillin therapy. It has also been used in patients with chronic urinary tract infection due to *Ps. aeruginosa*. The dose in patients with normal renal function is 80 mg intramuscularly, three times a day, following a loading dose of approximately 4 mg/kg. The blood concentrations should be monitored in all patients.

Tobramycin

Tobramycin is derived from *Streptomyces tenebrarius*. At least seven antibacterial compounds have been isolated from this organism and tobramycin is the most active.

The antibacterial spectrum of tobramycin differs from that of gentamicin in that, against gentamicin-sensitive strains of *Pseudomonas*, tobramycin displays slightly greater activity – but shows less activity against some staphylococci.

Serum levels of tobramycin are similar to or slightly higher than those after a similar dose of gentamicin. Ototoxic effects in experimental animals are mainly on the vestibular branch.

Amikacin

Amikacin is the aminoglycoside that has the widest range of activity against antibiotic-resistant Gram-negative rods. This stems from the resistance to inactivation by almost all the modifying enzymes found in such bacteria. It has, however, less specific activity than gentamicin and its analogues. Therefore a larger dose than that of gentamicin has to be given for the same antibacterial effect. Because the toxicity of amikacin is about half that of gentamicin this increased dosage is possible. The dosage for adults is 15 mg/kg/day – compared with 6–8 mg/kg/day for gentamicin. The therapeutic range of peak blood levels is also twice as high as gentamicin. One expects to achieve peak levels of 25 mg/ℓ of amikacin. The side effects and toxicity are similar to those of other aminoglycosides. The use of amikacin is usually reserved for organisms found to be resistant to gentamicin.

Tetracyclines

Tetracyclines have a chemical structure consisting of four interconnected carbon rings with small side chains in which various substitutions have been made.

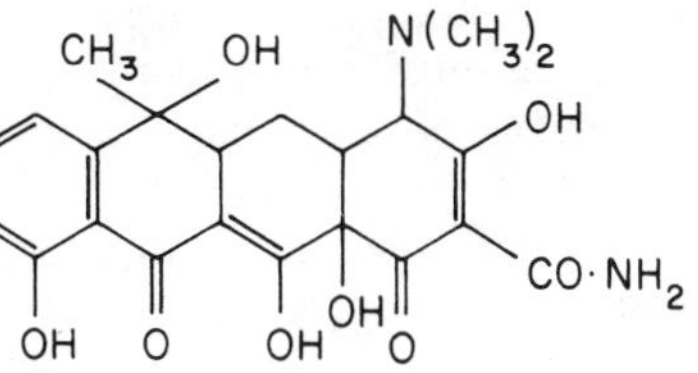

The three earliest members of the group were chlortetracycline, oxytetracycline, and tetracycline. Since then other substituents have been produced, such as demethylchlortetracycline, pyrrolidinomethyltetracycline, tetracycline-L-methylenelysine, methyleneoxytetracycline, chlormethylenecycline and deoxytetracycline.

The picture of tetracyclines is further confused by the proliferation of proprietary preparations of each category of tetracycline and the addition of other agents, for example, nystatin, to prevent side effects, or combined with other antibiotics to give broader activity. A recent issue of a prescribers' guide, for example, lists no fewer than 35 preparations of tetracylcines. This number of compounds suggests that tetracyclines are easy to manufacture and that they are effective and widely used antibiotics.

Fortunately, the understanding of the tetracyclines is made fairly easy because they exhibit almost identical antibacterial activity, and modifications to the side chains are made only to effect changes in their pharmacology. In most British hospitals the niceties of the pharmacological difference are usually (and probably correctly) ignored and a large batch of the cheapest available tetracycline is provided for the prescriber. Although widely used in Europe, the newer tetracyclines have not made much impact in Great Britain. Two that are worthy of note, however, are doxycycline and minocycline.

GENERAL PROPERTIES

Tetracyclines are poorly soluble in water, but the hydrochlorides are soluble and produce strongly acidic solutions. Chlortetracycline is more unstable in aqueous solution than the other two main compounds, losing most of its activity after incubation for 18 hours at 37°C.

Tetracyclines act by interfering with protein synthesis within the bacterial cell and are in consequence bacteriostatic in their action. There is antagonism *in vitro* between tetracycline and penicillins as the latter group can only act on actively dividing bacteria, but only isolated clinical cases of this antagonism *in vivo* have been reported.

ANTIBACTERIAL ACTIVITY

Tetracyclines are active against a wide range of organisms but some important species are resistant and after many years' use resistance is widespread among many species which were formerly sensitive.

Streptococci were fairly uniformly sensitive in 1950 but the incidence of tetracycline resistance in β-haemolytic streptococci is now as high as 50 per cent in some areas. The incidence of resistance in pneumococci is lower, but in some areas the incidence reaches 25 per cent. *Str. faecalis* strains in hospital patients are almost uniformly resistant but some strains in general practice are sensitive; 50 per cent of hospital strains of staphylococci are tetracycline resistant but outside hospitals most strains of staphylococci are still sensitive to the drug.

Some strains of *H. influenzae* are also tetracycline resistant. Minocycline differs in being active against many strains resistant to other tetracyclines. Sensitivity to minocycline has also been reported for tetracycline-resistant staphylococci, pneumococci, *H. influenzae* and for some strains of Gram-negative bacilli.

Gram-negative bacilli, with the exception of *Pr. mirabilis* and some strains of *Ps. aeruginosa*, were at one time sensitive but hospital strains of *E. coli, Klebsiella* and so on now show resistance in approximately 30 per cent of strains. Gram-positive bacilli remain sensitive to tetracyclines.

The very broad range of action of tetracyclines includes spirochaetes, chlamydia (psittacosis, lymphogranuloma venereum), rickettsia, and *H. influenzae*.

PHARMACOLOGY

The tetracyclines are absorbed from the gastrointestinal tract after oral administration, but in neutral or alkaline solutions, as are found in the intestine, tetracyclines tend to precipitate. Divalent ions such as calcium and iron also combine with tetracycline in the intestine to delay its absorption. Phosphate is often included with tetracycline preparations to counteract the latter effect. Blood levels tend to form a plateau rather than a peak and 20–40 per cent of the tetracycline in the serum is protein bound.

Tetracyclines are distributed widely in the tissues; levels in the fetus reach 50 per cent of the maternal level and concentrations in the CSF reach 10 per cent of the serum level. Tetracycline is deposited in bone especially in osteoblastic areas.

Concentrations in the bile are 10 times higher than in the blood and some of this tetracycline can be reabsorbed from the intestine. The main route of excretion is via the kidney.

Some of the newer tetracyclines are better absorbed than the standard tetracyclines allowing the use of smaller doses for a given blood level. For example, demethylchlortetracycline is approximately twice as well absorbed as tetracycline and a dose of 600 mg/day in divided dosage is adequate. Other compounds such as deoxytetracycline show delayed excretion by the kidney and a single dose per day is adequate.

When used parenterally, the standard tetracyclines are usually given by slow intravenous infusion. One of the newer tetracyclines, pyrrolidinomethyltetracycline, is not only highly soluble but of neutral pH and high doses can be given intramuscularly.

TOXICITY AND SIDE EFFECTS

High blood concentrations of tetracyclines cause liver damage. Fatal cases of liver failure have followed the parenteral administration of doses in excess of 2 g/day. Pregnant women appear to be especially prone to this toxic effect but there is no indication for exceeding 1 g/day even in non-pregnant patients and there are almost always alternative antibiotics available for use in pregnancy. Toxic effects have also been reported in patients with renal impairment in whom they have caused increasing renal failure, and therefore tetracyclines should not be given to such patients. Doxycycline has much less effect on renal function than other tetracyclines.

The effect of tetracycline on teeth is now well recognized: when the antibiotic is given during the formation of teeth, tetracycline is precipitated with the calcium in the tooth bud causing discoloration and hypoplasia. Primary or secondary teeth may be affected depending on whether the drug is given while the child is still *in utero* or afterwards; the risk is present until the child reaches 8 years of age.

The side effects of tetracycline on the gastrointestinal tract were recognized early. The effects range from mild nausea and diarrhoea to fulminating and fatal gastroenteritis. Two mechanisms are responsible; early symptoms are probably due to a direct irritant effect of the drug on the mucosa following precipitation in the small intestine; biliary–intestinal recirculation of the tetracycline may contribute to this. Symptoms arising after some days are more likely to be the result of superadded infections of the bowel by tetracycline-resistant organisms. The spectrum of tetracycline is so wide that in addition to suppressing the pathogens for which therapy was instituted, there is suppression of the essential normal flora of the gut. Staphylococcal enterocolitis is the most serious superinfection particularly when it occurs in postoperative surgical patients. Colonization by organisms such as *Candida albicans* can lead to protracted pruritus ani but rarely produces life-threatening infections. Minocycline has side effects peculiar to itself – headache, nausea, and vertigo – which appear to be dose related.

CLINICAL APPLICATIONS AND DOSAGE

Upper respiratory tract infections have *not* been an indication for tetracyclines since the appearance of resistant pneumococci and β-haemolytic streptococci, but they still are valuable in pneumonias caused by mycoplasma, chlamydia (psittacosis) and rickettsia. The commonest usage is in the treatment of chronic bronchitis. Other indications are brucellosis, cholera, leptospirosis, and trachoma. They are also valuable in intra-abdominal sepsis where a wide variety of Gram-negative and Gram-positive bacterial species are likely to be involved. As these organisms are not originally acquired in hospital they are also likely to be tetracycline sensitive.

The oral dosage of standard tetracyclines is 250 mg 6-hourly, but less of the newer compounds is required. Intravenously the dose should not exceed 1 g/day.

Chloramphenicol

Chloramphenicol is a broad-spectrum bacteriostatic antibiotic derived from an actinomycete.

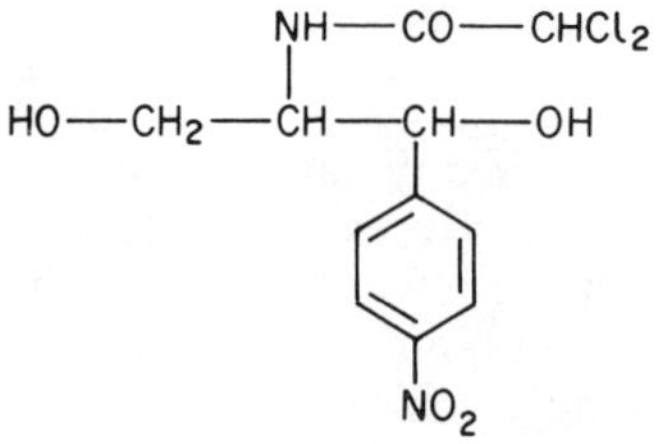

```
            NH—CO—CHCl2
            |
HO—CH2—CH—CH—OH
                 |
              (C6H4)
                 |
                NO2
```

It has a very simple structure based on a nitrophenol with a short side chain; it is readily synthesized and can now be manufactured without the use of the organism from which it was originally derived.

Chloramphenicol is a very stable compound moderately soluble in water.

ANTIBACTERIAL ACTIVITY

The antibacterial spectrum is very wide and is mediated by an inhibition of protein synthesis inside the bacterial cell. Almost all pathogens were originally sensitive to chloramphenicol but the activity against *Ps. aeruginosa* is marginal and penicillins are much more active against Gram-positive cocci. Important organisms which are more likely to be more sensitive to chloramphenicol than any other antibiotic include *Salmonella typhi* and other *Salmonella* species. *H. influenzae* and *Bordetella pertussis* are also highly sensitive. Like tetracyclines, chloramphenicol is active against organisms of the rickettsia and chlamydia groups.

PHARMACOLOGY

The absorption of chloramphenicol depends to a large extent on the form in which it is administered and the smaller the particle size of the powder, the better. The taste is bitter but can be masked by forming salts, such as the palmitate, which are hydrolysed in the gut releasing chloramphenicol for absorption.

Chloramphenicol is highly diffusible because of its small molecule and high concentrations are reached in the serous cavities, the cerebrospinal fluid, and the fetus. Small quantities also reach the bile. Excretion is by way of the urinary tract; there is glomerular filtration of the active antibiotic, but an acetylated breakdown product is secreted by the tubules and the majority of the chloramphenicol excreted in the urine is in this form – a form which is microbiologically inactive.

For parenteral use the succinate salt, which is readily soluble, is used either intramuscularly or intravenously. Like the palmitate, this is inactive but is hydrolysed *in vivo* to release chloramphenicol.

TOXICITY AND SIDE EFFECTS

Chloramphenicol was used for many years before two potentially lethal toxic effects were recognized. The frequency of marrow aplasia following chloramphenicol is unknown but the total number of cases of fatal aplastic anaemia in which chloramphenicol has been implicated is very large. While excessive doses were used in some of these cases, in others only a standard course of treatment was given. Chloramphenicol is a highly effective antibiotic but because of this lethal complication should never be used for minor infections. The incidence of aplastic anaemia following chloramphenicol varies somewhat in countries with similar reporting systems suggesting some variation in susceptibility between population groups.

The absorption and metabolism of chloramphenicol are inefficient in the newborn, particularly if premature, and toxic accumulation can occur unless very small doses are used. The symptoms of overdosage are flaccidity, ashen colour, and hypothermia, and fatal cases of this 'grey syndrome' have occurred in infants given chloramphenicol prophylactically. There is no evidence that chloramphenicol is of any clinical value given in this way. A reversible optic neuritis can occur if treatment is prolonged. Soreness of the mouth due to overgrowth of *Cand. albicans* is common with prolonged treatment.

CLINICAL APPLICATIONS AND DOSAGE

Chloramphenicol is the drug of choice for typhoid fever and other invasive salmonella infections. Drugs such as ampicillin or co-trimoxazole although active against *Salm. typhi* have not been as effective as chloramphenicol in clinical use. Initial doses may need to be as high as 500 mg 6-hourly but can be reduced to 250 mg 6-hourly after 3–5 days and can usually be discontinued after 10 days.

Meningitis due to *H. influenzae* and on occasion severe respiratory infections caused by this organism are also indications for chloramphenicol therapy, but in other infections alternative and less toxic antibiotics such as tetracycline are usually effective.

Erythromycin

Erythromycin is the most frequently used of a group of closely related macrolide antibiotics. Derived from *Streptomyces erythreus* it was the first of this group to be discovered and has a greater degree of activity than the other members. Solutions are stable at 5°C.

ANTIBACTERIAL ACTIVITY

The spectrum of activity of erythromycin is similar to that of benzylpenicillin, that is, Gram-positive and Gram-negative cocci and Gram-positive bacilli; Gram-negative bacilli are relatively resistant. The main differences from benzylpenicillin are in its antistaphylococcal activity but many penicillinase-producing staphylococci resistant to erythromycin readily emerge and in most large hospitals about 10 per cent of strains are resistant at present. Resistance among strains of pneumococci and haemolytic streptococci have also been reported but resistant organisms of these types are not widespread. Erythromycin has been little used in hospitals during the past 10–15 years and the number of resistant strains of bacteria has been slowly declining. The use of erythromycin is increasing because of its activity against *Legionella pneumophila* and *Campylobacter jejuni*.

PHARMACOLOGY

Erythromycin is not acid-stable and absorption after oral administration is not good even if enteric-coated capsules are used. Salts of erythromycin such as the propionate and the estolate are absorbed more readily. Excretion is partly into the bile but predominantly into the urinary tract. A proportion of the drug is demethylated and rendered inactive by the liver. For parenteral use salts derived from the gluconate esters can be given intravenously to produce high blood levels.

TOXICITY AND SIDE EFFECTS

Erythromycin is one of the safest of all antibiotics, with no serious toxicity. Prolonged use of the estolate produces abnormal liver function and some patients develop jaundice, abdominal pain, and fever. The reaction is reversible on stopping the drug but use of the estolate should not be continued for more than 10 days. Gastrointestinal symptoms appear in a few patients.

CLINICAL APPLICATIONS AND DOSAGE

The main use of erythromycin is as an alternative to benzylpenicillin either in patients who are hypersensitive to penicillin or in children who find penicillin unpalatable. It is also useful for staphylococcal infections if the strains are sensitive, and against many respiratory pathogens such as mycoplasma, chlamydia and legionella.

Lincomycin and clindamycin

Lincomycin, derived from *Streptomyces lincolnensis*, and its 7-chloro-derivative, clindamycin, differ mainly quantitatively and will therefore be considered together.

ANTIBACTERIAL ACTIVITY

The antibacterial activity of the lincomycins is rather unusual. They are highly active against streptococci, with the exception of most strains of *Str. faecalis*, and against staphylococci. About 5 per cent of hospital strains of staphylococci show appreciable resistance. Resistant strains of haemolytic streptococci have also been found but are also unusual. There are some unexpected resistances, gonococci and meningococci being resistant as are most Haemophilus strains. On the other hand, faecal Gram-negative anaerobes, that is Bacteroides and Veillonella are sensitive while Gram-negative aerobic bacilli from the bowel are resistant. There is partial cross-resistance also with the erythromycin group. Clindamycin is microbiologically more active than lincomycin.

PHARMACOLOGY

Both lincomycin and clindamycin are absorbed after oral administration but lincomycin less well than clindamycin. The drug is distributed to the body tissues and passes into the fetus, amniotic fluid, and breast milk. Appreciable amounts are found in the bone.

Only 10 per cent of the administered oral dose is recoverable from the urine.

For parenteral administration only lincomycin is available.

TOXICITY AND SIDE EFFECTS

Abdominal pain and diarrhoea have been associated with lincomycin since its first use. These effects were less marked with clindamycin and it was thought that the side effect problem had been solved. However, a much more serious condition, pseudomembranous enterocolitis, appeared and its association with these compounds now seems certain. The use of lincomycin has declined recently. Should a patient receiving lincomycin develop diarrhoea, the treatment should be stopped.

CLINICAL APPLICATIONS AND DOSAGE

One of the main uses of lincomycins is the treatment of staphylococcal infections, particularly osteomyelitis (when the high levels obtained in bone are helpful), and in hospital staphylococcal infections with strains resistant to other antibiotics. The other main use is in bacteroides infections which most commonly arise in association with abdominal and gynaecological surgery. Clindamycin appears to be superior in all respects to lincomycin. Oral dosage of lincomycin is 500 mg 6-hourly and of clindamycin is 150 mg 6-hourly. For intravenous use 600 mg lincomycin should be given 8-hourly in 150 ml of isotonic saline over a period of 30 minutes.

Other antibiotics active against staphylococci

Fusidic acid

Fusidic acid, isolated from *Fusidium coccineum*, has a steroid ring structure but has only antibacterial actions and no significant steroid effects. The sodium salt, sodium fusidate, is soluble in water.

Fusidic acid is highly active against staphylococci and, apart from hospitals in which large amounts are used topically, resistant strains are unusual. Neisseria and Gram-positive bacilli are also highly sensitive, but streptococci are relatively insensitive and Gram-negative bacilli are resistant.

Absorption and elimination of sodium fusidate is slow so that blood levels gradually build up on repeated administration. Food delays absorption and the drug is highly protein-bound in serum. A parenteral preparation is available.

Sodium fusidate is widely distributed in the body, with the exception of the CSF. There is evidence of penetration of the drug into the eye and into bones. Most of the drug is metabolized and only small amounts are excreted in the urine.

Some gastric irritation occurs and sodium fusidate is therefore usually given with food even though this delays absorption. No direct toxicity has been reported despite high blood levels, but occasionally jaundice has been associated with sodium fusidate therapy.

The primary use of sodium fusidate is in staphylococcal infections often in combination with a penicillin which delays the emergence of resistant strains. It is widely used in osteomyelitis and staphylococcal pneumonia. Oral dosage is 250 mg 6-hourly in adults.

Vancomycin

Vancomycin is a toxic antibiotic which is not absorbed from the gastrointestinal tract and can only be given intravenously; its use is therefore limited. Most strains of staphylococci and streptococci are sensitive to vancomycin and they do not easily acquire resistance.

Intravenous administration, although essential, may produce thrombophlebitis. High blood levels produce deafness and as the main route of excretion is via the kidney, patients with renal impairment need careful monitoring of the serum concentration.

Vancomycin is used mainly for severe staphylococcal infections such as endocarditis and septicaemia resulting from infection of the arteriovenous shunt used for chronic renal dialysis. Dosage varies but ranges from 0.5 g to 1 g every 12 hours intravenously.

Rifampicin

Streptomyces mediterranei is the organism that has yielded the rifamycins, a group of antibiotics which differs from all the others. Of these compounds, only rifamycin B has so far been obtained in a stable form. Chemical modification of the nucleus has produced methylpiperazinyliminomethylrifamycin (rifampicin). It is a highly coloured, crystalline substance with a complex chemical formula.

ANTIBACTERIAL ACTIVITY

Rifampicin is highly active against *Myco. tuberculosis*, including strains resistant to streptomycin and other agents. High activity is also shown against staphylococci and streptococci, although the effect on *Str. faecalis* is marginal. A naturally occurring resistant staphylococcus has not been reported. Neisseria are fully sensitive. Gram-negative bacilli are less sensitive, the MIC being rather higher than the blood levels of the drug usually achieved. Rifampicin is also active against most anaerobic Gram-negative bacilli including bacteroides. Some synergy is shown with tetracycline and erythromycin, and antagonism to the penicillins. Acquisition of resistance occurs readily *in vitro* and *in vivo*.

PHARMACOLOGY

Rifampicin is well absorbed despite the high molecular weight, but negligible amounts cross the placenta. Excretion appears to be mainly by way of the biliary tract and high levels in bile have been recorded. Part of the dose is excreted into the urine where high levels are also found.

TOXICITY AND SIDE EFFECTS

In short-term therapy, side effects are unusual. In long-term therapy, hepatic toxicity has appeared with jaundice, nausea, and abnormal tests of function. The mechanism is via the formation of rifampicin-dependent antibodies and the mechanism is stimulated by high dosage and intermittent therapy (once or twice weekly doses). The reaction is unusual if the dose is below 600 mg/day, especially if given continuously. Haematological abnormalities have also been reported on occasions.

CLINICAL APPLICATION AND DOSAGE

Because of the readiness with which resistance to rifampicin emerges, there are strong arguments for reserving this drug solely for the treatment of tuberculosis. However, it has also been used to good effect for biliary tract infections because of the exceptional levels in the bile and it has been successfully used for severe staphylococcal infections.

Rifampicin dosage varies with individual regimens of treatment in tuberculosis; for acute infections a daily dose of 450 mg in divided doses is common.

Polymyxins

These antibiotics are not isolated from fungi but from a Gram-positive soil bacillus – *Bacillus aerosporus* (or *B. polymyxa*). Five separate polymyxins have been isolated which are active against Gram-negative bacilli but only two, polymyxins B and E (colistin), are used clinically. They are cyclic polypeptides and are available as either sulphate or sulphomethyl salts.

ANTIBACTERIAL ACTIVITY

The polymyxins are active against almost all Gram-negative bacilli including *Ps. aeruginosa, Salmonella* and *Shigella* species but excluding *Proteus* strains, all of which are resistant. *Vibrio cholerae* is also sensitive but not the El Tor vibrio. Development of resistance is not a problem. Gram-positive organisms are resistant.

PHARMACOLOGY AND TOXICITY

The polymyxins are not absorbed from the gastrointestinal tract and are therefore administered parenterally. The main route of excretion is via the urinary tract and high blood levels may occur in patients with renal impairment. The sulphomethate derivatives are excreted more rapidly than the sulphate by the kidney. Toxic effects are confined to the CNS and to the kidneys; the former give rise to circumoral paraesthesia and dizziness while renal function impairment has been demonstrated in volunteers and in patients. However, if therapy is well controlled the symptoms are mild and the renal changes reversible. The sulphomethate salt is less toxic but also microbiologically less active than the sulphate.

CLINICAL APPLICATIONS AND DOSAGE

The main uses of polymyxins are in resistant urinary tract infections, particularly with *Ps. aeruginosa*, in non-invasive salmonella and shigella infections (when it is given orally) and as a topical application in superficial skin lesions colonized with *Ps. aeruginosa*. They were also much used for treating undiagnosed Gram-negative septicaemia before the advent of gentamicin and carbenicillin.

The parenteral dose of colistin sulphomethate is 3–5 million units a day intramuscularly in divided doses.

Metronidazole

Metronidazole is the most frequently used of a group of nitroimidazoles. For many years it was used solely for protozoan infections, especially *Trichomonas vaginalis*. It was also found effective in treating Vincent's angina, which is a mixed spirochaetal and anaerobic infection. The activity of metronidazole against anaerobes was unrecognized until the mid-1960s and even then the activity was in the main regarded as an interesting side reaction to its antiprotozoal effects. The antianaerobic activity came into prominence when clindamycin was linked to enterocolitis. At that period in 1973–74 there was a paucity of effective drugs active against *Bact. fragilis* and metronidazole has since then held a leading place in the treatment of infections caused by obligate anaerobic bacteria.

Metronidazole only acts against obligate anaerobes and has no action on facultative anaerobes; even microaerophilic cocci are unaffected by this compound. Metronidazole passes freely into bacterial cells where it interferes with the anaerobic processes involved in protein synthesis. The biochemical mechanisms are complex and involve electron transport proteins such as ferredoxin.

The majority of *Bacteroides* strains, including *Bact. fragilis* and related species, are inhibited by 0.5 mg/ℓ or less of metronidazole and anaerobic cocci by 0.25 mg/ℓ or less. These levels are readily reached in the blood after oral administration of 200 mg or by 1–2 g rectally. Because many of the patients with anaerobic infections require parenteral therapy intravenous preparations containing 500 mg doses are also now available. When metronidazole was used mainly for the treatment of trichomoniasis relatively small doses were given for short periods but higher doses appear to be given for anaerobic infections. The only untoward effect reported as a result of increased dosage or prolonged administration has been the development of peripheral neuritis. The activity against anaerobes has been found especially useful in bacteroides infections, and has been widely used in sepsis of the chest, abdomen, and pelvis. The value of perioperative prophylaxis for the prevention of anaerobic sepsis following abdominal surgery is well recognized.

Compounds used in urinary tract infections

Nitrofurantoin

Nitrofurantoin is a synthetic nitrofuran which is well absorbed after oral administration and although fairly rapidly broken down in the body the unmetabolized portion which escapes into the urine remains active. This activity is most effective against *E. coli* and *Str. faecalis* and most strains of these organisms are sensitive particularly if the infection arises outside hospital. *Ps. aeruginosa* and many *Klebsiella* strains are resistant. Although *Pr. mirabilis* often appears sensitive, the alkaline pH produced by these organisms in the urine considerably reduces the activity of the drug.

Side effects such as nausea and vomiting are common with high doses; prolonged therapy may cause a peripheral neuropathy and should be avoided. In renal failure, accumulation of toxic metabolites may occur.

The drug is only used for urinary tract infections with sensitive organisms in a dose of 50–100 mg every 6 hours by mouth.

Nalidixic acid

Nalidixic acid is a synthetic naphthyridine-carboxylic acid which is well absorbed orally and excreted into the urine in high concentrations. The antibacterial activity is confined to the commoner Gram-negative bacilli – *E. coli, Pr. mirabilis*, and *Klebsiella* species. Gram-positive bacteria and *Ps. aeruginosa* are resistant. Acquisition of resistance occurs readily in the laboratory and may occur clinically during treatment with nalidixic acid.

Toxic effects of the drug to the nervous system have been seen in the newborn and young children producing convulsions and distended fontanelles, and it is therefore contraindicated in infants and pregnant women. It has less marked side effects on the gastrointestinal tract than nitrofurantoin.

The dose in urinary tract infections is 1 g every 6 hours by mouth.

Analogues of nalidixic acid

Two closely related analogues of nalidixic acid have been introduced, oxolinic acid and cinoxacin. Both are absorbed more rapidly and excreted more slowly than is nalidixic acid, resulting in measurable levels of the compound in the blood and urine. Oxolinic acid is the more active but appears to stimulate the CNS, producing excitability and insomnia. Several other analogues of nalidixic acid active against a wide range of Gram-negative organisms, including *Ps. aeruginosa*, are currently under trial.

Hexamine and mandelic acid

These two agents preceded all other antibacterial agents and still have some limited used in urinary infections. They are well absorbed, both separately or combined as hexamine mandelate, and are excreted into the urine. Both are only active at an acid pH when hexamine is degraded to formaldehyde and mandelic acid also becomes active. They are sometimes used in low dosage for prolonged prophylactic therapy or to treat urinary candidiasis. The dose of hexamine mandelate is 1 g every 6 hours by mouth.

Antifungal agents

Nystatin

The first of the polyene antibiotics was nystatin isolated from *Streptomyces noursei* in 1957. Nystatin is poorly soluble and only available as a suspension; it is not active against bacteria but affects most fungi, especially *Cand. albicans*.

Nystatin is not absorbed from the intestine and is mostly recoverable from the faeces; it is also not absorbed after deposition into muscles and it is used therefore purely as a topical application. No resistance has been encountered among *Candida* species and it is effective against thrush infections of the mouth, gastrointestinal tract, skin, and vagina.

Amphotericin

Isolated from *Streptomyces nodosus* this polyene not only has higher activity than nystatin against fungi but also forms salts which are to some extent soluble. This enables it to be given parenterally for systemic infections with candida and other fungi. Small amounts are absorbed from the gastrointestinal tract and excretion into the urine is slow. For treatment of severe fungal infections such as histoplasmosis, cryptococcal meningitis, candida endocarditis, and other systemic fungal infections, the intravenous route is used. Passage into the CSF is negligible.

Toxicity of this compound is high, thrombophlebitis, fever, vomiting, anaemia, hypokalaemia, and renal damage all being prominent. Dosage needs careful calculation and depends on the blood level, the clinical response, and toxicity. The initial dose is 1 mg/day, building up to 25 mg/day on occasions.

Griseofulvin

Griseofulvin was isolated in 1939 from a penicillium, but was not introduced into clinical practice until about 20 years later, after it had been identified as the source of the 'curling factor' in conifers, and its antifungal activity had therefore been re-examined. It is a white powder supplied in the form of coarse or fine particles and is poorly soluble in water.

Griseofulvin inhibits the growth of most of the pathogenic fungi, particularly the dermatophytes, but is relatively inactive against bacteria. It is absorbed from the alimentary tract. Absorption is best if it is administered in the form of fine particles and it is assisted by a fatty diet. After absorption it is deposited in keratin while it is being formed, so that the antibiotic remains in the hair and nails and prevents the growth of fungi in these sites.

In large doses, griseofulvin is antimitotic and may also cause a disturbance of porphyrin metabolism. Neither of these side effects has been seen in man during therapy.

Griseofulvin by mouth is highly effective in the treatment of ringworm of the scalp and in skin infections due to *Trichophyton* species but interdigital infection (athlete's foot) tends to be resistant. In infection of the nails, although there is clinical improvement, the fungi are rarely eradicated. The oral dose is 0.25–0.5 g 12-hourly.

Flucytosine (5-Fluorocytosine)

This compound is derived from the pyrimidine base cytosine and is highly active against most strains of *Cand. albicans*, *Torulopsis* and *Cryptococcus* species. It is absorbed well after oral administration and excreted in the urine in an active form. Toxicity to the bone marrow and liver has been recorded. Although not in itself nephrotoxic, in the presence of renal impairment the drug accumulates and thus should be given in smaller dosage.

Clinical uses of the drug include treatment of urinary infection due to *Candida* or *Torulopsis* species and systemic mycoses such as candida endocarditis and cryptococcal infections. Treatment failures may occur due to resistance of a fungus being present prior to, or arising during, therapy. During treatment, blood levels should be monitored if there is any impairment of renal function. The oral dose is 200 mg/kg/day divided into four doses. An intravenous infusion containing 2.5 g flucytosine in 250 ml is available for the treatment of severely ill patients. Blood levels should not be allowed to exceed 80 mg/ℓ.

5-Fluorocytosine and amphotericin may act synergistically in the treatment of some systemic fungal infections.

Clotrimazole

Clotrimazole is a tritylimidazole derivative which has been shown to inhibit a wide range of both filamentous and yeast-like fungi including candida, cryptococci, *Aspergillus* species, and almost all dermatophytes of medical importance.

An oral preparation is available and has been shown to be well absorbed from the alimentary tract. It has been used to treat systemic infections such as urinary candidiasis and pulmonary aspergillosis, although its value in these situations has yet to be established. There is a high incidence of side effects which include gastrointestinal and mental disturbances. These may be severe and necessitate discontinuing treatment. The dosage is 60–120 mg/kg/day given in three or four divided doses.

The drug is also available in the form of a 1 per cent cream for the treatment of superficial infections such as the dermatomycoses caused by yeasts or dermatophytes, or for pityriasis versicolor. Vaginal tablets have been produced for the local treatment of candidiasis.

Other imidazoles

Two further imidazole derivatives, miconazole and econazole have been developed. Their spectrum of activity against fungal species is similar to that of clotrimazole and their relative advantages have yet to be established.

Antiviral agents

Agents capable of attacking viruses have not been as easily found as those attacking bacteria and the main uses of the compounds so far discovered have been in prophylaxis.

Idoxuridine

Idoxuridine (IDU) is sparingly soluble in water but soluble in dimethyl sulphoxide. The main activity is shown against *Herpesvirus hominis* and its chief use is as a topical agent for herpetic lesions of the skin, conjunctiva, and mucous membranes. IDU is applied in 5–40 per cent solutions and the lesion is kept continually moistened with the drug. Its main value is in herpetic keratitis. Cases of herpetic encephalitis have also been treated but owing to the poor solubility of the drug and its rapid deactivation in the body it is administered in high dosage, up to 1 g/kg into the carotid artery.

Amantidine

The mode of action of amantidine is to block the uptake of viruses into mammalian cells; the main viruses blocked in this way are influenza A and C and rubella viruses. Prophylactic oral administration of 100 mg every 12 hours has been used in the treatment of contacts of influenza A sufferers and reduction in the incidence of cases has been reported.

Cytosine arabinoside

Cytosine arabinoside is a purine analogue and acts by inhibiting nucleic acid synthesis. It was originally developed as an anti-tumour agent. In cell culture it is effective against a number of DNA viruses such as those causing vaccinia, herpes simplex, and varicella/zoster.

It has been used to treat generalized varicella/zoster in patients with a depressed immune response. However, its value in this situation has not been established. Its main toxic manifestation is bone marrow depression. The drug is administered as a rapid intravenous infusion in a dose of 2–4 mg/kg/day, although this may have to be adjusted in the light of the clinical response.

Adenine arabinoside

Adenine arabinoside is another purine analogue which has been investigated as a potential antiviral agent. Like cytosine arabinoside, it has been used in the treatment of disseminated varicella/zoster infections in the immunosuppressed and there is evidence that it may be more effective in limiting the condition. It also produces less bone marrow depression than cytosine arabinoside. The dosage is 10 mg/kg/day.

An eye ointment containing adenine arabinoside is also available and has been shown to be effective in the treatment of herpetic ulceration of the cornea.

Acycloguanosine

The antiherpetic activity of this compound has created much current interest. The mode of action appears to be very specifically related to virus metabolism. The antiviral moiety is the phosphorylated form of acycloguanosine and a virus-induced enzyme is responsible for bringing about phosphorylation. This means that the active substance is produced more avidly in virus-infected cells than in uninfected cells. The phosphorylated compound has an inhibitory effect on DNA polymerases of both type I and type II *Herpesvirus hominis*.

The pharmacokinetics of the compound indicate that the agent could be used parenterally for the treatment of disseminated herpes infection in man.

Abraham, E. P. (1971) *Biographical memoirs of Fellows of the Royal Society,* **17,** 255
Hare, R. (1970) *The Birth of Penicillin.* London: Allen and Unwin

Further reading

Garrod, L. P., Lambert, H. P. and O'Grady, F. (Eds) (1981) *Antibiotics and Chemotherapy*, 5th Edn. Edinburgh and London: Churchill Livingstone
Kucers, A. and Bennett, J. (1982) *The Use of Antibiotics. A Comprehensive Review with Clinical Emphasis,* 3rd Edn. London: Heinemann

20

Electrolytes and infusion fluids

The following account concerns the administration of intravenous fluids to surgical patients. In recent years, the emphasis has swung away from the concept that 'balance' must be preserved above all (that is, that intake and output must be matched). More importance is now accorded to maintenance of circulatory haemodynamics; this is achieved by continuous monitoring of the filling pressures of the right and left ventricles and holding these pressures within predetermined limits. This is well illustrated in relation to the blood volume: instead of expressing this as so many millilitres per kilogram of body weight or square metres of body surface area, it is defined as the volume of blood which maintains an adequate filling pressure of both sides of the heart in the presence of normal vasomotor tone. As Bell (1972) put it, 'a normal blood volume is not necessarily, in all patients and at all times, the optimum blood volume'.

Caution needs to be exercised if this approach is used for controlling the administration of crystalloid solutions as very large positive balances will always cause a progressive fall in the colloid osmotic pressure (COP) of the plasma, and there are well-documented cases of pulmonary oedema occurring in the presence of normal left ventricular filling pressure (Stein *et al.*, 1975).

Fundamental concepts of physical chemistry

Molar solutions

The sum of the atomic weights of the elements of a compound constitutes the molecular weight of that compound. The molecular weight in grams is referred to as a mole; if this is dissolved in 1 litre of water a molar solution will be obtained. Such a solution will therefore contain one thousandth of a mole (1 millimole) in 1 millilitre. Thus a millimole of any substance is the molecular weight of that substance (which may be an element or a compound) expressed in milligrams.

Valency

This is the combining power of an atom or radical with reference to hydrogen. Most inorganic elements or radicals which are of importance in the body fluids are monovalent, for example Na^+, K^+, NH_4^+ and Cl^-. Divalent and trivalent elements or radicals occur in relatively small concentrations, for example Ca^{2+}, Mg^{2+}, SO_4^{2-}, and PO_4^{3-}, and have little significant effect on osmotic activity.

Equivalent weight

The term equivalent weight is a shortened version of gram equivalent weight, which is the weight in grams of a substance which will combine with or displace one gram of hydrogen. Such a substance may be an atom, a molecule, or an ion and if the valency is one the equivalent weight is equal to its unit weight, that is atomic, molecular, or ionic weight. The equivalent weight of divalent units is half their unit weight. In extracellular fluid (ECF) the concentration of sodium and chloride expressed in moles per litre would be 0.14 and 0.1, respectively; it is more convenient to multiply by 1000, thus obtaining 140 and 100 millimoles or milliequivalents per litre. Note that equivalence implies that the substance can combine with or displace hydrogen; if substances such as urea or dextrose are under consideration, the term millimole alone is applicable and millimoles and milliequivalents are only interchangeable when applied to monovalent elements or radicals.

Osmotic pressure

If one mole of a compound such as urea or dextrose, neither of which dissociates in solution, is dissolved in 22.4 litres of water it will exert an osmotic pressure of 1 atm (760 mmHg, 101.3 kPa). Thus a normal solution of such a compound will exert an osmotic pressure of 22.4 atm, and this amount of the substance is referred to as 1 osmol. A milliosmole is one thousandth of this and, accordingly, exerts an osmotic pressure of

$$\frac{22.4 \times 760}{1000} = 17\,\text{mmHg}\ (2.3\,\text{kPa})$$

Osmotic pressure is a function of the absolute number of particles in solution irrespective of their weight. Therefore, a molar solution of a highly dissociated compound such as NaCl will exert nearly double the osmotic pressure of a molar solution of a non-electrolyte. In fact, no salt is completely dissociated and the degree of dissociation is governed by its osmotic coefficient. This is the factor by which the 'ideal' (assuming complete dissociation) concentration must be multiplied to obtain actual concentration. The osmotic coefficient of 0.9 per cent NaCl at body temperature is 0.93; isotonic saline theoretically contains $2 \times 154 = 308$ mosmol/ℓ, whereas the actual concentration of osmotically active particles is $308 \times 0.93 = 286$ mosmol/ℓ.

Tonicity

This is a clinical term describing an aqueous solution in which cells neither shrink nor swell. It follows that the solute of such a solution must be one that does not penetrate the cell membrane. Solutions of urea or potassium chloride may be described as iso-osmotic with body fluids but they cannot be isotonic.

Because of the preponderance of sodium outside the cells it is directly responsible for nearly half the total osmolality of plasma and ECF. The osmolality of plasma can normally be obtained by doubling the sodium concentration and adding 10 mosmol.

Oncotic activity

This is another clinical term which shares with oncology derivation from a Greek word meaning a lump or swelling. Oncotic solutions contain solutes that do not readily leave the capillaries because their molecules have molecular weights which are in the range 20 000–70 000. Such large molecules exert COP and therefore retain water or attract movement of water into the circulation. Note that the total osmotic activity is small and that, as in the case of albumin, it is the intravascular confinement of the large molecules which is important. A 10 per cent solution of a solute with a molecular weight of 40 000 would contain 100 g/ℓ. Each millimole is 40 g so that its osmolality is 2.5 mosmol/ℓ. Synthetic oncotic preparations always contain another solute such as dextrose or saline in isotonic concentration.

Millimoles, milliequivalents and milliosmoles

One millimole of a compound in solution may form varying numbers of milliequivalents and milliosmoles depending upon the valency and dissociation of its constituents, as illustrated in *Table 20.1*.

Table 20.1 Examples of the interrelationships between millimoles, milliequivalents, and milliosmoles

Millimoles	*Milliequivalents*	*Milliosmoles*
1 mmol NaCl	→ 1 mEq Na^+	→ 1 mosmol Na^+
	+ 1 mEq Cl^-	→ 1 mosmol Cl^-
1 mmol Dextrose	—	→ 1 mosmol dextrose
1 mmol Na_2SO_4	→ 2 mEq Na^+	→ 2 mosmol Na^+
	+ 2 mEq SO_4^{2-}	→ 1 mosmol SO_4^{2-}

Gases

A mole of any gas (at STP) will occupy 22.4 litres and a millimole therefore comprises 22.4 ml: thus 8–10 mmol of carbon dioxide are excreted per minute by the lungs.

Definitions

mole = molecular weight of a substance in grams.

valency = number of hydrogen atoms which enter into combination with one atom or radical.

equivalent weight = weight in grams of a substance which combines with or displaces 1 g of hydrogen;

$$\text{equivalent weight} = \frac{\text{molecular weight}}{\text{valency}};$$

osmole = amount of a substance which exerts an osmotic pressure of 22.4 atm when dissolved in 1 litre of water.

$$\left.\begin{array}{l}\text{millimole}\\ \text{milliequivalent}\\ \text{milliosmole}\end{array}\right\} = \text{one thousandth of} \left\{\begin{array}{l}\text{mole}\\ \text{equivalent}\\ \text{osmole}\end{array}\right.$$

osmolarity = concentration in osmoles (or milliosmoles) per litre *of a solution*;

osmolality = concentration in osmoles (or milliosmoles) per kilogram *of water* [for plasma (normally 93 per cent water) the difference is normally small and unimportant, but occasionally very large discrepancies occur between osmolarity and osmolality of plasma which are therapeutically important].

Water

The regulation of water balance in health depends mainly upon the sensation of thirst and upon the action of antidiuretic hormone (ADH) of the posterior pituitary. The water requirement of an adult at rest is 2–3 ℓ/day; this, if it cannot be taken by mouth, is given as 5 per cent dextrose intravenously. The dextrose, in addition to making the solution iso-osmotic, provides sufficient carbohydrate to reduce protein breakdown to a minimum. This protein-sparing effect is achieved by the daily provision of 80 g of carbohydrate.

The requirement for water is closely related to the output of urea and electrolytes by the kidney. If a high nitrogen intake is given by parenteral fluids, the resultant urea excretion will necessitate a higher water intake than is appropriate to the low calorie provision of common fluid maintenance schedules.

Distribution of body water

The figures in *Table 20.2*, taken from Edelman and colleagues (1958), show the average water content at different ages, expressed as a percentage of the body weight.

Table 20.2 Average water content (per cent of body weight) by age

Children			*Men*				*Women*			
0–1 mth	1–12 mths	1–10 yrs	10–16	17–39	40–59	60+	10–16	17–39	40–59	60+
75.7	64.5	61.7	58.9	60.6	54.7	51.5	57.3	50.2	46.7	45.5

Water content progressively decreases with age and is much less in fat subjects. In order to plan any fluid replacement, it is useful to know the approximate volume of the total body water (TBW): it sufficiently accurate to halve the weight in kilograms to obtain the TBW in litres. Appropriate corrections for age, obesity, and sex can then be made.

The total body water is divided into cell water and extracellular water (ECF). Studies using radioactive isotopes have revealed that a sizeable pool of ECF resides in the skeleton and in dense connective tissue such as ligaments and cartilage. This pool was not penetrated by the earlier substances used to measure the ECF and was therefore assigned to the cells. In health, the ratio of cell to extracellular water in an adult is approximately 55:45 (Edelman and Leibman, 1959).

The intravascular part of the ECF is chemically similar to the remainder of the ECF apart from its much higher content of protein. Its volume is about 3 litres and when selective loss of plasma occurs it must be replaced with plasma or a plasma substitute.

Water losses

Skin and lungs

Loss of water vapour from the skin and lungs is inevitable: the amount is independent of the body's need to conserve water and of control of ADH, varying slightly with the hydration of the patient, the rate and depth of breathing, and the humidity of the air. It can be taken as 1 litre per day in an afebrile patient.

Water is produced by the oxidative catabolism of fat (1 ml/g), carbohydrate (0.6 ml/g) and amino acids (0.4 ml/g). In health this amounts to about 300 ml per day. After surgery there is enhanced breakdown of fat and a loss of intracellular muscle protein. The principal solutes holding water within the cells are the proteins and when they leave the cells water will accompany them; this endogenous water is sodium-free and it will enter the extracellular compartment. It must be taken into account when fluid balance is computed (Orloff and Hutchin, 1972). The net unmeasured loss of an afebrile surgical patient is in the range 500–750 ml/day for the first 72 hours after operation.

Renal water excretion

For a variable time after trauma, the kidney is subjected to the effect of ADH released in response to mechanisms which override the normal osmoreceptor control. 'Free' water (which in this context means water entering the body unaccompanied by sodium) cannot therefore be excreted as hypotonic urine and its only channels of escape are the skin and the lungs. This increased ADH activity usually lasts for 2–3 days after major surgery, occasionally longer. The high plasma levels of the hormone fall gradually during this time. If an exogenous solute such as mannitol is given, an osmotic diuresis will result but the urine will not become hypotonic.

During the period of ADH release the intake of 'free' water should not exceed 1.5–2 litres; this can conveniently be given as 2–2.5 litres of 4 per cent dextrose in 0.18 per cent saline.

Water depletion

Pure water depletion is relatively uncommon and occurs as a result of a condition that stops water intake. The usual causes are oesophageal obstruction, prolonged unconsciousness, and states of great weakness. It is the only likely cause of a raised plasma sodium concentration.

Water intoxication

Mild overhydration is common in surgical patients and is likely to pass unrecognized unless it progresses and results in a restless disorientated state with twitching and finally convulsions. The plasma [Na] is low, 120 mmol/ℓ or less, and the cause of the symptoms is cerebral cellular overhydration. Mild forms call for no more than restriction of water intake; actual intoxication confirmed by a plasma [Na] below 120 mmol/ℓ should be treated with hypertonic saline. Five per cent saline (0.85 mmol/ml) should be used and not more than 120 ml (approximately 100 mmol of sodium) should be given over 20 minutes. This may be repeated until the plasma [Na] is 120–125 mmol/ℓ; the effect is dramatic in contrast to the effects of isotonic saline which should never be given.

Cerebral oedema and intracellular dehydration

Deprivation of oxygen from any cause will, if protracted, cause oedema of the cerebral cells. This oedema fluid can be withdrawn from the cells by any substance that remains in the ECF and exerts osmotic attraction. Hypertonic solutions of urea or mannitol are given intravenously for this purpose.

Urea

Urea, 30 per cent, in 10 per cent invert sugar is a most efficient agent in reducing brain volume. Given intravenously the dose is 0.5 g/kg body weight. At least 15–20 minutes should be taken over the infusion. Brain shrinkage occurs within 20 minutes and the effect lasts several hours. Urea has the disadvantage that it slowly penetrates the white matter and therefore causes 'rebound' swelling. It is seldom used now.

Mannitol

Twenty per cent mannitol is used; the dose for a patient with no cardiovascular disease is 1 g/kg body weight given in 20–30 minutes. On a weight basis the osmotic effect of mannitol is one third that of urea but mannitol remains extracellular and is equally effective.

Precautions

As with all hypertonic fluids, great care must be taken to ensure that they are given into a vein and do not leak into the tissues. It is important to pass a catheter or express urine manually from the bladder. Haemolysis is liable to occur if these fluids are given too rapidly, and they both cause considerable expansion of the plasma volume.

Electrolytes

Electrolytes are atoms or molecules carrying either a positive or a negative charge and which therefore migrate to the cathode or anode when placed in an electrical field. The term 'electrolyte' is by common usage applied to undissociated molecules of acids, bases, and salts, but strictly speaking should be reserved for their active form as dissociated ions in an aqueous solution.

Sodium chloride, at concentrations occurring in the body, is highly dissociated:

$$NaCl \rightleftharpoons Na^+ + Cl^-$$

Thus a solution of NaCl in water will contain a very small number of NaCl molecules and large numbers of Na^+ and Cl^- ions.

Osmotic balance

A clear understanding of the behaviour of the body cells in response to osmotic forces is essential. This is described in two papers (Wynn, 1957; Edelman *et al.*, 1958) which unify many of the previously apparently conflicting observations on osmotically active ions in the intracellular fluid (ICF) and ECF in surgical patients.

Reduced to its simplest terms, this states that there is no sustained osmotic gradient between the cells and the ECF. The osmolarity of the cells is dependent on K^+, just as the osmolarity of the ECF is dependent on Na^+, and it assigns the same osmotic effect to the two ions. Thus, if it were possible to introduce 100 mmol of K^+ into the ICF, the resultant water shift would raise the plasma [Na]. This rise would be of the same order as would follow the introduction of 100 mmol of Na^+ into the ECF.

The other corollary of practical importance is that the osmotic effect of either Na^+ or K^+ must be calculated as if it were being distributed throughout the TBW and not the compartment in which the ion is predominantly found. This may be illustrated by the result to be expected if 2 litres of isotonic saline (154 mmol/ℓ) are given to a patient with a plasma [Na] of 124 mmol/ℓ and a TBW of 28 litres. The only part of the saline to exert an osmotic change will be the 30 mmol/ℓ by which its concentration exceeds the patient's plasma [Na]. Thus, 60 mmol in all will be given and its osmotic effect distributed through 30 litres of TBW, raising the plasma [Na] by 2 mmol/ℓ to 126 mmol/ℓ. This ignores simultaneous changes in water and potassium balance but it illustrates that isotonic saline is unlikely to have much effect on plasma [Na] when this is low.

Sodium

Average concentration in plasma and ECF	140 mmol/ℓ
Average concentration in ICF	8 mmol/ℓ
Total body content is about 42 mmol/kg body weight	

Distribution

In a 70 kg adult, $42 \times 70 = 3000$ mmol

3000 mmol → ⅓ or about 1000 mmol inexchangeable (in bone)
3000 mmol → ⅔ or about 2000 mmol exchangeable

Of the total body sodium, some 60 per cent, or 1800 mmol, is in the part of the ECF, including the plasma, concerned with rapid losses of the ion.

Sodium turnover

Intake of sodium depends chiefly on the amount of salt added to the food in cooking. It varies from 100–200 mmol per day on a European diet: renal excretion maintains sodium balance, the chief controlling factor being the adrenal hormone aldosterone. When sodium intake ceases, normal kidneys cease to excrete sodium after 72–96 hours.

The plasma [Na] is maintained with great constancy at 140 ± 5 mmol/ℓ in health. Low plasma [Na], less than 130 mmol/ℓ, is a common finding postoperatively, and it must be appreciated that hyponatraemia may be accompanied by increased, normal, or reduced total amounts of extracellular sodium. Thus, a patient with a plasma [Na] of 130 mmol/ℓ may be oedematous with double his normal amount of exchangeable sodium, dying from salt and water loss, or convalescing normally from an operation. Hyponatraemia may be due to:

1. Loss of sodium
2. Loss of potassium
3. Water retention
4. Combinations of 1, 2 and 3.

The usual causes in surgical patients not losing sodium are water retention associated with potassium depletion. Such patients do not require isotonic sodium chloride, and plasma [Na] levels must be interpreted with all the above factors in mind. The whole subject has been well reviewed by Danowski, Fergus and Mateer (1955), and the practical implications were clearly described in an excellent paper by Moore (1962).

Sodium depletion

Sodium lost from the body is necessarily accompanied by water and anions, chiefly chloride or bicarbonate ions. Often the patient continues to drink and thus a depletion of sodium occurs relatively greater than the water loss. This is the common depletion which occurs in surgical patients; the channel of fluid loss is usually obvious but several litres of ECF may be translocated into the intestinal lumen and wall in intestinal obstruction and cause profound circulatory collapse with little or no history of vomiting or diarrhoea.

Sodium depletion may occur preoperatively as a result of overt or occult losses from the gastrointestinal tract, or postoperatively when sodium-containing fluids are lost by gastric aspiration, or from various 'ostomies', and have been replaced with salt-free fluids.

Preoperative losses

These can only be assessed by careful appraisal of information derived from the history, examination, and biochemical data. The hallmark of severe sodium depletion is circulatory failure in an obviously ill patient with sunken eyes, a dry wrinkled tongue, and loss of tissue elasticity. The hands, feet and face are cold, the pulse is very rapid and sometimes impalpable, and the mean blood pressure is low. There is usually rapid laboured breathing and in severe cases cyanosis of the lips and ears due to circulatory stagnation.

These are indications for a rapid infusion of fluid containing sodium in isotonic concentration. Isotonic (0.9 per cent) saline is the fluid of choice when gastric juice has been lost as a result of pyloric obstruction but in most other circumstances Ringer/lactate is more appropriate. Large volumes of saline will expand the ECF and contribute no bicarbonate thus producing a 'dilutional acidosis' (Christensen, 1962). When more than 1.5 litres of saline are given rapidly, every fourth unit should consists of isotonic (1.4 per cent) sodium bicarbonate unless the patient is known to be alkalotic as a result of loss of gastric hydrochloric acid. Each 500 ml of saline or Ringer/lactate should be given every 10 minutes until the peripheral vasoconstriction disappears and the systolic blood pressure reaches 100 mmHg (13.3 kPa). This usually happens after 1.5 litres have been given but more may be required and the rate must be reduced to 500 ml every 30 minutes after the first 1.5 litres. Most patients do not require such therapy but the few who do are in danger of their lives and must be treated boldly, with due allowance for old age and associated disease.

The blood changes that are most constant are the rise in the concentration of urea, often to 15 mmol/ℓ or more, and of haemoglobin. The rise in haemoglobin concentration is a direct result of the fall in extracellular volume of the only tissue in which it can be accurately and simply measured. If both these changes are present, they indicate that both sodium and water have been lost and Ringer/lactate or isotonic saline should be given. If a 5 per cent dextrose solution is given, it will produce a temporary improvement which is followed by relapse: sodium loss is associated with shift of water from the ECF into the cells and hypotonic or salt-free infusions will aggravate this.

Postoperative losses

The postoperative period is characterized by diminished renal ability to excrete sodium. If, as commonly happens, water is retained in excess of sodium, the plasma [Na] will fall although the total body content of sodium is increasing. This has been called the 'sodium paradox' by Moore (1954). This diminished ability to excrete sodium may last 5 days, both its duration and intensity being variable, but generally increasing with the extensiveness of the operation. It will also be more marked if operative blood loss is not replaced. The daily sodium requirement during this period is 75–100 mmol. This can either be provided by 500 ml of Ringer/lactate or isotonic saline, or by adding about 30 mmol of sodium to each litre of the daily water intake. In practice this is conveniently achieved by prescribing the daily requirements as dextrose 4 per cent/saline 0.18 per cent – the so-called fifth normal saline in dextrose. The knowledge that sodium retention is inevitable in the immediate postoperative period must not be allowed to prevent sodium replacement of extrarenal body fluid losses. Replacement of all such losses should be with an equal volume of either saline or Ringer/lactate. Saline (0.9 per cent) is used whenever the loss is of gastric juice, otherwise Ringer/lactate is to be preferred. If losses exceed 1.5 ℓ/day they should be analysed and appropriate amounts of Na^+, K^+, and HCO_3^- given to replace them accurately.

Postoperatively, a plasma [Na] of 125–130 mmol/ℓ is commonly seen, particularly in patients who have not been given potassium. If there is no channel of sodium loss and there are no signs of sodium depletion, such patients should not be given saline. Whenever very low plasma [Na] is reported, particularly in intensive care units, it should be confirmed by measurement of plasma osmolality. If the total osmolality corresponds approximately to twice the reported sodium concentration plus 10, then the hyponatraemia is true and may be managed as described under water intoxication above. Five per cent saline (0.85 mmol/ml) is appropriate in these circumstances; not more than 100 mmol (120 ml) should be given and the plasma [Na] re-estimated. It may be repeated until a level of 125 mmol/ℓ is regained, after which isotonic saline should be given to replace measured losses. A wide discrepancy between osmolarity and osmolality is usually due to triglycerides which can reach concentrations of 180 mmol/ℓ in the plasma (Bell, Hilton and Walker, 1972). Anion 'gaps' of 20–40 mmol/ℓ may be due to lactic acidosis. If there is evidence of potassium loss, potassium should be given with the saline as hypertonic saline infusion aggravates potassium depletion.

Sodium requirements

Sodium requirements may be summarized as follows:

1. No abnormal losses, 75–100 mmol/day;
2. Extrarenal losses up to 1.5 litres daily;
   (a) due to loss of gastric HCl – replace with equal volumes of isotonic saline in addition to the daily requirements;
   (b) other losses – replace with equal volumes of Ringer/lactate in addition to daily requirements;
3. Large extrarenal losses. Measure accurately and analyse for Na^+, K^+, HCO_3^- and Cl^-. Replace with appropriate mixtures of isotonic saline, 5 per cent dextrose and isotonic sodium bicarbonate.

Potassium

Average concentration in plasma and ECF	3.5–5 mmol/ℓ
Average concentration in ICF	150 mmol/ℓ

Distribution

In cells	98.6 per cent
In ECF (excluding plasma)	1 per cent
In plasma	0.4 per cent

Intake and output

About 70–100 mmol/day of potassium are ingested in an average diet. A similar amount is excreted, 90 per cent by the kidneys.

All patients lose potassium in large but variable amounts from the moment they cease to eat: the actual amount varies, but may be taken as 50 mmol/day and is often more. Operation itself and the infusion of saline greatly increase this loss. Renal conservation of potassium is much less efficient than that of sodium and even when there is a large overall depletion of potassium, it may be found in the urine in 5–10 times its plasma concentration. A plasma [K] of less than 3.5 mmol/ℓ is usually associated with potassium depletion, but if the plasma [K] is within normal limits of 3.5–5.0 mmol/ℓ it is no indication that potassium depletion does not exist. The predominant channel of potassium loss is the urine and alimentary losses have an average [K] of 10 mmol/ℓ but, if they are very large, their electrolyte content should be determined and accurately replaced. When K^+ leaves the cells, it is replaced partly by Na^+ and partly by other cations, one of which is H^+. In this way potassium depletion is associated with acidosis of the ICF and alkalosis of the ECF, so that a high [HCO_3] in the plasma may indicate potassium depletion even if the plasma [K] is within the normal range.

Potassium depletion is now known to depress renal tubular function as one of its earliest effects: the kidneys become progressively less able to secrete a concentrated urine and the glomerular filtration rate is also lowered. If the patient survives after prolonged potassium depletion, irreversible structural changes occur in the renal tubules. Severe potassium depletion causes profound muscular weakness and ultimately death.

Both experimental and clinical experience suggests that acidosis increases the 'penetration' of hypokalaemia so that a very low plasma [K] in a patient alkalotic as a result of pyloric stenosis will rarely cause symptoms.

Administration

Oral route

Potassium should be given intravenously only if it cannot be given by mouth. It is now recognized that potassium depletion may be refractory to treatment unless chloride is given at the same time. *Slow K* is a wax-based, slow-release preparation containing 8 mmol each of K^+ and Cl^- per tablet. *Kloref* is a tablet which effervesces in water and contains 6.7 mmol each of K^+ and Cl^- per tablet.

Intravenous route

Administration of potassium is now routine in medical and surgical fluid schedules and has engendered an attitude that it is harmless. The concentration of potassium is often 30–40 mmol/ℓ and anaesthetists must beware of patients who come to theatre with such intravenous infusions running. The potassium-containing pack should be discarded and the giving set flushed with a potassium-free fluid before induction. It is only justifiable to give potassium during surgery if there is a specific indication to do so and the ECG is being monitored. The following criteria should be fulfilled for the routine use of intravenous potassium:

1. Potassium should be withheld during and immediately after surgery;
2. The state of the circulation must be such that the kidneys can be expected to function normally;
3. Neither respiratory nor metabolic acidosis must be present.

The simplest method is to add 1 g of KCl to each 500 ml of fluid infused. Each gram of KCl contains 13.4 mmol of K^+, and 4 g of KCl a day is sufficient to prevent depletion and 8 g of KCl a day to treat established depletions. Whenever an infusion contains K^+, the prescriber should clearly state in writing the rate at which it is to be given. Not more than 20 mmol should ordinarily be given in 2 hours and each 500 ml infused should never have more than 1.5 g of KCl (40 mmol/ℓ) added to it.

The plasma [K] should be measured daily: if the above criteria are observed, it is unnecessary to take ECG records. If potassium is given more rapidly, ECG monitoring is essential. Signs to look for are an increasing amplitude and peaking of the T waves, alterations in the P waves, and widening of the ventricular complexes.

Treatment of hyperkalaemia
Rapid reduction of plasma [K] levels which are dangerous (above 7 mmol/ℓ) can be achieved by the intravenous injection of 25–50 g of dextrose as a 50 per cent solution, together with 12–24 units of soluble insulin. If the patient is anuric and is being transferred to a kidney unit a slow infusion of hypertonic sodium lactate or sodium bicarbonate should be given. One-third molar solutions are suitable (3.5 per cent sodium lactate or 2.8 per cent sodium bicarbonate). If the patient is anuric and being transferred for haemodialysis, a slow infusion of one-third molar (2.8 per cent) sodium bicarbonate will tend to prevent plasma [K] from rising. Fifty to 100 ml of 10 per cent calcium gluconate should be added unless the patient is digitalized; 500 ml of this solution should be infused over 6 hours.

Polystyrene sulphonate resins are an effective means of reducing high plasma [K]. They are usually given as retention enemas in a dose of 0.5 g/kg. Calcium and sodium resins are available and unless there is a contraindication to the use of calcium, it is to be preferred.

Magnesium

Average plasma concentration	1.75–2.5 mmol/ℓ
Average ICF concentration	26 mmol/ℓ

The daily intake of magnesium is 12–15 mmol. Like potassium, it is predominantly an intracellular ion and plasma concentrations do not necessarily reflect the intracellular [Mg]. Levels of less than 0.5 mmol/ℓ are likely to be accompanied by signs of neuromuscular dysfunction, of which tetany is a common manifestation (Paymaster, 1976).

Parenteral fluids, if they have to be continued for more than a week, should contain 10 mmol/day. It can be added from ampoules of magnesium sulphate (Macarthy) which are supplied as follows:
1 g in 10 ml (containing 4.07 mmol Mg^{2+})
5 g in 10 ml (containing 20.4 mmol Mg^{2+})

Phosphorus

Hypophosphataemia is a well-recognized result of parenteral feeding regimens which rely on hypertonic dextrose and insulin. The normal plasma concentration of phosphate is 2 mmol/ℓ and signs of phosphate deficiency are unlikely unless the plasma [HPO_4] falls below 0.8 mmol/ℓ. Sheldon and Grzyb (1975) recommend that for every 1000 calories, 20–25 mmol of HPO_4^{2-} should be given. Many proprietary preparations contain phosphates. If it is wished to add phosphate it can be done either from an ampoule of potassium phosphate (Macarthy) which contains 5 mmol of HPO_4^{2-} and 10 mmol of K^+, or from a Boots Polyfusor 'Phosphates' which contains 100 mmol/ℓ of PO_4^{3-}, 162 mmol/ℓ of Na^+, and 19 mmol/ℓ of K^+.

Acidosis and alkalosis

Hydrogen ion regulation

Nomenclature

An acid is a substance capable of dissociating into one or more hydrogen ions and an anion; it is therefore a hydrogen ion donor. A base is a substance that combines with hydrogen ions and is therefore a hydrogen ion acceptor. Thus an acid HB will dissociate,

$$HB \rightleftharpoons H^+ + B^-$$

B^- is known as the congugate base of the acid HB and the acid and base are known as a conjugate pair. The law of mass action states that, in any chemical

---

Nomenclature

H^+	= hydrogen ion. Synonyms: hydrion; proton.
[ ]	= concentration of. Unless otherwise specified, the concentration in gram-molecules per litre is implied.
Acid	= substance capable of donating H^+ in aqueous solution.
Base	= substance capable of accepting H^+ in aqueous solution.
Alkali	= substance capable of releasing OH^- in aqueous solutions.
K	= dissociation constant. Synonym: equilibrium constant.

For acid $HB \rightleftharpoons H^+ + B^-$, $K = \frac{[H^+][B^-]}{HB}$. The larger is K, the stronger is the acid.

$$pH = \frac{1}{\log [H^+]} \text{ or } -\log [H^+].$$

$$pK = \frac{1}{\log K} \text{ or } -\log K.$$ The smaller is pK, the stronger is the acid.

α	= solubility constant of CO_2 at 38°C, i.e. the factor by which the P_{CO_2} in mmHg is multiplied in order to convert it to mmol per litre of dissolved CO_2.
P_{CO_2}	= partial pressure of CO_2. Unless otherwise specified, the partial pressure in arterial blood is implied.
M	= molar, i.e. 1 gram-molecule per litre.
$M \times 10^{-3}$	= millimolar (or milliequivalent for a univalent ion).
$M \times 10^{-6}$	= micromolar (or microequivalent for a univalent ion).
$M \times 10^{-9}$	= nanomolar (or nanoequivalent for a univalent ion).

reaction, the ratio of the reacting masses at equilibrium remains constant; thus, for the acid HB,

$$HB \rightleftharpoons H^+ + B^-$$

Therefore,

$$\frac{[H^+] \times (B^-]}{[HB]} = K$$

$$[H^+] = \frac{K[HB]}{[B^-]}$$

or

$$[H^+] = \frac{K[\text{undissociated acid}]}{[\text{conjugate base}]}$$

Thus, the hydrogen ion concentration of a solution containing a weak acid equals a constant multiplied by the ratio of the concentration of undissociated acid to conjugate base.

The ECF can be regarded as a mixture of weak acids and their corresponding sodium salts, which are for practical purposes completely ionized. If carbonic acid, which is a weak acid, and its highly dissociated sodium salt are present in solution, the conjugate base HCO_3^- will practically all result from the dissociation of the salt, and the small amount of HCO_3^- formed by dissociation of the acid can be ignored. The equation may thus be written,

$$[H^+] = K'\frac{[\text{acid}]}{[\text{salt}]} = K'\frac{[\text{acid}]}{[\text{conjugate base}]} = \frac{K'[H_2CO_3]}{[HCO_3^-]}$$

This is the Henderson approximation equation, in which K' (called K prime) differs slightly from K by incorporating small corrections. It is an equation of fundamental importance as it indicates how the degree of ionization of the acid is governed by the concentration of its conjugate base provided by its sodium salt.

Buffers

The weak acid and its salt constitute a buffer pair because they have the effect of maintaining the hydrogen ion concentration relatively constant when a strong acid is added to it.

In order of importance, the buffer pairs of the ECF are:

Acid	*Conjugate base*
Carbonic (H_2CO_3)	Bicarbonate (HCO_3^-)
Plasma protein (HPr)	Protein anion (Pr^-)
Dihydrogen phosphate (NaH_2PO_4)	Monohydrogen phosphate (Na_2HPO_4)

Buffering in whole blood. In whole blood the haemoglobin of the red cells and, to a much smaller extent, the proteins of plasma together equal the buffering capacity of bicarbonate. These two conjugate bases constitute the buffer bases of Singer and Hastings (1948).

When acids other than carbonic acid are added to the blood, the buffer base concentration will fall (if Pco_2 remains constant).

$$HCl + H_2CO_3 + NaHCO_3 \rightarrow NaCl + 2H_2CO_3$$

The hydrogen ions remaining in solution will result from the dissociation of the weak acid H_2CO_3 instead of the very strong acid HCl. The small increase in HCO_3^- resulting from dissociation of the acid will be more than offset by the disappearance of HCO_3^- resulting from substitution of the weak conjugate base Cl^- for the strong base HCO_3^-.

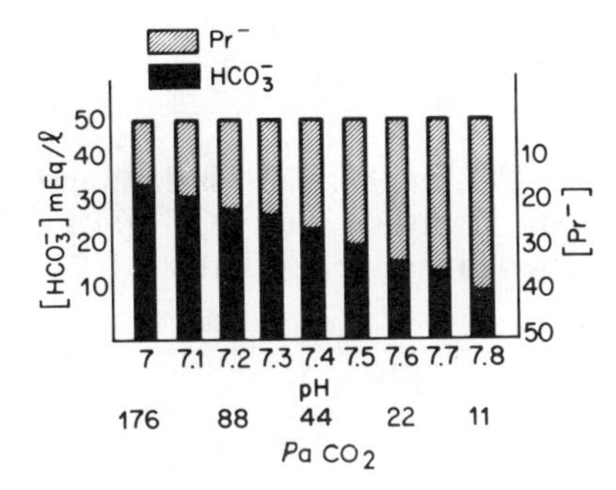

Figure 20.1 Alteration to components of total buffer base as pH is changed by changes in $Paco_2$. Note (1) the equal amounts of Pr^- and HCO_3^- at normal values of pH and $Paco_2$; (2) the increase in HCO_3^- as pH falls and $Paco_2$ rises; (3) the increase in Pr^- (predominantly due to haemoglobin) as the $Paco_2$ falls; (4) the constancy of $Pr^- + HCO_3^-$ when pH changes as a result of variations of $Paco_2$. (After Singer and Hastings, 1948, reproduced by courtesy of the authors and Editor of *Medicine*, Baltimore.)

Buffering in whole blood when $Paco_2$ *varies.* If $Paco_2$ alters there will be no alteration in the total buffer base concentration, but there will be a change in the contribution of its two components. This is well shown in *Figure 20.1*. The changes may be expressed as follows:

In red cells $\quad CO_2 + H_2O \rightleftharpoons H_2CO_3 \rightleftharpoons H^+ + HCO_3^-$

$$\begin{array}{c}\upharpoonleft\downharpoonright \\ Hb^- \rightleftharpoons H.Hb\end{array}$$

In plasma $\quad CO_2 + H_2O \rightleftharpoons H_2CO_3 \rightleftharpoons H^+ \rightleftharpoons HCO_3^-$

$$\begin{array}{c}\upharpoonleft\downharpoonright \\ Pr^- \rightleftharpoons HPr\end{array}$$

Nanoequivalents

Campbell (1962) has described a simple method of expressing $[H^+]$ in suitable units. The secretion of the oxyntic cells of the gastric mucosa is found to have a pH of between 2 and 1; this means that the concentration of hydrogen ions in gram equivalents is from $1/10^2$ to $1/10^1$; converting this into milliequivalents (multiplying by 1000) reveals a concentration of from 10–100 mEq/ℓ. Hydrogen ions therefore exist in gastric juice in concentrations which are applicable to other electrolytes. Campbell has suggested that if suitable units are chosen, the hydrogen ion concentration in ECF can equally well be expressed in absolute numbers. In man the pH of blood seldom reaches 8 or decreases below 7; expressed differently, $[H^+]$ varies between $1/10^8$ and $1/10^7$ gram equivalents per litre. One gram equivalent constitutes 10^9 nanoequivalents, so that these limits of hydrogen ion concentration become

$$\frac{1}{10^8} \times 10^9 \text{ and } \frac{1}{10^7} \times 10^9 = 10 \text{ and } 100\,\text{nEq}/\ell\text{, respectively.}$$

Returning to the Henderson equation:

$$[H^+] = K' \frac{[H_2CO_3]}{[HCO_3^-]}$$

K' is found to equal 8×10^{-7} gram equivalents per litre or $8 \times 10^{-7} \times 10^9 = 800\,\text{nEq}/\ell$. The equation may then be written as

$$[H^+] = 800 \frac{[H_2CO_3]}{[HCO_3^-]} \text{nEq}/\ell$$

The numerator $[H_2CO_3]$ is a fixed proportion of the CO_2 in physical solution, and this is itself determined by the product of the partial pressure of CO_2 and its solubility constant at 38°C (α). When $P\text{co}_2$ is expressed in mmHg, the latter is 0.03, so that the equation may then be written as

$$[H^+] = 800 \times \frac{0.03 P\text{co}_2}{[HCO_3^-]} = 24 \frac{P\text{co}_2}{[HCO_3^-]}$$

This simple equation clearly shows the relationship between $P\text{co}_2$ and HCO_3^- as determinants of the hydrogen ion concentration of the body fluids. *Figure 20.2* shows $[H^+]$ plotted in nanoequivalents against pH. The curve is very much steeper on the acidic side of pH 7.4, and it illustrates that the body is appreciably more tolerant of absolute increases in $[H^+]$ than it is of decreases in $[H^+]$.

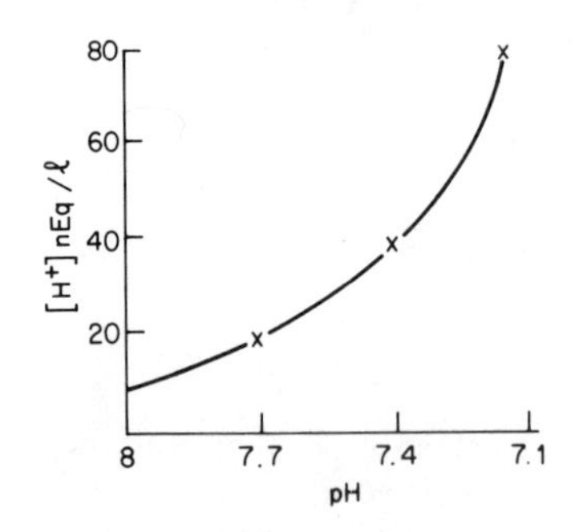

Figure 20.2 Change of H^+ with changes in pH. A fall in pH of 0.3 unit from 7.4 to 7.1 results in twice the change in H^+ that a rise in pH of 0.3 unit from 7.4 to 7.7 produces. (After Davenport, 1960, reproduced by courtesy of the author and University of Chicago Press.)

The Henderson–Hasselbalch equation

The Henderson approximation equation has been shown to be a simply derived expression of the law of mass action. Hasselbalch conceived the idea of expressing $[H^+]$ in the pH scale first described by Sørensen in which $\text{pH} = -\log[H^+]$ and $\text{p}K' = -\log K'$. The steps in the conversion are:

$$[H^+] = K' \frac{[\text{undissociated acid}]}{[\text{conjugate base}]} = K' \frac{[H_2CO_3]}{[HCO_3^-]}$$

$$\log [H^+] = \log K' + \log \frac{[H_2CO_3]}{HCO_3^-]}$$

$$-\log [H^+] = -\log K' - \log \frac{[H_2CO_3]}{[HCO_3^-]}$$

$$= -\log K' + \log \frac{[HCO_3^-]}{[H_2CO_3]}$$

$$pH = pK' + \log \frac{[HCO_3^-]}{[H_2CO_3]}$$

The expression $[HCO_3^-]$ is derived as follows. The total CO_2 content of whole blood is measured. This is derived mostly from CO_2 extracted from HCO_3^- and to a small extent from dissolved CO_2. The dissolved CO_2 is subtracted from the total. Thus the equation may be written:

$$pH = pK' + \log \frac{(\text{total } CO_2 - \alpha P\text{CO}_2)}{\alpha P\text{CO}_2}$$

It will be seen from the Henderson equation, or either of the other two equations derived from it, that $[H^+]$, $P\text{CO}_2$ and $[HCO_3^-]$ are so related that if any two are known there is a unique value for the third which can be simply calculated.

When whole blood is fully oxygenated and equilibrated at 38°C with a gas mixture containing CO_2 accurately adjusted so that its partial pressure is 40 mmHg (5.3 kPa), the standard bicarbonate is obtained (Astrup and colleagues, 1960).

Limitations of standard bicarbonate

Schwartz and Relman (1963) have criticized the use of the standard bicarbonate. It must be appreciated that any sustained change in either $P\text{CO}_2$ or $[HCO_3^-]$ will be followed by an alteration in the same direction of whichever component is not the prime mover. This can best be illustrated by reference to Campbell's equation:

$$[H^+] = 24 \frac{P\text{CO}_2}{[HCO_3^-]}$$

It can readily be seen that this secondary or compensatory change will reduce or even nullify the effect of the primary change on $[H^+]$. Thus a patient with emphysema and a $P\text{CO}_2$ of 65 mmHg (8.7 kPa) may have a pH which is normal; this implies that $[HCO_3^-]$ must have risen above the small increase due to the rise in $P\text{CO}_2$ itself, and a measurement of standard bicarbonate would reveal a higher than normal figure. If, however, the rise in $[HCO_3^-]$ is the primary change, as it would be when hydrogen ions are lost in large amounts as a result of pyloric stenosis, the standard bicarbonate will also be raised. It therefore gives no indication of the treatment required if taken by itself unless it has changed as a primary and sole result of a non-respiratory cause. If the change is due to renal excretion or retention of bicarbonate secondary to a change in ventilation it will, if taken by itself, tend to indicate quite inappropriate therapy. The patient must be seen and his disease diagnosed before the standard bicarbonate is evaluated.

Alterations in alveolar ventilation very rapidly change the arterial P_{CO_2} and levels of 15–20 mmHg (2–2.65 kPa) can be attained in 10–20 minutes of vigorous hyperventilation; if CO_2 is totally prevented from leaving the body as it is in so-called apnoeic diffusion oxygenation, the P_{CO_2} rises at a rate of 3–5 mmHg (0.4–0.6 kPa) per minute and the pH will fall to 7 or less after about 30 minutes. Renal compensatory changes are far slower and take from 1 to 3 days to become fully established. During anaesthesia, acids other than carbonic may accumulate in the blood independently of renal function. Any period of tissue hypoxia may be expected to be followed by some degree of metabolic acidosis and this is particularly evident after an episode of cardiac arrest.

Metabolic alkalosis cannot occur during anaesthesia unless bicarbonate or a precursor of bicarbonate such as lactate is given.

In recent years, automated systems have largely replaced the Astrup method. These employ calibration solutions of known pH, P_{CO_2} and P_{O_2} which are read on specific electrodes. A microprocessor stores the calibrated data, corrects the sample readings and calculates derived values, including base deficit.

Blood gas analysis

Direct determination of pH and P_{CO_2} became routine after introduction of an interpolation technique on small samples by Astrup and his colleagues (1960). This utilizes a plot of P_{CO_2} on a logarithmic scale against pH, which, with certain derived curves, has become familiar as the Siggaard-Andersen Nomogram (Siggaard-Andersen, 1962). One of these, the base excess curve, has generated the quantity-base deficit – which is most commonly employed as the basis of therapy.

It used to be contended that base deficit could be taken as the amount of bicarbonate necessary to restore the deficit in a litre of ECF. Extracellular fluid was taken to be 30 per cent of the body weight, so the total deficit became:

$$0.3 \times \text{body weight in kg} \times \text{base deficit per litre.}$$

This arithmetical approach is now out of favour for several reasons: there may be discrepancies between the *in vitro* and *in vivo* behaviour of blood as mentioned in the next section; the metabolic production of H^+ ions is a dynamic process capable of very rapid alterations without exogenous infusion of bicarbonate; and, finally, it is now appreciated that the more severe the deficit, the more important it is to restore it gradually with repeated measurements of pH, P_{CO_2} and standard bicarbonate. There is no place in extreme acidosis (concentrations of standard bicarbonate below 10 mmol/ℓ) for calculation of the theoretical total base deficit and infusion of molar sodium bicarbonate with the aim of total correction in a single infusion.

Whole-body response to acute rise in CO_2
Flenley (1971) has pointed out that in acute respiratory acidosis the Astrup method is valid for the measurement of $P\text{CO}_2$ but that it may introduce a significant error when 'base excess' is taken as a guide to therapy. This is because the response to an acute rise in $P\text{CO}_2$ *in vitro* differs from the response in the whole body. The rise in bicarbonate when blood is equilibrated in a tonometer with increasing partial pressures of CO_2 is appreciably greater (*see Figure 20.1*) than in the same blood in the body (Prys-Roberts, Kelman and Nunn, 1966). This is due to the bicarbonate generated as a result of buffering by haemoglobin being diluted throughout the ECF which itself has negligible buffering mechanisms for carbonic acid. Stoker and colleagues (1972) have shown that in certain circumstances the difference between the *in vitro* and the *in vivo* CO_2 response curves could result in the administration of 85 mEq of bicarbonate to correct a non-existent 'base deficit'. This would represent the addition of nearly 200 mosmol/ℓ of solutes to the ECF and might clearly be undesirable in a patient, for instance after open-heart surgery.

When the $P\text{CO}_2$ is known to be acutely raised, the base deficit should not be calculated from the simple formula given above. In such circumstances apparent base deficits of less than 5 mEq/ℓ need no correction; larger deficits are an indication for giving 50–100 mEq of sodium bicarbonate and repeated blood analyses.

Solutions used for correcting pH changes

The ionic composition of intravenous fluids is given in *Table 20.3*.

Sodium lactate
Sodium lactate is no longer available and sodium bicarbonate, which is now available in concentrations from sixth molar (isotonic) to molar, should be used instead.

Sodium bicarbonate
The molecular weight is 84, and therefore a molar solution contains 8.4 per cent and an isotonic solution (M/6) 1.4 per cent. It is available in the following strengths:

1.4 per cent containing 166 mmol/ℓ HCO_3^-
4.2 per cent containing 500 mmol/ℓ HCO_3^-
8.4 per cent containing 1000 mmol/ℓ HCO_3^-.

The half molar (4.2 per cent) solution is generally to be preferred and 0.5–1 mmol/kg body weight can be given and the pH and standard bicarbonate reassessed.

Calcium chloride
Calcium chloride is a potent acidifying salt and is also intensely sclerosing if injected into the tissues. It is not in the *British National Formulary*, but is available in ampoules of 13.4 per cent $CaCl_2 . 2H_2O$, which have the same calcium content as 20 per cent $CaCl_2 . 6H_2O$ and 10 per cent anhydrous $CaCl_2$.

Ammonium chloride
Ammonium chloride has been used for the correction of refractory alkalosis. It is available in ampoules containing 1 g in 5 ml. It is seldom indicated and should be

Table 20.3 Ionic composition of intravenous fluids

	Na^+ mmol/ℓ	*K^+* mmol/ℓ	*Cl^-* mmol/ℓ	*HCO_3^- or lactate* mmol/ℓ	*Ca^{2+}* mmol/ℓ	*Remarks*
Isotonic saline, 0.9 per cent	154		154			
1 M saline, 5.85 per cent	1000		1000			Should usually be diluted; reassess when 200 mmol given
M/6, 1.4 per cent sodium bicarbonate	166			166		
1 M, 8.4 per cent sodium bicarbonate	1000			1000		
1-g ampoule of potassium chloride		13.4	13.4			2 g added to each 500 ml is maximum safe amount
Hartmann Ringer/lactate	131	5.0	112	29	2.0	Amounts of K^+ and Ca^{2+} are insufficient to replace deficits of these ions

Useful data
1 g of ammonium chloride contains 18.7 mmol of ammonia
1 g of calcium chloride ($CaCl_2.2H_2O$) contains 6.8 mmol Ca^{2+}
1 g of calcium gluconate contains 4.5 mmol of Ca^{2+}
1 g of sodium chloride contains 17.1 mmol of Na^+
1 g of sodium lactate contains 8.9 mmol of Na^+
1 g of sodium bicarbonate contains 11.9 mmol of HCO_3^-

1 ml of any molar solution of an electrolyte contains 1 mmol of cation and 1 mmol of anion.
One-sixth molar solutions (166 mmol/ℓ) of electrolytes are approximately isosmotic with body fluids.
One-third molar solutions of non-electrolytes such as dextrose are approximately isotonic.

given in the same way as sodium bicarbonate, with frequent measurement of pH and standard bicarbonate. It should not be given to patients with hepatic failure and alkalosis.

Hydrochloric acid
The commonest cause of severe metabolic alkalosis is loss of hydrochloric acid as a result of pyloric or high jejunal obstruction. It is compounded by loss of potassium, mainly in the urine. The resulting hypochloraemic alkalosis can nearly always be rectified by the kidneys if sufficient sodium and potassium chloride are given; this may require 4–5 litres of isotonic saline and 500–600 mmol of potassium in the first 24 hours. Other causes of profound alkalosis may be seen in intensive care units and have been reported in some states of shock, in liver failure, and orthotopic liver transplants (Editorial, 1974).

If refractory and persistent alkalosis is encountered there is a case for the cautious infusion of hydrochloric acid. A molar solution of HCl can be prepared by any pharmacy which has facilities for autoclaving fluids for injection; 100–150 ml of this solution can replace a similar volume of 5 per cent dextrose in a 500 ml pack and be infused slowly (Beach and Sherwood Jones, 1971). As with infusion of bicarbonate for acidosis, frequent measurements of pH and standard bicarbonate are essential and not more than 100 mEq of H^+ should be infused without reassessing the effect.

Plasma substitutes

Fluid that has a viscosity and colloid osmotic pressure similar to that of plasma can be used to replace plasma or whole blood within certain limits. There are at present only two types of preparations which can be used, the dextrans and the gelatins. Dextrans have the advantage that they can be produced with higher average molecular weights and their intravascular persistence can therefore be longer. The incidence of anaphylactoid reactions to dextrans is related to the molecular weight and Ring and Messmer (1977) reported the same incidence for dextran 70 as for the best of the gelatins.

The disadvantages of the dextrans are that they enter the cells of the reticuloendothelial system and they have definite effects on platelet function and fibrin structure which tend to result in increased bleeding. They also interfere with cross-matching.

Gelatins, so far as is known, are inert in the body. They do not enter the cells of the reticuloendothelial system, nor do they have an effect on bleeding or coagulation other than that consequent upon dilution of normal plasma clotting factors.

Dextran

Dextran is a plasma substitute which is produced by the action of selected strains of *Leuconostoc mesenteroides* on sucrose. By controlling the hydrolysis, glucose chains of the desired average molecular weight can be selected. The renal threshold for dextran molecules is about 50 000 and the most appropriate molecular weight for dextran as a plasma volume expander is 70 000–110 000. The size of the molecules fluctuates about a mean, the smaller ones being excreted by the kidneys in a few hours. The remainder leave the blood at a uniform rate of about one-third per day (Maycock, 1954) and enter the tissues and particularly the cells of the reticuloendothelial system. All the administered dextran molecules are believed to be metabolized eventually, but the precise route is not known.

Preparations

High molecular weight dextrans

Dextran 110 (*BP*), average molecular weight 110 000

Dextran 70 (*BP*), average molecular weight 70 000

Although both these preparations are listed in the *British National Formulary 1981*, dextran 110 is very seldom used now and should be regarded as obsolete.

Dextran 70 is available in either 0.9 per cent saline or 5 per cent dextrose. There would seem to be no indication for giving the 5 per cent dextrose preparation if one is replacing plasma which contains 140 mmol/ℓ of sodium.

Dextran 70 is an effective substitute for whole blood or plasma. Vickers, Heath and Dunlap (1969) showed that it was as effective as stored blood in maintaining blood volume for up to 3 days after surgery. Blood must be taken for cross-matching before dextran is given and it is advisable, because of its effect on clotting, to restrict the volume given to 1 litre.

Low molecular weight dextran (dextran 40). Dextran with an average molecular weight of 40 000 is available as a 10 per cent solution in either 0.9 per cent saline or 5 per cent dextrose. It was originally marketed with emphasis on the rheological benefits it was held to confer. It was therefore advocated in the management of any condition in which tissue perfusion was critical. The evidence that it did prevent red cell sludging and improve flow to grafts and ischaemic limbs was strong but not unquestioned. Some of the observed increases in blood flow were probably due to dilution and no greater than could be seen with appropriate volumes of crystalloid solutions (Dormandy, 1971). Data and Nies (1974) reviewed the clinical use of dextran 40 and contended that it had no significant advantage over other plasma substitutes.

Low molecular weight dextran and renal failure. There are numerous reports linking the development of acute renal failure with the administration of dextran 40. The smaller molecules are very rapidly excreted by the kidneys and concentrations as high as 40 g/100 ml of urine are seen. This results in very viscous urine. Feest (1976) described six cases of acute renal failure associated with dextran 40 and thought it was probably the commonest cause of drug-induced renal failure. It should not be given when there is any reason to doubt renal function and urine output should be maintained above 40 ml/hour.

Antithrombotic properties of dextran

Both dextran 40 and dextran 70 have been used to prevent postoperative venous thrombosis. Dextran alters normal platelet function and tends to prevent platelet aggregation; it also alters the structure and chemical stability of fibrin and facilitates fibrinolysis by plasmin. Although dextran in doses of up to 1.5 g/kg body weight induces no measurable changes in the clotting mechanism, it does prolong the bleeding time and it should not be used in neurosurgery or other operations when this would be particularly undesirable. The antithrombotic effect is a property of the dextran molecule and unaffected by its molecular weight. Dextran 40 offers no advantages over dextran 70 for this purpose as the average molecular weight of colloid remaining in the circulation 24 hours after infusion of dextran 40 is 80 000 (Arturson and Wallenius, 1964). Five hundred millilitres of dextran 70 should be infused before surgery starts and the same volume repeated daily for 2–3 days postoperatively.

Gelatins

Gelatin preparations are obtained from bovine collagen which is treated in different ways in order to obtain a fluid solution of gelatin. This has colloid osmotic activity and viscosity which make it a suitable plasma substitute. The use of gelatin solutions is certain to increase as a result of the demands for fractionation of whole blood.

There are two preparations at present available in the UK: Gelofusine and Haemaccel.

Molecular weight of gelatin solutions

Unlike albumin, the molecular weights of all synthetic colloid solutions vary widely and for gelatin solutions the range is from 5000–50 000. The average molecular weight can be expressed in two ways, the weight average M_w, or the number average M_n. M_w in such solutions is always higher than M_n, but M_n is the determinant of colloid osmotic activity. The molecular weights shown in *Table 20.4* are the average M_n of the products.

Although the average molecular weights of the gelatins would lead one to expect very rapid renal excretion, the half-life in the circulation is claimed to be 4–6 hours and there is extensive clinical experience of both products on the Continent which shows them to be very effective plasma substitutes.

Anaphylactoid reactions

Although at first it was claimed that gelatins were 'non-antigenic' there is now no doubt that they can cause anaphylactoid reactions. Gelofusine is a succinylated gelatin whereas Haemaccel is urea-linked and their composition is different (*Table 20.4*). The balance of published reports at present favours the succinylated preparation as being the less likely to cause serious anaphylactoid reactions. In a 17-year study of reactions to over 100 000 units of this preparation, Lundsgaard-Hansen and Tschirren (1979) reported one fatality and seven grade III reactions. This is a significantly lower incidence than Ring and Messmer (1977) reported for dextran 70.

Table 20.4 Constituents of the two preparations of gelatin at present available in the UK

	Gelofusine	*Haemaccel*
Synonyms	Succinylated gelatin Physiogel Modified fluid gelatin	Urea-linked gelatin Polygeline
Average molecular weight (M_n)	22 600	24 500
Gelatin	40 g/ℓ	35 g/ℓ
Sodium	154 mmol/ℓ	145 mmol/ℓ
Potassium	0.4 mmol/ℓ	5.1 mmol/ℓ
Magnesium	0.4 mmol/ℓ	—
Calcium	0.4 mmol/ℓ	6.26 mmol/ℓ
Carbonate	20–30 mmol/ℓ	—
Chloride	125 mmol/ℓ	145 mmol/ℓ

Mixing drugs with intravenous infusions

Drugs are often added to intravenous infusions; surveys have found that a sizeable proportion have drugs added to the container and that many have more than one drug added. Some of the problems involved are insufficiently recognized. A drug may be unstable in solution in the infusion fluid and lose activity rapidly, or it may be incompatible with the infusion fluid or with another drug added to it.

Addition of a drug to an infusion solution requires special skill and care, and is preferably carried out by a pharmacist. Infusions should be clearly labelled with the identity and amount of drug added, together with the time and date of addition. It is important to mix the intravenous infusion and the added drug very thoroughly particularly with drugs such as potassium chloride in which layering can occur due to the density of the preparation. They should be given in the minimum time compatible with the clinical state of the patient. An infusion bottle should not be left up longer than about 8 hours.

The stability of a drug solution for intravenous administration depends on the formulation of the drug and its nature, the pH and temperature of the infusion solution to which it is added, and for how long the solution is stored and exposed to light and air. Loss of activity is especially likely to occur if the infusion lasts a long time or if prepared mixtures are stored before infusion. Antibiotics, notably some semisynthetic penicillins, break down rapidly in aqueous solution; their stability can be markedly affected by changes in pH, and the polymers that form on storage can conjugate with protein and amino acids to form potentially allergenic complexes.

Incompatibility between drug formulations in aqueous solution is commonly caused by changes in pH occurring when solutions are mixed. At the new pH the solubility or stability of one or more components may be altered, resulting in precipitation or partial decomposition. Gross physical changes may occur when drugs are added to intravenous fat emulsions or saturated solutions, such as 20 per cent mannitol.

Many drugs are insoluble in water. Those that are weak acids are therefore presented as sodium or potassium salts, and those that are weak bases as hydrochlorides, sulphates, and so on, to make them soluble; the former tend to produce solutions of high pH and the latter solutions of low pH. When a solution of a drug is added to an infusion fluid of different pH or an acidic drug mixed with a basic one, free acid or base may be precipitated or the pH may be shifted outside the optimum range for maximum stability. Such precipitation may be influenced by the order or the manner in which solutions are mixed, and often progresses over several hours. When two or more drugs are to be given in an infusion, each must be reconstituted and added separately to the infusion vehicle. If there is any change in colour or clarity of a solution during administration the infusion must be stopped at once.

Blood and solutions containing carbohydrates or amino acids provide highly nutrient media for the multiplication of bacteria and it is better to add nothing to them. The adoption of four basic rules would go far to limit the complications associated with contamination of infusions.

1. The giving set should be changed whenever clear fluids are to follow blood, protein, or amino acid solutions, or fat emulsions;
2. The giving set should be changed every 24 hours when only dextrose or electrolyte solutions are being given;

3. During prolonged blood transfusions the giving set should be changed every 6–8 hours;
4. All procedures relating to intravenous therapy should be carried out using strict aseptic techniques.

It is wise to change the giving set before infusing a drug solution, particularly after blood. Manufacturers now can provide much more data on the stability and compatibility of drugs and infusion fluids and should always be consulted in the first instance. As a general rule drugs should not be added to large volumes (500–1000 ml) of infusion solutions unless therapeutically necessary. There is less risk of bacterial contamination or chemical or physical interaction if drugs are administered by an intravenous bolus, from a burette, through the septum of the giving set, or as a 'piggy-back' infusion from a mini-bag through the infusion line. To reach therapeutic levels of the drug in blood and tissues these methods of administration are often to be preferred. Unless data on compatibility are available it is wise not to add more than one drug to one infusion (*British National Formulary 1981, Number 2*).

Some comments on the properties of commonly used intravenous solutions are listed in *Table 20.5*. *Table 20.6* is a list of drugs that may be given intravenously and the solutions and other drugs with which they are incompatible.

Table 20.5 Intravenous fluids as vehicles for infusing drugs

Solution	*Comments*
Dextrose Dextrose – saline Laevulose	The pH ranges from 3.5–6.5. Weak acids may be precipitated from solutions of their salts, particularly methicillin, novobiocin, sulphonamides, and barbiturates. Ampicillin and methicillin should be infused within 4 hours. **Do not add:** Aminophylline, barbiturates, cyanocobalamin, erythromycin, hydrocortisone, kanamycin, novobiocin, sulphonamides, warfarin.
Sodium chloride	Usually slightly acidic or neutral. Suitable for infusing many drugs. **Do not add:** Alcohol, amphotericin.
Compound sodium lactate (Hartmann's)	**Do not add:** Amphotericin, novobiocin, suxamethonium, tetracyclines, or any calcium salt.
Dextrans	Slightly acidic. Suitable for infusing many drugs but they may degrade acid-labile drugs, bind drugs or form drug complexes.
Mannitol	Saturated solutions containing 20 per cent or more may crystallize out when drugs or electrolytes (e.g. potassium chloride) are added. **Do not add (to any strength):** Corticotrophin, barbiturates, noradrenaline, metaraminol, suxamethonium, tetracyclines.
Sodium bicarbonate	Slightly alkaline. **Do not add:** Tetracyclines (which contain ascorbic acid), barbiturates, calcium salts, corticotrophin, hydrocortisone, insulin, methicillin, narcotics, noradrenaline, procaine, streptomycin, vancomycin, Parentrovite.
Amino acids	Slightly acidic. Contaminating micro-organisms are more likely to multiply than in other intravenous solutions. **Do not add any drugs.** (Insulin may be added to total parenteral nutrition regimens containing amino acids.)
Fat emulsions	Addition of drugs may crack emulsion or cause aggregation of fat globules. Some specially formulated preparations (e.g. Vitlipid) are available. Heparin *may* be added.

Table 20.6 pH, unsuitable infusion vehicles and incompatible mixtures given by infusion

Drug	*pH*	*Comments on infusion solution*	*Incompatible mixtures*
Aminophylline	7–9.5	Unstable in acid solutions, e.g. dextrose	Insulin, phenothiazines, tetracyclines
Amphotericin	5	Infuse in dextrose solutions only; protect containers from light	Avoid adding any drugs, all of which may cause precipitation
Atropine	3	Do not mix with alkaline solutions	Frusemide, sodium bicarbonate, sulphonamides
Calcium salts	6–8.2		Blood, cardiac glycosides, phenothiazines, phosphate injections, prednisolone, streptomycin, tetracycline
Cephalosporins			
Cephaloridine	3.5–6	May be added to saline or dextrose without significant loss of potency over 12 hours	Barbiturates, calcium gluconate, erythromycin, polymyxins, tetracyclines, THAM, phenylephrine
Cephalothin	5.2		
Chlorothiazide	4		Phenothiazines
Chloramphenicol	6–7.5	Stable in dextrose or saline	Ascorbic acid, erythromycin, hydrocortisone solutions, penicillins, phenothiazines, sulphonamides, tetracyclines
Digoxin	6.7–7.3	Do not dilute	Calcium or magnesium salts
Dipyridamole	2.8	Avoid adding to dextran solutions and sodium bicarbonate solutions	Heparin
Erythromycin	7.5		Acidic and alkaline solutions, barbiturates, cephalosporins, chloramphenicol, colistin, heparin, metaraminol, novobiocin, penicillins, phenothiazines, streptomycin, tetracyclines, Parentrovite
Frusemide	8.8–9.3	Must not be added to very acid solutions; direct intramuscular or intravenous injection recommended	All other drugs
Gentamicin	4–5	Should be given by bolus injection	
Heparin	6–7	Do not add to acidic solutions	Phenothiazines, erythromycin, gentamicin, hydrocortisone, kanamycin, novobiocin, streptomycin, tetracyclines, vancomycin

Hyaluronidase	4–7	Use mixture immediately	Adrenaline, alkaline solutions, heavy metals, heparin
Hydrocortisone hemisuccinate	7–8	May produce transient paraesthesia if injected too rapidly; avoid highly acidic or alkaline solutions	Ampicillin, calcium salts, cephalothin, chloramphenicol, colistin, heparin, kanamycin, novobiocin, phenothiazines, tetracyclines, vancomycin, Parentrovite
Insulin	3–5	Must not be added to strongly alkaline solutions	Aminophylline, barbiturates, sodium bicarbonate, sulphadiazine
Iron dextran	5.2–6.5		Sulphonamides
Isoprenaline	2–9	Avoid sodium bicarbonate and other alkaline solutions	All alkaline drugs
Kanamycin	6		Amphotericin, calcium salts, cephalothin, gentamicin, heparin, hydrocortisone, methohexitone, nitrofurantoin, penicillins, phenobarbitone, phenytoin, prochlorperazine, sulphonamides
Lignocaine	6.6–7		Barbiturates, sulphonamides
Lincomycin	6		Erythromycin, novobiocin, penicillins, phenytoin, sulphonamides
Methyldopa	4		Barbiturates, sulphonamides, tetracyclines
Methotrexate	4	For large doses use only water for injection BP since addition to isotonic saline would result in a hypertonic solution	
Orciprenaline	3–4	Must not be added to sodium bicarbonate	Avoid alkaline drugs and heavy metal salts
Penicillins			
Ampicillin	8–10	Potency reduced 10 per cent over 4 hours in solutions containing dextrose	Ascorbic acid, barbiturates, chloramphenicol, erythromycin, gentamicin, heparin, hydrocortisone, kanamycin, lincomycin, phenothiazines, streptomycin, sulphonamides, tetracyclines
Benzylpenicillin	5–7	Unstable in dextrose solutions	Chloramphenicol, phenothiazines, gentamicin, heparin, hydroxyzine, lincomycin, metaraminol, phenytoin, polymyxin B, tetracyclines, vancomycin, vitamin B, vitamin E

Table 20.6 *continued*

Drug	*pH*	*Comments on infusion solution*	*Incompatible mixtures*
Carbenicillin	6–8	Insufficient blood levels result from addition to infusion bottle; breaks down to benzylpenicillin on standing	Chloramphenicol, erythromycin, gentamicin, lincomycin, tetracyclines
Cloxacillin Flucloxacillin	5–7	Stable for 12 hours in solution	Erythromycin, gentamicin, polymyxin B, tetracyclines
Methicillin	7–8	Stable for 6–8 hours in solution	Phenothiazines, erythromycin, gentamicin, heparin, hydrocortisone, kanamycin, levallorphan, metaraminol, methohexitone, sulphonamides, tetracyclines, vancomycin
Pentazocine	4–4.8		Frusemide, potassium chloride, sodium bicarbonate
Phenothiazines Chlorpromazine Promazine Promethazine Prochlorperazine	5–6		Aminophylline, amphotericin, barbiturates, chloramphenicol, chlorothiazide, ethamivan, heparin, hydrocortisone, penicillins, sulphonamides, Parentrovite
Phenytoin	12	Dissolved in special solvent. Do not dilute	Do not add any other drugs
Phosphate injections		Avoid solutions containing calcium	Calcium gluconate and calcium chloride
Polymyxins Colistin Polymyxin B	6.5–7.5		Do not mix with drugs of very high or low pH, e.g. ascorbic acid, barbiturates, cephalosporins, penicillins, sulphonamides, tetracyclines. Also avoid amphotericin, chlorothiazide, heparin
Potassium chloride	7	Dilute the concentrate (1.5 g/10 ml) with at least 40 times its volume with either saline or dextrose	Amphotericin
Practolol	5.5–6		Ampicillin, barbiturates, frusemide, sodium bicarbonate, sulphonamides
Prednisolone sodium phosphate	7.5–9		Calcium salts, phenothiazines, polymyxin B
Reserpine	3–4	Must not be added to sodium bicarbonate	Chlorothiazide
Sodium bicarbonate	7.5–8.5		Calcium and magnesium salts, corticotrophin, insulin, narcotics, noradrenaline

Sodium iodide	7.5–9	Avoid acidic solutions	Narcotics, noradrenaline, procaine
Streptomycin	5–5.5		Amphotericin, ampicillin, barbiturates, chloramphenicol, heparin, sulphonamides, tetracyclines
Succinylcholine	3–4.5	Must not be added to sodium bicarbonate	Barbiturates
Sulphonamides Sulphadiazine Sulphadimidine	8.5– 10.5	Avoid acidic solutions; incompatible with dextrose and fructose solutions	Amiphenazole, chloramphenicol, hydralazine, insulin, iron dextran, lignocaine, lincomycin, metaraminol, methicillin, methyldopa, narcotics, noradrenaline, phenothiazines, procaine, streptomycin group, tetracyclines, vancomycin
Tetracyclines Chlortetracycline Oxytetracycline Tetracycline	 3–4 2–3 2–3	Stable 8–12 hours in solution; incompatible with the calcium in Hartmann's solution	Aminophylline, amphotericin, barbiturates, calcium salts, cephalosporins, chloramphenicol, erythromycin, heparin, hydrocortisone, novobiocin, penicillins, phenothiazines, phenytoin, polymyxins, sulphonamides, Parentrovite
Thiopentone	10–11		Insulin, methylamphetamine, morphine, pethidine, phenothiazines, polymyxins, procaine, sodium bicarbonate
Trimetaphan	5–6		Alkaline solutions, barbiturates, gallamine, tubocurarine
Vitamins B and C (Pabrinex, Parentrovite)	4–5		Aminophylline, amphotericin, barbiturates, chloramphenicol, erythromycin, heparin, hydrocortisone, novobiocin, penicillins, phenothiazines, polymyxins, sulphonamides, tetracyclines
Warfarin	7.2–8.3		Avoid strongly basic and acidic drugs

Arturson, G. and Wallenius, G. (1964) The renal clearance of dextran of different molecular sizes in normal humans. *Scandinavian Journal of Clinical Laboratory Investigation,* **16,** 81
Astrup, P., Jørgensen, K., Andersen, O. S. and Engel, K. (1960) The acid–base metabolism – a new approach. *Lancet,* **1,** 1035
Beach, F. X. M. and Sherwood Jones, E. (1971) Metabolic alkalosis treated with intravenous hydrochloric acid. *Postgraduate Medical Journal,* **47,** 516
Bell, H. E. (1972) Clinical assessment of postoperative blood volume. *Lancet,* **2,** 659
Bell, J. A., Hilton, P. J. and Walker, G. (1972) Severe hyponatraemia in hyperlipaemic diabetic ketosis. *British Medical Journal,* **4,** 709
Campbell, E. J. M. (1962) RIpH. *Lancet,* **1,** 681
Christensen, H. N. (1962) General concepts of neutrality regulation. *American Journal of Surgery,* **103,** 286
Danowski, T. S., Fergus, E. B. and Mateer, F. M. (1955) The low salt syndromes. *Annals of Internal Medicine,* **43,** 643
Data, J. L. and Nies, A. S. (1974) Drugs five years later: Dextran 40. *Annnals of Internal Medicine,* **81,** 500
Davenport, H. W. (1960) *The ABC of Acid Base Chemistry*. Chicago: University of Chicago Press
Dormandy, J. A. (1971) Influence of blood viscosity on blood flow and the effect of low molecular weight dextran. *British Medical Journal,* **4,** 716
Edelman, I. S., Leibman, J., O'Meara, M. P. and Birkenfeld, L. W. (1958) Interrelations between serum sodium concentration, serum osmolarity and total exchangeable sodium, total exchangeable potassium and total body water. *Journal of Clinical Investigation,* **37,** 1236
Edelman, I. S. and Leibman, J. (1959) Anatomy of body water and electrolytes. *American Journal of Medicine,* **27,** 256
Editorial (1974) Hydrochloric acid for metabolic alkalosis. *Lancet,* **1,** 720
Editorial (1977) Hypophosphataemia. *Lancet,* **2,** 122
Feest, T. G. (1976) Low molecular weight dextran: a continuing cause of acute renal failure. *British Medical Journal,* **2,** 1300
Flenley, D. C. (1971) Another non-logarithmic acid–base diagram. *Lancet,* **1,** 961
Lundsgaard-Hansen, P. and Tschirren, B. (1979) Anaphylactoid reactions to 102,787 units of modified fluid gelatin. Paper presented to workshop on Immunologic Aspects of the Side Effects of Plasma Substitutes. German Society of Research in Allergy and Immunity. Weisbaden, F. R. G. 27th April 1979
Maycock, W. d'A. (1954) Plasma substitutes. *British Medical Bulletin,* **10,** 29
Moore, F. D. (1954) The low sodium syndromes of surgery. An outline for practical management. *Journal of the American Medical Association,* **154,** 379
Moore, F. D. (1962) Regulation of the serum sodium concentration. *American Journal of Surgery,* **103,** 302
Moore, F. D., Haley, H. B., Bering, E. A., Brooks, L. and Edelman, I. S. (1952) Further observations on total body water. II. Changes of body composition in disease. *Surgery, Gynecology and Obstetrics,* **95,** 155
Orloff, M. J. and Hutchin, P. (1972) Fluid and electrolyte response to trauma and surgery. In *Clinical Disorders of Fluid and Electrolyte Metabolism,* 2nd Edition, p. 1065, Ed. Maxwell, M. H. and Kleeman, C. R. New York: McGraw-Hill
Paymaster, N. J. (1976) Magnesium metabolism: a brief review. *Annals of the Royal College of Surgeons of England,* **58,** 310
Prys-Roberts, C., Kelman, G. R. and Nunn, J. F. (1966) Determination of the *in-vivo* carbon dioxide titration curve in anaesthetized man. *British Journal of Anaesthesia,* **38,** 500
Ring, J. and Messmer, K. (1977) Incidence and severity of anaphylactoid reactions to colloid substitutes. *Lancet,* **1,** 466
Schwartz, W. B. and Relman, A. S. (1963) A critique of the parameters used in the evaluation of acid-base disorders. *New England Journal of Medicine,* **268,** 1382
Sheldon, G. F. and Grzyb, S. (1975) Phosphate depletion and repletion: relation to parenteral nutrition and oxygen transport. *Annals of Surgery,* **182,** 683
Siggaard-Andersen, O. (1962) The pH–log P_{CO_2} blood and acid-base nomogram revised. *Scandinavian Journal of Clinical and Laboratory Investigation,* **14,** 598
Singer, R. B. and Hastings, A. B. (1948) An improved clinical method for the estimation of disturbances of the acid–base balance of human blood. *Medicine,* **27,** 223
Stein, L., Beraud, J-J., Morissetts, M., da Luz, P., Weil, M. H. and Shubin, H. (1975) Pulmonary edema during volume infusion. *Circulation,* **52,** 483

Stoker, J. B,. Kappagoda, C.T., Grimshaw, V. A. and Linden, R. J. (1972) A new method for assessing states of acute acidaemia in man. *Clinical Science,* **42,** 455

Vickers, M. D., Heath, M. L. and Dunlap, D. (1969) A comparison of Macrodex and stored blood as replacement for blood loss during planned surgery. I. Blood volume maintenance. *British Journal of Anaesthesia,* **41,** 676

Wynn, V. (1957) Osmotic behaviour of the body cells in man. Significance of changes of plasma-electrolyte levels in body-fluid disorder. *Lancet,* **2,** 1212

Appendix:

Drug name equivalents, UK and USA

In most instances trade names are those of preparations that contain only the single ingredient. In some instances trade names are not listed where they are so numerous as to be unhelpful, e.g. aspirin and adrenaline.

Lists were compiled from *Martindale, The Extra Pharmacopoeia,* 28th edn, (1982), Pharmaceutical Press: London; *The American Drug Index,* 27th edn, (1983), Lippincott: Philadelphia; *Monthly Index of Medical Specialities,* November (1983): London.

UK approved name *UK trade name(s)*	US approved name *US trade name(s)*
Acebutolol *Sectral*	Acebutolol
Acepifylline *Etophylate*	Acepifylline *Etophylate*
Acetazolamide *Diamox*	Acetazolamide *Diamox, Hydrazol*
Acetylcysteine *Airbron*	Acetylcysteine *Mucomyst*
Acycloquanosine (*see* Acyclovir)	
Acyclovir *Zovirax*	Acyclovir *Zovirax*
Adenine arabinoside (*see* Vidarabine)	
Adrenaline	Epinephrine
Albuterol (*see* Salbutalol)	
Alcuronium *Alloferin*	
Alfacalcidol *One-Alpha*	
Allobarbitone	Allobarbital
Aloxiprin *Palaprin*	Aloxiprin *Palaprin*
Alphadolone	Alfadolone
Alphaxalone *Althesin*	Alfaxalone
Alphaprodine	Alphaprodine *Nisentil*
Alprenolol	
Amantadine *Symmetrel*	Amantadine *Symmetrel*
Ambenonium *Mytelase*	Ambenonium *Mytelase*
Amethocaine *Minims Amethocaine*	Tetracaine *Pontocaine*
Amidopyrine	
Amikacin *Amikin*	Amikacin *Amikin*

UK approved name *UK trade name(s)*	US approved name *US trade name(s)*
Amiloride *Midamor*	Amiloride *Midamor*
Aminophylline *Phyllocontin*	Aminophylline *Phyllocontin, Panamin, Lixaminol, Aminodur, Somaphyllin*
Amiodarone *Cordarone*	
Amitriptyline *Domical, Lentizol, Limbritol, Saroten, Tryptizol*	Amitriptyline *Elavil, Elegen, Endep*
Amoxycillin *Amoxil*	Amoxicillin *Amoxil, Polymox, Robamox, Sumox, Trimox, Utimox, Wymox*
Amphotericin *Fungilin, Fungizone*	Amphotericin *Fungizone*
Ampicillin *Amfipen, Vidopen, Penbritin*	Ampicillin *Omnipen, Roampicillin, Amcill, Ameril, Pensyn, Polycillin, Principen, Totacillin, Penbritin, Pfizerpen*
Amyl nitrite	Amyl nitrite *Vaporole, Aspirols*
Amylobarbitone *Amytal*	Amobarbital *Amytal, Pulvule*
Apomorphine	Amomorphine
Aprotinin *Trasylol*	Aprotinin *Trasylol*
Atenolol *Tenormin*	Atenolol *Tenormin*
Azapropazone *Rheumox*	
Azlocillin *Securopen*	
Bacampicillin *Ambaxin*	Bacampicillin *Spectrobid*
Barbitone	Barbital *Veronal, Medinal, Embinal*
Benapryzine	
Bendrofluazide *Aprinox, Berkozide, Centyl, Neo-Naclex*	Bendroflumethiazide *Naturetin*
Benorylate *Benoral*	
Benoxaprofen *Opren*	Benoxaprofen *Oraflex*
Benzathine penicillin *Penidural*	Benzathine penicillin *Permapen*
Benzhexol *Artane*	Benzhexol *Artane, Trinol*
Benzocaine	Benzocaine
Benztropine *Cogentin*	Benztropine *Cogentin*

UK approved name *UK trade name(s)*	US approved name *US trade name(s)*
Benzylpenicillin *Crystapen*	Penicillin G *Hyasorb, Paclin, Pentids, Pfizerpen, Lanacillin, Cryspen, Duracillin*
Betamethasone *Betnelan, Betnesol, Betnovate*	Betamethasone *Diprosone, Celestone, Valisone*
Bethanechol *Myotonine*	Bethanechol *Duvoid, Myotonachol, Urecholine, Vesicholine*
Bethanidine *Esbatal*	Bethanidine *Esbatal*
Bretylium *Bretylate*	Bretylium *Bretylol, Bretylate, Darenthin*
Bromhexine *Bisolvomycin, Bisolvon*	Bromhexine *Bisolvon*
Bromocryptine *Parlodel*	Bromocryptine *Parlodel*
Bumetanide *Burinex*	Bumetanide *Burinex*
Bupivacaine *Marcain*	Bupivacaine *Marcaine, Sensorcaine*
Buprenorphine *Temgesic*	
Butobarbitone *Soneryl*	Butabarbital *Butalen, Butazem, Butisol, Expansatol, Soduben, Medarsed*
Butorphanol	Butorphanol *Stadol*
Butyl aminobenzoate	Butamben *Butesin*
Caffeine	Caffeine *No Doz*
Calcitriol *Rocaltrol*	Calcitriol *Rocaltrol*
Captopril *Capoten*	Captopril *Capoten*
Carbachol *Isopto Carbachol*	Carbachol *Carbacel, Murocarb, Miostat Intraocular*
Carbamazepine *Tegretol*	Carbamazepine *Tegretol*
Carbenicillin *Pyopen*	Carbenicillin *Pyopen, Geopen, Geocillin*
Carbidopa in *Sinemet*	Carbidopa in *Sinemet*
Carbimazole *Neo-Mercazole*	 *Bimazole, Neo-Mercazole*
Carboxymethylcysteine *Mucodyne, Mucolex*	Carboxymethylcysteine *Mucodyne, Thiodril*
Carfecillin *Uticillin*	
Cefaclor *Distaclor*	Cefaclor *Ceclor*
Cefotaxime *Claforan*	

UK approved name *UK trade name(s)*	US approved name *US trade name(s)*
Cefoxitin *Mefoxin*	Cefoxitin
Cefsoludin *Monaspor*	
Cefuroxime *Zinacef*	
Cephalexin *Ceporex, Keflex*	Cephalexin *Keflex, Ceporex*
Cephaloridine *Ceporin*	Cephaloridine *Loridine*
Cephalothin *Keflin*	Cephalothin *Keflin*
Cephazolin *Kefzol*	Cephazolin *Kefzol*
Cephradine *Velosef*	Cephradine *Velosef, Anspor, Eskasef*
Chloral hydrate *Noctec*	Chloral hydrate *Noctec, Aquachloral, Rectules, Oradrate, Felsules, Somnos*
Chloramphenicol *Chloromycetin, Kemicetine, Minims Chloramphenicol, Sno phenicol*	Chloramphenicol *Amphicol, Antibiopto, Chloromycetin, Econochlor, Mychel, Ophthoclor, Kemicetine, Paraxin, Chlorcetin*
Chlorazepate *Tranxene*	Chlorazepate *Azene, Tranxene*
Chlordiazepoxide *Librium*	Chlordiazepoxide *A-Poxide, Librium, Screen, Libritabs, SK-Lygen, Zetran, Chlordiazachel*
Chlormethiazole *Heminevrin*	Chlormethiazole *Heminevrin*
	Chloroprocaine *Nesacaine*
Chlorothiazide *Saluric*	Chlorothiazide *Diuril*
Chlorpheniramine *Piriton*	Chlorpheniramine *Chlor-4, Chlor Niramine, Chlormene, Chlorspan, Chlortab, Chlor-Trimeton, Histaspan, Phenetron, Panahist, Histacon, Teldrin*
Chlorpromazine *Largactil*	Chlorpromazine *Promachlor, Thorazine, Terpium, Sonazine, Promaz, Chlorizine*
Chlorpropamide *Diabinese, Melitase*	Chlorpropamide *Diabinese*
Chlortetracycline *Aureomycin*	Chlortetracycline *Aureomycin*
Chlorthalidone *Hygroton*	Chlorthalidone *Hygroton, Combipres*
Chymotrypsin *Chymar*	Chymotrypsin *Catarase, Avazyme*
Cimetidine *Tagamet*	Cimetidine *Tagamet*

UK approved name *UK trade name(s)*	US approved name *US trade name(s)*
Cinchocaine *Nupercaine*	Dibucaine *Nupercaine, Dulzit*
Cinnarizine *Stugeron*	Cinnarizine *Stugeron, Mitronal*
Cinoxacin *Cinobac*	Cinoxacin *Cinobac*
Clavulanic acid in *Augmentin*	
Clindamycin *Dalacin*	Clindamycin *Cleocin, Dalacin*
Clomipramine *Anafranil*	Clomipramine *Anafranil*
Clonazepam *Rivotril*	Clonazepam *Clonopin*
Clonidine *Catapres, Dixarit*	Clonidine *Catapres, Dixarit*
Clopenthixol *Clopixol*	Clopenthixol *Sordinol*
Clotrimazole *Canesten*	Clotrimazole *Gyne-Lotrimin, Lotrimin Myclex*
Cloxacillin *Orbenin*	Cloxacillin *Cloxapen, Tegopen*
Colistin *Colomycin*	Colistin *Coly-Mycin, Colomycin*
Cortisone *Cortelan, Cortistab, Cortisyl*	Cortisone *Cortone, Cortistan*
Co-trimoxazole *Bactrim, Comox, Chemotrim, Spetrin, Nodilon*	Co-trimoxazole *Bactrim, Septra, Spetrin*
Cyclizine *Valoid*	Cyclizine *Marzine, Valoid*
Cyclobarbitone *Phanodorm*	Cyclobarbital
Cyclopenthiazide *Navidrex*	Cyclopenthiazide *Navidrex*
Cyclopentolate *Minims Cyclopentolate, Mydrilate*	Cyclopentolate *Cyclogyl*
Cycloserine	Cycloserine *Seromycin*
Cyproheptadine *Periactin*	Cyproheptadine *Periactin*
Dantrolene *Dantrium*	Dantrolene *Dantrium*
Debrisoquine *Declinax*	
Demethylchlortetracycline (*see* Demeclocyclin)	
Demeclocyclin *Ledermycin*	Demeclocyclin *Declomycin*
Deoxycortone	Deoxycorticosterone *Doca, Percorten*
Deoxytetracycline (*see* Doxycycline)	
Deptropine *Brontina*	Deptropine *Brontina*

UK approved name *UK trade name(s)*	US approved name *US trade name(s)*
Desipramine *Pertofran*	Desipramine *Norpramin, Pertofrane*
Desmopressin *DDAVP*	Desmopressin *DDAVP*
Dexamethasone *Decadron, Oradexon*	Dexamethasone *Decadron, Dexadron, Dexone, Dezone, Hexadrol, Savacort-D, Maxidex*
Dexamphetamine *Dexedrine*	Dexamphetamine *Dexedrine, Dexamped, Oxydess, Diphylets*
Dextromoramide *Palfium*	Dextromoramide *Palfium, Jetrium*
Dextropropoxyphene	Propoxyphene *Darvon, Dolene, Myospaz, Proxagesic, Stogesic, Wygesic*
Diazepam *Atensine, Diazemuls, Evacalm, Solis, Valium*	Diazepam *Valium*
Diazoxide *Eudemine*	Diazoxide *Proglycem, Hyperstat*
Dichloralphenazone *Paedo-Sed, Welldorm*	Dichloralphenazone *Welldorm, Fenzol*
	Dicloxacillin *Dynapen, Dycill, Pathocil, Veracillin*
Dicyclomine *Merbentyl*	Dicyclomine *Benacol, Bentyl, Pasmin, Stannitol, Merbentyl, Wyovin*
Diflunisal *Dolobid*	Diflunisal *Dolobid*
Digoxin *Lanoxin*	Digoxin *Lanoxin, Masoxin*
Dihydrocodeine *DF-118*	
Dihydroergotamine *Dihydergot*	Dihydroergotamine *DHE 45*
Dimenhydrinate *Dramamine, Gravol*	Dimenhydrinate *Dimenate, Dramocen Dramamine, Marmine, Signate, Traveltabs*
Diphenhydramine *Benadryl*	Diphenhydramine *Lensen, Valdrene, Wehydryl Benylin, Histin, T-Dryl*
Dipipanone *Diconal*	Dipipanone *Pipadone*
Diprophylline *Silbephylline, Neutraphylline*	Diprophylline *Isophylline*
Dipyridamole *Persantin*	Dipyridamole *Persantine*
Disoprofol *Diprovan*	
Disopyramide *Dirythmin, Rythmodan*	Disopyramide *Rhymodan*

UK approved name *UK trade name(s)*	US approved name *US trade name(s)*
Distigmine *Ubretid*	Distigmine *Ubretid*
Disulfiram *Antabuse*	Disulfiram *Antabuse*
Dobutamine *Dobutrex*	Dobutamine *Dobutrex, Inotrex*
Dopamine *Intropin*	Dopamine *Intropin, Dopostat*
Dothiepin *Prothaiden*	Dothiepin *Prothiaden*
Doxapram *Dopram*	Doxapram *Dopram*
Doxycycline *Doxatet, Nordox, Vibramycin*	Doxycycline *Vibramycin, Vibra-Tabs*
Droperidol *Droleptan*	Droperidol *Inapsine*
Econazole *Ecostatin, Gyno-Pevaryl, Pevaryl*	
Ecothiopate *Phospholine*	Ecothiopate *Phospholine*
Edrophonium *Tensilon*	Edrophonium *Tensilon*
Enflurane *Ethrane*	Enflurane *Ethrane*
Epicillin	Epicillin *Dexacillin*
Ergometrine *Syntometrine*	Ergonovine *Ergotrate*
Ergotamine *Cafergot, Lingraine, Migril*	Ergotamine *Ergomar, Ergostat, Gynergen*
Erythromycin *Erymsin, Erythromid, Ilotycin*	Erythromycin *Ilotycin, E-Mycin, Robimycin*
Erythromycin estolate *Ilosone*	Erythromycin estolate *Ilosone*
Erythromycin ethylsuccinate *Erythroped*	Erythromycin ethylsuccinate *EES, E-Mycin-E, Erythrocin, Pediamycin, Wyamycin E*
Erythromycin stearate *Erythrocin*	Erythromycin stearate *Erythrocin, Dowmycin, Erypar, Ethril, SK-Erythromycin*
Etamiphylline *Millophylline*	Etamiphylline *Milliophylline*
Ethacrynic acid *Edecrin*	Ethacrynic acid *Edecrin*
Ethambutol *Myambutol*	Ethambutol *Myambutol*
Ethamivan *Clairvan*	Ethamivan *Vandid*
Ethamsylate *Dicynene*	Ethamsylate
Ethionamide	Ethionamide *Trecator*
Ethosuximide *Emeside, Zarontin*	Ethosuximide *Zarontin*

UK approved name *UK trade name(s)*	US approved name *US trade name(s)*
Etidocaine	Etidocaine *Duranest*
Etomidate *Hypnomidate*	
Fazadinium *Fazadon*	
Felypressin *Octapressin*	Felypressin *Octapressin*
Fenclofenac *Flenac*	
Fenfluramine *Ponderax*	Fenfluramine *Pondimin, Ponderax*
Fenoprofen *Fenopron, Progesic*	Fenoprofen
Fentanyl *Sublimaze*	Fentanyl *Sublimaze, Innovar*
Feprazone *Methrazone*	
Flucloxacillin *Floxapen*	
Flucytosine *Albocon*	Flucytosine *Ancobon*
Fludrocortisone *Florinef*	Fludrocortisone *Florinef*
Flufenamic acid *Meralen*	
Flupenthixol *Depixol, Fluanxol*	Flupenthixol *Depixol*
Flurazepam *Dalmane*	Flurazepam *Dalmane*
Flurbiprofen *Froben*	
Fluphenazine *Modecate, Moditen*	Fluphenazine *Permitil, Prolixin*
Framycetin *Framygen, Soframycin*	Framycetin *Framygen, Soframycin*
Frusemide *Diumide, Dryptal, Frusetic, Lasix*	Furosemide *Lasix*
Fusidic acid *Fucidin*	
Gallamine *Flaxedil*	Gallamine *Flaxedil*
Gentamicin *Alcomicin, Cidomycin, Garamycin, Genticin, Gentigan, Minims Gentamicin*	Gentamicin *Garamycin, Genoptic Bristagen, Apogen*
Glibenclamide *Daonil, Euglucon*	Glibenclamide *Daonil, Euglucon*
Glutethimide *Doriden*	Glutethimide *Doriden, Dorimide, Rolathimide*
Glyceryl Trinitrate *Nitrocontin, Nitrolingual Percutol, Sustac, Tridil Nitrocine*	Nitroglycerin *Cardabid, Nitrocap, Nitrobid Nitroglyn, Nitrol, Nitrong, Nitro-Lyn, Nitrospan, Nitrostat, Trates*

UK approved name	UK trade name(s)	US approved name	US trade name(s)
Glycopyrronium	*Robinul*	Glycopyrronium	*Robinul*
Griseofulvin	*Fulcin, Grissovin*	Griseofulvin	*Fulvicin, Grifulvin, Grisactin*
Guanethidine	*Ismelin*	Guanethidine	*Ismelin*
Guanoclor	*Vatensol*		
Haloperidol	*Fortunan, Haldol, Serenace*	Haloperidol	*Haldol*
Halothane	*Fluothane*	Halothane	*Fluothane*
Hexafluorenium		Hexafluorenium	*Mylaxen*
Hexamine mandelate	*Hiprex, Mandelamine*	Methenamine mandelate	*Mandelamine, Renelate, Thendelate, Mandalay*
Hexobarbitone		Hexobarbital	*Sombulex*
Homatropine	*Minims Homatropine*	Homatropine	*Homatrocel, Murocoll*
Hydralazine	*Apresoline*	Hydralazine	*Apresoline, Dralzine, Hydralyn*
Hydrochlorothiazide	*Esidrex, HydroSaluric*	Hydrochlorothiazide	*Chlorizide, Delco-Retic, Esidrix, Hydrozide, Hydro Diuril, Hyperetic, Thiuretic, Hydromal, Oretic, Ro-Hydrazide, SK-Hydrochlorthiazide, Diu-Scrip*
Hydroflumethiazide	*Hydrenox*	Hydroflumethiazide	*Salutensin*
Hyoscine	*Buscopan, Minims Hyoscine*	Scopolamine	
Hyoscine methobromide		Methscopolamine bromide	*Pamine*
Ibuprofen	*Brufen, Ibo-Slo*	Ibuprofen	*Motrin*
Idoxuridine	*Dendrid, Idoxene, Kerecid, Ophthalmadine*	Idoxuridine	*Stoxil, Dendrid, Herplex*
Imipramine	*Tofranil*	Imipramine	*Tofranil, Imavate*
Indapamide	*Natrilix*		
Indomethacin	*Mobilan, Imbrilon, Indocid,*	Indomethacin	*Indocin*
Indoramin	*Baratol*		
Ipratropium	*Atrovent*	Ipratropium	*Atrovent*
Iprindole	*Prondol*		
Iproniazid	*Marsilid*	Iproniazid	*Marsilid*
Isoetharine	*Numotac*	Isoetharine	*Bronkometer, Bronkosol*

UK approved name	*UK trade name(s)*	US approved name	*US trade name(s)*
Isoflurane		Isoflurane	*Forane*
Isoniazid	*Rimifon*	Isoniazid	*Niconyl, Nydrazid, Panazid, Rolazid, Triniad, Laniazid*
Isoprenaline	*Aleudrin, Iso-Autohaler, Medihaler, Saventrine*	Isoproterenol	*Medihaler, Aerolone, Isuprel Norisodrine, Proternol*
Isosobide	*Cedocard, Isoket, Isodil, Soni-Slo, Sorbichew, Sorbid, Vascardin*	Isosorbide	*Isodril, Dilatrate, Iso-Bid, Iso-D, Sorbitrate, Sorquad*
Isoxsuprine	*Defencin, Duvadilan*	Isoxsuprine	*Rolisox, Vasodilan*
Kanamycin	*Kannasyn, Kantrex*	Kanamycin	*Kantrex, Kannasyn*
Ketamine	*Ketalar*	Ketamine	*Ketalar, Ketaject*
Ketoprofen	*Alrheumat, Orudis, Oruvail*		
Labetolol	*Trandate*		
Latamoxef	*Moxalactam, Lauromacrogol*		
Levallorphan	*Lorfan*	Levallorphan	*Lorfan*
Levodopa	*Brocadopa, Larodopa*	Levodopa	*Larodopa, Levopa, Parda, Bendopa*
Levorphanol	*Dromoran*	Levorphanol	*Levo-Dromoran*
Lignocaine	*Xylocard, Xylocaine*	Lignocaine	*Xylocaine, Anestacon, Dolicaine, Stanacaine, Rocaine, Ardecaine*
Lincomycin	*Lincocin*	Lincomycin	*Lincocin*
Liothyronine	*Tertroxin*	Liothyronine	*Cytomel*
Lorazepam	*Almazine, Ativan*	Lorazepam	*Ativan*
Lypressin	*Pitressin, Syntopressin*	Lypressin	*Diapid*
Mafenide	*Sulfamylon, Sulfomyl*	Mafenide	*Sulfamylon*
Malathion	*Derbac, Prioderm*		
Mannitol	*Osmitrol*	Mannitol	*Osmitrol*
Maprotiline	*Ludiomil*		
Mecamylamine	*Inversine*	Mecamylamine	*Inversine*
Mecillinam	*Selexidin*		

UK approved name *UK trade name(s)*	US approved name *US trade name(s)*
Meclozine	Meclizine
Ancoloxin	*Antivert, Bonine, Lamine, Vertrol*
Medazepam	Medazepam
Nobrium	
Mefenamic acid	Mefenamic acid
Ponstan	*Ponstel*
Mefruside	
Baycaron	
Mephentermine	Mephentermine
	Wyamine
Mepivacaine	Mepivacaine
Chlorocain	*Carbocaine*
Meprobamate	Meprobamate
Equanil, Milonorm, Miltown	*Miltown, Mecrocon, Meprospan SK-Bamate, Tranmep, Bamate*
Mepyramine	Pyrilamine
	Pyma, Pyristan
Metaraminol	Metaraminol
Aramine	*Aramine*
Methacholine	Methacholine
Amechol	*Mecholyl*
Methadone	Methadone
Physeptone	*Dolophine*
Methaqualone	Methaqualone
	Mequin, Parest, Quaalude
Mithimazole	Methimazole
	Tapazole, Thiamazole
Methicillin	Methicillin
Celbenin	*Celbenin, Azapen, Staphcillin*
Methohexitone	Methohexital
Brietal	*Brevital*
Methotrexate	Methotrexate
Emtexate	*Mexate*
Methotrimeprazine	Methotrimeprazine
	Levoprome
Methoxamine	Methoxamine
Vasoxine	
Methoxyflurane	Methoxyflurane
Penthrane	*Penthrane*
Methylamphetamine	Methamphetamine
	Desoxyn, Methampex
Methyldopa	Methyldopa
Aldomet, Dopamet	*Aldoril, Aldomet*
Methylene Blue	Methylene Blue
	Urolene Blue
Methylphenidate	Methylphenidate
Ritalin	*Ritalin*
Methyprylone	Methyprylon
Noludar	*Noludar*
Methysergide	Methysergide
Deseril	*Sansert*
Metoclopramide	Metoclopramide
Maxolon, Primperan, Metox	*Reglan*
Metolazone	Metalozone
Metenix	*Zaroxolyn*

UK approved name	UK trade name(s)	US approved name	US trade name(s)
Metronidazole	*Flagyl, Zadstat*	Metronidazole	*Flagyl, Metryl*
Metyrapone	*Metopirone*	Metyrapone	*Metopirone*
Mexiletine	*Mexitil*		
Mezlocillin	*Baypen*		
Mianserin	*Bolvidon, Norval*		
Miconazole	*Daktarin, Monistat*	Miconazole	*Monistat*
Minocycline	*Minocin*	Minocycline	*Minocin*
Nadolol	*Corgard*	Nadolol	*Corgard*
Nafcillin	*Nafcil*	Nafcillin	*Unipen, Nafcil*
Nalidixic acid	*Uriben, Negram*	Nalidixic acid	*NegGram*
Naloxone	*Narcan*	Naloxone	*Narcan*
Naphazoline		Naphazoline	*Clear Eyes, Naphcon, Privine Vasocon*
Naproxen	*Naprosyn, Synflex*	Naproxen	*Naprosyn, Anaprox*
Nefopam	*Acupan*	Nefopam	
Neomycin	*Kaomycin, Minims Neomycin, Mycifradin, Myciguent, Nivemycin*	Neomycin	*Mycifradin, Myciguent, Neobiotic*
Neostigmine	*Prostigmin*	Neostigmine	*Prostigmin*
Netilmicin	*Netillin*	Netilmicin	*Netromycin*
Nicoumalone	*Sinthrome*		
Nifedipine	*Adalat*	Nifedipine	*Procardia*
Nikethamide		Nikethamide	*Coramine*
Nitrazepam	*Mogadon, Nitrados, Somnite, Surem, Unisomnia*		
Nitrofurantoin	*Berkfurin, Macrodantin, Furadantin*	Nitrofurantoin	*Furadantin, Macrodantin, Urotoin, Nitrofor, Nitrex, Trantoin*
Nomifensine	*Merital*	Nomifensine	*Merital*
Nystatin	*Nystavescent, Nystan*	Nystatin	*Mycostatin, Nilstat*
Orciprenaline	*Alupent*	Orciprenaline	*Alupent*

UK approved name	*UK trade name(s)*	US approved name	*US trade name(s)*
Orphenadrine	*Disipal, Norflex*	Orphenadrine	*Norflex, Flexor, Flexon*
		Oxacillin	*Bactocill, Prostaphlin*
Oxazepam	*Serenid*	Oxazepam	
Oxprenolol	*Slow-Pren, Trasicor*		
Oxybuprocaine	*Opulets benoxinate, Minims benoxinate*	Benoxinate	*Dorsacaine*
		Oxymorphone	*Numorphan*
Oxyphenbutazone	*Tandacote, Tanderil*	Oxyphenbutazone	*Oxalid, Tandearil*
Oxytocin	*Syntocinon*	Oxytocin	*Syntocinon, Pitocin*
Pancuronium	*Pavulon*	Pancuronium	*Pavulon*
Papaverine		Papaverine	*Cerebid, Cerespan, Dylate, Kavrin, Myobid, Pavabid, Pava Caps, Pavadyl, Pavacen, Pavakey, Pavatran, Pava-Wol, Therapav, Vasal, Vasocap, Vasopan*
p-Aminobenzoic acid		p-Aminobenzoic acid	*Pabafilm, Presun, Pabanol*
Paracetamol		Acetaminophen	
Paraldehyde		Paraldehyde	*Paral*
Pargyline	*Eutonyl*	Pargyline	*Eutonyl*
Pemoline	*Ronyl, Volital*	Pemoline	*Cylert*
Pentaerythritol tetranitrate	*Cardicap, Mycardol, Peritrate*	Pentaerythritol tetranitrate	*Peritrate, Duotrate, El-Petn, Metranil, Pentafin, Pentritol, Pentryate, Tentrate, Tranite, Vasolate*
Pentazocine	*Fortral*	Pentazocine	*Talwin*
Pentobarbitone	*Nembutal*	Pentobarbital	*Nembutal*
Pethidine		Meperidine	*Demerol*
Perhexiline	*Pexid*		
Perphenazine	*Fentazin*	Perphenazine	*Trilafon*
Phenazocine	*Narphen*		
Phenazone		Antipyrine	
Phenelzine	*Nardil*	Phenelzine	*Nardil*

UK approved name *UK trade name(s)*	US approved name *US trade name(s)*
Phenethicillin *Broxil*	Phenethicillin *Chemipen*
Phenindione *Dindevan*	Phenindione *Hedulin, Eridione*
Phenobarbitone *Luminal, Parabal*	Phenobarbital *Luminal, Sedadrops, Orprine*
Phenoperidine *Operidine*	
Phenoxybenzamine *Dibenyline*	Phenoxybenzamine *Dibenzyline*
Phenoxymethylpenicillin *Apsin VK, Co-Caps Penicillin VK, Crystapen V, Distaquine V-K, Stabillin V-K, V-Cil-K*	Penicillin V *V-Cillin, Betapen-VK, Dowpen VK, Ledercillin VK, Bopen, Penapar VK, Pen-Vee-K, Pfizerpen VK, Robicillin VK, Ro-Cillin VK, Uticillin VK, V-Cillin K, Veetids*
Phentolamine *Rogtitine*	Phentolamine *Regitine, Rogitine*
Phenylbutazone *Butazolidin, Butacote*	Penylbutazone *Butazolidin, Azolid*
Phenytoin *Epanutin*	Phenytoin *Dilantin, Diphenylan, Ekko, Dihycon*
Phthalylsulphathiazole *Thalazole*	Phthalylsulfathiazole *Sulfathalidine*
Physostigmine	Physostigmine *Isopto-Eserine, Miocel*
Phytomenadione *Konakion*	Phytonadiol *Konakion, Aguamephyton, Mephyton*
Pilocarpine *Isopto Carpine, Sno pilo, Ocusert Pilo*	Pilocarpine *Almocarpine, Mi-Pilo, Pilocar, Pilocel, Piloptic*
Pimozide *Orap*	
Pindolol *Visken*	Pindolol *Visken*
Piperidolate *Dactil*	Piperidolate
Piritramide *Dipidolor*	
Pivampicillin *Pondocillin*	
Pivmecillinam *Selexid*	
Polymixin *Aerosporin*	Polymixin *Aerosporin*
Practolol *Eraldin*	
Pralidoxime	Pralidoxime *Protopam*
Prazosin *Hypovase*	Prazosin *Minpress, Minizide*

UK approved name *UK trade name(s)*	US approved name *US trade name(s)*
Prednisolone *Deltastab, Codelsol Precortisyl, Predenema, Prednesol, Predsol, Sintisone*	Prednisolone *Delta-Cortef, Meti-Drem, Prednis, Ropred, Sterane, Ulacort, Econpred, Meticortelone, Savacort, Hydeltrasol, Inflamase, Metreton*
Prednisone *Decortisyl*	Prednisone *Delta-Dome, Deltasone, Lisacort, Meticorten, Orasone, Sterapred*
Prenalterol *Hyprenan, Varbian*	
Prenylamine *Synadrin*	
Prilocaine *Citanest*	Prilocaine *Citanest*
Primidone *Mysoline*	Primidone *Mysoline*
Probenecid *Benemid*	Probenecid *Benemid, Benacen, Probalan, Robenecid*
Procainamide *Pronestyl*	Procainamide *Pronestyl, Procan, Procapan*
Procaine Penicillin *Depocillin*	Penicillin G Procaine *Crysticillin, Duracillin, Pfizerpen AS, Wycillin*
Prochlorperazine *Stemetil, Vertigon,*	Prochlorperazine *Compazine*
Progesterone *Cyclogest*	Progesterone *Progestin, Gesterol, Femotrone, Lipo-Lutin, Prorone*
Promazine *Sparine*	Promazine *Sparine*
Promethazine *Phenergan, Avomine*	Promethazine *Phenergan, Fellozine, Ganphen, Phencen, Phenerex, Phenerhist, Remsed, Prorex*
Propantheline *Pro-banthine*	Propantheline *Pro-Banthine, Norpanth, Robantaline, Ropanth, Spastil*
Propanidid *Epontol*	Propanidid *Epontol*
	Propiomazine *Largon*
Propranolol *Berkolol, Inderal*	Propanolol *Inderal*
Propylthiouracil	Propylthiouracil *Propacil*
Proxymetacaine *Ophthaine*	Proxymetacaine *Ophthaine, Proparacaine,*
Pyrazinamide *Zinamide*	Pyrazinamide *Zinamide*
Pyridostigmine *Mestinon*	Pyridostigmine *Mestinon, Regona*

UK approved name	*UK trade name(s)*	US approved name	*US trade name(s)*
Quinalbarbitone	*Seconal*	Secobarbital	*Seconal*
Quinethazone		Quinethazone	*Hydromox*
Quinidine	*Kiditard, Kinidin*	Quinidine	*Duraguin, Quinaglute, Cin-Quin, Quinidex, Quinora*
Ranitidine	*Zantac*		
Reserpine	*Serpasil*	Reserpine	*Serpasil, Rau-Sed, Tensin Reserjen, Reserpoid, Sandril Serpate, Vio-Serpine*
Rifampicin	*Rifadin, Rimactane*	Rifampin	*Rifadin, Rimactane*
Ritodrine	*Yutopar*		*Yutopar*
Salbutamol	*Ventolin*	Albuterol	*Ventolin*
Sissomicin		Sisomicin	
Sodium cromoglycate	*Intal, Lomusol, Nalcrom, Opticrom, Rynacrom*	Cromolyn Sodium	*Intal*
Sodium nitroprusside	*Nipride*	Sodium nitroprusside	*Nipride, Keto-Diastix, Nitropress*
Sodium salicylate		Sodium salicylate	*Uracel, Alysine*
Sodium thiosulphate		Sodium thiosulfate	
Sodium valproate	*Epilim*	Valproic acid	*Depakene*
Sotalol	*Beta-Cardone, Sotacor*		*Beta-Cardone, Sotacor*
Spectinomycin	*Trobicin*	Spectinomycin	*Trobicin*
Spironolactone	*Aldactone, Diatensec, Spiroctan*	Spironolactone	*Aldactone*
Streptokinase	*Varidase*	Streptokinase	*Streptase, Kabikinase*
Sulindac	*Clinoril*	Sulindac	*Clinoril*
Sulphadiazine		Sulfadiazine	*Microsulfon, Neo-Quinette*
Sulphadimidine	*Sulphamethazine*	Sulfamethazine	*Neotrizine*
Sulphfurazole	*Gantrisin*	Sulfisoxazole	*Gantrisin, G-Sox, Koro-Sulf, SK-Spoxazole, Sosal, Soxa, Sulfagan, Sulfizin, Velmatrol,*
Sulphamethizole	*Urolucosil*	Sulfamethizole	*Microsul, Proklar-M, Thiosulfil*
Sulphamethoxazole		Sulfamethoxazole	*Gantanol*
Sulphamethoxydiazine		Sulfamethoxydiazine	*Sulla*

UK approved name *UK trade name(s)*	US approved name *US trade name(s)*
Sulphamethoxypyridazine *Lederkyn*	
Sulphasalazine *Salazopyrin*	Sulfasalazine *Azulfidine, SAS-500, Salazopyrin, Sulcolon*
Sulphinpyrazone *Anturan*	Sulfinpyrazone *Anturane*
Sulthiame *Ospolot*	
Suxamethonium *Anectine, Brevidil, Scoline*	Succinylcholine *Anectine, Quelicin, Sucostrin, Pintop*
Talampicillin *Talpen*	
Temazepam *Euhypnos, Normison*	Temazepam *Restoril*
Terbutaline *Bricanyl*	Terbutaline *Brethine*
Tetracosactrin *Synacthen*	Tetracosactrin *Synacthen, Cosyntropin*
Thiopentone *Intravel*	Thiopental *Pentothal*
Thiopropazate *Dartalan*	
Thioridazine *Melleril*	Thioridazine *Mellaril*
Thromboplastin *Tachostyptan*	
Thyrotrophin *Thytropar*	Thyrotrophin *Thytropar*
Ticarcillin *Ticar*	Ticarcillin *Ticar*
Timolol *Betim, Blocadren, Timoptol*	Timolol *Blocadren*
Tobramycin *Nebcin, Tobralex*	Tobramycin *Nebcin, Tobrex, Hyporet*
Tolazoline *Priscol*	Tolazoline *Priscoline, Tazol, Tolzol, Toloxan*
Tolbutamide *Pramidex, Rastinon*	Tolbutamide *Orinase*
Tolmetin *Tolectin*	Tolmetin *Tolectin*
Tranylcypromine *Parnate*	Tranylcyoromine *Parnate*
Triamcinolone *Adcortyl, Kenalog, Ledercort*	Triamcinolone *Kenalog, Aristocort, Tri-Kort, Tramacin, Triam-A*
Triamterene *Dytac*	Triamterene *Dyrenium*
Trichloroethylene *Trilene*	
Triclofos	Triclofos *Triclos*
Trifluoperazine *Stelazine*	Trifluoperazine *Stelazine*

UK approved name *UK trade name(s)*	US approved name *US trade name(s)*
Trimeprazine *Vallergan*	Trimeprazine *Temaril*
Trimetaphan *Arfonad*	Trimethaphan *Arfonad*
Trimethoprim *Ipral, Monotrim, Syraprim, Trimopan*	Trimethoprim *Proloprim, Trimpex*
Triprolidine *Actidil*	Triprolidine *Actidil*
Trypsin *Trypure*	Trypsin
Tubocurarine *Tubarine*	Tubocurarine *Metubine*
Vancomycin *Vancocin*	Vancomycin *Vancocin*
Verapamil *Cordilox*	
Vidarabine *Vira-A*	Vidarabine *Vira-A*
Viloxazine *Vivalan*	Viloxazine *Vivalan*
Warfarin *Marevan*	Warfarin *Coumadin, Panwarfin, Marevan*
Xipamide *Diurexan*	
Zomepirac *Zomax*	Zomepirac *Zomax*

UK NAMES

Approved name	*Trade name*
Acebutolol	*Sectral*
Acepifylline	*Etophylate*
Acetazolamide	*Diamox*
Acetylcysteine	*Airbron*
Acyclovir	*Zovirax*
Alcuronium	*Alloferin*
Alfacalcidol	*One-Alpha*
Aloxiprin	*Palaprin*
Alphaxalone	*Althesin*
Amantadine	*Symmetrel*
Ambenonium	*Mytelase*
Amethocaine	*Minims Amethocaine*
Amikacin	*Amikin*
Amiloride	*Midamor*
Aminophylline	*Phyllocontin*
Amiodarone	*Cordarone*
Amitriptyline	*Domical*
	Lentizol
	Limbritol
	Saroten
	Tryptizol
Amoxycillin	*Amoxil*
Amphotericin	*Fungilin*
	Fungizone
Ampicillin	*Amfipen*
	Penbritin
	Vidopen
Amylobarbitone	*Amytal*
Aprotinin	*Trasylol*
Atenolol	*Tenormin*
Azapropazone	*Rheumox*
Azlocillin	*Securopen*
Bacampicillin	*Ambaxin*
Bendrofluazide	*Aprinox*
	Berkozide
	Centyl
Benorylate	*Benoral*
Benoxaprofen	*Opren*
Benzathine penicillin	*Penidural*
Benzhexol	*Artane*
Benztropine	*Cogentin*
Benzylpencillin	*Crystapen*
Betamethasone	*Betnelan*
	Betnesol
	Betnovate
Bethanechol	*Myotonine*
Bethanidine	*Esbatal*
Bretylium	*Bretylate*
Bromhexine	*Bisolvomycin*
	Bisolvon
Bromocryptine	*Parlodel*
Bumetanide	*Burinex*
Bupivacaine	*Marcain*
Buprenorphine	*Temgesic*
Butobarbitone	*Soneryl*
Calcitriol	*Rocaltrol*
Captopril	*Capoten*
Carbachol	*Isopto Carbachol*
Carbamazepine	*Tegretol*
Carbenicillin	*Pyopen*
Carbimazole	*Neo-Mercazole*
Carboxymethyl-cysteine	*Mucodyne*
	Mucolex
Carfecillin	*Uticillin*
Cefaclor	*Distaclor*
Cefotaxime	*Claforan*
Cefoxitin	*Mefoxin*
Cefsoludin	*Monaspor*
Cefuroxime	*Zinacef*
Cephalexin	*Ceporex*
Cephaloridine	*Ceporin*
Cephalothin	*Keflin*
Cephazolin	*Kefzol*
Cephradine	*Velosef*
Chloral hydrate	*Noctec*
Chloramphenicol	*Chloromycetin*
	Kemicetine
	Minims Chloramphenicol
	Sno Phenicol
Chlorazepate	*Tranxene*
Chlordiazepoxide	*Librium*
Chlormethiazole	*Heminevrin*
Chlorothiazide	*Saluric*
Chlorpheniramine	*Piriton*
Chlorpromazine	*Largactil*
Chlorpropamide	*Diabinese*
	Melitase
Chlortetracycline	*Aureomycin*
Chlorthalidone	*Hygroton*
Chymotrypsin	*Chymar*
Cimetidine	*Tagamet*
Cinchocaine	*Nupercaine*
Cinnarizine	*Stugeron*
Cinoxacin	*Cinobac*
Clindamycin	*Dalacin*
Clomipramine	*Anafranil*
Clonazepam	*Rivotril*
Clonidine	*Catapres*
	Dixarit
Clopenthixol	*Clopixol*
Clotrimazole	*Canesten*
Cloxacillin	*Orbenin*
Co-trimoxazole	*Bactrim*
	Chemotrim
	Comox
	Nolidon
	Septrin
Colistin	*Colomycin*
Cortisone	*Cortelan*
	Cortistab
	Cortisyl
Cyclizine	*Valoid*

UK NAMES

Approved name	*Trade name*
Cyclobarbitone	*Phanodorm*
Cyclopenthiazide	*Navidrex*
Cyclopentolate	*Minims Cyclopentolate*
	Mydrilate
Cyproheptadine	*Periactin*
Dantrolene	*Dantrium*
Debrisoquine	*Declinax*
Demeclocyclin	*Ledermycin*
Deptropine	*Brontina*
Desipramine	*Pertofran*
Desmopressin	*DDAVP*
Dexamethasone	*Decadron*
	Oradexon
Dexamphetamine	*Dexedrine*
Dextromoramide	*Palfium*
Diazepam	*Atensine*
	Diazemuls
	Evacalm
	Solis
	Valium
Diazoxide	*Eudemine*
Dichloralphenazone	*Paedo-Sed*
	Welldorm
Dicyclomine	*Merbentyl*
Diflunisal	*Dolobid*
Digoxin	*Lanoxin*
Dihydrocodeine	*DF-118*
Dihydroergotamine	*Dihydergot*
Dimenhydrinate	*Dramamine*
Diphenhydramine	*Benadryl*
Dipipanone	*Diconal*
Diprophylline	*Neutraphylline*
	Silbephylline
Dipyridamole	*Persantin*
Disoprofol	*Diprovan*
Disopyramide	*Dirythmin*
	Rythmodan
Distigmine	*Ubretid*
Disulfiram	*Antabuse*
Dobutamine	*Dobutrex*
Dopamine	*Intropin*
Dothiepin	*Prothiaden*
Doxapram	*Dopram*
Doxycycline	*Doxatet*
	Nordon
	Vibramycin
Droperidol	*Droleptan*
Econazole	*Ecostatin*
	Gyno-Pevaryl
	Pevaryl
Ecothiopate	*Phospholine*
Edrophonium	*Tensilon*
Enflurane	*Ethrane*
Ergometrine	*Syntometrine*
Ergotamine	*Cafergot*
	Lingraine
	Migril
Erythromycin	*Erymsin*
	Erythromid
	Ilotycin
Erythromycin estolate	*Ilosone*
Erythromycin ethyl-succinate	*Erythroped*
Erythromycin stearate	*Erythrocin*
Etamiphylline	*Millophylline*
Ethacrynic acid	*Edecrin*
Ethambutol	*Myambutol*
Ethamivan	*Clairvan*
Ethamsylate	*Dicynene*
Ethosuximide	*Emeside*
	Zarontin
Etomidate	*Hypnomidate*
Fazadinium	*Fazadon*
Felypressin	*Octapressin*
Fenclofenac	*Flenac*
Fenfluramine	*Ponderax*
Fenoprofen	*Fenopron*
	Progesic
Fentanyl	*Sublimaze*
Feprazone	*Methrazone*
Flucloxacillin	*Floxapen*
Flucytosine	*Albocon*
Fludrocortisone	*Florinef*
Flufenamic acid	*Meralen*
Flupenthixol	*Depixol*
	Fluanxol
Fluphenazine	*Modecate*
	Moditen
Flurazepam	*Dalmane*
Flurbiprofen	*Froben*
Framycetin	*Framygen*
	Soframycin
Frusemide	*Diumide*
	Dryptal
	Frusetic
	Lasix
Fusidic acid	*Fucidin*
Gallamine	*Flaxedil*
Gentamicin	*Alcomicin*
	Garamycin
	Minims Gentamicin
Gentamycin	*Cidomycin*
	Genticin
	Gentigan
Glibenclamide	*Daonil*
	Euglucon
Glutethimide	*Doriden*
Glyceryl Trinitrate	*Nitrocine*
	Nitrocontin
	Nitrolingual
	Percutol
	Sustac
	Tridil

UK NAMES

Approved name	*Trade name*	*Approved name*	*Trade name*
Glycopyrronium	*Robinul*	Levallorphan	*Lorfan*
Griseofulvin	*Fulcin*	Levodopa	*Brocadopa*
	Grisovin		*Larodopa*
Guanethidine	*Ismelin*	Levorphanol	*Dromoran*
Guanoclor	*Vatensol*	Lignocaine	*Xylocaine*
Haloperidol	*Fortunan*		*Xylocard*
	Haldol	Lincomycin	*Lincocin*
	Serenace	Liothyronine	*Tertroxin*
Halothane	*Fluothane*	Lorazepam	*Almazine*
Hexamine mandelate	*Hiprex*		*Ativan*
	Mandelamine	Lypressin	*Pitressin*
Homatropine	*Minims Homatropine*		*Syntopressin*
Hydralazine	*Apresoline*	Mafenide	*Sulfamylon*
Hydrochlorothiazide	*Esidrex*		*Sulfomyl*
	HydroSaluric	Malathion	*Derbac*
Hydroflumethiazide	*Hydrenox*		*Prioderm*
Hyoscine	*Buscopan*	Mannitol	*Osmitrol*
	Minims Hyoscine	Maprotiline	*Ludiomil*
Ibuprofen	*Brufen*	Mecamylamine	*Inversine*
	Ibo-Slo	Mecillinam	*Selexidin*
Idoxuridine	*Dendrid*	Meclozine	*Ancoloxin*
	Idoxene	Medazepam	*Nobrium*
	Kerecid	Mefenamic acid	*Ponstan*
	Ophthalmadine	Mefruside	*Baycaron*
Imipramine	*Tofranil*	Mepivacaine	*Chlorocain*
Indapamide	*Natrilix*	Meprobamate	*Eguanil*
Indomethacin	*Imbrilon*		*Milonorm*
	Indocid		*Miltown*
Indoramin	*Baratol*	Metaraminol	*Aramine*
Ipratropium	*Atrovent*	Methacholine	*Amechol*
Iprindole	*Prondol*	Methadone	*Physeptone*
Iproniazid	*Marsilid*	Methicillin	*Celbenin*
Isoetharine	*Numotac*	Methohexitone	*Brietal*
Isoniazid	*Rimifon*	Methotrexate	*Emtexate*
Isoprenaline	*Aleudrin*	Methoxamine	*Vasoxine*
	Iso-Autohaler	Methoxyflurane	*Penthrane*
	Medihaler	Methyldopa	*Aldomet*
	Saventrine		*Dopamet*
Isosorbide	*Cedocard*	Methylphenidate	*Ritalin*
	Isodil	Methyprylone	*Noludar*
	Isoket	Methysergide	*Deseril*
	Soni-Slo	Metoclopramide	*Maxolon*
	Sorbichew		*Metox*
	Sorbid		*Primperan*
	Vascardin	Metolazone	*Metenix*
Isoxsuprine	*Defencin*	Metronidazole	*Flagyl*
	Duvadilan		*Zadstat*
Kanamycin	*Kannasyn*	Metyrapone	*Metopirone*
	Kantrex	Mexiletine	*Mexitil*
Ketamine	*Ketalar*	Mezlocillin	*Baypen*
Ketoprofen	*Alrheumat*	Mianserin	*Bolvidon*
	Orudis		*Norval*
	Oruvail	Miconazole	*Daktarin*
Labetolol	*Trandate*		*Monistat*
Latamoxef	*Lauromacroqol*	Minocycline	*Minocin*
	Moxalactam	Nadolol	*Corgard*

UK NAMES

Approved name	*Trade name*
Nafcillin	*Nafcil*
Nalidixic acid	*Negram*
	Uriben
Naloxone	*Narcan*
Naproxen	*Naprosyn*
	Synflex
Nefopam	*Acupan*
Neomycin	*Kaomycin*
	Minims Neomycin
	Mycifradin
	Myciguent
	Nivemycin
Neostigmine	*Prostigmin*
Netilmicin	*Netillin*
Nicoumalone	*Sinthrome*
Nifedipine	*Adalat*
Nitrazepam	*Mogadon*
	Nitrados
	Somnite
	Surem
	Unisomnia
Nitrofurantoin	*Berkfurin*
	Furadantin
	Macrodantin
Nomifensine	*Merital*
Nystatin	*Nystan*
	Nystavescent
Orciprenaline	*Alupent*
Orphenadrine	*Disipal*
	Norflex
Oxazepam	*Serenid*
Oxprenolol	*Slow-Pren*
	Trasicor
Oxybuprocaine	*Minims benoxinate*
	Opulets benoxinate
Oxyphenbutazone	*Tandacote*
	Tanderil
Oxytocin	*Syntocinon*
Pancuronium	*Pavulon*
Pargyline	*Eutonyl*
Pemoline	*Ronyl*
Pentaerythritol tetranitrate	*Cardicap*
	Mycardol
	Peritrate
Pentazocine	*Fortral*
Perhexiline	*Pexid*
Perphenazine	*Fentazin*
Phenazocine	*Narphen*
Phenelzine	*Nardil*
Phenethicillin	*Broxil*
Phenindione	*Dindevan*
Phenobarbitone	*Luminal*
	Parabal
Phenoperidine	*Operidine*
Phenoxybenzamine	*Dibenyline*
Phenoxymethylpenicillin	*Apsin VK*
	Co-Caps Penicillin VK
	Crystapen V
	Distaquine V-K
	Stabillin V-K
	V-Cil-K
Phentolamine	*Rogitine*
Phenylbutazone	*Butacote*
	Butazolidin
Phenytoin	*Epanutin*
Phthalylsulphathiazole	*Thalazole*
Phytomenadione	*Konakion*
Pilocarpine	*Isopto Carpine*
	Ocusert Pilo
	Sno Pilo
Pimozide	*Orap*
Pindolol	*Visken*
Piperidolate	*Dactil*
Piritramide	*Dipidolor*
Pivampicillin	*Pondocillin*
Pivmecillinam	*Selexid*
Polymixin	*Aerosporin*
Practolol	*Eraldin*
Prazosin	*Hypovase*
Prednisolone	*Codelsol*
	Deltastab
	Precortisyl
	Predenema
	Prednesol
	Predsol
	Sintisone
Prednisone	*Decortisyl*
Prenalterol	*Hyprenan*
	Varbian
Prenylamine	*Synadrin*
Prilocaine	*Citanest*
Primidone	*Mysoline*
Probenecid	*Benemid*
Procainamide	*Pronestyl*
Procaine Penicillin	*Depocillin*
Prochlorperazine	*Stemetil*
	Vertigon
Progesterone	*Cyclogest*
Promazine	*Sparine*
Promethazine	*Avomine*
	Phenergan
Propanidid	*Epontol*
Propantheline	*Pro-banthine*
Propranolol	*Berkolol*
	Inderal
Proxymetacaine	*Ophthaine*
Pyrazinamide	*Zinamide*
Pyridostigmine	*Mestinon*
Quinalbarbitone	*Seconal*

UK NAMES

Approved name	*Trade name*	*Approved name*	*Trade name*
Quinidine	*Kiditard*	Tetracosactrin	*Synacthen*
	Kinidin	Thiopentone	*Intraval*
Ranitidine	*Zantac*	Thiopropazate	*Dartalan*
Reserpine	*Serpasil*	Thioridazine	*Melleril*
Rifampicin	*Rifadin*	Thromboplastin	*Tachostyptan*
	Rimactane	Thyrotrophin	*Thytropar*
Ritodrine	*Yutopar*	Ticarcillin	*Ticar*
Salbutamol	*Ventolin*	Timolol	*Betim*
Sodium cromoglycate	*Intal*		*Blocadren*
	Lomusol		*Timoptol*
	Nalcrom	Tobramycin	*Nebcin*
	Opticrom		*Tobralex*
	Rynacrom	Tolazoline	*Priscol*
Sodium nitroprusside	*Nipride*	Tolbutamide	*Pramidex*
Sodium valproate	*Epilim*		*Rastinon*
Sotalol	*Beta-Cardone*	Tolmetin	*Tolectin*
	Sotacor	Tranylcypromine	*Parnate*
Spectinomycin	*Trobicin*	Triamcinolone	*Adcortyl*
Spironolactone	*Aldactone*		*Kenalog*
	Diatensec		*Ledercort*
	Spiroctan	Triamterene	*Dytac*
Streptokinase	*Varidase*	Trichloroethylene	*Trilene*
Sulindac	*Clinoril*	Trifluoperazine	*Stelazine*
Sulphadimidine	*Sulphamethazine*	Trimeprazine	*Vallergan*
Sulphamethizole	*Urolucosil*	Trimetaphan	*Arfonad*
Sulphamethoxy-pyridazine	*Lederkyn*	Trimethoprim	*Ipral*
			Monotrim
Sulphasalazine	*Salazopyrin*		*Syraprim*
Sulphfurazole	*Gantrisin*	Triprolidine	*Actidil*
Sulphinpyrazone	*Anturan*	Trypsin	*Trypure*
Sulthiame	*Ospolot*	Tubocurarine	*Tubarine*
Suxamethonium	*Brevidil*	Vancomycin	*Vancocin*
	Scoline	Verapamil	*Cordilox*
Suxamethonium	*Anectine*	Vidarabine	*Vira-A*
Talampicillin	*Talpen*	Viloxazine	*Vivalan*
Temazepam	*Euhypnos*	Warfarin	*Marevan*
	Normison	Xipamide	*Diurexan*
Terbutaline	*Bricanyl*	Zomepirac	*Zomax*

UK NAMES

Trade name	*Approved name*	*Trade name*	*Approved name*
Actidil	Triprolidine	*Bolvidon*	Mianserin
Acupan	Nefopam	*Bretylate*	Bretylium
Adalat	Nifedipine	*Brevidil*	Suxamethonium
Adcortyl	Triamcinolone	*Bricanyl*	Terbutaline
Aerosporin	Polymixin	*Brietal*	Methohexitone
Airbron	Acetylcysteine	*Brocadopa*	Levodopa
Albocon	Flucytosine	*Brontina*	Deptropine
Alcomicin	Gentamicin	*Broxil*	Phenethicillin
Aldactone	Spironolactone	*Brufen*	Ibuprofen
Aldomet	Methyldopa	*Burinex*	Bumetanide
Aleudrin	Isoprenaline	*Buscopan*	Hyoscine
Alloferin	Alcuronium	*Butacote*	Phenylbutazone
Almazine	Lorazepam	*Butazolidin*	Phenylbutazone
Alrheumat	Ketoprofen	*Cafergot*	Ergotamine
Althesin	Alphaxalone	*Canesten*	Clotrimazole
Alupent	Orciprenaline	*Capoten*	Captopril
Ambaxin	Bacampicillin	*Cardicap*	Pentaerythritol tetra-nitrate
Amechol	Methacholine		
Amfipen	Ampicillin	*Catapres*	Clonidine
Amikin	Amikacin	*Cedocard*	Isosorbide
Amoxil	Amoxycillin	*Celbenin*	Methicillin
Amytal	Amylobarbitone	*Centyl*	Bendrofluazide
Anafranil	Clomipramine	*Ceporex*	Cephalexin
Ancoloxin	Meclozine	*Ceporin*	Cephaloridine
Anectine	Suxamethonium	*Chemotrim*	Co-trimoxazole
Antabuse	Disulfiram	*Chlorocain*	Mepivacaine
Anturan	Sulphinpyrazone	*Chloromycetin*	Chloramphenicol
Apresoline	Hydralazine	*Chymar*	Chymotrypsin
Aprinox	Bendrofluazide	*Cidomycin*	Gentamycin
Apsin VK	Phenoxymethylpenicillin	*Cinobac*	Cinoxacin
Aramine	Metaraminol	*Citanest*	Prilocaine
Arfonad	Trimetaphan	*Claforan*	Cefotaxime
Artane	Benzhexol	*Clairvan*	Ethamivan
Atensine	Diazepam	*Clinoril*	Sulindac
Ativan	Lorazepam	*Clopixol*	Clopenthixol
Atrovent	Ipratropium	*Co-Caps Penicillin VK*	Phenoxymethylpencillin
Aureomycin	Chlortetracycline		
Avomine	Promethazine	*Codelsol*	Prednisolone
Bactrim	Co-trimoxazole	*Cogentin*	Benztropine
Baratol	Indoramin	*Colomycin*	Colistin
Baycaron	Mefruside	*Comox*	Co-trimoxazole
Baypen	Mezlocillin	*Cordarone*	Amiodarone
Benadryl	Diphenhydramine	*Cordilox*	Verapamil
Benemid	Probenecid	*Corgard*	Nadolol
Benoral	Benorylate	*Cortelan*	Cortisone
Berkfurin	Nitrofurantoin	*Cortistab*	Cortisone
Berkolol	Propranolol	*Cortisyl*	Cortisone
Berkozide	Bendrofluazide	*Crystapen*	Benzylpencillin
Beta-Cardone	Sotalol	*Crystapen V*	Phenoxymethylpencillin
Betim	Timolol	*Cyclogest*	Progesterone
Betnelan	Betamethasone	*DDAVP*	Desmopressin
Betnesol	Betamethasone	*DF-118*	Dihydrocodeine
Betnovate	Betamethasone	*Dactil*	Piperidolate
Bisolvomycin	Bromhexine	*Daktarin*	Miconazole
Bisolvon	Bromhexine	*Dalacin*	Clindamycin
Blocadren	Timolol	*Dalmane*	Flurazepam

UK NAMES

Trade name	*Approved name*	*Trade name*	*Approved name*
Dantrium	Dantrolene	*Erythrocin*	Erythromycin stearate
Daonil	Glibenclamide	*Erythromid*	Erythromycin
Dartalan	Thiopropazate	*Erythroped*	Erythromycin ethyl-succinate
Decadron	Dexamethasone		
Declinax	Debrisoquine	*Esbatal*	Bethanidine
Decortisyl	Prednisone	*Esidrex*	Hydrochlorothiazide
Defencin	Isoxsuprine	*Ethrane*	Enflurane
Deltastab	Prednisolone	*Etophylate*	Acepifylline
Dendrid	Idoxuridine	*Eudemine*	Diazoxide
Depixol	Flupenthixol	*Euglucon*	Glibenclamide
Depocillin	Procaine Penicillin	*Euhypnos*	Temazepam
Derbac	Malathion	*Eutonyl*	Pargyline
Deseril	Methysergide	*Evacalm*	Diazepam
Dexedrine	Dexamphetamine	*Fazadon*	Fazadinium
Diabinese	Chlorpropamide	*Fenopron*	Fenoprofen
Diamox	Acetazolamide	*Fentazin*	Perphenazine
Diatensec	Spironolactone	*Flagyl*	Metronidazole
Diazemuls	Diazepam	*Flaxedil*	Gallamine
Dibenyline	Phenoxybenzamine	*Flenac*	Fenclofenac
Diconal	Dipipanone	*Florinef*	Fludrocortisone
Dicynene	Ethamsylate	*Floxapen*	Flucloxacillin
Dihydergot	Dihydroergotamine	*Fluanxol*	Flupenthixol
Dindevan	Phenindione	*Fluothane*	Halothane
Dipidolor	Piritramide	*Fortral*	Pentazocine
Diproven	Disoprofol	*Fortunan*	Haloperidol
Dirythmin	Disopyramide	*Framygen*	Framycetain
Disipal	Orphenadrine	*Froben*	Flurbiprofen
Distaclor	Cefaclor	*Frusetic*	Frusemide
Distaquine V-K	Phenoxymethylpenicillin	*Fucidin*	Fusidic acid
Diumide	Frusemide	*Fulcin*	Griseofulvin
Diurexan	Xipamide	*Fungilin*	Amphotericin
Dixarit	Clonidine	*Fungizone*	Amphotericin
Dobutrex	Dobutamine	*Furadantin*	Nitrofurantoin
Dolobid	Diflunisal	*Gantrisin*	Sulphfurazole
Domical	Amitriptyline	*Garamycin*	Gentamicin
Dopamet	Methyldopa	*Genticin*	Gentamycin
Dopram	Doxapram	*Gentigan*	Gentamycin
Doriden	Glutethimide	*Grisovin*	Griseofulvin
Doxatet	Doxycycline	*Gyno-Pevaryl*	Econazole
Dramamine	Dimenhydrinate	*Haldol*	Haloperidol
Droleptan	Droperidol	*Heminevrin*	Chlormethiazole
Dromoran	Levorphanol	*Hiprex*	Hexamine mandelate
Dryptal	Frusemide	*Hydrenox*	Hydroflumethiazide
Duvadilan	Isoxsuprine	*HydroSaluric*	Hydrochlorothiazide
Dytac	Triamterene	*Hygroton*	Chlorthalidone
Ecostatin	Econazole	*Hypnomidate*	Etomidate
Ededrin	Ethacrynic acid	*Hypovase*	Prazosin
Emeside	Ethosuximide	*Hyprenan*	Prenalterol
Emtexate	Methotrexate	*Ibo-Slo*	Ibuprofen
Entonox	Nitrous oxide	*Idoxene*	Idoxuridine
Epanutin	Phenytoin	*Ilosone*	Erythromycin estolate
Epilim	Sodium valproate	*Ilotycin*	Erythromycin
Epontol	Propanidid	*Imbrilon*	Indomethacin
Equanil	Meprobamate	*Inderal*	Propranolol
Eraldin	Practolol	*Inocid*	Indomethacin
Erymsin	Erythromycin	*Intal*	Sodium cromoglycate

UK NAMES

Trade name	*Approved name*	*Trade name*	*Approved name*
Intraval	Thiopentone	*Metopirone*	Metyrapone
Intropin	Dopamine	*Metox*	Metoclopramide
Inversine	Mecamylamine	*Mexitil*	Mexiletine
Ipral	Trimethoprim	*Midamor*	Amiloride
Ismelin	Guanethidine	*Migril*	Ergotamine
Iso-Autohaler	Isoprenaline	*Millophylline*	Etamiphylline
Isodil	Isosorbide	*Milonorm*	Meprobamate
Isoket	Isosorbide	*Miltown*	Meprobamate
Isopto Carbachol	Carbachol	*Minims Amethocaine*	Amethocaine
Isopto Carpine	Pilocarpine	*Minims Chloramphenicol*	Chloramphenicol
Kannasyn	Kanamycin		
Kantrex	Kanamycin	*Minims Cyclopentolate*	Cyclopentolate
Kaomycin	Neomycin		
Keflin	Cephalothin	*Minims Gentamicin*	Gentamicin
Kefzol	Cephazolin	*Minims Homatropine*	Homatropine
Kemicetine	Chloramphenicol	*Minims Hyoscine*	Hyoscine
Kenalog	Triamcinolone	*Minims Neomycin*	Neomycin
Kerecid	Idoxuridine	*Minims benoxinate*	Oxybuprocaine
Ketalar	Ketamine	*Minocin*	Minocycline
Kiditard	Quinidine	*Modecate*	Fluphenazine
Kinidin	Quinidine	*Moditen*	Fluphenazine
Konakion	Phytomenadione	*Mogadon*	Nitrazepam
Lanoxin	Digoxin	*Monaspor*	Cefosludin
Largactil	Chlorpromazine	*Monistat*	Miconazole
Larodopa	Levodopa	*Monotrim*	Trimethoprim
Lasix	Frusemide	*Moxalactam*	Latamoxef
Lauromacrogol	Latamoxef	*Mucodyne*	Carboxymethylcysteine
Ledercort	Triamcinolone	*Mucolex*	Carboxymethylcysteine
Lederkyn	Sulphamethoxypyridazine	*Myambutol*	Ethambutol
		Mycardol	Pentaerythritol tetranitrate
Ledermycin	Demeclocyclin		
Lentizol	Amitriptyline	*Mycifradin*	Neomycin
Librium	Chlordiazepoxide	*Myciguent*	Neomycin
Limbritol	Amitriptyline	*Mydrilate*	Cyclopentolate
Lincocin	Lincomycin	*Myotonine*	Bethanechol
Lingraine	Ergotamine	*Mysoline*	Primidone
Lomusol	Sodium cromoglycate	*Mytelase*	Ambenonium
Lorfan	Levallorphan	*Nafcil*	Nafcillin
Ludiomil	Maprotiline	*Nalcrom*	Sodium cromoglycate
Luminal	Phenobarbitone	*Naprosyn*	Naproxen
Macrodantin	Nitrofurantoin	*Narcan*	Naloxone
Mandelamine	Hexamine mandelate	*Nardil*	Phenelzine
Marcain	Bupivacaine	*Narphen*	Phenazocine
Marevan	Warfarin	*Natrilix*	Indapamide
Marsilid	Iproniazid	*Navidrex*	Cyclopenthiazide
Maxolon	Metoclopramide	*Nebcin*	Tobramycin
Medihaler	Isoprenaline	*Negram*	Nalidixic acid
Mefoxin	Cefoxitin	*Neo-Mecazole*	Carbimazole
Melitase	Chlorpropamide	*Netillin*	Netilmicin
Melleril	Thioridazine	*Neutraphylline*	Diprophylline
Meralen	Flufenamic acid	*Nipride*	Sodium nitroprusside
Merbentyl	Dicyclomine	*Nitrados*	Nitrazepam
Merital	Nomifensine	*Nitrocine*	Glyceryl Trinitrate
Mestinon	Pyridostigmine	*Nitrocontin*	Glyceryl Trinitrate
Metenix	Metolazone	*Nitrolingual*	Glyceryl Trinitrate
Methrazone	Feprazone	*Nivemycin*	Neomycin

UK NAMES

Trade name	*Approved name*	*Trade name*	*Approved name*
Nobrium	Medazepam	*Pramidex*	Tolbutamide
Noctec	Chloral hydrate	*Precortisyl*	Prednisolone
Nolidon	Co-trimoxazole	*Predenema*	Prednisolone
Noludar	Methyprylone	*Prednesol*	Prednisolone
Nordon	Doxycycline	*Predsol*	Prednisolone
Norflex	Orphenadrine	*Prioderm*	Malathion
Normison	Temazepam	*Priscol*	Tolazoline
Norval	Mianserin	*Pro-banthine*	Propantheline
Numotac	Isoetharine	*Progesic*	Fenoprofen
Nupercaine	Cinchocaine	*Prondol*	Iprindole
Nystan	Nystatin	*Pronestyl*	Procainamide
Nystavescent	Nystatin	*Prostigmin*	Neostigmine
Octapressin	Felypressin	*Prothiaden*	Dothiepin
Ocusert Pilo	Pilocarpine	*Primperan*	Metoclopramide
One-Alpha	Alfacalcidol	*Pyopen*	Carbenicillin
Operidine	Phenoperidine	*Rastinon*	Tolbutamide
Ophthaine	Proxymetacaine	*Rheumox*	Azapropazone
Ophthalmadine	Idoxuridine	*Rifadin*	Rifampicin
Opren	Benoxaprofen	*Rimactane*	Rifampicin
Opticrom	Sodium cromoglycate	*Rimifon*	Isoniazid
Opulets benoxinate	Oxybuprocaine	*Ritalin*	Methylphenidate
Oradexon	Dexamethasone	*Rivotril*	Clonazepam
Orap	Pimozide	*Robinul*	Glycopyrronium
Orbenin	Cloxacillin	*Rocaltrol*	Calcitriol
Orudis	Ketoprofen	*Rogitine*	Phentolamine
Oruvail	Ketoprofen	*Ronyl*	Pemoline
Osmitrol	Mannitol	*Rynacrom*	Sodium cromoglycate
Ospolot	Sulthiame	*Rythmodan*	Disopyramide
Paedo-Sed	Dichloralphenazone	*Salazopyrin*	Sulphasalazine
Palaprin	Aloxiprin	*Saluric*	Chlorothiazide
Palfium	Dextromoramide	*Saroten*	Amitriptyline
Parabal	Phenobarbitone	*Saventrine*	Isoprenaline
Parlodel	Bromocryptine	*Scoline*	Suxamethonium
Parnate	Tranylcypromine	*Seconal*	Quinalbarbitone
Pavulon	Pancuronium	*Sectral*	Acebutolol
Pentritin	Ampicillin	*Securopen*	Azlocillin
Penidural	Benzathine penicillin	*Selexid*	Pivmecillinam
Penthrane	Methoxyflurane	*Selexidin*	Mecillinam
Percutol	Glyceryl Trinitrate	*Septrin*	Co-trimoxazole
Periactin	Cyproheptadine	*Serenace*	Haloperidol
Peritrate	Pentaerythritol tetra-	*Serenid*	Oxazepam
	nitrate	*Serpasil*	Reserpine
Persantin	Dipyridamole	*Silbephylline*	Diprophylline
Pertofran	Desipramine	*Sinthrome*	Nicoumalone
Pevaryl	Econazole	*Sintisone*	Prednisolone
Pexid	Perhexiline	*Slow-Pren*	Oxprenolol
Phanodorm	Cyclobarbitone	*Sno Phenicol*	Chloramphenicol
Phenergan	Promethazine	*Sno pilo*	Pilocarpine
Phospholine	Ecothiopate	*Soframycin*	Framycetin
Phyllocontin	Aminophyllin	*Solis*	Diazepam
Physeptone	Methadone	*Somnite*	Nitrazepam
Piriton	Chlorpheniramine	*Soneryl*	Butobarbitone
Pitressin	Lypressin	*Soni-Slo*	Isosorbide
Ponderax	Fenfluramine	*Sorbichew*	Isosorbide
Pondocillin	Pivampicillin	*Sorbid*	Isosorbide
Ponstan	Mefenamic acid	*Sotacor*	Sotalol

UK NAMES

Trade name	*Approved name*	*Trade name*	*Approved name*
Sparine	Promazine	*Tridil*	Glyceryl Trinitrate
Spiroctan	Spironolactone	*Trilene*	Trichloroethylene
Stabillin V-K	Phenoxymethylpenicillin	*Trobicin*	Spectinomycin
Stelazine	Trifluoperazine	*Tryptizol*	Amitriptyline
Stemetil	Prochlorperazine	*Trypure*	Trypsin
Stugeron	Cinnarizine	*Tubarine*	Tubocurarine
Sublimaze	Fentanyl	*Ubretid*	Distigmine
Sulfamylon	Mafenide	*Unisomnia*	Nitrazepam
Sulfomyl	Mafenide	*Uriben*	Nalidixic acid
Sulphamethazine	Sulphadimidine	*Urolucosil*	Sulphamethizole
Surem	Nitrazepam	*Uticillin*	Carfecillin
Sustac	Glyceryl Trinitrate	*V-Cil-K*	Phenoxymethylpencillin
Symmetrel	Amantadine	*Valium*	Diazepam
Synacthen	Tetracosactrin	*Vallergan*	Trimeprazine
Synadrin	Prenylamine	*Valoid*	Cyclizine
Synflex	Naproxen	*Vancocin*	Vancomycin
Syntocinon	Oxytocin	*Varbian*	Prenalterol
Syntometrine	Ergometrine	*Varidase*	Streptokinase
Syntopressin	Lypressin	*Vascardin*	Isosorbide
Syraprim	Trimethoprim	*Vasoxine*	Methoxamine
Tachostyptan	Thromboplastin	*Vatensol*	Guanoclor
Tagamet	Cimetidine	*Velosef*	Cephradine
Talpen	Talampicillin	*Ventolin*	Salbutamol
Tandacote	Oxyphenbutazone	*Vertigon*	Prochlorperazine
Tanderil	Oxyphenbutazone	*Vibramycin*	Doxycycline
Tegretol	Carbamazepine	*Vidopen*	Ampicillin
Temgesic	Buprenorphine	*Vira-A*	Vidarabine
Tenormin	Atenolol	*Visken*	Pindolol
Tensilon	Edrophonium	*Vivalan*	Viloxazine
Tertroxin	Liothyronine	*Welldorm*	Dichloralphenazone
Thalazole	Phthalylsulphathiazole	*Xylocaine*	Lignocaine
Thytropar	Thyrotrophin	*Xylocard*	Lignocaine
Ticar	Ticarcillin	*Yutopar*	Ritodrine
Timoptol	Timolol	*Zadstat*	Metronidazole
Tobralex	Tobramycin	*Zantac*	Ranitidine
Tofranil	Imipramine	*Zarontin*	Ethosuximide
Tolectin	Tolmetin	*Zinacef*	Cefuroxime
Trandate	Labetolol	*Zinamide*	Pyrazinamide
Tranxene	Chlorazepate	*Zomax*	Zomepirac
Trasicor	Oxprenolol	*Zovirax*	Acyclovir
Trasylol	Aprotinin		

US NAMES

Approved name	*Trade name*
Acepifylline	*Etophylate*
Acetazolamide	*Diamox*
	Hydrazol
Acetylcysteine	*Mucomyst*
Acyclovir	*Zovirax*
Albuterol	*Ventolin*
Aloxiprin	*Palaprin*
Alphaprodine	*Nisentil*
Amantadine	*Symmetrel*
Ambenonium	*Mytelase*
Amikacin	*Amikin*
Amiloride	*Midamor*
Aminophylline	*Aminodur*
	Lixaminol
	Panamin
	Phyllocontin
	Somaphyllin
Amitriptyline	*Elavil*
	Elegen
	Endep
Amobarbital	*Amytal*
	Pulvule
Amoxicillin	*Amoxil*
	Polymox
	Robamox
	Sumox
	Trimox
	Utimox
	Wymox
Amphotericin	*Fungizone*
Ampicillin	*Amcill*
	Ameril
	Omnipen
	Penbritin
	Pensyn
	Pfizerpen
	Polycillin
	Principen
	Roampicillin
	Totacillin
Amyl nitrite	*Aspirols*
	Vaporole
Aprotinin	*Trasylol*
Atenolol	*Tenormin*
Bacampicillin	*Spectrobid*
Barbital	*Embinal*
	Medinal
	Veronal
Bendroflumethiazide	*Naturetin*
Benoxaprofen	*Oraflex*
Benoxinate	*Dorsacaine*
Benzathine penicillin	*Permapen*
Benzhexol	*Artane*
	Trinol
Benztropine	*Cogentin*

Approved name	*Trade name*
Betamethasone	*Celestone*
	Diprosone
	Valisone
Bethanechol	*Duvoid*
	Myotonachol
Bethanechol	*Urecholine*
	Vesicholine
Bethanidine	*Esbatal*
Bretylium	*Bretylate*
	Bretylol
	Darenthin
Bromhexine	*Bisolvon*
Bromocryptine	*Parlodel*
Bumetanide	*Burinex*
Bupivacaine	*Marcaine*
	Sensorcaine
Butabarbital	*Butalen*
	Butazem
	Butisol
	Expansatol
	Medarsed
	Soduben
Butamben	*Butesin*
Butorphanol	*Stadol*
Caffeine	*No Doz*
Calcitriol	*Rocaltrol*
Captopril	*Capoten*
Carbachol	*Carbacel*
	Miostat Intraocular
	Murocarb
Carbamazepine	*Tegretol*
Carbenicillin	*Geocillin*
	Geopen
	Pyopen
Carbidopa	in *Sinemet*
Carbimazole	*Bimazole*
	Neo-Mercazole
Carboxymethyl-cysteine	*Mucodyne*
	Thiodril
Cefaclor	*Ceclor*
Cephalexin	*Ceporex*
	Keflex
Cephaloridine	*Loridine*
Cephalothin	*Keflin*
Cephazolin	*Kefzol*
Cephradine	*Anspor*
	Eskasef
	Velosef
Chloral hydrate	*Aguachloral*
	Felsules
	Noctec
	Oradate
	Rectules
	Somnos

US NAMES

Approved name	*Trade name*
Chloramphenicol	*Amphicol*
	Antibiopto
	Chlorcetin
	Chloromycetin
	Econochlor
	Kemicetine
	Mychel
	Ophthoclor
	Paraxin
Chlorazepate	*Azene*
Chlorazepate	*Tranxene*
Chlordiazepoxide	*A-Poxide*
	Chlordiazachel
	Libritabs
	Librium
	SK-Lygen
	Screen
	Zetran
Chlormethiazole	*Heminevrin*
Chloroprocaine	*Nesacaine*
Chlorothiazide	*Diuril*
Chlorpheniramine	*Chlor-4*
	Chlor-Trimeton
	Chlormene
	Chlorspan
	Chlortab
	Histacon
	Histaspan
	Panahist
	Phenetron
	Teldrin
Chlorpromazine	*Chlorzine*
	Promachlor
	Promaz
	Sonazine
	Terpium
	Thorazine
Chlorpropamide	*Diabinese*
Chlortetracycline	*Aureomycin*
Chlorthalidone	*Combipres*
	Hygroton
Chymotrypsin	*Avazyme*
	Catarase
Cimetidine	*Tagamet*
Cinnarizine	*Mitronal*
	Stugeron
Cinoxacin	*Cinobac*
Clindamycin	*Cleocin*
	Dalacin
Clomipramine	*Anafranil*
Clonazepam	*Clonopin*
Clonidine	*Catapres*
	Dixarit
Clopenthixol	*Sordinol*
Clotrimazole	*Gyne-Lotrimin*
	Lotrimin
	Myclex

Approved name	*Trade name*
Co-trimoxazole	*Bactrim*
	Septra
	Septrin
Cyclizine	*Marzine*
	Valoid
Cyclopenthiazide	*Navidrex*
Cyclopentolate	*Cyclogyl*
Cycloserine	*Seromycin*
Cyproheptadine	*Periactin*
Dantrolene	*Dantrium*
Demeclocyclin	*Declomycin*
Deoxycorticosterone	*Doca*
	Percorten
Deptropine	*Brontina*
Desipramine	*Norpramin*
	Pertofrane
Desmopressin	*DDAVP*
Dexamethasone	*Dexadron*
	Dexone
	Hexadrol
	Maxidex
	Savacort-D
Dexamphetamine	*Dexamped*
	Dexedrine
	Diphylets
	Oxydess
Dextromoramide	*Jetrium*
	Palfium
Diazepam	*Valium*
Diazoxide	*Hyperstat*
	Proglycem
Dibucaine	*Dulzit*
	Nupercaine
Dichloralphenazone	*Fenzol*
	Welldorm
Dicloxacillin	*Dycill*
	Dynapen
	Pathocil
	Veracillin
Dicyclomine	*Benacol*
	Bentyl
	Merbentyl
	Pasmin
	Stannitol
	Wyovin
Diflunisal	*Dolobid*
Digoxin	*Lanoxin*
	Masoxin
Dihydroergotamine	*DHE 45*
Dimenhydrinate	*Dimenate*
	Dramamine
	Dramocen
	Marmine
	Signate
	Traveltabs

US NAMES

Approved name	*Trade name*
Diphenhydramine	*Benylin*
	Histine
	Lensen
	T-Dryl
	Valdrene
	Wehydryl
Dipipanone	*Pipadone*
Diprophylline	*Isophylline*
Dipyridamole	*Persantine*
Disopyramide	*Rhymodan*
Distigmine	*Ubretid*
Disulfiram	*Antabuse*
Dobutamine	*Dobutrex*
	Inotrex
Dopamine	*Dopostat*
	Intropin
Dothiepin	*Prothiaden*
Doxapram	*Dopram*
Doxycycline	*Vibra-Tabs*
	Vibramycin
Droperidol	*Inapsine*
Ecothiopate	*Phospholine*
Edrophonium	*Ethrane*
	Tensilon
Enflurane	*Ethrane*
Epicillin	*Dexacillin*
Ergonovine	*Ergotrate*
Ergotamine	*Ergomar*
	Ergostat
	Gynergen
Erythromycin	*E-Mycin*
	Ilotycin
	Robimycin
Erythromycin estalate	*Ilosone*
Erythromycin ethylsuccinate	*E-Mycin-E*
	EES
	Erythrocin
	Pediamycin
	Wyamycin E
Erythromycin stearate	*Dowmycin*
	Erypar
	Erythrocin
	Ethril
	SK-Erythromycin
Etamiphylline	*Millophylline*
Ethacrynic acid	*Edecrin*
Ethambutol	*Myambutol*
Ethamivan	*Vandid*
Ethionamide	*Trecator*
Ethosuximide	*Zarontin*
Etidocaine	*Duranest*
Felypressin	*Octapressin*
Fenfluramine	*Ponderax*
	Pondimin
Fentanyl	*Innovar*
	Sublimaze
Flucytosine	*Ancobon*
Fludrocortisone	*Florinef*
Flupenthixol	*Depixol*
Fluphenazine	*Permitil*
	Prolixin
Flurazepam	*Dalmane*
Framycetin	*Framygen*
	Soframycin
Furosemide	*Lasix*
Gallamine	*Flaxedil*
Gentamicin	*Apogen*
	Bristagen
	Garamycin
	Genoptic
Glibenclamide	*Daonil*
	Euglucon
Glutethimide	*Doriden*
	Dorimide
	Rolathimide
Glycopyrronium	*Robinul*
Griseofulvin	*Fulvicin*
	Grifulvin
Griseofulvin	*Grisac*
	Grisactin
Guanethidine	*Ismelin*
Haloperidol	*Haldol*
Halothane	*Fluothane*
Hexafluorenium	*Mylaxen*
Hexobarbital	*Sombulex*
Homatropine	*Homatrocel*
	Murocoll
Hydralazine	*Apresoline*
	Dralzine
	Hydralyn
Hydrochlorothiazide	*Chlorzide*
	Delco-Retic
	Diu-Scrip
	Esidex
	Hydro Diuril
	Hydromal
	Hydrozide
	Hyperetic
	Oretic
	Ro-Hydrazide
	SK-Hydrochlorthiazide
	Thiuretic
Hydroflumethiazide	*Salutensin*
Ibuprofen	*Motrin*
Idoxuridine	*Dendrid*
	Herplex
	Stoxil

US NAMES

Approved name	*Trade name*
Imipramine	*Imavate*
	Tofranil
Ipratropium	*Atrovent*
Iproniazid	*Marsilid*
Isoetharine	*Bronkometer*
	Bronkosol
Isoflurane	*Forane*
Isoniazid	*Laniazid*
	Niconyl
	Nydrazid
	Panazid
	Rolazid
	Triniad
Isoproterenol	*Aerolone*
	Isuprel
	Medihaler
	Norisodrine
	Proternol
Isosorbide	*Dilatrate*
	Iso-Bid
	Iso-D
	Isodril
	Sorbitrate
	Sorquad
Isoxsuprine	*Rolisox*
	Vasodilan
Kanamycin	*Kannasyn*
	Kantrex
Ketamine	*Ketaject*
	Ketalar
Levallorphan	*Lorfan*
Levodopa	*Bendopa*
	Larodopa
	Levopa
	Parda
Levorphanol	*Levo-Dromoran*
Lidocaine	*Anestacon*
	Ardecaine
	Dolicaine
	Rocaine
	Stanacaine
	Xylocaine
Lincomycin	*Lincocin*
Liothyronine	*Cytomel*
Lorazepam	*Ativan*
Lypressin	*Diapid*
Mafenide	*Sulfamylon*
Mannitol	*Osmitrol*
Mecamylamine	*Inversine*
Meclizine	*Antivert*
	Bonine
	Lamine
	Vertrol
Mefenamic acid	*Ponstel*
Meperidine	*Demerol*
Mephentermine	*Wyamine*
Mepivacaine	*Carbocaine*
Meprobamate	*Bamate*
	Mecrocon
	Meprospan
	Miltown
	SK-Bamate
	Tranmep
Metaraminol	*Aramine*
Methacholine	*Mecholyl*
Methadone	*Dolophine*
Methamphetamine	*Desoxyn*
	Methampex
Methaqualone	*Meguin*
	Parest
	Quaalude
Methenamine mandelate	*Mandalay*
	Mandelamine
	Renelate
	Thendelate
Methicillin	*Azapen*
	Celbenin
	Staphcillin
Methimazole	*Tapazole*
	Thiamazole
Methohexital	*Brevital*
Methotrexate	*Mexate*
Methotrimeprazine	*Levoprome*
Methoxyflurane	*Penthrane*
Methscopolamine bromide	*Pamine*
Methyldopa	*Aldomet*
	Aldoril
Methylene Blue	*Urolene Blue*
Methylphenidate	*Ritalin*
Methyprylon	*Noludar*
Methysergide	*Sansert*
Metoclopramide	*Reglan*
Metolazone	*Zaroxolyn*
Metronidazole	*Flagyl*
	Metryl
Metyrapone	*Metopirone*
Miconazole	*Monistat*
Minocycline	*Minocin*
Nadolol	*Corgard*
Nafcillin	*Nafcil*
	Unipen
Nalidixic acid	*NegGram*
Naloxone	*Narcan*
Naphazoline	*Clear Eyes*
	Naphcon
	Privine
	Vasocon

US NAMES

Approved name	*Trade name*
Naproxen	*Anaprox*
	Naprosyn
Neomycin	*Mycifradin*
	Myciguent
	Neobiotic
Neostigmine	*Prostigmin*
Netilmicin	*Netromycin*
Nifedipine	*Procardia*
Nikethamide	*Coramine*
Nitrofurantoin	*Furadantin*
	Macrodantin
	Nitrex
	Nitrofor
	Trantoin
	Urotoin
Nitroglycerin	*Cardabid*
	Nitro-Lyn
	Nitrobid
	Nitrocap
	Nitroglyn
	Nitrol
	Nitrong
	Nitrospan
	Nitrostat
	Trates
Nomifensine	*Merital*
Nystatin	*Mycostatin*
	Nilstat
Orciprenaline	*Alupent*
Orphenadrine	*Flexon*
	Flexor
	Norflex
	Oxacillin
Oxacillin	*Bactocill*
	Prostaphlin
Oxymorphone	*Numorphan*
Oxyphenbutazone	*Oxalid*
	Tandearil
Oxytocin	*Pitocin*
	Syntocinon
Pancuronium	*Pavulon*
Papaverine	*Cerebid*
	Cerespan
	Dylate
	Kavrin
	Myobid
	Pava Caps
	Pava-Wol
	Pavabid
	Pavacen
	Pavadyl
	Pavakey
	Pavatran
	Therapay
Papaverine	*Vasal*
	Vasocap
	Vasopan
Paraldehyde	*Paral*
Pargyline	*Eutonyl*
Pemoline	*Cylert*
Penicillin G	*Cryspen*
	Duracillin
	Hyasorb
	Lanacillin
	Paclan
	Pentids
Penicillin G Procaine	*Crysticillin*
	Duracillin
	Pfizerpen AS
	Wycillin
Penicillin V	*Betapen-VK*
	Bopen
	Dowpen VK
	Ledercillin VK
	Pen-Vee-K
	Penapar VK
	Pfizerpen VK
	Robicillin VK
	Uticillin VK
	V-Cillin
	V-Cillin K
	Veetids
Pentaerythritol tetranitrate	*Duotrate*
	El-petn
	Metranil
	Pentafin
	Pentritol
	Pentryate
	Peritrate
	Tentrate
	Tranite
	Vasolate
Pentazocine	*Talwin*
Pentobarbital	*Nembutal*
Perphenazine	*Trilafon*
Phenelzine	*Nardil*
Phenethicillin	*Chemipen*
Phenindione	*Eridione*
	Hedulin
Phenobarbital	*Luminal*
	Orprine
	Seladrops
Phenoxybenzamine	*Dibenzyline*
Phentolamine	*Regitine*
	Rogitine
Phenylbutazone	*Azolid*
	Butazolidin
Phenytoin	*Dihycon*
	Dilantin
	Diphenylan
	Ekko

US NAMES

Approved name	*Trade name*	*Approved name*	*Trade name*
Phthalylsulfathiazole	*Sulfathalidine*	Promethazine	*Prorex*
Physostigmine	*Isopto-Eserine*		*Remsed*
	Miocel	Propanidid	*Epontol*
Phytonadiol	*Aquamephyton*	Propantheline	*Norpanth*
	Konakion		*Pro-Banthine*
	Mephyton		*Robantaline*
Pilocarpine	*Almocarpine*		*Ropanth*
	Mi-Pilo		*Spastil*
	Pilocar	Propiomazine	*Largon*
	Pilocel	Propoxyphene	*Darvon*
	Piloptic		*Dolene*
Pindolol	*Visken*		*Myospaz*
Polymixin	*Aerosporin*		*Proxagesic*
Pralidoxime	*Protopam*		*Stogesic*
Prazosin	*Minizide*		*Wygesic*
	Minpress	Propranolol	*Inderal*
Prednisolone	*Delta-Cortef*	Propylthiouracil	*Propacil*
	Econpred	Proxymetacaine	*Ophthaine*
	Hydeltrasol		*Proparacaine*
	Inflamase	Pyrazinamide	*Zinamide*
	Meti-Drem	Pyridostigmine	*Mestinon*
	Meticortelone		*Regona*
	Metreton	Pyrilamine	*Pyma*
	Prednis		*Pyristan*
	Ropred		
	Savacort	Quinethazone	*Hydromox*
	Sterane	Quinidine	*Cin-Quin*
	Ulacort		*Duraquin*
Prednisone	*Delta-Dome*		*Quinaglute*
	Deltasone		*Quinidex*
	Lisacort		*Quinora*
	Meticorten		
	Orasone	Reserpine	*Rau-Sed*
	Sterapred		*Reserjen*
Prilocaine	*Citanest*		*Reserpoid*
Primidone	*Mysoline*		*Sandril*
Probenecid	*Benacen*		*Serpasil*
	Benemid		*Serpate*
	Probalan		*Tensin*
	Robenecid		*Vio-Serpine*
Procainamide	*Procan*	Rifampin	*Rifadin*
	Procapan		*Rimactane*
	Pronestyl	Ritodrine	*Yutopar*
Prochlorperazine	*Compazine*		
Progesterone	*Femotrone*	Secobarbital	*Seconal*
	Gesterol	Sodium nitroprusside	*Keto-Diastix*
	Lipo-Lutin		*Nipride*
	Progestin		*Nitropress*
	Prorone	Sodium salicylate	*Alysine*
Promazine	*Sparine*		*Uracel*
Promethazine	*Fellozine*	Sotalol	*Beta-Cardone*
	Ganphen		*Sotacor*
Promethazine	*Phencen*	Spectinomycin	*Trobicin*
	Phenerex	Spironolactone	*Aldactone*
	Phenergan	Streptokinase	*Kabikinase*
	Phenerhist		*Streptase*

US NAMES

Approved name	*Trade name*
Succinylcholine	*Anectine*
	Pintop
	Quelicin
	Sucostrin
Sulfadiazine	*Microsulfon*
	Neo-Quinette
Sulfamethazine	*Neotrizine*
Sulfamethizole	*Microsul*
	Proklar-M
	Thiosulfil
Sulfamethoxazole	*Gantanol*
Sulfamethoxydiazine	*Sulla*
Sulfasalazine	*Azulfidine*
	SAS-500
	Salazopyrin
	Sulcolon
Sulfinpyrazone	*Anturane*
Sulfisoxazole	*G-Sox*
	Gantrisin
	SK-Spoxazole
	Sosal
	Soxa
	Sulfagan
	Sulfizin
	Velmatrol
Sulindac	*Clinoril*
Temazepam	*Restoril*
Terbutaline	*Brethine*
Tetracaine	*Pontocaine*
Tetracosactrin	*Cosyntropin*
	Synacthen
Thiopental	*Pentothal*
Thioridazine	*Mellaril*
Thyrotrophin	*Thytropar*
Ticarcillin	*Ticar*
Timolol	*Blocadren*
Tobramycin	*Hyporet*
	Nebcin
	Tobrex
Tolazoline	*Priscoline*
	Tazol
	Toloxan
	Tolzol
Tolbutamide	*Orinase*
Tolmetin	*Tolectin*
Tranylcypromine	*Parnate*
Triamcinolone	*Aristocort*
	Kenalog
	Tramacin
	Tri-Kort
	Triam-A
Triamterene	*Dyrenium*
Triclofos	*Triclos*
Trifluoperazine	*Stelazine*
Trimeprazine	*Temaril*
Trimethaphan	*Arfonad*
Trimethoprim	*Proloprim*
	Trimpex
Triprolidine	*Actidil*
Tubocurarine	*Metubine*
Valproic acid	*Depakene*
Vancomycin	*Vancocin*
Vidarabine	*Vira-A*
Viloxazine	*Vivalan*
Warfarin	*Coumadin*
	Marevan
	Panwarfin
Zomepirac	*Zomax*
p-Aminobenzoic acid	*Pabafilm*
	Pabanol
	Presun

US NAMES

Trade name	*Approved name*	*Trade name*	*Approved name*
Actidil	Triprolidine	*Bisolvon*	Bromhexine
Aerolone	Isoproterenol	*Blocadren*	Timolol
Aerosporin	Polymixin	*Bonine*	Meclizine
Aldactone	Spironolactone	*Bopen*	Penicillin V
Aldomet	Methyldopa	*Brethine*	Terbutaline
Aldoril	Methyldopa	*Bretylate*	Bretylium
Almocarpine	Pilocarpine	*Bretylol*	Bretylium
Alupent	Orciprenaline	*Brevital*	Methohexital
Alysine	Sodium salicylate	*Bristagen*	Gentamicin
Amcill	Ampicillin	*Bronkometer*	Isoetharine
Ameril	Ampicillin	*Bronkosol*	Isoetharine
Amikin	Amikacin	*Brontina*	Deptropine
Aminodur	Aminophylline	*Burinex*	Bumetanide
Amoxil	Amoxicillin	*Butalen*	Butabarbital
Amphicol	Chloramphenicol	*Butazem*	Butabarbital
Amytal	Amobarbital	*Butazolidin*	Phenylbutazone
Anafranil	Clomipramine	*Butesin*	Butamben
Anaprox	Naproxen	*Butisol*	Butabarbital
Ancobon	Flucytosine	*Capoten*	Captopril
Anectine	Succinylcholine	*Carbacel*	Carbachol
Anestacon	Lidocaine	*Carbocaine*	Mepivacaine
Anspor	Cephradine	*Cardabid*	Nitroglycerin
Antabuse	Disulfiram	*Catapres*	Clonidine
Antibiopto	Chloramphenicol	*Catarase*	Chymotrypsin
Antivert	Meclizine	*Ceclor*	Cefaclor
Anturane	Sulfinpyrazone	*Celbenin*	Methicillin
Apogen	Gentamicin	*Celestone*	Betamethasone
Apresoline	Hydralazine	*Ceporex*	Cephalexin
Aquachloral	Chloral hydrate	*Cerebid*	Papaverine
Aquamephyton	Phytonadiol	*Cerespan*	Papaverine
Aramine	Metaraminol	*Chemipen*	Phenethicillin
Ardecaine	Lidocaine	*Chlor Niramine*	Chlorpheniramine
Arfonad	Trimethaphan	*Chlor-4*	Chlorpheniramine
Aristocort	Triamcinolone	*Chlor-Trimeton*	Chlorpheniramine
Artane	Benzhexol	*Chlorcetin*	Chloramphenicol
Aspirols	Amyl nitrite	*Chlordiazachel*	Chlordiazepoxide
Ativan	Lorazepam	*Chlormene*	Chlorpheniramine
Atrovent	Ipratropium	*Chloromycetin*	Chloramphenicol
Aureomycin	Chlortetracycline	*Chlorspan*	Chlorpheniramine
Avazyme	Chymotrypsin	*Chlortab*	Chlorpheniramine
Azapen	Methicillin	*Chlorzide*	Hydrochlorothiazide
Azene	Chlorazepate	*Chlorzine*	Chlorpromazine
Azolid	Phenylbutazone	*Cin-Quin*	Quinidine
Azulfidine	Sulfasalazine	*Cinobac*	Cinoxacin
Bactocill	Oxacillin	*Citanest*	Prilocaine
Bactrim	Co-trimoxazole	*Clear eyes*	Naphazoline
Bamate	Meprobamate	*Cleocin*	Clindamycin
Benacen	Probenecid	*Clinoril*	Suldinac
Benacol	Dicyclomine	*Clonopin*	Clonazepam
Bendopa	Levodopa	*Cogentin*	Benztropine
Benemid	Probenecid	*Combipres*	Chlorthalidone
Bentyl	Dicyclomine	*Compazine*	Prochlorperazine
Benylin	Diphenhydramine	*Coramine*	Nikethamide
Beta-Cardone	Sotalol	*Corgard*	Nadolol
Betapen-VK	Penicillin V	*Cosyntropin*	Tetracosactrin
Bimazole	Carbimazole	*Coumadin*	Warfarin

US NAMES

Trade name	Approved name
Cryspen	Penicillin G
Crysticillin	Penicillin G Procaine
Cyclogyl	Cyclopentolate
Cylert	Pemoline
Cytomel	Liothyronine
DDAVP	Desmopressin
DHE 45	Dihydroergotamine
Dalacin	Clindamycin
Dalmane	Flurazepam
Dantrium	Dantrolene
Daonil	Glibenclamide
Darenthin	Bretylium
Darvon	Propoxyphene
Declomycin	Demeclocyclin
Delco-Retic	Hydrochlorothiazide
Delta-Cortef	Prednisolone
Delta-Dome	Prednisone
Deltasone	Prednisone
Demerol	Meperidine
Dendrid	Idoxuridine
Depakene	Valproic acid
Depixol	Flupenthixol
Desoxyn	Methamphetamine
Dexacillin	Epicillin
Dexadron	Dexamethasone
Dexamped	Dexamphetamine
Dexedrine	Dexamphetamine
Dexone	Dexamethasone
Diabinese	Chlorpropamide
Diamox	Acetazolamide
Diapid	Lypressin
Dibenzyline	Phenoxybenzamine
Dihycon	Phenytoin
Dilantin	Phenytoin
Dilatrate	Isosorbide
Dimenate	Dimenhydrinate
Diphenylan	Phenytoin
Diphylets	Dexamphetamine
Diprosone	Betamethasone
Diu-Scrip	Hydrochlorothiazide
Diuril	Chlorothiazide
Dixarit	Clonidine
Dobutrex	Dobutamine
Doca	Deoxycorticosterone
Dolene	Propoxyphene
Dolicaine	Lidocaine
Dolobid	Diflunisal
Dolophine	Methadone
Dopostat	Dopamine
Dopram	Doxapram
Doriden	Glutethimide
Dorimide	Glutethimide
Dorsacaine	Benoxinate
Dowmycin	Erythromycin stearate
Dowpen VK	Penicillin V
Dralzine	Hydralazine
Dramamine	Dimenhydrinate
Dramocen	Dimenhydrinate
Dulzit	Dibucaine
Duotrate	Pentaerythritol tetranitrate
Duracillin	Penicillin G
Duranest	Etidocaine
Duraquin	Quinidine
Duvoid	Bethanechol
Dycill	Dicloxacillin
Dylate	Papaverine
Dynapen	Dicloxacillin
Dyrenum	Triamterene
E-Mycin	Erythromycin
E-Mycin-E	Erythromycin ethylsuccinate
EES	Erythromycin ethylsuccinate
Econochlor	Chloramphenicol
Econpred	Prednisolone
Edecrin	Ethacrynic acid
Ekko	Phenytoin
El-petn	Pentaerythritol tetranitrate
Elavil	Amitriptyline
Elegen	Amitriptyline
Embinal	Barbital
Endep	Amitriptyline
Epontol	Propanidid
Ergomar	Ergotamine
Ergostat	Ergotamine
Ergotrate	Ergonovine
Eridione	Phenindione
Erypar	Erythromycin stearate
Erythrocin	Erythromycin ethylsuccinate
Erythrocin	Erythromycin stearate
Esbatal	Bethanidine
Esidex	Hydrochlorothiazide
Eskasef	Cephradine
Ethrane	Edrophonium
Ethril	Erythromycin stearate
Etophylate	Acepifylline
Euglucon	Glibenclamide
Eutonyly	Pargyline
Expansatol	Butabarbital
Fellozine	Promethazine
Felsules	Chloral hydrate
Femotrone	Progesterone
Fenzol	Dichloralphenazone
Flagyl	Metronidazole
Flaxedill	Gallamine
Flexon	Orphenadrine
Flexor	Orphenadrine
Florinef	Fludrocortisone
Fluothane	Halothane

US NAMES

Trade name	*Approved name*	*Trade name*	*Approved name*
Forane	Isoflurane	*Isuprel*	Isoproterenol
Framygen	Framycetin	*Jetrium*	Dextromoramide
Iulvicin	Griseofulvin	*Kabikinase*	Streptokinase
Fungizone	Amphotericin	*Kannasyn*	Kanamycin
Furadantin	Nitrofurantoin	*Kantrex*	Kanamycin
G-Sox	Sulfisoxazole	*Kavrin*	Papaverine
Ganphen	Promethazine	*Keflex*	Cephalexin
Gantanol	Sulfamethoxazole	*Keflin*	Cephalothin
Gantrisin	Sulfisoxazole	*Kefzol*	Cephazolin
Garamycin	Gentamicin	*Kemicetine*	Chloramphenicol
Genoptic	Gentamicin	*Kenalog*	Triamcinolone
Geocillin	Carbenicillin	*Ketaject*	Ketamine
Geopen	Carbenicillin	*Ketalar*	Ketamine
Gesterol	Progesterone	*Keto-Diastix*	Sodium nitroprusside
Grifulvin	Griseofulvin	*Konakion*	Phytonadiol
Grisac	Griseofulvin	*Lamine*	Meclizine
Grisactin	Griseofulvin	*Lanacillin*	Penicillin G
Gyne-Lotrimin	Clotrimazole	*Laniazid*	Isoniazid
Gynergen	Ergotamine	*Lanoxin*	Digoxin
Haldol	Haloperidol	*Largon*	Propiomazine
Hedulin	Phenindione	*Larodopa*	Levodopa
Heminevrin	Chlormethiazole	*Lasix*	Furosemide
Herplex	Idoxuridine	*Ledercillin VK*	Penicillin V
Hexadrol	Dexamethasone	*Lensen*	Diphenhydramine
Histacon	Chlorpheniramine	*Levo-Dromoran*	Levorphanol
Histapan	Chlorpheniramine	*Levopa*	Levodopa
Histine	Diphenyhydramine	*Levoprome*	Methotrimeprazine
Homatrocel	Homatropine	*Libritabs*	Chlordiazepoxide
Hyasorb	Penicillin G	*Librium*	Chlordiazepoxide
Hydeltrasol	Prednisolone	*Lincocin*	Lincomycin
Hydralyn	Hydralazine	*Lipo-Lutin*	Progesterone
Hydrazol	Acetazolamide	*Lisacort*	Prednisone
Hydro Diuril	Hydrochlorothiazide	*Lixaminol*	Aminophylline
Hydromal	Hydrochlorothiazide	*Lorfan*	Levallorphan
Hydromox	Quinethazone	*Loridine*	Cephaloridine
Hydrozide	Hydrochlorothiazide	*Lotrimin*	Clotrimazole
Hygroton	Chlorthalidone	*Luminal*	Phenobarbital
Hyperetic	Hydrochlorothiazide	*Macrodantin*	Nitrofurantoin
Hyperstat	Diazoxide	*Mandalay*	Methenamine mandelate
Hyporet	Tobramycin	*Mendelamine*	Methenamine mandelate
Ilosone	Erythromycin estolate	*Marcaine*	Bupivacaine
Ilotycin	Erythromycin	*Marevan*	Warfarin
Imavate	Imipramine	*Marmine*	Dimenhydrinate
Inapsine	Droperidol	*Marsilid*	Iproniazid
Inderal	Propranolol	*Marzine*	Cyclizine
Inflamase	Prednisolone	*Masoxin*	Digoxin
Innovar	Fentanyl	*Maxidex*	Dexamethasone
Inotrex	Dobutamine	*Mecholyl*	Methacholine
Intropin	Dopamine	*Mecrocon*	Meprobamate
Inversine	Mecamylamine	*Medarsed*	Butabarbital
Ismelin	Guanethidine	*Medihaler*	Isoproterenol
Iso-Bid	Isosorbide	*Medinal*	Barbital
Iso-D	Isosorbide	*Mellaril*	Thioridazine
Isodril	Isosorbide	*Mephyton*	Phytonadiol
Isophylline	Diprophylline	*Meprospan*	Meprobamate
Isopto-Eserine	Physostigmine	*Mequin*	Methaqualone

US NAMES

Trade name	*Approved name*
Merbentyl	Dicyclomine
Merital	Nomifensine
Mestinon	Pyridostigmine
Methampex	Methamphetamine
Meti-Drem	Prednisolone
Meticortelone	Prednisolone
Meticorten	Prednisone
Metopirone	Metyrapone
Metranil	Pentaerythritol tetranitrate
Metreton	Prednisolone
Metryl	Metronidazole
Metubine	Tubocurarine
Mexate	Methotrexate
Mi-Pilo	Pilocarpine
Microsul	Sulfamethizole
Microsulfon	Sulfadiazine
Midamor	Amiloride
Millophylline	Etamiphylline
Miltown	Meprobamate
Minizide	Prazosin
Minocin	Minocycline
Minpress	Prazosin
Miocel	Physostigmine
Miostat Intraocular	Carbachol
Mitronal	Cinnarizine
Monistat	Miconazole
Motrin	Ibuprofen
Mucodyne	Carboxymethylcysteine
Mucomyst	Acetylcysteine
Murocarb	Carbachol
Murocoll	Homatropine
Myambutol	Ethambutol
Mychel	Chloramphenicol
Mycifradin	Neomycin
Myciguent	Neomycin
Myclex	Clotrimazole
Mycostatin	Nystatin
Mylaxen	Hexafluorenium
Myobid	Papaverine
Myospaz	Propoxyphene
Myotonachol	Bethanechol
Mysoline	Primidone
Mytelase	Ambenonium
Nafcil	Nafcillin
Naphcon	Naphazoline
Naprosyn	Naproxen
Narcan	Naloxone
Nardil	Phenelzine
Naturetin	Bendroflumethiazide
Navidrex	Cyclopenthiazide
Nebcin	Tobramycin
NegGram	Nalidixic acid
Nembutal	Pentobarbital
Neo-Mercazole	Carbimazole
Neo-Quinette	Sulfadiazine

Trade name	*Approved name*
Neobiotic	Neomycin
Neotrizine	Sulfamethazine
Nesacaine	Chloroprocaine
Netromycin	Netilmicin
Niconyl	Isoniazid
Nilstat	Nystatin
Nipride	Sodium nitroprusside
Nisentil	Alphaprodine
Nitrex	Nitrofurantoin
Nitro-Lyn	Nitroglycerin
Nitrobid	Nitroglycerin
Nitrocap	Nitroglycerin
Nitrofor	Nitrofurantoin
Nitroglyn	Nitroglycerin
Nitrol	Nitroglycerin
Nitrong	Nitroglycering
Nitropress	Sodium nitroprusside
Nitrospan	Nitroglycerin
Nitrostat	Nitroglycerin
No Doz	Caffeine
Noctec	Chloral hydrate
Noludar	Methyprylon
Norflex	Orphenadrine
Norisodrine	Isoproterenol
Norpanth	Propantheline
Norpramin	Desipramine
Numorphan	Oxymorphone
Nupercaine	Dibucaine
Nydrazid	Isoniazid
Octapressin	Felypressin
Omnipen	Ampicillin
Ophthaine	Proxymetacaine
Ophthoclor	Chloramphenicol
Oradrate	Chloral hydrate
Oraflex	Benoxaprofen
Orasone	Prednisone
Oretic	Hydrochlorothiazide
Orinase	Tolbutamide
Orprine	Phenobarbital
Osmitrol	Mannitol
Oxacillin	Orphenadrine
Oxalid	Oxyphenbutazone
Oxydess	Dexamphetamine
Pabafilm	p-Aminobenzoic acid
Pabanol	p-Aminobenzoic acid
Paclan	Penicillin G
Palaprin	Aloxiprin
Palfium	Dextromoramide
Pamine	Methscopolamine bromide
Panahist	Chlorpheniramine
Panamin	Aminophylline
Panazid	Isoniazid
Panwarfin	Warfarin
Paral	Paraldehyde
Paraxin	Chloramphenicol

US NAMES

Trade name	*Approved name*	*Trade name*	*Approved name*
Parda	Levodopa	*Pondimin*	Fenfluramine
Parest	Methaqualone	*Ponstel*	Mefenamic acid
Parlodel	Bromocryptine	*Pontocaine*	Tetracaine
Parnate	Tranylcypromine	*Prednis*	Prednisolone
Pasmin	Dicyclomine	*Presun*	p-Aminobenzoic acid
Pathocil	Dicloxacillin	*Principen*	Ampicillin
Pava Caps	Papaverine	*Priscoline*	Tolazoline
Pava-Wol	Papaverine	*Privine*	Naphazoline
Pavabid	Papaverine	*Pro-Banthine*	Propantheline
Pavacen	Papaverine	*Probalan*	Probenecid
Pavadyl	Papaverine	*Procan*	Procainamide
Pavakey	Papaverine	*Procapan*	Procainamide
Pavatran	Papaverine	*Procardia*	Nifedipine
Pavulon	Pancuronium	*Progestin*	Progesterone
Pediamycin	Erythromycin ethyl-succinate	*Proglycem*	Diazoxide
		Proklar-M	Sulfamethizole
Pen-Vee-K	Penicillin V	*Prolixin*	Fluphenazine
Penapar VK	Penicillin V	*Proloprim*	Trimethoprim
Penbritin	Ampicillin	*Promachlor*	Chlorpromazine
Pensyn	Ampicillin	*Promaz*	Chlorpromazine
Pentafin	Pentaerythritol tetra-nitrate	*Pronestyl*	Procainamide
		Propacil	Propylthiouracil
Penthrane	Methoxyflurane	*Proparacaine*	Proxymetacaine
Pentids	Penicillin G	*Prorex*	Promethazine
Pentothal	Thiopental	*Prorone*	Progesterone
Pentritol	Pentaerythritol tetra-nitrate	*Prostaphlin*	Oxacillin
		Prostigmin	Neostigmine
Pentryate	Pentaerythritol tetra-nitrate	*Proternol*	Isoproterenol
		Prothiaden	Dothiepin
Percorten	Deoxycorticosterone	*Protopam*	Pralidoxine
Periactin	Cyproheptadine	*Proxagesic*	Propoxyphene
Peritrate	Pentaerythritol tetra-nitrate	*Pulvule*	Amobarbital
		Pyma	Pyrilamine
Permapen	Benzathine penicillin	*Pyopen*	Carbenicillin
Permitil	Fluphenazine	*Pyristan*	Pyrilamine
Persantine	Dipyridamole	*Quaalude*	Methaqualone
Pertofrane	Desipramine	*Quelicin*	Succinylcholine
Pfizerpen	Ampicillin	*Quinaglute*	Quinidine
Pfizerpen AS	Penicillin G Procaine	*Quinidex*	Quinidine
Pfizerpen VK	Penicillin V	*Quinora*	Quinidine
Phencen	Promethazine	*Rau-Sed*	Reserpine
Phenerex	Promethazine	*Rectules*	Chloral hydrate
Phenergan	Promethazine	*Regitine*	Phentolamine
Phenerhist	Promethazine	*Reglan*	Metoclopramide
Phenetron	Chlorpheniramine	*Regona*	Pyridostigmine
Phospholine	Ecothiopate	*Remsed*	Promethazine
Phyllocontin	Aminophylline	*Renelate*	Methenamine mandelate
Pilocar	Pilocarpine	*Reserjen*	Reserpine
Pilocel	Pilocarpine	*Reserpoid*	Reserpine
Piloptic	Pilocarpine	*Restoril*	Temazepam
Pintop	Succinylcholine	*Rhymodan*	Disopyramide
Pipadone	Dipipanone	*Rifadin*	Rifampin
Pitocin	Oxytocin	*Rimactane*	Rifampin
Polycillin	Ampicillin	*Ritalin*	Methylphenidate
Polymox	Amoxicillin	*Ro-Hydrazide*	Hydrochlorothiazide
Ponderax	Fenfluramine	*Roampicillin*	Ampicillin

US NAMES

Trade name	*Approved name*
Robamox	Amoxicillin
Robantaline	Propantheline
Robenecid	Probenecid
Robicillin VK	Penicillin V
Robimycin	Erythromycin
Robinul	Glycopyrronium
Rocaine	Lidocaine
Rocaltrol	Calcitriol
Rogitine	Phentolamine
Rolathimide	Glutethimide
Rolazid	Isoniazid
Rolisox	Isoxsuprine
Ropanth	Propantheline
Ropred	Prednisolone
SAS-500	Sulfasalazine
Sk-Bamate	Meprobamate
SK-Erythromycin	Erythromycin stearate
SK-Hydrochlorthiazide	Hydrochlorothiazide
SK-Lygen	Chlordiazepoxide
SK-Spoxazole	Sulfisoxazole
Salazopyrin	Sulfasalazine
Salutensin	Hydroflumethiazide
Sandril	Reserpine
Sansert	Methysergide
Savacort	Prednisolone
Savacort-D	Dexamethasone
Screen	Chlordiazepoxide
Seconal	Secobarbital
Seladrops	Phenobarbital
Sensorcaine	Bupivacaine
Septra	Co-trimoxazole
Septrin	Co-trimoxazole
Seromycin	Cycloserine
Serpasil	Reserpine
Serpate	Reserpine
Signate	Dimenhydrinate
Soduben	Butabarbital
Soframycin	Framycetin
Somaphyllin	Aminophylline
Sombulex	Hexobarbital
Somnos	Chloral hydrate
Sonazine	Chlorpromazine
Sorbitrate	Isosobide
Sordinol	Clopenthixol
Sorquad	Isosorbide
Sosal	Sulfisoxazole
Sotacor	Sotalol
Soxa	Sulfisoxazole
Sparine	Promazine
Spastil	Propantheline
Spectrobid	Bacampicillin
Stadol	Butorphanol
Stanacaine	Lidocaine
Stannitol	Dicyclomine
Staphcillin	Methicillin
Stelazine	Trifluoperazine
Sterane	Prednisolone
Sterapred	Prednisone
Stogesic	Propoxyphene
Stoxil	Idoxuridine
Streptase	Streptokinase
Stugeron	Cinnarizine
Sublimaze	Fentanyl
Sucostrin	Succinylcholine
Sulcolon	Sulfasalazine
Sulfagan	Sulfisoxazole
Sulfamylon	Mafenide
Sulfathalidine	Phthalylsulfathiazole
Sulfizin	Sulfisoxazole
Sulla	Sulfamethoxydiazine
Sumox	Amoxicillin
Symmetrel	Amantadine
Synacthen	Tetracosactrin
Syntocinon	Oxytocin
T-Dryl	Diphenhydramine
Tagamet	Cimetidine
Talwin	Pentazocine
Tandearil	Oxyphenbutazone
Tapazole	Methimazole
Tazol	Tolazoline
Tegretol	Carbamazepine
Teldrin	Chlorpheniramine
Temaril	Trimeprazine
Tenormin	Atenolol
Tensilon	Edrophonium
Tensin	Reserpine
Tentrate	Pentaerythritol tetranitrate
Terpium	Chlorpromazine
Thendelate	Methenamine mandelate
Therapav	Papaverine
Thiamazole	Methimazole
Thiodril	Carboxymethylcysteine
Thiosulfil	Sulfamethizole
Thiuretic	Hydrochlorothiazide
Thorazine	Chlorpromazine
Thytropar	Thyrotrophin
Ticar	Ticarcillin
Tobrex	Tobramycin
Tofranil	Imipramine
Tolectin	Tolmetin
Toloxan	Tolazoline
Tolzol	Tolazoline
Totacillin	Ampicillin
Tramacin	Triamcinolone
Tranite	Pentaerythritol tetranitrate
Tranmep	Meprobamate
Trantoin	Nitrofurantoin
Tranxene	Chlorazepate
Trasylol	Aprotinin

US NAMES *Trade name*	*Approved name*	*Trade name*	*Approved name*
Trates	Nitroglycerin	*Vasolate*	Pentaerythritol tetra-nitrate
Traveltabs	Dimenhydrinate		
Trecator	Ethionamide	*Vasopan*	Papaverine
Tri-Kort	Triamcinolone	*Veetids*	Penicillin V
Triam-A	Triamcinolone	*Velmatrol*	Sulfisoxazole
Triclos	Triclofos	*Velosef*	Cephradine
Trilafon	Perphenazine	*Ventolin*	Albuterol
Trimox	Amoxicillin	*Veracillin*	Dicloxacillin
Trimpex	Trimethoprim	*Veronal*	Barbital
Triniad	Isoniazid	*Vertrol*	Meclizine
Trinol	Benzhexol	*Vesicholine*	Bethanechol
Trobicin	Spectinomycin	*Vibra-Tabs*	Doxycycline
Ubretid	Distigmine	*Vibramycin*	Doxycycline
Ulacort	Prednisolone	*Vio-Serpine*	Reserpine
Unipen	Nafcillin	*Vira-A*	Vidarabine
Uracel	Sodium salicylate	*Visken*	Pindolol
Urecholine	Bethanechol	*Vivalan*	Viloxazine
Urolene Blue	Methylene Blue	*Wehydryl*	Diphenhydramine
Urotoin	Nitrofurantoin	*Welldorm*	Dichloralphenazone
Uticillin VK	Penicillin V	*Wyamine*	Mephentermine
Utimox	Amoxicillin	*Wyamycin E*	Erythromycin ethyl-succinate
V-Cillin	Penicillin V		
V-Cillin K	Penicillin V	*Wycillin*	Penicillin G Procaine
Valdrene	Diphenhydramine	*Wygesic*	Propoxyphene
Valisone	Betamethasone	*Wymox*	Amoxicillin
Valium	Diazepam	*Wyovin*	Dicyclomine
Valoid	Cyclizine	*Xylocaine*	Lidocaine
Vancocin	Vancomycin	*Yutopar*	Ritodrine
Vandid	Ethamivan	*Zarontin*	Ethosuximide
Vaporole	Amyl nitrite	*Zaroxolyn*	Metolazone
Vasal	Papaverine	*Zetran*	Chlordiazepoxide
Vasocap	Papaverine	*Zinamide*	Pyrazinamide
Vasocon	Naphazoline	*Zomax*	Zomepirac
Vasodilan	Isoxsuprine	*Zovirax*	Acyclovir

Index